KT-392-232
WS
304
NEW

Withdrawn

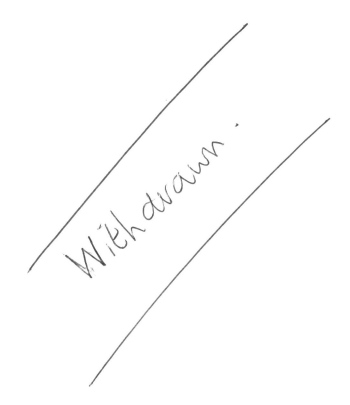

THE NEWBORN LUNG
Neonatology Questions and Controversies

THE NEWBORN LUNG
Neonatology Questions and Controversies

Series Editor

Richard A. Polin, MD
Professor of Pediatrics
College of Physicians and Surgeons
Columbia University
Vice Chairman for Clinical and Academic Affairs
Department of Pediatrics
Director, Division of Neonatology
Morgan Stanley Children's Hospital of NewYork-Presbyterian
Columbia University Medical Center
New York, New York

Other Volumes in the Neonatology Questions and Controversies Series

---

GASTROENTEROLOGY AND NUTRITION

HEMATOLOGY, IMMUNOLOGY AND INFECTIOUS DISEASE

HEMODYNAMICS AND CARDIOLOGY

NEPHROLOGY AND FLUID/ELECTROLYTE PHYSIOLOGY

NEUROLOGY

THE NEWBORN LUNG

Neonatology Questions and Controversies

Eduardo Bancalari, MD
Professor of Pediatrics, Obstetrics and Gynecology
Director, Division of Neonatology
Department of Pediatrics
University of Miami
Miller School of Medicine
Chief Newborn Service
Jackson Memorial Hospital
Miami, Florida

Consulting Editor
Richard A. Polin, MD
Professor of Pediatrics
College of Physicians and Surgeons
Columbia University
Vice Chairman for Clinical and Academic Affairs
Department of Pediatrics
Director, Division of Neonatology
Morgan Stanley Children's Hospital of NewYork-Presbyterian
Columbia University Medical Center
New York, New York

SECOND EDITION

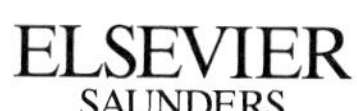

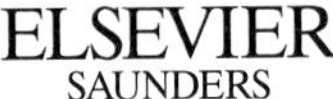

1600 John F. Kennedy Blvd.
Ste 1800
Philadelphia, PA 19103-2899

The Newborn Lung Neonatology Questions and Controversies, Second Edition ISBN: 978-1-4377-2682-4

Notices

Knowledge and best practice in this field are constantly changing. As new research and experience broaden our understanding, changes in research methods, professional practices, or medical treatment may become necessary.

Practitioners and researchers must always rely on their own experience and knowledge in evaluating and using any information, methods, compounds, or experiments described herein. In using such information or methods they should be mindful of their own safety and the safety of others, including parties for whom they have a professional responsibility.

With respect to any drug or pharmaceutical products identified, readers are advised to check the most current information provided (i) on procedures featured or (ii) by the manufacturer of each product to be administered, to verify the recommended dose or formula, the method and duration of administration, and contraindications. It is the responsibility of practitioners, relying on their own experience and knowledge of their patients, to make diagnoses, to determine dosages and the best treatment for each individual patient, and to take all appropriate safety precautions.

To the fullest extent of the law, neither the Publisher nor the authors, contributors, or editors, assume any liability for any injury and/or damage to persons or property as a matter of products liability, negligence or otherwise, or from any use or operation of any methods, products, instructions, or ideas contained in the material herein.

Library of Congress Cataloging-in-Publication Data

The newborn lung : neonatology questions and controversies / [edited by] Eduardo Bancalari ; consulting editor, Richard A. Polin. – 2nd ed.
p. ; cm. – (Neonatology questions and controversies)
Includes bibliographical references and index.
ISBN 978-1-4377-2682-4 (hardback)
I. Bancalari, Eduardo. II. Polin, Richard A. (Richard Alan), 1945- III. Series: Neonatology questions and controversies.
[DNLM: 1. Infant, Newborn, Diseases. 2. Lung Diseases. 3. Infant, Newborn. 4. Lung–growth & development. 5. Respiration Disorders. WS 421]
Lc classification not assigned
618.92′2–dc23

2012001602

Senior Content Strategist: Stefanie Jewell-Thomas
Content Development Specialist: Lisa Barnes
Publishing Services Managers: Catherine Albright Jackson/Hemamalini Rajendrababu
Project Managers: Sara Alsup/Divya Krish
Designer: Ellen Zanolle

Printed in the United States

Last digit is the print number: 9 8 7 6 5 4 3 2 1

Contributors

Steven H. Abman, MD
Professor, Department of Pediatrics
University of Colorado Health Sciences Center
Director, Pediatric Heart Lung Center
The Children's Hospital
Aurora, Colorado
Management of the Infant with Severe Bronchopulmonary Dysplasia

Eduardo Bancalari, MD
Professor of Pediatrics, Obstetrics and Gynecology
Director, Division of Neonatology
Department of Pediatrics
University of Miami
Miller School of Medicine
Chief Newborn Service, Jackson Memorial Hospital
Miami, Florida
Patent Ductus Arteriosus and the Lung: Acute Effects and Long-Term Consequences
New Developments in the Pathogenesis and Prevention of Bronchopulmonary Dysplasia
Hypoxemic Episodes in the Premature Infant: Causes, Consequences, and Management
Patient-Ventilator Interaction
Strategies for Limiting the Duration of Mechanical Ventilation
Automation of Respiratory Support

Vineet Bhandari, MD, DM
Yale University School of Medicine
Department of Pediatrics
Division of Perinatal Medicine
New Haven, Connecticuit
Genetic Influences in Lung Development and Injury

Waldemar A. Carlo, MD
Edwin M. Dixon Professor of Pediatrics
Director, Division of Neonatology
University of Alabama at Birmingham
Birmingham, Alabama
Oxygenation Targeting and Outcomes in Preterm Infants: The New Evidence

Nelson Claure, MSc, PhD
Research Associate
Professor of Pediatrics
Director, Neonatal Pulmonary Research Laboratory
Department of Pediatrics
Division of Neonatology
University of Miami
Miller School of Medicine
Miami, Florida
Patent Ductus Arteriosus and the Lung: Acute Effects and Long-Term Consequences
Hypoxemic Episodes in the Premature Infant: Causes, Consequences, and Management
Patient-Ventilator Interaction
Strategies for Limiting the Duration of Mechanical Ventilation
Automation of Respiratory Support

Peter G. Davis, MD, FRACP, MBBS
Professor, Neonatology
The Royal Women's Hospital
Melbourne, Australia
Noninvasive Respiratory Support: An Alternative to Mechanical Ventilation in Preterm Infants

Lex W. Doyle, MD, MSc
Head, Clinicial Research Development
Research Office
The Royal Women's Hospital
Professor of Neonatal Paediatrics
Departments of Obstetrics and Gynaecology
The University of Melbourne
Honorary Fellow
Critical Care and Neurosciences
Murdoch Children's Research Institute
Victoria, Australia
Long-Term Pulmonary Outcome of Preterm Infants

Samir Gupta, MD, FRCPCH
Senior Lecturer
School of Medicine and Health
Durham University
Co-Director
Research and Development
University Hospital of North Tees
Stockton-Cleveland, United Kingdom
Oxygenation Targeting and Outcomes in Preterm Infants: The New Evidence

Alan H. Jobe, MD, PhD
Professor of Pediatrics
Pulmonary Biology, Neonatology
Cincinnati Children's Hospital Medical Center
Cincinnati, Ohio
Perinatal Events and Their Influence on Lung Development and Function

Suhas G. Kallapur, MD
Associate Professor of Pediatrics
Division Of Neonatology and Pulmonary Biology
Cincinnati Children's Hospital Medical Center
Cincinnati, Ohio
Perinatal Events and Their Influence on Lung Development and Function

Roberta L. Keller, MD
Assistant Professor of Clinical Pediatrics
Pediatrics/Neonatology
University of California, San Francisco
Director
Neonatal ECMO Program
University of California, San Francisco
Benioff Children's Hospital
San Francisco, California
Management of the Infant with Congenital Diaphragmatic Hernia

Girija G. Konduri, MD
Professor of Pediatrics and Chief of Neonatology
Pediatrics
Medical College of Wisconsin
Staff Neonatologist
Children's Hospital of Wisconsin
Milwaukee, Wisconsin
The Role of Nitric Oxide in Lung Growth and Function

Boris W. Kramer, MD, PhD
Maastricht University Medical Center
Department of Pediatrics
Maastricht, The Netherlands
Perinatal Events and Their Influence on Lung Development and Function

Brett J. Manley, MBBS, FRACP
Neonatal Research Fellow
Department of Newborn Research
The Royal Women's Hospital
Department of Obstetrics and Gynaecology
The University of Melbourne
Murdoch Children's Research Institute
Melbourne, Australia
Noninvasive Respiratory Support: An Alternative to Mechanical Ventilation in Preterm Infants

Colin J. Morley, MD, FRACP, FRCPCH
Professor Neonatal Research
Royal Women's Hospital
Melbourne, Australia
Noninvasive Respiratory Support: An Alternative to Mechanical Ventilation in Preterm Infants

Cristina T. Navarrete, MD
Assistant Professor of Clinical Pediatrics
Division of Neonatology
Department of Pediatrics
University of Miami
Miami, Florida
Influence of Nutrition on Neonatal Respiratory Outcomes

Leif D. Nelin, MD
Director, Center for Perinatal Research
Research Institute at Nationwide Children's Hospital
Professor, Pediatrics
The Ohio State University
Columbus, Ohio
Management of the Infant with Severe Bronchopulmonary Dysplasia

Paul T. Schumacker, PhD
Patrick M. Magoon Distinguished Professor
Northwestern University Feinberg School of Medicine
Chicago, Illinois
Hypoxia and Hyperoxia: Effects on the Newborn Pulmonary Circulation

Ilene R.S. Sosenko, MD
Professor of Pediatrics
Department of Pediatrics/Neonatology
University of Miami
Miller School of Medicine
Miami, Florida
Influence of Nutrition on Neonatal Respiratory Outcomes
Patent Ductus Arteriosus and the Lung: Acute Effects and Long-Term Consequences
New Developments in the Pathogenesis and Prevention of Bronchopulmonary Dysplasia

Christian P. Speer, MD, FRCPE
Professor, University Children's Hospital
Wuerzburg, Germany
Surfactant Replacement: Present and Future

Robin H. Steinhorn, MD
Professor and Vice Chair of Pediatrics
Northwestern University Feinberg School of Medicine
Chicago, Illinois
Hypoxia and Hyperoxia: Effects on the Newborn Pulmonary Circulation

Cleide Suguihara, MD, PhD
Associate Professor of Pediatrics
Director, Molecular & Cell Biology Neonatology Research Lab
University of Miami Health Systems
Miami, Florida
Role of Stem Cells in Neonatal Lung Injury

David Sweet, MD, FRCPCH
Regional Neonatal Unit
Royal Maternity Hospital
Belfast, Ireland
Surfactant Replacement: Present and Future

Win Tin, MD
Department of Neonatal Medicine
The James Cook University Hospital
Middlesbrough, England
Oxygenation Targeting and Outcomes in Preterm Infants: The New Evidence

Rose Marie Viscardi, MD
Professor, Department of Pediatrics
University of Maryland School of Medicine
Baltimore, Maryland
Prenatal and Postnatal Microbial Colonization and Respiratory Outcome in Preterm Infants

Stephen Wedgwood, PhD
Research Assistant Professor, Pediatrics
Northwestern University
Chicago, Illinois
Hypoxia and Hyperoxia: Effects on the Newborn Pulmonary Circulation

Shu Wu, MD
Associate Professor of Clinical Pediatrics
Department of Pediatrics
University of Miami School of Medicine
Miami, Florida
Molecular Bases for Lung Development, Injury, and Repair

Myra H. Wyckoff, MD
Associate Professor
Department of Pediatrics
University of Texas Southwestern Medical Center
Director of Newborn Resuscitation Services
Parkland Health and Hospital Systems
Dallas, Texas
Respiratory and Cardiovascular Support in the Delivery Room

Karen C. Young, MD
Assistant Professor of Pediatrics
Pediatrics/Neonatology
University of Miami Miller School of Medicine
Miami, Florida
Role of Stem Cells in Neonatal Lung Injury

Series Foreword

Richard A. Polin, MD

"Medicine is a science of uncertainty and an art of probability."

William Osler

Controversy is part of everyday practice in the NICU. Good practitioners strive to incorporate the best evidence into clinical care. However, for much of what we do, the evidence is either inconclusive or does not exist. In those circumstances, we have come to rely on the teachings of experienced practitioners who have taught us the importance of clinical expertise. This series, "Neonatology Questions and Controversies," provides clinical guidance by summarizing the best evidence and tempering those recommendations with the art of experience.

To quote David Sackett, one of the founders of evidence-based medicine:

> *Good doctors use both individual clinical expertise and the best available external evidence and neither alone is enough. Without clinical expertise, practice risks become tyrannized by evidence, for even excellent external evidence may be inapplicable to or inappropriate for an individual patient. Without current best evidence, practice risks become rapidly out of date to the detriment of patients.*

This series focuses on the challenges faced by care providers who work in the NICU. When should we incorporate a new technology or therapy into everyday practice, and will it have positive impact on morbidity or mortality? For example, is the new generation of ventilators better than older technologies such as CPAP, or do they merely offer more choices with uncertain value? Similarly, the use of probiotics to prevent necrotizing enterocolitis is supported by sound scientific principles (and some clinical studies). However, at what point should we incorporate them into everyday practice given that the available preparations are not well characterized or proven safe? A more difficult and common question is when to use a new technology with uncertain value in a critically ill infant. As many clinicians have suggested, sometimes the best approach is to do nothing and "stand there."

The "Questions and Controversies" series was developed to highlight the clinical problems of most concern to practitioners. The editors of each volume (Drs. Bancalari, Oh, Guignard, Baumgart, Kleinman, Seri, Ohls, Maheshwari, Neu, and Perlman) have done an extraordinary job in selecting topics of clinical importance to everyday practice. When appropriate, less controversial topics have been eliminated and replaced by others thought to be of greater clinical importance. In total, there are 56 new chapters in the series. During the preparation of the *Hemodynamics and Cardiology* volume, Dr. Charles Kleinman died. Despite an illness that would have caused many to retire, Charlie worked until near the time of his death. He came to work each day, teaching students and young practitioners and offering his wisdom and expertise to families of infants with congenital heart disease. We are dedicating the second edition of the series to his memory. As with the first edition, I am indebted to the exceptional group of editors who chose the content and edited each of the volumes. I also wish to thank Lisa Barnes (content development specialist at Elsevier) and Judy Fletcher (global content development director at Elsevier), who provided incredible assistance in bringing this project to fruition.

Preface

The increasing survival of very premature infants has produced major challenges for neonatologists and pediatricians because these infants have immaturity of multiple organ systems that predisposes them to long-term sequelae. Despite remarkable progress in newborn care, respiratory problems continue to prevail as one of the most important threats during the newborn period. Much of the progress in respiratory care has been achieved through research leading to a better understanding of the processes involved in normal and deranged development of the respiratory system. Several recent and important clinical trials have also addressed some of the more pressing issues in neonatal respiratory care.

For this second edition of *The Newborn Lung*, we have been able to engage as authors some of the leading clinicians and scientists from around the world who have been responsible for many of the recent advances in respiratory care of the newborn.

The aim of this book is to address those aspects that are more relevant and controversial or those in which there has been recent progress. Several chapters deal primarily with developmental issues in pulmonary biology, while others address some of the important challenges facing the clinician responsible for the care of infants with respiratory failure.

I am very grateful to all of the contributors to this book for their willingness to share their knowledge and experience, and I am certain the reader will share my appreciation for the outstanding quality of each of the chapters.

Eduardo Bancalari, MD

Contents

SECTION A

Normal and Abnormal Lung Development

CHAPTER 1 Molecular Bases for Lung Development, Injury, and Repair 3
Shu Wu, MD

CHAPTER 2 Genetic Influences in Lung Development and Injury 29
Vineet Bhandari, MD, DM

CHAPTER 3 Perinatal Events and Their Influence on Lung Development and Function 57
Alan H. Jobe, MD, PhD, Suhas G. Kallapur, MD, and Boris W. Kramer, MD, PhD

CHAPTER 4 Hypoxia and Hyperoxia: Effects on the Newborn Pulmonary Circulation 91
Stephen Wedgwood, PhD, Paul T. Schumacker, PhD, and Robin H. Steinhorn, MD

CHAPTER 5 The Role of Nitric Oxide in Lung Growth and Function 111
Girija G. Konduri, MD

SECTION B

Lung Injury—Bronchopulmonary Dysplasia

CHAPTER 6 Prenatal and Postnatal Microbial Colonization and Respiratory Outcome in Preterm Infants 135
Rose Marie Viscardi, MD

CHAPTER 7 Influence of Nutrition on Neonatal Respiratory Outcomes 163
Cristina T. Navarrete, MD, and Ilene R.S. Sosenko, MD

CHAPTER 8 Patent Ductus Arteriosus and the Lung: Acute Effects and Long-Term Consequences 181
Eduardo Bancalari, MD, Ilene R.S. Sosenko, MD, and Nelson Claure, MSc, PhD

CHAPTER 9 Role of Stem Cells in Neonatal Lung Injury 197
Karen C. Young, MD, and Cleide Suguihara, MD, PhD

CHAPTER 10 New Developments in the Pathogenesis and Prevention of Bronchopulmonary Dysplasia 217
Ilene R.S. Sosenko, MD, and Eduardo Bancalari, MD

CHAPTER 11 Long-Term Pulmonary Outcome of Preterm Infants 235
Lex W. Doyle, MD, MSc

SECTION C

Management of Respiratory Failure

CHAPTER 12 Respiratory and Cardiovascular Support in the Delivery Room 247
Myra H. Wyckoff, MD

CHAPTER 13 Noninvasive Respiratory Support: An Alternative to Mechanical Ventilation in Preterm Infants 265
Peter G. Davis, MD, FRACP, MBBS, Colin J. Morley, MD, FRACP, FRCPCH, and Brett J. Manley, MBBS, FRACP

CHAPTER 14 Surfactant Replacement: Present and Future 283
Christian P. Speer, MD, FRCPE, and David Sweet, MD, FRCPCH

CHAPTER 15 Oxygenation Targeting and Outcomes in Preterm Infants: The New Evidence 301
Win Tin, MD, Waldemar A. Carlo, MD, and Samir Gupta, MD, FRCPCH

CHAPTER 16 Hypoxemic Episodes in the Premature Infant: Causes, Consequences, and Management 329
Nelson Claure, MSc, PhD, and Eduardo Bancalari, MD

CHAPTER 17 Patient-Ventilator Interaction 339
Eduardo Bancalari, MD, and Nelson Claure, MSc, PhD

CHAPTER 18 Strategies for Limiting the Duration of Mechanical Ventilation 355
Eduardo Bancalari, MD, and Nelson Claure, MSc, PhD

CHAPTER 19 Automation of Respiratory Support 367
Nelson Claure, MSc, PhD, and Eduardo Bancalari, MD

CHAPTER 20 Management of the Infant with Congenital Diaphragmatic Hernia 381
Roberta L. Keller, MD

CHAPTER 21 Management of the Infant with Severe Bronchopulmonary Dysplasia 407
Steven H. Abman, MD, and Leif D. Nelin, MD

SECTION A

Normal and Abnormal Lung Development

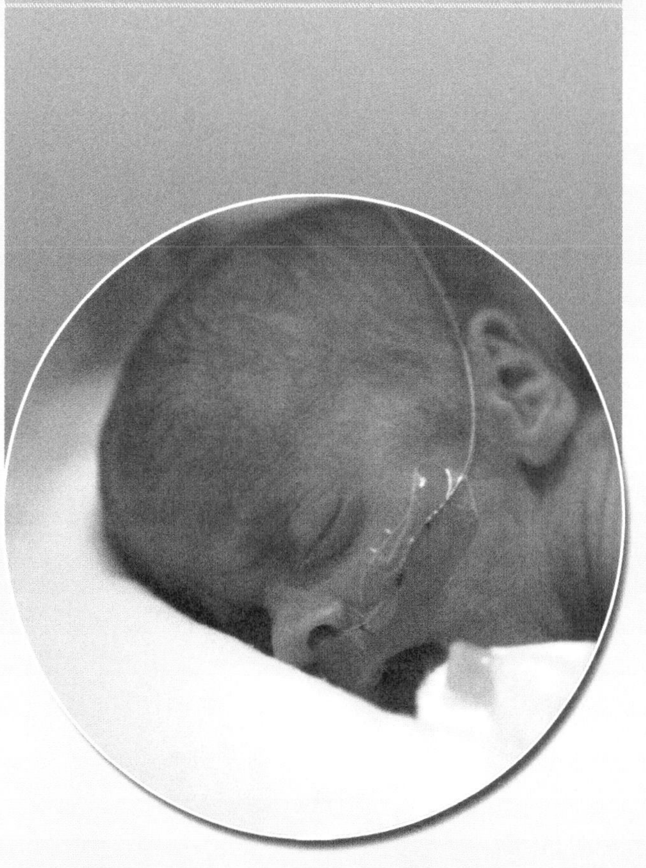

CHAPTER 1

Molecular Bases for Lung Development, Injury, and Repair

Shu Wu, MD

1

- **Stages of Lung Development**
- **Molecular Regulation of Lung Bud Initiation and Tracheal-Esophageal Separation**
- **Epithelial-Mesenchymal Interactions Control Branching Morphogenesis**
- **Regulatory Mechanisms of Alveologenesis**
- **Regulation of Pulmonary Vascular Development**
- **Lung Injury and Repair: Disruption of Normal Lung Development**

The first breath taken by newborns after birth transitions them from fetal to neonatal life. Successful transition depends on the lung to transport oxygen from the atmosphere into the bloodstream and to release carbon dioxide from the bloodstream into the ambient air. This exchange of gases takes place in the alveoli, the terminal units of the lung, which consist of an epithelial layer surrounded by capillaries, and supported by extracellular matrix (ECM). The alveolocapillary barrier should be as thin as possible and should cover as large a surface area as possible to maximize the area over which gas exchange can take place. The human lung achieves a final gas diffusion surface of 70 m^2 in area with 0.2 mm in thickness by young adulthood and is capable of supporting systemic oxygen consumption ranging between 250 mL/min at rest to 5500 mL/min during maximal exercise.[1-4] To facilitate the development of such a large, diffusible interface of the epithelial layer with the circulation, the embryonic lung undergoes branching morphogenesis to form a vast network of branched airways and subsequent formation and multiplication of alveoli by septation during the late stage of fetal development.[1] By the time the full-term infant is born, there are about 50 million alveoli in the lungs, which provide sufficient gas exchange for the beginning of extrauterine life.[4-6] Postnatally, alveoli continue to grow in size and number by septation to form approximately 300 million units in the adult lung.[4-6] A matching capillary network develops in close apposition to the alveolar surface beginning in the middle to late stage of fetal development and continuing through postnatal development, which can accommodate pulmonary blood flow rising from 4 L/min at rest to 40 L/min during maximal exercise.[1,3]

Our understanding of basic lung developmental processes has been significantly improved though extensive studies in mouse molecular genetics and genomics. It is well recognized that these developmental processes are regulated by diverse signaling crosstalks between the airway epithelium and surrounding mesenchyme, which are highly coordinated by growth factors, transcriptional factors, and ECM residing in the lung microenvironment. Specific temporal-spatial cell proliferation, differentiation, migration, and apoptosis orchestrated by these interplays give rise to the complex lung structure that prepares for the first breath. Genetic mutations, physical forces, intrauterine infection, and particularly premature birth can disrupt these developmental processes, thus resulting in defective lungs in the neonate, which can lead to respiratory failure and death.

Bronchopulmonary dysplasia (BPD) is a chronic lung disease of premature infants that is increasingly being recognized as a developmental arrest of the immature lung caused by injurious stimuli such as mechanical ventilation, oxygen exposure, and intrauterine or postnatal infections.[7] Data from extensive animal studies suggest that dysregulation of those key signaling pathways in normal lung development may play an important role in neonatal lung injury and repair and subsequent development of BPD. Therefore, fundamental knowledge about lung developmental processes and their cellular and molecular regulatory mechanisms is essential to an understanding of the molecular basis of lung injury and repair. This understanding may lead to much needed novel therapeutic strategies in managing neonatal lung diseases, particularly BPD.

This chapter provides a brief overview of normal lung developmental processes, the key signaling pathways and proposed models in regulating lung budding, branching morphogenesis, alveolarization, and vascular development, and how injury from mechanical ventilation and oxygen exposure modulates some of these key pathways, thus affecting neonatal lung development in the context of prematurity.

Stages of Lung Development

Human lung development begins as formation of airway primordia in the embryonic period and subsequently undergoes branching morphogenesis to form the conducting airway, with expansion of the terminal airways in combination with epithelial cell differentiation and vascular development to form the alveoli. On the basis of histologic appearances, lung development is classically divided into five overlapping stages: embryonic, pseudoglandular, canalicular, saccular, and alveolar (Fig. 1-1).[1,8] Distinctive histologic and structural changes in each stage of lung development have been well described, although the regulatory mechanisms that are responsible for these changes are not fully understood. There are striking similarities in the stages of lung development in humans and mice. In fact, most of the current knowledge of lung developmental biology is acquired from mouse molecular genetic and genomic studies. This section reviews the key events in each of the lung developmental stages in humans and mice with a goal of better understanding of the regulatory mechanisms during these processes.

Embryonic Stage

The embryonic stage of human lung development spans from 4 to 7 weeks of gestation (wk). At the beginning of this stage, the lung originates as the laryngotracheal groove from the ventral surface of the primitive foregut. The proximal portion of the laryngotracheal groove separates dorsoventrally from the primitive esophagus to form the tracheal rudiment, which gives rise to the left and right main bronchi by branching into the ventrolateral mesenchyme derived from the splanchnic mesoderm. Subsequently, the right main bronchus branches to form three lobar bronchi, and the left main bronchus branches to form two lobar bronchi, giving rise to the three-lobe right lung and two-lobe left lung. The embryonic stage of mouse lung development occurs from embryonic day 9 (E9) to E14, which begins as the formation of two endodermal buds from the ventral side of the primitive foregut. The single foregut tube then separates into the trachea containing the two primary lung buds and esophagus by means of inward movement of lateral mesodermal ridges, which proceeds in a posterior to anterior direction. The two primary lung buds subsequently grow and branch into the splanchnic mesenchyme, with the right bud giving rise to four lobar bronchi and the left bud giving rise to a single lobar bronchus. During this stage, the trachea, primary bronchi, and major airways are lined with undifferentiated columnar epithelium.

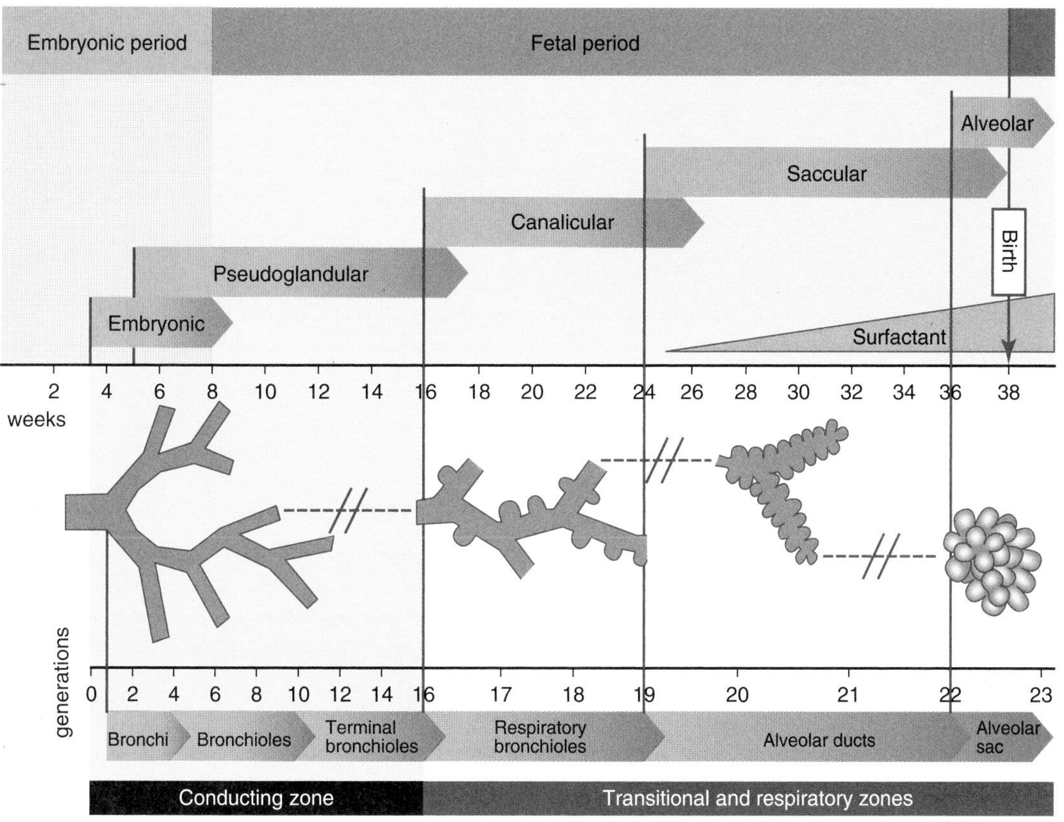

Figure 1-1 Scheme of stages and key events in human lung development. Human lung development begins with the formation of lung buds at 4 weeks of gestation. Trachea and major bronchi are formed by the end of the embryonic stage. The conducting airways are formed during the pseudoglandular stage up to the level of terminal bronchioles. Respiratory bronchioles are formed during the canalicular stage. The alveolar ducts are formed during the saccular stage. Alveolarization begins at around 36 weeks of gestation and continues during the first few years of childhood. (Modified from Online course in embryology for medicine students developed by the universities of Fribourg, Lausanne and Bern (Switzerland). www.embryology.ch/anglais/rrespiratory/phasen07.html.)

Pseudoglandular Stage

During the pseudoglandular stage (5 to 17 wk in humans, E14 to E16.5 in mice), the airway epithelial tubules undergo reproducible, bilaterally asymmetrical and stereotypical branching to form a treelike structure, which gives rise to 16 generations of conducting airways up to the level of terminal bronchioles.[1] There is also proximal airway epithelial differentiation with the appearance of basal cells, goblet cells, pulmonary neuroendocrine cells, ciliated cells, and nonciliated columnar (Clara) cells. The surrounding mesenchymal cells differentiate into fibroblasts, myofibroblasts, smooth muscle cells, and chondrocytes to form muscle and cartilage around the proximal airways. The vascular growth is in close proximity to the airway branching during this stage. By the end of the pseudoglandular stage, the conducting airways and their accompanying pulmonary and bronchial arteries are developed in the pattern corresponding to that found in the adult lung.

Canalicular Stage

During the canalicular stage (16 to 26 wk in humans, E16.5 to E17.5 in mice), the terminal bronchioles continue to branch to form the final seven generations of the respiratory tree that supply air. The respiratory bronchioles branch out from the terminal bronchioles to form the future acini, an action that is accompanied by increasing development of the capillary bed, the beginning of alveolar type II epithelial (AT II) cell differentiation to synthesize surfactant proteins, and the thinning of the surrounding mesenchymal tissues. The lung appears "canalized" as capillaries begin to arrange themselves around the air space and come into close apposition to the overlying epithelium. At sites of apposition, thinning of the epithelium occurs to form the first sites of the air-blood barrier. Thus, if a fetus is born at around 24 wk, the end of the canalicular stage, these primitive acini have the capacity to perform some gas exchange with or without respiratory support.

Saccular Stage

The saccular stage in humans spans from 24 to 36 wk. During this stage, clusters of thin-walled saccules appear in the distal lung to form the alveolar ducts, the last generation of airways prior to the development of alveoli. Small mesenchymal ridges are developed on the saccule walls to form the initial stage of septation. The capillaries form a bilayer "double capillary network" within the relatively broad and cellular intersaccular septa. The AT II cells are further differentiated and become functionally mature with the ability to produce surfactant. Also, the alveolar type I epithelial (AT I) cells are differentiated from the AT II cells at the sites opposing the capillaries for gas exchange. The interstitium between the air spaces becomes thinner as the result of decreased deposition of collagen fibers. Furthermore, elastic fibers are deposited in the interstitium, which lays the foundation for subsequent septation and formation of alveoli. The process of saccular formation in mice is quite similar to that in humans; however, the timing of the saccular stage in mice begins at E17.5 and continues up to postnatal day (P) 5.

Alveolar Stage

During the alveolar stage (36 wk to childhood in humans, P5 to P30 in mice), the saccules are subdivided by the ingrowth of ridges or crests known as secondary septa. The AT II and AT I cells continue to differentiate. Postnatally, the alveoli continue to multiply by increasing secondary septa. Between birth and adulthood, the alveolar surface area expands nearly 20-fold.[9] Early in this stage, the capillary network is in a double pattern in alveolar septa. Postnatally, with the process of alveolar septation and thinning of the primary septa, the matching capillary network undergoes a maturational process, with the double capillary network fusing into a single layer to assume the form present in the adult lung.[9] Thus, the capillary volume is increased by 35-fold from birth to adulthood.[9] The alveolar stage of mouse lung development is completely a postnatal event. The newborn mouse lung is in the saccular stage, which is similar to that found in the human fetal lung at 26 to 32 wk. Mouse alveologenesis begins around P5 and continues up to P30. This postnatal pattern of mouse alveolar development provides an excellent model system for mechanistic studies in understanding neonatal lung injury and repair in preterm infants.

Molecular Regulation of Lung Bud Initiation and Tracheal-Esophageal Separation

The processes and molecular regulators for lung bud initiation and tracheal-esophageal separation are not well established. However, mouse models have demonstrated that localized domain expression of key transcription factors as well as growth factors is essential during these processes (Fig. 1-2). Nkx2.1—also known as thyroid transcription factor 1(TTF-1)—is the earliest known transcriptional factor that is expressed in endodermal cells in the prospective lung/tracheal region of the anterior foregut.[10,11] Deletion of the Nkx2.1 gene in mice results in abnormal lung formation with two main bronchi that give rise to cystic structures.[11] Additional studies have also demonstrated that Nkx2.1 is essential for differentiation of distal lung epithelial cells and for expression of surfactant protein C (SP-C).[12] Studies have now indicated that expression of Nkx2.1 in the foregut endoderm is regulated by wingless/int (Wnt)-β-catenin signaling. Combined loss of Wnt2 and Wnt2b, which are expressed in the mesoderm surrounding the anterior foregut, or of

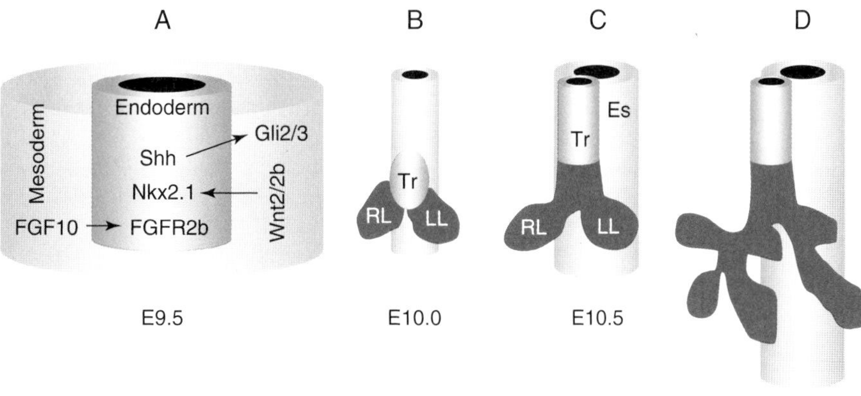

Figure 1-2 Scheme of lung bud initiation and tracheal-esophageal separation in mice. Lung bud initiation on the foregut endoderm is controlled by a temporal-spatial expression of transcription factors and growth factors. **A,** At embryonic day (E) E9.5, the factor Nkx2.1 is expressed in the foregut endoderm, which specifies future trachea and lung development. This Nkx2.1 expression is regulated by Wnt2/2b, expressed in the mesoderm. Sonic Hedgehog, Shh, expressed in the endoderm, and its signaling transducers, Gli2/3, expressed in the mesoderm, are required for lung budding. Fibroblast growth factor 10 (FGF10), expressed in mesoderm, and the FGF receptor 2b (FGFR2b), expressed in endoderm, are required for lung budding. **B,** At E10, primitive trachea (Tr), right lung bud (RL), and left lung bud (LL) appear on the ventral face of the foregut. **C,** At E10.5, distinct tracheal and esophageal (Es) tubes emerge from the foregut tube. **D,** AT E11.5, the trachea and esophagus are separated, being connected only at the larynx. The right lung bud gives rise to right main bronchus and subsequently four lobar bronchi, and the left lung bud gives rise to the single left lobar bronchus by branching into the ventrolateral mesenchyme derived from the splanchnic mesoderm.

β-catenin in the endoderm leads to loss of Nkx2.1 expression and failure of foregut separation.[13,14]

Sonic hedgehog (Shh) is expressed in the ventral foregut endoderm as early as E9.5 and appears to mediate early signaling between the endoderm and mesoderm.[15-17] Shh mediates its effects via GLI–Kruppel family member (Gli) 2/3 transcriptional factors that are present in the mesoderm. Mice with a targeted deletion of Shh gene have foregut defects with tracheoesophageal atresia/stenosis, tracheoesophageal fistula, and tracheal and lung anomalies.[18] The homozygous Gli 2 null ($Gli2^{-/-}$) mice have unilobar left and right lungs[19] and $Gli3^{-/-}$ mice present with reductions in shape and size of pulmonary segmental branches.[20] However, compound null mutations of both Gli2 and Gli3 in mice result in a more severe foregut phenotype with complete agenesis of the esophagus, trachea, and lung.[19]

Besides transcription factors, signaling mediated by fibroblast growth factor-10 (FGF10) and its receptor 2b (FGFR2b) is crucial for lung bud initiation. FGF10 belongs to an increasingly large and complex family of growth factors that signal through four cognate tyrosine kinases' FGFRs.[1] FGF10 is a chemotactic and proliferation factor for lung endoderm that is expressed in the mesenchyme at the prospective sites of lung bud formation.[21-23] The essential role of FGF10 in lung bud initiation is highlighted by the findings that deletion of FGF10 gene results in lung agenesis in mice.[24-26] Although $FGFR2b^{-/-}$ mice form an underdeveloped lung bud, it soon undergoes apoptosis.[27] This has been attributed to FGF10-mediated activation of FGFR1b, a receptor that also binds to FGF10, but with much lower affinity.[28]

Our understanding of the critical signals required for initial lung budding and tracheal-esophageal separation is incomplete, and many other factors are likely to be involved. Knowledge gained from mice molecular genetic and genomic studies will likely provide new insights into human congenital anomalies such as lung or tracheal agenesis, esophageal atresia, and tracheoesophageal fistula.

Epithelial-Mesenchymal Interactions Control Branching Morphogenesis

Following the formation of primary lung buds, the airway epithelial tubules undergo branching morphogenesis to form the respiratory tree. Although the process of airway branching morphogenesis is still far from being fully understood, the interactions between epithelium and mesenchyme orchestrated by compartmental transcriptional factors, growth factors, and ECM have long been known to play a critical role. This involves FGF10, Shh, bone morphogenetic protein (BMP), transforming growth factor β (TGF-β), Wnts, and retinoic acid (RA).[29] These molecules express in specific temporal, spatial, and cellular fashions, and together, these signaling pathways coordinate reciprocal interactions between the epithelium and mesenchyme that control cell proliferation, differentiation, survival, and ultimately the number and size of airway branches (Fig. 1-3).

FGF10-FGFR2b Signaling: Driving Force for Branching Morphogenesis

At the early stages of branching morphogenesis, FGF10 is expressed in the mesenchyme surrounding the distal lung bud tip, whereas FGFR2b is expressed at high levels along the entire proximal-distal axis of the airway endoderm.[30,31] Extensive in vitro studies have demonstrated the critical role of FGF10 in stimulating budding in mouse embryonic lung explants. In mesenchyme-free embryonic lung bud cultures, addition of recombinant FGF10 to culture medium induces budding.[21,32] Furthermore, placing a FGF10-soaked heparin bead either in mesenchyme-free or in whole lung bud cultures induces bud elongation toward the FGF10 bead.[33] These in vitro data combined with in vivo data showing lung agenesis in FGF10 mutant mice indicate a critical role for FGF10 in driving branching morphogenesis. However, spatial-temporal expression as well as the signaling activity of FGF10 needs to be precisely regulated during branching morphogenesis, which will ultimately control the specific sites of budding, bud elongation, and branching.

Control of FGF10-FGFR2b Signaling by Shh and Sprouty

The exchange of signals between the growing bud and the surrounding mesenchyme establishes feedback responses that control the size and shape of the bud during branching. Shh, which is highly expressed in the distal lung epithelium, has been proposed to play a role in controlling localized FGF10 expression in the mesenchyme surrounding the distal lung bud tip (Fig. 1-3). In lung explant cultures, expression of FGF10 is inhibited by Shh.[34] In Shh transgenic mice, FGF10 expression is downregulated in the lungs.[16] Furthermore, in $Shh^{-/-}$ mice, FGF10 expression is no longer restricted to the focal mesenchyme surrounding the distal bud but becomes widespread throughout the distal mesenchyme.[35]

Another antagonistic mechanism that interacts with FGF10 signaling occurs through the Sprouty (Spry) pathway.[36] In the developing mouse lung, Spry2 is present at the tips of the growing epithelial buds, but Spry4 is expressed in the surrounding distal lung mesenchyme. FGF10 induces Spry2 expression in lung epithelium.[37] Interestingly, reducing Spry2 activity results in increased branching in lung explant cultures.[38] In contrast, overexpression of Spry2 or misexpression of Spry4 in the distal lung epithelium of transgenic mice severely impairs branching.[37,39] It is possible that Spry2 acts as a FGF10-dependent inhibitor of branching morphogenesis.

BMP Signaling: Controversial Role in Regulating Branching Morphogenesis

The BMP family contains more than 20 members that have been shown to regulate many developmental processes, including lung development, and BMP4 is the best studied in lung branching morphogenesis. BMP4, the type I receptor of BMP4, activin-like kinase 3 (Alk3), and the BMP signaling transducer, Smad1, are present

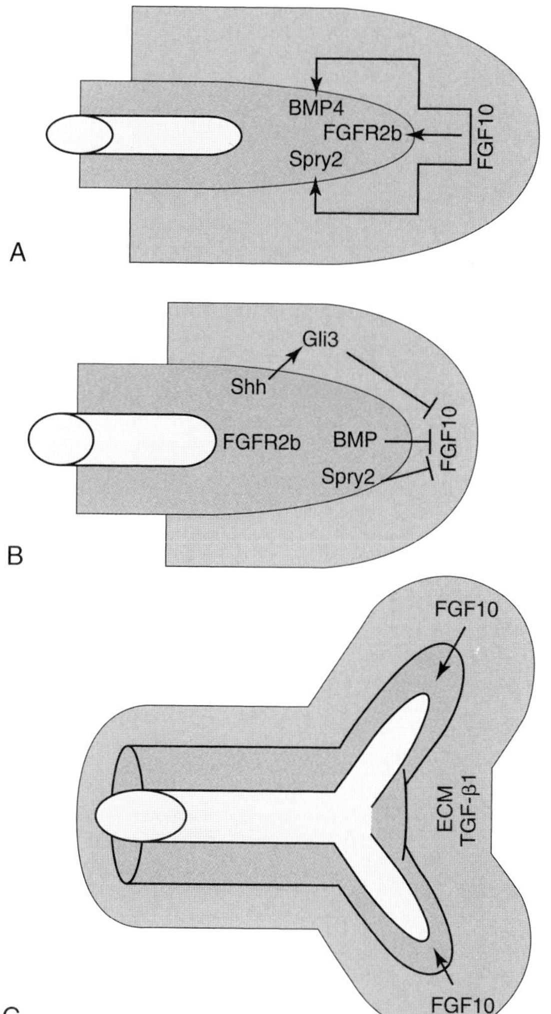

Figure 1-3 Models of branching morphogenesis in mice. **A,** Lung budding is induced by the localized expression of FGF10 in the distal mesenchyme, which acts on FGFR2b, which is expressed in epithelium. At the same time, FGF10 also induces expression of bone morphogenetic protein 4 (BMP4) and the protein Sprouty 2 (Spry2) in epithelium. **B,** As the buds elongate, increased expression of Spry2 in epithelium negatively regulates FGF signaling and inhibits its budding. Increased BMP4 expression in epithelium may also inhibit budding. The Shh, expressed in the epithelium and acting on signaling transducer Gli3, which is expressed in the mesenchyme, inhibits FGF and FGFR2b expression, thus inhibiting budding. **C,** FGF10 increases laterally to form new foci of lung buds that create a cleft. Transforming growth factor beta 1 (TGF-β1), expressed in the subepithelial mesenchyme, increases deposition of extracellular matrix (ECM) in the cleft areas that become the branching points.

1

in both the epithelium and mesenchyme of the embryonic lung during early branching morphogenesis.[40-43] Transgenic overexpression of BMP4 in the distal epithelium causes abnormal lung morphogenesis with cystic terminal sacs.[42] Interestingly, blockage of endogenous BMP4 in embryonic mouse lung epithelium results in abnormal lung development with dilated terminal sacs, similar to those observed in BMP4 transgenic mice.[44] Furthermore, conditional deletion of Alk3 in embryonic lung epithelium causes retardation of branching morphogenesis.[45] These findings suggest that balanced BMP4 signaling is important for in vivo lung branching morphogenesis, although the precise mechanisms remain unclear. In mesenchyme-intact embryonic lung bud cultures, BMP4 is expressed in high levels in distal epithelial buds, near mesenchymal FGF10 expressing cells when buds are elongating, and recombinant BMP4 stimulates branching.[33,34,46] However, in mesenchyme-free embryonic lung bud cultures, addition of FGF10 to the culture media induces budding and also BMP4 expression, whereas recombinant BMP4 inhibits FGF10-induced budding in these cultures.[33] Thus, BMP4 may affect lung bud branching through both autocrine and paracrine mechanisms.

TGF-β Signaling Inhibits Branching

Members of the TGF-β family, TGF-β1, TGF-β2, and TGF-β3, have also been implicated in regulation of lung branching morphogenesis.[47-52] During lung branching morphogenesis, TGF-β1 gene is expressed in the mesenchyme adjacent to the epithelium.[48] However, TGF-β1 protein accumulates in stalks and in regions between buds, where ECM components collagen I, collagen III, and fibronectin are also present. TGF-$\beta1^{-/-}$ mice demonstrate severe pulmonary inflammation,[49] whereas TGF-β2 gene mutation results in embryonic lethality around E14.5 with abnormal branching morphogenesis.[50] TGF-$\beta3^{-/-}$ mice have cleft palate, retarded lung development, and neonatal lethality.[51,52] In contrast, overexpression of TGF-β1 in embryonic lung epithelium decreases airway and vascular development as well as epithelial cell differentiation.[53,54] Many in vitro studies have demonstrated that exogenous TGF-β1 severely inhibits embryonic lung branching and epithelial differentiation but stimulates mesenchymal differentiation by inducing ectopic expression of α smooth muscle actin (α-SMA) and collagen.[55-57] TGF-β1 also markedly inhibits FGF10 expression in lung explant culture.[34] Abrogation of TGF-signaling transducers Smad2, Smad3, and Smad4 also significantly affects branching.[58] Cumulatively, TGF-β signaling may be part of a mechanism that prevents FGF10 from being expressed in the mesenchyme of bud stalks or in more proximal regions of the lung. At these sites, TGF-β could also induce synthesis of ECM and prevent budding locally (Fig. 1-3).

Wnt Signaling: Autocrine and Paracrine Effects on Branching Morphogenesis

The Wnt family constitutes a large family of secreted glycoproteins with highly conserved cysteine residues.[59-62] Wnt ligands bind to the membrane receptors, frizzled (FZD) and low-density lipoprotein receptor–related protein (LRP) 5 or LRP6, thus activating a diverse array of intracellular signaling, target gene transcriptions, and cellular responses.[59-62] The canonical Wnt signaling is the one best studied that involves nuclear translocation of β-catenin, which then interacts with members of T cell–specific transcription factor (Tcf)/lymphoid enhancer–binding factor (Lef) family to induce target gene transcription.[59,62] Several Wnt ligands, receptors, and components of the canonical pathway, such as β-catenin and Tcf/Lef transcription factors, are expressed in a highly cell-specific fashion in the developing lung.[63-67] The role of Wnt/β-catenin signaling in branching morphogenesis is further elucidated by studies of mouse mutagenesis as well as embryonic lung explant cultures. Epithelial-specific overexpression of Wnt5a results in decreased branching morphogenesis and increased enlargement of distal air spaces.[68] Lungs with these features have increased FGF signaling in the mesenchyme but decreased Shh signaling in the epithelium. In addition, targeted deletion of Wnt5a leads to overexpansion of distal airways and expanded interstitium, accompanied by greater Shh expression.[69] Epithelium-specific deletion of β-catenin or overexpression of Wnt inhibitor dickkopf1 (Dkk1) results in disruption of distal airway development and expansion of proximal airways.[70] Furthermore, inhibition of Wnt signaling by Dkk1 in vitro also leads to disruption of branching morphogenesis and defective formation of pulmonary vascular network in embryonic lung explants.[71] However, increased branching morphogenesis has also been observed in embryonic lung explants when β-catenin is reduced by antisense morpholino knockdown, whereas treatment with Wnt3a-conditioned medium represses growth and proliferation of embryonic lung explants.[72] Clearly, the mechanisms by which Wnt signaling regulates lung branching morphogenesis are very complex. They may be related to the facts that multiple Wnt ligands exist in the embryonic lung and that Wnt signaling is known to regulate epithelial and mesenchymal cell biology in an autocrine and paracrine fashion. In addition, canonical-β-catenin and noncanonical Wnt signaling pathways probably both play a role in lung branching morphogenesis. Furthermore, how Wnt signaling interacts with other key signaling pathways, such as FGF, Shh, and BMP, remains unknown.

Summary

Lung branching morphogenesis is controlled by epithelium-mesenchyme interactions that are orchestrated by a network of groups of transcriptional factors, growth factors, and ECM. Apart from what has already been reviewed, many other molecules may also play a role in lung branching morphogenesis, such as integrins[73-77] and matrix metalloproteinases (MMPs) that are dynamically expressed during lung development.[78,79] Along with airway tubule budding, elongation, and branching, specific cell differentiation occurs in the endodermal and mesenchymal compartments. Perhaps the regulatory mechanisms are even more complex as to proximal-distal patterning, establishing cell fate as well as maintaining progenitor cells. The physical forces, such as intraluminal fluid pressure, also play an important role in branching morphogenesis and, ultimately, alveolar formation. Understanding the mechanisms of how the fluid is produced and how the fluid pressure is sensed and maintained has clinical implications in understanding congenital pulmonary hypoplasia, which is caused by physical occupation of the thorax, such as by congenital diaphragmatic hernia and congenital lung masses. More importantly, this understanding may help with formulation of fetal therapies to enhance lung development.

Regulatory Mechanisms of Alveologenesis

During the saccular stage, the walls of the saccules, the primary septa, are tightly associated with the vascular plexus, with ECM rich in elastin, and with as yet poorly defined mesenchymal cell types, including precursors of myofibroblasts. The endoderm begins to differentiate into two main specialized cell types of the future AT II and AT I cells. During alveolarization the sacs are subdivided by the ingrowth of secondary septa. Both myofibroblast progenitors and endothelial cells migrate into these crests, and a scaffold of matrix proteins is deposited, enriched in elastin at the tip. One can clearly see that the development of secondary septa and formation of alveoli involve highly coordinated interactions among multiple cell lineages, myofibroblasts, epithelial cells, and microvascular endothelial cells and proper deposition of ECM, particularly elastin. In contrast to the extensive knowledge gained about the regulatory mechanisms in branching morphogenesis, it has been challenging to identify the molecular mechanisms that regulate cell proliferation, differentiation, and migration as well as ECM deposition in alveologenesis. Part of the reason is that mouse mutagenesis profoundly affects the earliest stages of lung development, thus resulting in cessation of lung development and/or death prior to the initiation of sacculation and alveolarization. Nevertheless, several signaling pathways have been proposed to play a role in regulating alveolar development.

Myofibroblast Differentiation and Elastin Deposition: Key to Alveolar Septation

Alveolar myofibroblasts have long been recognized to play an essential role in alveolar septation, and platelet-derived growth factor (PDGF) is probably one of the most important factors regulating myofibroblast differentiation. It has been proposed that myofibroblasts are differentiated from alveolar interstitial lipofibroblasts, which "traffic" lipids and store retinoids.[80] Confocal microscopy has revealed that lipofibroblasts with high lipid content are located at the bases of alveolar septa and express low levels of PDGF receptor α(PDGFRα).[81] The same study showed that cells expressing high levels of PDGFRα have the characteristic of myofibroblasts located at the alveolar entry ring. Myofibroblasts have the morphology of fibroblasts but they express α-SMA and contain contractile elements.[82-84] They also produce tropoelastin, the soluble precursor of elastin.[85] Elastin is assembled by crosslinking of tropoelastin under the action of lysyl oxidase in the ECM environment.[86] PDGF subunit A (PDGF-A), a strong chemoattractant for fibroblasts, is produced by alveolar epithelial cells.[87] The importance of PDGF-A, myofibroblasts, and elastin in alveolar septation was demonstrated by early studies in PDGF-$A^{-/-}$ mice. In these mice, a profound deficiency in alveolar myofibroblasts and associated bundles of elastin fibers resulted in absence of secondary septa and definitive alveoli.[87,88] Interestingly, the loss of myofibroblasts and elastin was limited to the lung parenchyma, not occurring in vascular and bronchial smooth muscle cells, indicating the

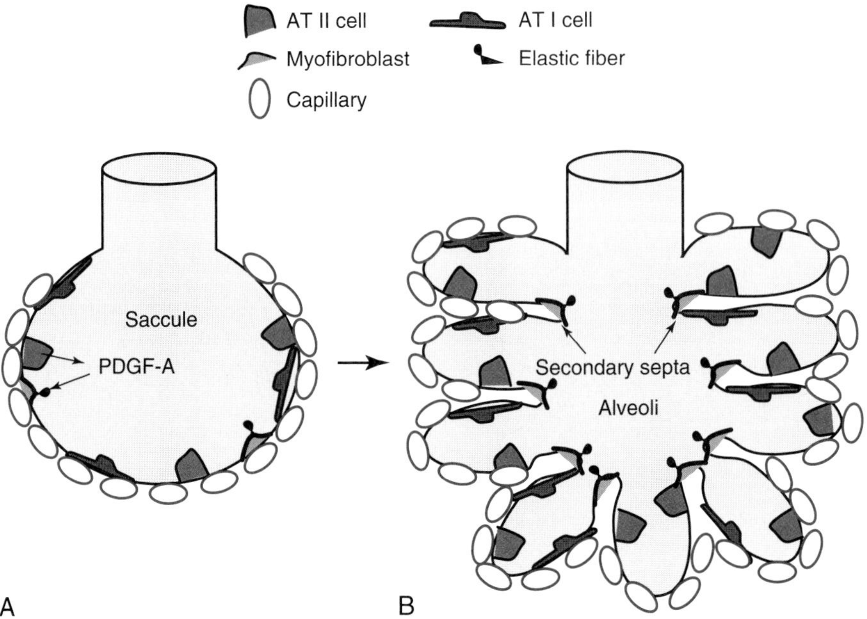

Figure 1-4 Model of alveolarization. **A,** During the later saccular stage, there is increased myofibroblast differentiation and elastin synthesis, stimulated by platelet-derived growth factor subunit A (PDGF-A), which is produced by alveolar type II epithelial (AT II) cells. **B,** During alveolar development, these myofibroblasts produce elastic fibers and migrate toward the alveolar air spaces. The AT II cells, AT I cells, and capillaries move together with the myofibroblasts into the alveolar air spaces to become the secondary septa.

specificity of myofibroblast differentiation and elastin deposition in alveolar septa. It has been suggested that in the absence of PDGF-A, alveolar myofibroblasts or their precursors fail to migrate to the sites where elastin deposition and septation should occur. Furthermore, this migration to the sites of septal budding is not a random phenomenon; conversely, a morphogen gradient would be needed to tightly regulate PDGF-A production, myofibroblast differentiation and migration, and elastin deposition, thus providing instruction for the precise and specific localization of septa (Fig. 1-4).

Many other molecules have been suggested as playing roles in alveolarization by directly or indirectly affecting PDGF signaling, myofibroblast differentiation and migration, and elastin assembly. Increasing data have shown that members of the FGF family play important roles not only in branching morphogenesis but also in alveolarization. Multiple FGFs and FGFRs are expressed in the lung during late stage of fetal development. The critical role for the FGF pathway in alveolar development was demonstrated by a study showing that the lungs of FGFR3/FGFR4 double-mutant mice failed to undergo secondary septation.[89] Retinoic acid is known to be involved not just in early lung morphogenesis but also in alveolar development. Synthesizing enzymes, receptors, and signaling transducers of RA are abundant during alveolar septation. Mice with deletions of RA receptors fail to form normal alveoli.[90] Precisely how RA signaling regulates alveolarization is not well understood. There is evidence for RA crosstalking with PDGF and FGF signaling.[91-94] RA and endogenous retinoids enhance tropoelastin gene expression in rat lung fibroblasts and fetal lung explants.[95,96]

VEGF Signaling Mediates Alveolar Epithelial-Endothelial Interaction in Alveolarization

There is growing evidence that epithelial-endothelial interaction plays an important role in alveolarization. During alveolar development, the extensive capillary network runs parallel to the vast alveolar epithelium, generating functional alveolar structure. The temporal and spatial relationship between the alveolar epithelium and capillary endothelium suggests that their development has to be exquisitely coordinated. Indeed, vascular endothelial growth factor (VEGF) is probably one of the most important angiogenic factors known to play a key role during this process.[97,98] VEGF has the ability to stimulate proliferation, migration, differentiation, and tube formation in endothelial cells. These stimulatory effects are elicited by the binding of VEGF to the two high-affinity VEGF receptors, VEGF receptor 1 (VEGFR1), or Flt-1, and VEGFR2, or Flk-1, on endothelial cells.[97] During normal mouse lung development, various VEGF isoforms (VEGF120, VEGF164, VEGF188) are present in AT II cells, and their expression increases during later canalicular and saccular stages, when most of the vessel growth occurs in the lung.[99] In contrast, VEGFR1 and VEGFR2 are expressed in the adjacent endothelial cells.[100,101] Targeted deletion of the VEGF gene in respiratory epithelium results in an almost complete absence of pulmonary capillaries, and this defective vascular formation is associated with a defect in primary septal formation.[102] Interestingly, these structural defects are coupled with suppression of epithelial proliferation and decreased hepatocyte growth factor (HGF) expression in endothelial cells. Furthermore, targeted deletion of HGF receptor gene in epithelium led to a septation defect similar to that seen in VEGF-deleted lungs. These data highlight the mechanism by which VEGF and HGF signaling pathways orchestrate the reciprocal interactions between airway epithelium and the surrounding endothelium in developing septation. Additional experiments have also demonstrated that inhibition of VEGF signaling by VEGFR inhibitor SU5416 and VEGFR-neutralizing antibodies results in disruption of both angiogenesis and alveolarization.[103-105] Nitric oxide (NO) is known to mediate VEGF angiogenic activity. In a neonatal rat model, SU5416 was shown to downregulate expression of endothelial NO synthase protein and NO production, suggesting a role for NO in mediating VEGF's effect on alveolarization.[104] In contrast, inhaled NO improves alveolar development and pulmonary hypertension in VEGFR inhibitor–treated rats.[106] Further evidence of the importance of NO in alveolarization and vascularization was demonstrated by the combination of disruption of alveolarization and paucity of distal arteries observed in NO synthase–deficient fetal and neonatal mice.[107,108]

There is a great need for improving our understanding of the regulatory mechanisms of alveologenesis. More animal models are needed to better define the crosstalk among alveolar epithelium, endothelium, myofibroblasts, and ECM during alveolar development. This may lead to discovery of novel signaling pathways and a deeper understanding of the interactions among the known pathways in regulation of alveolar septation and vasculogenesis.

Regulation of Pulmonary Vascular Development

The lung vasculature comprises the pulmonary and bronchial vascular systems. The pulmonary system consists of pulmonary arteries that carry blood to the alveolar capillary network to be oxygenated; oxygenated blood returns through pulmonary veins back to the heart. The bronchial system supplies oxygen and nutrients to the nonrespiratory portion of the lung, including the bronchial walls and perihilar region. In contrast to the extensive studies and reviews of the regulatory mechanisms of branching morphogenesis, the molecular bases of pulmonary vascular development are not well understood. Yet pulmonary vascular development is increasingly recognized as being controlled by epithelium-endothelium as well as endothelium-mesenchyme crosstalks.

Vascular Morphogenesis

It is generally believed that early pulmonary vascular development involves three processes to establish a circulatory network: angiogenesis, vasculogenesis, and fusion. *Angiogenesis* is defined as formation of new blood vessels from preexisting ones by sprouting. The new vessels sprout via a well-defined program: degradation of the basement membrane, differentiation of endothelial cells, formation of solid sprouts of endothelial cells connecting neighboring vessels, and restructuring of each sprout into a luminal line by endothelial cells that is integrated into the vascular network.[109] *Vasculogenesis* is defined as de novo formation of blood vessels from angioblasts or endothelial precursor cells arising in the mesodermal mesenchyme. The proximal and distal vessels fuse to establish the luminal connection via a lytic process.[110] Earlier studies by deMello and colleagues[110] indicated that the proximal vessels are generated by angiogenesis, whereas the distal vessels are formed by vasculogenesis during lung morphogenesis. These researchers analyzed serial sections of human embryos and suggested that the same processes occur during human lung formation.[111] However, this concept has been challenged by multiple additional studies. Work from Schachtner and associates[112] suggested that vasculogenesis is primarily responsible for both proximal and distal vascular formation during lung development. Studies by Hall and coworkers[113] in human embryos have also indicated that intrapulmonary arteries originate from a continuous expansion and coalescence of a primary capillary plexus that would form by vasculogenesis during pseudoglandular stage; they have also indicated that the pulmonary veins are formed by the same mechanism. Parera and colleagues[114] have proposed distal angiogenesis as a new concept for early pulmonary vascular morphogenesis. Most recently, Schwarz and associates[115] have proposed that initial pulmonary vessel formation within the mesenchyme is predominately angiogenic.

VEGF-Mediated Epithelial-Endothelial Interaction in Vascular Development

VEGF is one of the most important angiogenic factors regulating vascular development of the lung. During lung development in the mouse embryo, VEGF is expressed in lung mesenchyme and epithelium from E12.5 to E14.5 and then becomes increasingly restricted to epithelium after E14.5.[99,116] Flk-1 (VEGFR2) is abundantly detected in mesenchyme surrounding the developing lung buds from E9.5 to E13.5, with decreased expression from E17.5 to E18.5.[100] This high expression of Flk-1 is associated with active endothelial cell proliferation, and knockdown of Flk-1 by antisense oligonucleotides inhibits endothelial cell proliferation and tube branching. In contrast, Flt-1 (VEGFR1) expression is low from E9.5 to E13.5 and is increased from E14.5 to E18.5. The greater expression of Flt-1 is associated with reduced endothelial cell proliferation, and inhibition of Flt-1 promotes endothelial cell proliferation and tube branching. Moreover, inhibition of Flt-1 also promotes Flk-1 expression. Studies in rat embryonic lung explant cultures have shown that lung bud epithelium determines the level and pattern of expression of Flk-1 in the mesenchyme.[117] The critical role of VEGF signaling in embryogenesis is highlighted by the fact that individual knockouts for VEGF, Flk-1, and Flt-1 result in embryonic lethality prior to the development of the lung capillary plexus.[118-121] Mice with expression of only the non–heparin-binding VEGF120 isoform have significant defects in pulmonary vascular development.[122] Conditional overexpression of VEGF164 in distal lung epithelial cells is reported to disrupt peripheral vascular net assembly and arrest branching of airway tubules.[123] These data suggest that tightly controlled expression of VEGF isoforms and levels is critical to normal pulmonary vascular development. Growing data indicate that VEGF signaling is differentially regulated by FGF9 and Shh signaling during mouse lung development.[124] Mesenchymal expression of VEGF is regulated by gain- and loss-of-function of FGF9, and VEGF is required for FGF9-induced pulmonary blood vessel formation.[124] Shh, on the other hand, regulates the pattern of VEGF expression rather than the level, because loss of Shh signaling did not affect VEGF expression in subepithelial mesenchyme but did decrease VEGF expression in submesothelial mesenchyme.

Additional Angiogenic Factors in Vascular Development

Angiopoietin (Ang)/Tie (tyrosin kinase with immunoglobulin and EGF-like domain) signaling is also known to play an important role in vascular morphogenesis and homeostasis.[125-127] Ang1through Ang4 are members of the Ang family and they primarily bind to Tie2, one of the two receptor tyrosine kinases predominantly expressed in vascular endothelial cells.[128-130] Ang/Tie signaling is known to play a primary role in the later stages of vascular development and in adult vasculature, where they control remodeling and stabilization of vessels.[127,131] Ang1 appears to work in complementary fashion with VEGF during early vascular development. VEGF appears to initiate vascular formation, and Ang1 promotes subsequent vascular remodeling, maturation, and stabilization, perhaps, in part, by supporting interactions between endothelial cells and surrounding support cells and ECM. The role of Ang1/Tie2 in developmental angiogenesis is highlighted by the early embryonic lethality and significant abnormal vascular development observed in offspring of Ang1$^{-/-}$, Tie1$^{-/-}$, Tie2$^{-/-}$, and Tie1/Tie2$^{-/-}$ mice.[132-134] Although the vessels are formed in these mice, they have decreased complexity and sprouting and increased dilation and rupture. In contrast, Ang2$^{-/-}$ mice lack embryonic vascular defects but have impaired lymphatic development.[135] Thus, Ang2 is not requisite during embryonic vascular development but, instead, is necessary during subsequent, postnatal vascular remodeling. The specific role of Ang/Tie2 signaling in pulmonary vascular development is poorly understood. Studies have shown that Ang1 is expressed in lungs of newborn mice and that its expression is increased from P1 to P14, whereas Ang2 is abundantly expressed at birth and decreases as Ang1 increases.[136] Transgenic overexpression of a potent form of Ang1 protein, COMP-Ang1, in lung epithelium resulted in 50% lethality at birth due to respiratory failure. The alveolar and vascular structures were abnormal in the affected mice.[136] Thus, precise regulation of Tie2 signaling through an Ang1 and Ang2 expression switch is important to construct the mature lung vascular network required for normal lung development. There are studies suggesting that Ang1 plays a role in pulmonary hypertension, on the basis of the fact that overexpression of Ang1 causes severe pulmonary hypertension and Ang1 is increased in lungs of patients with pulmonary hypertension.[137,138] However, cell-based Ang1 gene transfer protects against monocrotaline-induced experimental pulmonary hypertension.[139]

The Eph family of receptor tyrosine kinases and their membrane-tethered ligands, known as *ephrins,* also play an important role in vascular development. Ephrin-B2 is expressed on arterial and lymphatic endothelial cells as well as perivascular cells, and its receptor, EphB4, is largely confined to venous and lymphatic endothelial cells.[140] This differential expression of ephrin/Eph may direct commitment of vessels to arteries, veins, or lymphatics. The final vascular response to ephrin-B2 engagement with its receptors on adjacent cells is adapted by bidirectional signaling interactions with endothelial cells and between endothelial cells and adjacent nonendothelial cells.[141,142] Gene targeting studies have established several class B Eph family members as key regulators of embryonic vascular development. Targeted disruption of ephrin-B2, EphB4, or combined deficiency in the receptors EphB2 and EphB3 in mice results in embryonic lethality and angiogenic defects.[140-144] Despite strong genetic evidence that class B Eph/ephrin plays an essential role in vasculogenesis, its role in pulmonary vascular development is largely unknown. Studies have also shown that ephrin-B2 is expressed on the epithelial layers during pseudoglandular and canalicular stages of mouse lung development and in capillary network during the saccular stage.[145] EphB2, EphB4, and EphA4, receptors for ephrin-B2, are present in endothelial cells. Ephrin-B1 is expressed on vasculature and interstitial cells during early stages of secondary septation. Thus these complex expression patterns among ephrins and Ephs indicate that they may coordinate interactions between lung epithelial-endothelial as well as endothelial-interstitial compartments. Indeed, mice homozygous for the hypomorphic knockin allele of ephrin-B2, encoding mutant ephrin-B2, show severe postnatal lung defects, including an almost complete absence of alveoli and disorganized elastic matrix.[145]

Other angiogenic signaling pathways, such as Notch, Wnt and midkine, are likely involved in pulmonary vascular development.[9,146] More studies are needed to define the regulatory mechanisms of these important pathways as well as the interactions among the pathways during normal and abnormal lung vascular morphogenesis.

Lung Injury and Repair: Disruption of Normal Lung Development

With its vast airway and alveolar epithelium open to the atmosphere, the newborn lung is at a great risk for harmful environmental insults, such as oxidative stress, physical forces, and infective agents. These environmental challenges put the lung under constant threat of injury, repair, and remodeling processes. The lungs of full-term neonates have a great ability to overcome various injuries, to generate needed repair and remodeling processes, and ultimately to maintain and/or restore normal lung architecture and normal lung function. When premature delivery occurs, particularly between 24 and 28 wk, the lungs of the preterm infants are in the late canalicular to early saccular stage. Alveolarization has not yet begun, and surfactant production is minimal. These lungs are at great risk for injury, altered development, and BPD.

Over the past four decades, with the improvement in neonatal intensive care, introduction of exogenous surfactant therapy, and development of advanced ventilator strategies, the survival of extremely premature infants has been significantly enhanced. At the same time, the incidence of BPD has risen. BPD is increasingly being recognized as developmental arrest of the immature lung caused by injurious stimuli such as mechanical ventilation, oxygen exposure, and intrauterine or postnatal infection. Larger and simplified alveoli and decreased vascular growth are the key pathologic features observed in the lungs of infants dying of BPD.[7] The combination of decreased vascular growth and excessive pulmonary vascular remodeling leads to pulmonary hypertension, which significantly contributes to the morbidity and mortality of these infants.[9] Yet the underlying cellular and molecular mechanisms are poorly defined. The higher incidence of BPD has not only provided us with tremendous challenge in managing these patients but has also shown the need for better understanding of the molecular basis of neonatal lung injury and repair. Experimental models of BPD have utilized larger animals such as baboons and sheep as well as smaller animals such as rats and mice. These studies attempt to create a BPD model by exposing immature baboons and sheep or neonatal rats and mice to noxious stimuli such as mechanical ventilation, hyperoxia, and infection. Extensive data generated from these studies indicate that the key signaling pathways that regulate normal lung development can be disrupted by injurious stimuli in the immature lung, and this disruption appears to play an important role in the pathogenesis of BPD. Although many growth factors have been shown to be involved in neonatal lung injury, it is clear that TGF-β and VEGF are probably the two most important growth factors studied to date (Fig. 1-5).

Increased TGF-β Signaling in Neonatal Lung Injury and Bronchopulmonary Dysplasia

More than a decade ago, Kotecha and associates[147] showed that higher levels of total and bioactive TGF-β were detected in bronchoalveolar lavage (BAL) fluid from preterm infants in whom BPD subsequently developed. Since then, cumulative data from both clinical and animal studies have indicated a critical role for dysregulated TGF-β signaling in neonatal lung injury, deranged repair, and pathogenesis of BPD. One study has shown that increased TGF-β concentration in amniotic fluid of preterm deliveries is correlated with histologic severity of chorioamnionitis, subsequent development of BPD, and duration of oxygen therapy in preterm infants.[148] In fetal sheep, chorioamnionitis-associated antenatal inflammation increases TGF-β levels and induces Smad2 phosphorylation, indicating activation of TGF-β signaling.[149] In preterm lambs, long-term mechanical ventilation increases TGF-β expression in the lung, which is associated with dysregulated pulmonary elastin synthesis and disrupted alveolar development.[150] In oxygen-exposed newborn mice, increased

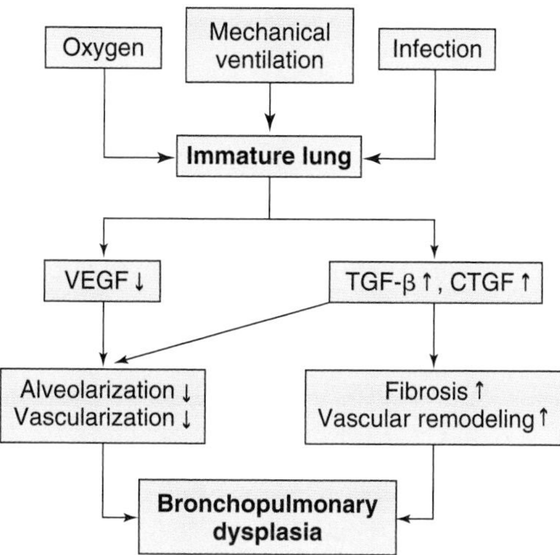

Figure 1-5 Schematic illustrating the involvement of dysregulated vascular endothelial growth factor (VEGF) and transforming growth factor β (TGF-β) in the pathogenesis of bronchopulmonary dysplasia. CTGF, connective tissue growth factor; ↑, increased; ↓, decreased.

TGF-β signaling is responsible for aberrant lysyl oxidase expression, which may impede the matrix remodeling that is required for normal alveolarization.[151] Additional studies confirmed that hyperoxia upregulates TGF-β in neonatal mice.[152] Furthermore, primary AT II cells isolated from oxygen-exposed mice were more susceptible to TGF-β–induced apoptosis, and oxygen exposure enhanced TGF-β–induced production of ECM components, including type I collagen, tropoelastin, and tenascin-C.[152]

Studies in transgenic mouse models further support that increasing lung expression of TGF-β disrupts alveolar development. For example, overexpression of TGF-β in respiratory epithelium under the control of human surfactant protein C (SFPTC) gene promoter resulted in arrested lung development at the pseudoglandular stage and perinatal death at E18.5.[153] There was decreased epithelial cell differentiation, as indicated by inhibition of Clara cell secretory protein (CCSP) and pro-surfactant protein C expression in the transgenic lungs. Expression of α-SMA and collagen I was also altered in the transgenic lungs. To solve the problem of prenatal death, a later study used a triple transgenic construct to overexpress bioactive TGF-β under the control of CCSP promoter and doxycyclin.[154] Induction of TGF-β expression from P7 to P14 resulted in larger alveoli with thick and hypercellular septa, increased proliferation in α-SMA–positive cells in the septa, and abnormal capillary development.

Although increased TGF-β signaling is overwhelmingly linked to clinical as well as animal models of BPD, there have been very few studies examining the therapeutic potential of TGF-β antagonism in neonatal lung injury. Nakanishi and coworkers[155] injected a TGF-β–neutralizing antibody to pregnant mice at E17 and E19 and then exposed the newborn pups to 85% oxygen for 10 days.[155] They found that treatment with TGF-β–neutralizing antibody significantly attenuated hyperoxia-induced Smad2 activation and improved alveolar development, ECM assembly, and microvascular development. In another study, treatment with rosiglitazone, a peroxisome proliferator–activated receptor-γ agonist, blocked hyperoxia-induced activation of TGF-β signaling and prevented alveolar damage.[156] Whether TGF-β inhibition would be beneficial in preventing BPD is yet to be determined. Given the exceptionally broad range of biologic activity ascribed to TGF-β and its fundamental physiologic roles, nonselective TGF-β blockade could have undesired consequences. Complete abrogation of TGF-β signaling could lead to loss of immune tolerance, spontaneous autoimmunity, and defective tissue repair.[157] Therefore, identification of the downstream mediators and pathways of TGF-β may enhance our mechanistic understanding of neonatal lung injury and repair and provide effective targets for preventing or treating BPD.

Connective tissue growth factor (CTGF), a multimodular matrix-associated protein, is thought to be a downstream mediator and coactivator of TGF-β and plays an important role in tissue development and remodeling.[158-162] CTGF expression can also be induced by other factors involved in tissue remodeling, such as angiotensin II, endothelin, mechanical forces, and oxygen exposure.[163-166] Upon stimulation, CTGF is secreted into the extracellular environment where it interacts with distinct cell surface receptors, growth factors, and ECM. The principal CTGF receptors are the heterodimeric cell surface integrin complexes.[167] CTGF can also bind to Wnt coreceptors, LPR5 and LPR6, thus activating Wnt signaling.[168] In addition to its ability to bind to integrins and LRPs, CTGF can also bind to growth factors in ECM, thus modulating diverse signaling pathways. Binding of CTGF to TGF-β enhances dimerization of TGF-β to its receptor, thus facilitating TGF-β signaling.[169] In contrast, binding of CTGF to VEGF decreases VEGF interaction with its receptor, thus inhibiting VEGF angiogenic activity.[170] Furthermore, CTGF can also bind to BMP, leading to inhibition of BMP signaling.[169]

Historically, CTGF is best known for its fibroproliferative effect and is implicated in various forms of adult lung fibrosis.[168] Growing evidence indicates that CTGF plays an important role in embryonic lung development. CTGF is expressed in distal airway epithelium during embryonic lung development.[171] In mouse embryonic lung explant cultures, expression of CTGF is upregulated by TGF-β and CTGF inhibits branching morphogenesis.[172] $CTGF^{-/-}$ mice die soon after birth with respiratory failure.[173] These mice display severe rib cage malformations, and their lungs are hypoplastic with reduced cell proliferation and increased apoptosis, suggesting that CTGF deficiency may disrupt the normal processes of embryonic lung development.[173,174]

The clinical relevance of CTGF in BPD is suggested by a study demonstrating increased CTGF in bronchoalveolar lavage fluid from premature infants with BPD.[175] The role of CTGF in neonatal lung development and remodeling has been examined in multiple studies, results of which indicate that long-term exposure to hyperoxia increases CTGF expression in lungs of neonatal mice and rats.[152,166] In addition, injurious mechanical ventilation with high tidal volume upregulates CTGF expression in newborn rat and lamb lungs.[165,176] Utilizing conditional transgenic mouse models, two studies have investigated the functional role of CTGF in neonatal lung development. Overexpression of CTGF in respiratory epithelial cells under the control of the CCSP gene promoter resulted in thickened alveolar septa and decreases in alveolarization and capillary density in neonatal mice.[177] These structural changes were associated with dysregulated gene expression of elastin-assembling molecules and disorganized deposition of elastin in the alveolar septa. Overexpression of CTGF in AT II cells under the control of SFTPC gene promoter not only disrupted alveolarization and decreased vascular density but also induced pulmonary vascular remodeling and pulmonary hypertension in neonatal mice.[178] These pathologic changes have striking similarities to those observed in clinical BPD and hyperoxia-induced rodent models of BPD. In addition, treatment with a CTGF-neutralizing antibody significantly improved alveolar and vascular development and decreased pulmonary vascular remodeling and pulmonary hypertension in hyperoxia-induced lung injury in neonatal rats.[179] The efficacy of CTGF antibody in this study was confirmed by multiple studies in adult patients as well as adult animal models with various fibrotic disorders, including lung fibrosis caused by radiation exposure and bleomycin treatment.[180,181]

Decreased VEGF Signaling in Neonatal Lung Injury and Bronchopulmonary Dysplasia

A growing body of data has shown that lung VEGF expression is decreased in clinical BPD as well as experimental models of BPD. Preterm infants in whom BPD subsequently develops have lower VEGF concentration in their tracheal aspirates (TAs) than those in whom BPD does not develop.[182] Expression of VEGF and VEGFR1 is decreased in lung autopsy specimens from preterm infants dying with BPD and that is correlated with decreased expression of platelet endothelial cell adhesion molecule (PECAM) in alveolar capillary endothelial cells.[183] However, infants who have undergone long-term ventilation were found to have increased total pulmonary microvascular endothelial volume and PECAM expression, suggesting increased angiogenesis.[184] These increases were attributed to brisk endothelial cell proliferation. Subsequent studies have shown that although VEGF and its receptors were decreased in ventilated lungs from preterm infants, endoglin, a hypoxia-inducible TGF-β coreceptor and important regulator of angiogenesis, was increased.[185] This finding suggests that BPD is associated with a shift from traditional angiogenic growth factors to alternative regulators that may contribute to BPD-associated microvascular dysangiogenesis.

Extensive studies in animal models of BPD were conducted to explore how VEGF signaling is regulated and whether enhancing VEGF signaling could protect against alveolar and vascular damage. Exposure to hyperoxia decreases lung VEGF expression in neonatal rabbits and rodents and in preterm baboons and lambs.[186-190] Hyperoxia also decreases VEGFR1 and VEGFR2 expression in neonatal rats and mice and in preterm baboons.[187,150,190] Mechanical ventilation has been shown to decrease VEGF and VEGFR expression in newborn mice and preterm baboons.[150,189] In addition to hyperoxia and mechanical ventilation, endotoxin exposure can modulate VEGF expression in immature lungs. Exposure of pregnant rats to endotoxin on E20 and E21 significantly increased lung VEGF and VEGFR2 gene expression in their offspring at P2 to P14.[191] These molecular changes were associated with alterations in gene expression of lysyl oxidase, fibulin, PDGFRα, and morphologic changes with fewer and larger alveoli, fewer secondary septa, and decreased peripheral vessel density. Although these data indicate that the timing, the length, and the type of lung injuries variably modulate VEGF signaling, the underlying mechanisms are poorly understood.

Given the increasing recognition of the importance of VEGF signaling in normal lung development and injury, investigations have tested the therapeutic potential of modulating VEGF signaling in experimental models of BPD. In a newborn rat model of BPD, treatment with recombinant VEGF during and after hyperoxia enhanced both vascular and alveolar development.[192,193] Adenovirus-mediated VEGF gene therapy improved survival, promoted lung angiogenesis, and prevented alveolar damage in hyperoxia-induced lung injury in newborn rats.[194] In these studies, increased VEGF also induced immature and leaky capillaries and lung edema. In a study using a transgenic mouse model, overexpression of VEGF in respiratory epithelial cells resulted in pulmonary hemorrhage, hemosiderosis, and air space enlargement in neonatal mice.[195] These adverse outcomes of capillary leakage and hemorrhage suggest the importance of tightly regulated angiogenesis in neonatal lung development and injury repair, as well as the complexity of enhancing angiogenesis as a therapeutic approach to treat BPD. It was proposed that VEGF may work with other angiogenic factors, such as angiopoietins, to form stabilized vessels during development. This hypothesis was supported by the data showing that combined VEGF and Ang1 gene therapy reduced capillary leakage and improved vascular and alveolar development in neonatal rats during hyperoxia.[194]

Imbalance of MMPs and Tissue Inhibitors of Metalloproteinases in Neonatal Lung Injury and Bronchopulmonary Dysplasia

ECM components, particularly collagens, are the major constituents of alveolar basement membrane. Normal ECM remodeling is important not only for the integrity of alveolar structure but also for alveolar septation. MMPs are a family of proteolytic enzymes that can degrade ECM components, thus leading to ECM remodeling during physiologic and pathologic processes.[196] MMPs are secreted as zymogens (pro-MMPs) that require proteolysis for activation, and their activities are tightly controlled by specific tissue inhibitors of metalloproteinases (TIMPs).[197] TIMP2 is the specific inhibitor of MMP2 (gelatinase A), and TIMP1 is the specific inhibitor of MMP9 (gelatinase B) but with overlapping inhibitory activities on other MMPs. MMP2 is secreted mainly by noninflammatory cells such as epithelial cells, endothelial cells, and fibroblasts. In contrast, MMP9 is produced by inflammatory cells, including macrophages and neutrophils.[198] MMP2 and MMP9 have the ability to degrade collagen IV, the major component of lung basement membrane. MMP1 and MMP8 are collagenases that break down type I collagen, the major structural protein of ECM.[198]

Extensive data indicate that MMPs play an important role in normal lung development, whereas imbalances of MMPs/TIMPs are implicated in neonatal lung injury and pathogenesis of BPD. Studies in baboons have shown that MMP1, MMP2, MMP8, and MMP9 are differentially expressed during lung development.[199] Hyperoxia exposure caused an increase in lung MMP9 expression in preterm baboons that was associated with changes in alveolar structure.[199] Hyperoxia exposure also increased MMP2, MMP9, type I collagen, and tropoelastin expression and caused alveolar enlargement in wild-type mice.[200] However, $MMP9^{-/-}$ mice were resistant to hyperoxia-induced alveolar damage as well as expression of type I collagen and tropoelastin, suggesting an important role for MMP9 in hyperoxia-induced neonatal lung injury.[200] Many studies have been conducted in preterm infants to investigate the potential role of MMPs/TIMPs in the pathogenesis of BPD, with conflicting results.[201-204] Increased MMP8 levels in TAs from preterm infants during the first 5 days of life is associated with increased risk for development of BPD.[201] Premature infants with BPD and intraventricular hemorrhage have higher MMP9 and MMP2 levels but lower MMP2 levels in their plasma.[202] Higher ratio of MMP9 to TIMP1 in TAs is observed in infants with BPD.[203] However, when data are controlled for gestational age, the imbalance of MMP9 with TIMP1 appears not to be a predictor for BPD.[204]

Conclusions

Lung developmental processes involve lung bud initiation, branching morphogenesis, saccular formation, alveolar septation, and accompanying vascular development, which begin in the embryonic period and continue through the fetal and postnatal periods. These dynamic processes are tightly regulated by epithelium-mesenchyme crosstalks orchestrated by groups of transcriptional factors, growth factors, and ECM components. Temporally and spatially regulated specific cell differentiation, proliferation, and survival and ECM deposition give rise to the complex lung structure. To add to the complexity of these interdependent cell-cell as well as cell-ECM interactions, the need to form a coordinated air passage system and blood circulating system in the lung is paramount and unmatched by any other organ system. Furthermore, airway epithelium is exposed to the atmosphere and puts the newborn lung at a great risk for injury. Significant progress has been made in our understanding of basic lung developmental processes and identification of some of the regulatory pathways through mouse molecular genetic and genomic studies. We have also discovered that many of the signaling pathways that control normal lung development are also key players in animal models of neonatal lung injury and BPD. However, there are still many unanswered questions as to how these pathways affect human lung development, injury, and repair, particularly BPD pathogenesis. Whether disruption of these pathways in the immature lung can be reversed and whether the structural defects observed in BPD can be regenerated through modulation of these pathways are also unknown. Thus, future studies are needed to clarify the interactions of these key regulatory pathways and to identify novel signaling in animal and human lung development. Such studies may provide new insights into BPD pathogenesis, prevention, and therapy.

References

1. Warburton D, Schwarz M, Tefft D, et al. The molecular basis of lung morphogenesis. *Mech Dev.* 2000;92:55-81.
2. Weibel ER. Design and development of the mammalian lung. In: *The Pathway of Oxygen*. London: Harvard University Press; 1984:211.

3. Comore JH. *Physiology of Respiration*. Chicago: Year Book; 1965:11-16.
4. Jeffery PK, Hislop AA. Embryology and growth. In: Gibson GJ, Geddes DM, Costabel U, et al, eds. *Respiratory Medicine*. Saunders; 2003:50-63.
5. Angus GE, Thurlbeck WM. Number of alveoli in the human lung. *J Appl Physiol*. 1972;32: 483-485.
6. Thurlbeck WM. Postnatal growth and development of the lung. *Am Rev Respir Dis*. 1975;3: 803-844.
7. Husain AN, Siddiqui NH, Stocker JT. Pathology of arrested acinar development in post surfactant bronchopulmonary dysplasia. *Hum Pathol*. 1998;29:710-717.
8. Burri PH. Lung development and pulmonary angiogenesis. In: Gaultier C, Bourbon JR, Post M, eds. *Lung Development*. New York: Oxford University Press; 1999:122-151.
9. Abman SH, Baker C, Balasubramaniam V. Growth and development of the lung circulation: mechanisms and clinical implications. In: Bancalari E, Polin RA, eds. *The Newborn Lung*. Saunders Elsevier; 2008:50-72.
10. Kimura S, Hara Y, Pineau T, et al. The T/ebp null mouse: thyroid-specific enhancer-binding protein is essential for the organogenesis of the thyroid, lung, ventral forebrain, and pituitary. *Genes Dev*. 1996;10:60-69.
11. Minoo P, Su G, Drum H, et al. Defects in tracheoesophageal and lung morphogenesis in Nkx2.1$^{-/-}$ mouse embryos. *Dev Biol*. 1999;209:60-71.
12. Kelly SC, Bachurski CJ, Burhans MS, Glasser SW. Transcription of the lung-specific surfactant protein C gene is mediated by thyroid transcript factor 1. *J Biol Chem*. 1996;271:6881-6888.
13. Goss AM, Tian T, Tsukiyama T, et al. Wnt2/2b and β-catenin signaling are necessary and sufficient to specify lung progenitors in the foregut, *Dev Cell*. 2009;17:290-298.
14. Harris-Johnson KS, Domyan ET, Vezina CM, Sun X. Beta-Catenin promotes respiratory progenitor identity in mouse foregut. *Proc Natl Acad Sci USA*. 2009;106:16287-16292.
15. Bitgood MJ, McMahon AP. Hedgehog and BMP genes are coexpressed at many diverse sites of cell-cell interaction in the mouse embryo. *Dev Biol*. 1995;172:126-138.
16. Bellusci S, Furuta Y, Rush MG, et al. Involvement of Sonic hedgehog (Shh) in mouse embryonic lung growth and morphogenesis. *Development*. 1997;124:53-63.
17. Urase K, Mukasa T, Irigashi H, et al. Spatial expression of Sonic hedgehog in the lung epithelium during branching morphogenesis. *Biochem Biophys Res Commun*. 1996;225:161-166.
18. Chiang C, Litingtung Y, Lee E, et al. Cyclopia and defective axial patterning in mice lacking Sonic hedgehog gene function. *Nature*. 1996 Oct 3;383:407-413.
19. Motoyama J, Liu J, Mo R, et al. Essential function of Gli2 and Gli3 in the formation of lung, trachea and esophagus. *Nat Genet*. 1998;20:54-57.
20. Grindley JC, Bellusci S, Perkins D, Hogan BL. Evidence for the involvement of the Gli gene family in embryonic mouse lung development. *Dev Biol*. 1997;188:337-348.
21. Bellusci S, Grindley J, Emoto H, et al. Fibroblast growth factor 10 (FGF10) and branching morphogenesis in the embryonic lung. *Development*. 1997;124:4867-4878.
22. Park WY, Miranda B, Lebeche D, et al. FGF-10 is chemotactic factor for distal epithelial buds during lung development. *Dev Biol*. 1998;201:125-134.
23. Cardoso WV, Lu J. Regulation of early lung morphogenesis: questions, facts and controversies. *Development*. 2006;133:1611-1624.
24. Min H, Danilenko DM, Scully SA, et al. FGF-10 is required for both limb and lung development and exhibits striking functional similarity to Drosophila branchless. *Gene Dev*. 1998;12: 3156-3161.
25. Sekine K, Ohuchi H, Fukiwara M, et al. FGF10 is essential for limb and lung formation. *Nat Genet*. 1999;21:138-141.
26. Rawins EL, Hogan BL. Intercellular growth factor signaling and the development of mouse tracheal submucosal glands. *Dev Dyn*. 2005;233;1378-1385.
27. De Moerlooze L, Spencer-Dene B, Revest J, et al. An important role of the IIIb isoform of fibroblast growth factor receptor (FGFR2) in mesenchymal-epithelial signaling during mouse organogenesis. *Development*. 2000;127:483-492.
28. Lu W, Luo Y, Kan M, Mckeehan WL. Fibroblast growth factor-10. A second candidate stromal to epithelial cell andromedin in prostate. *J Biol Chem*. 1999;274:12827-12834.
29. Morrisey EE, Hogan BLM. Preparing for the first breath: genetic and cellular mechanisms in lung development. *Developmental Cell*. 2010;18:8-23.
30. Peters KG, Chen WG, Williams LT. Two FGF receptors are differentially expressed in epithelial and mesenchymal tissue during limb formation and organogenesis. *Development*. 1992;114:233-243.
31. Cardoso WV, Itoh A, Nogawa H, et al. FGF-1 and FGF-7 induce distinct patterns of growth and differentiation in embryonic lung epithelium. *Dev Dyn*. 1997;208:398-405.
32. Bellusci S, Grindley J, Emoto H, et al. Fibroblast growth factor 10 (FGF10) and branching morphogenesis in the embryonic mouse lung. *Development*. 1997;124:4867-4878.
33. Weaver M, Dunn NR, Hogan BL. Bmp4 and FGF10 play opposing roles during lung bud morphogenesis. *Development*. 2000;127:2695-2704.
34. Lebeche D, Malpel S, Cardoso WV. Fibroblast growth factor interactions in the developing lung. *Mech Dev*. 1999;86(2):125-136.
35. Pepicelli CV, Lewis P, McMahon A. Sonic hedgehog regulates branching morphogenesis in the mammalian lung. *Cur Biol*. 1998;8:1083-1086.
36. Kim HJ, Bar-Sagi D. Modulation of signaling by Sprouty: a developing story. *Nat Rev Mol Cell Biol*. 2004;5:441-450.

37. Mailleux AA, Tefft D, Ndiaye D, et al. Evidence that Sprouty2 functions as an inhibitor of mouse embryonic lung growth and morphogenesis. *Mech Dev.* 2001:102:81-94.
38. Tefft JD, Lee M, Smith S, et al. Coserved function of mSpry-2, a murine homolog of Drosophila Sprouty, which negatively modulates respiratory organogenesis. *Curr Biol.* 1999;9:219-222.
39. Perl AK, Hokuto I, Impagnatiello MA, et al. Temporal effects of Sprouty on lung morphogenesis. *Dev Biol.* 2003;258:154-168.
40. Weaver M, Yingling JM, Dunn NR, et al. Bmp signaling regulates proximal-distal differentiation of endoderm in mouse lung development. *Development.* 1999;126:4005-4015.
41. Weaver M, Batts L, Hogan BL. Tissue interactions pattern the mesenchyme of the embryonic mouse lung. *Dev Biol.* 2003;258:169-184.
42. Bellusci S, Henderson R, Winnier G, et al. Evidence from normal expression and targeted misexpression that bone morphogenetic protein (Bmp-4) plays a role in mouse embryonic lung morphogenesis. *Development.* 1996;122:1693-1702.
43. Chen C, Chen H, Sun J, et al. Smad1 expression and function during mouse embryonic lung branching morphogenesis. *Am J Physiol Lung Cell Mol Physiol.* 2005;288:L1033-1039.
44. Eblaghie MC, Reedy M, Oliver T, et al. Evidence that autocrine signaling through BMPR1a regulates the proliferation, survival and morphogenetic behavior of distal lung epithelial cells. *Dev Biol.* 2006;291:67-82.
45. Sun J, Chen H, Chen C, et al. Prenatal lung epithelial cell-specific abrogation of Alk3-bone morphogenetic protein signaling causes neonatal respiratory distress by disrupting distal airway formation. *Am J Pathol.* 2008;172:571-582.
46. Bragg AD, Moses HL, Serra R. Signaling to the epithelium is not sufficient to mediate all the effects of transforming growth factor beta and bone morphogenetic protein 4 on mouse embryonic lung development. *Mech Dev.* 2001;109;13-26.
47. Heine UI, Munoz EF, Flanders KC, et al. Colocalization of TGF-beta1 and collagen I and III, fibronectin and glycosaminoglycans during lung branching morphogenesis. *Development.* 1990; 109:29-36.
48. Pelton RW, Johnson MD, Perkett EA, et al. Expression of transforming growth factor-beta 1, -beta 2, and -beta 3 mRNA and protein in the murine lung. *Am J Respir Cell Mol Biol.* 1991;5:522-530.
49. McLennan IS, Poussart Y, Koishi K. Development of skeletal muscles in transforming growth factor-beta 1 (TGF-beta1) null-mutant mice. *Dev Dyn.* 2000;217:250-256.
50. Bartram U, Molin DG, Wisse LJ, et al. Double-outlet right ventricle and overriding tricuspid valve reflect disturbances of looping, myocardialization, endocardial cushion differentiation, and apoptosis in TGF-beta(2)knockout mice. *Circulation.* 2001;103:2745-2752.
51. Kaartinen V, Voncken JW, Shuler C, et al. Abnormal lung development and cleft palate in mice lacking TGF-beta 3 indicates defects of epithelial-mesenchymal interaction. *Nat Genet.* 1995;11: 415-421.
52. Shi W, Heisterkamp N, Groffen J, et al. TGF-beta3-null mutation does not abrogate fetal lung maturation in vivo by glucocorticoids. *Am J Physiol.* 1999;277:L1205-L1213.
53. Zhou L, Dey CR, Wert SE, Whitsett JA. Arrested lung morphogenesis in transgenic mice bearing an SP-C-TGF-beta 1 chimeric gene. *Dev Biol.* 1996;175:227-238.
54. Zeng X, Gray M, Stahlman MT, Whitsett JA. TGF-beta1 perturbs vascular development and inhibits epithelial differentiation in fetal lung in vivo. *Dev Dyn.* 2001;221:289-301.
55. Serra R, Pelton RW, Moses HL. TGF beta 1 inhibits branching morphogenesis and N-myc expression in lung bud organ cultures. *Development.* 1994;120(8):2153-2161.
56. Serra R, Moses HL. pRb is necessary for inhibition of N-myc expression by TGF-beta 1 in embryonic lung organ cultures. *Development.* 1995;121:3057-3066.
57. Wu S, Peng J, Duncan MR, et al. ALK-5 mediates endogenous and TGF-beta1-induced expression of connective tissue growth factor in embryonic lung. *Am J Respir Cell Mol Biol.* 2007 May;36: 552-561.
58. Zhao J, Lee M, Smith S, Warburton D. Abrogation of Smad3 and Smad2 or of Smad4 gene expression positively regulates murine embryonic lung branching morphogenesis in culture. *Dev Biol.* 1998 Feb 15;194:182-195.
59. Konigshoff M, Eickelberg O. Wnt signaling in lung disease: a failure or a regeneration signaling? *Am J Respir Cell Mol Biol.* 2010;42:21-31.
60. Logan CY, Nusse R. The WNT signaling pathway in development and disease. *Annu Rev Cell Dev Biol.* 2004;20:781-810.
61. Dale TC. Signal transduction by the WNT family of ligands. *Biochem J.* 1998;329:209-223.
62. Moon RT, Kohn AD, De Ferrari GV, Kaykas A. WNT and beta-catenin signalling: Diseases and therapies. *Nat Rev Genet.* 2004;5:691-701.
63. Lako M, Strachan T, Bullen P, et al. Isolation, characterization and embryonic expression of WNT11, a gene which maps to 11q13.5 and has possible roles in the development of skeleton, kidney and lung. *Gene.* 1998;219:101-110.
64. Zakin LD, Mazan S, Maury M, et al. Structure and expression of Wnt13, a novel mouse Wnt2 related gene. *Mech Dev.* 1998;73:107-116.
65. Tebar M, Destree D, de Vree WJ, Have-Opbroek AA. Expression of Tcf/Lef and sfrp and localization of beta-catenin in the developing mouse lung. *Mech Dev.* 2001;109:437-440.
66. Levay-Young BK, Navre M. Growth and developmental regulation of WNT-2 (IRP) gene in mesenchymal cells of fetal lung. *Am J Physiol.* 1992;262:L672-L683.
67. Wu S, Jiang YQ, Lu MM, Morrisey EE. Wnt7b regulates mesenchymal proliferation and vascular development in the lung. *Development.* 2002;129:4831-4842.

A

68. Li C, Hu L, Xiao J, et al. Wnt5a regulates SHH and FGF10 signaling during lung development. *Dev Biol*. 2005;287:86-97.
69. Li C, Xiao J, Hormi K, et al. Wnt5a participates in distal lung morphogenesis. *Dev Biol*. 2002;248: 68-81.
70. Wu S, Guttentag S, Wang Z, et al. Wnt/beta-catenin signaling acts upstream of n-myc, BMP4, and FGF signaling to regulate proximal-distal patterning in the lung. *Dev Biol*. 2005;283: 226-239.
71. De Langhe SP, Sala FG, Del Moral PM, et al. Dickkopf-1 (DKK1) reveals that fibronectin is a major target of Wnt signaling in branching morphogenesis of the mouse embryonic lung. *Dev Biol*. 2005;277:316-331.
72. Dean CH, Miller LA, Smith AN, et al. Canonical Wnt signaling negatively regulates branching morphogenesis of the lung and lacrimal gland. *Dev Biol*. 2005;286:270-286.
73. Roman J, Little CW, McDonald JA. Potential role of RGD-binding integrins in mammalian lung branching morphogenesis. *Development*. 1991;112:551-558.
74. Wu JE, Santoro SA. Differential expression of integrin alpha subunits supports distinct roles during lung branching morphogenesis. *Dev Dyn*. 1996;206:169-181.
75. Kreidberg JA, Donovan MJ, Goldstein SL, et al. Alpha 3 beta 1 integrin has a crucial role in kidney and lung organogenesis. *Development*. 1996;122:3537-3547.
76. Coraux C, Meneguzzi G, Rousselle P, et al. Distribution of laminin 5, integrin receptors, and branching morphogenesis during human fetal lung development. *Dev Dyn*. 2002;225:176-185.
77. Benjamin JT, Gaston DC, Halloran BA, et al. The role of integrin alpha8beta1 in fetal lung morphogenesis and injury. *Dev Biol*. 2009;335:407-417.
78. Oblander SA, Zhou Z, Gálvez BG, et al. Distinctive functions of membrane type 1 matrix metalloproteinase (MT1-MMP or MMP-14) in lung and submandibular gland development are independent of its role in pro-MMP-2 activation. *Dev Biol*. 2005;277:255-269.
79. Greenlee KJ, Werb Z, Kheradmand F. Matrix metalloproteinases in lung: multiple, multifarious, and multifaceted. *Physiol Rev*. 2007;87:69-98.
80. Schultz CJ, Torres E, Londos C, Torday JS. Role of adipocyte differentiation-related protein in surfactant phospholipid synthesis by type II cells. *Am J Physiol Lung Cell Mol Physiol*. 2002;283:L288-L296.
81. McGowan SE, Grossmann RE, Kimani PW, Holmes AJ. Platelet-derived growth factor receptor-alpha-expressing cells localize to the alveolar entry ring and have characteristics of myofibroblasts during pulmonary alveolar septal formation. *Anat Rec (Hoboken)*. 2008;291:1649-1661.
82. Kapanci Y, Assimacopoulos A, Irle C, et al. "Contractile interstitial cells" in pulmonary alveolar septa: a possible regulator of ventilation-perfusion ratio? Ultrastructural, immunofluorescence, and in vitro studies. *J Cell Biol*. 1974;60:375-392.
83. Adler KB, Low RB, Leslie KO, et al. Contractile cells in normal and fibrotic lung. *Lab Invest*. 1989;60:473-485.
84. Leslie KO, Mitchell JJ, Woodcock-Mitchell JL, Low RB. Alpha smooth muscle actin expression in developing and adult human lung. *Differentiation*. 1990;44:143-149.
85. Berk JL, Franzblau C, Goldstein RH. Recombinant interleukin-1 beta inhibits elastin formation by a neonatal rat lung fibroblast subtype. *J Biol Chem*. 1991;266:3192-3197.
86. Kagan HM, Li W. Lysyl oxidase: properties, specificity, and biological roles inside and outside of cell. *J Cell Biochem*. 2003;88:660-672.
87. Lindahl P, Karlsson L, Hellstrom M, et al. Alveogenesis failure in PDGF-A-deficient mice is coupled to lack of distal spreading of alveolar smooth muscle cell progenitors during lung development. *Development*. 1997;124:3943-3953.
88. Boström H, Willetts K, Pekny M, et al. PDGF-A signaling is a critical event in lung alveolar myofibroblast development and alveogenesis. *Cell*. 1996;85:863-873.
89. Weinstein M, Xu X, Ohyama K, Deng CX. FGFR-3 and FGFR-4 function cooperatively to direct alveogenesis in the murine lung. *Development*. 1998;125:3615-3623.
90. McGowan S, Jackson SK, Jenkins-Moore M, et al. Mice bearing deletions of retinoic acid receptors demonstrate reduced lung elastin and alveolar numbers. *Am J Respir Cell Mol Biol*. 2000;23: 162-167.
91. Liebeskind A, Srinivasan S, Kaetzel D, Bruce M. Retinoic acid stimulates immature lung fibroblast growth via a PDGF-mediated autocrine mechanism. *Am J Physiol Lung Cell Mol Physiol*. 2000;279: L81-L90.
92. Chen H, Chang L, Liu H, et al. Effect of retinoic acid on platelet-derived growth factor and lung development in newborn rats. *J Huazhong Univ Sci Technolog Med Sci*. 2004;24:226-228.
93. Chailley-Heu B, Boucherat O, Barlier-Mur AM, Bourbon JR. FGF-18 is up-regulated in the postnatal rat lung and enhances elastogenesis in myofibroblasts. *Am J Physiol Lung Cell Mol Physiol*. 2005;288: L43-L51.
94. Perl AK, Gale E. FGF signaling is required for myofibroblast differentiation during alveolar regeneration. *Am J Physiol Lung Cell Mol Physiol*. 2009;297:L299-L308.
95. Liu B, Harvey CS, McGowan SE. Retinoic acid increases elastin in neonatal rat lung fibroblast cultures. *Am J Physiol Lung Cell Mol Physiol*. 1993;265:L430-L437.
96. McGowan SE, Doro MM, Jackson SK. Endogenous retinoids increase perinatal elastin gene expression in rat lung fibroblasts and fetal explants. *Am J Physiol*. 1997;273:L410-L416.
97. Ferrara N, Hauck K, Jakeman L, Leung DW. Molecular and biological properties of the vascular endothelial growth factor families of protein. *Endocr Rev*. 1992;13:18-32.

98. Stenmark KR, Abman SH. Lung vascular development: implication for the pathogenesis of bronchopulmonary dysplasia. *Annu Rev Physiol*. 2005;67:623-661.
99. Ng YS, Rohan R, Sunday ME, et al. Differential expression of VEGF isoforms in mouse during development and in the adult. *Dev Dyn*. 2001;220:112-121.
100. Millauer B, Wizigmann-Voos S, Schnurch S, et al. High affinity VEGF binding and developmental expression suggest Flk-1 as a major regulator of vasculogenesis and angiogenesis. *Cell*. 1993;72: 835-846.
101. Schachtner SK, Wang Y, Scott Boldwin H. Qualitative and quantitative analysis of embryonic pulmonary vessel formation. *Cell Mol Biol*. 2000;22:157-165.
102. Yamamoto Y, Shiraishi I, Dai P, et al. Regulation of embryonic lung vascular development by vascular endothelial growth factor receptors, Flk-1 and Flt-1. *The Anatomical Record*. 2007;290: 958-973.
103. Jakkula M, Le Cras TD, Gebb S, et al. Inhibition of angiogenesis decreases alveolarization in the developing rat lung. *Am J Physiol Lung Cell Mol Physiol*. 2000;279:L600-L607.
104. Le Cras TD, Markham NE, Tuder RM, et al. Treatment of newborn rats with a VEGF receptor inhibitor causes pulmonary hypertension and abnormal lung structure. *Am J Physiol Lung Cell Mol Physiol*. 2002;283:L555-L562.
105. McGrath-Morrow SA, Cho C, Cho C, et al. VEGF receptor 2 blockade disrupts postnatal lung development. *Am J Respir Cell Mol Biol*. 2005;32:420-427.
106. Tang JR, Markham NE, Lin YJ, et al. Inhaled nitric oxide attenuates pulmonary hypertension and improves lung growth in infant rats after neonatal treatment with a VEGF receptor inhibitor. *Am J Physiol Lung Cell Mol Physiol*. 2004;287(2):L344-L351.
107. Leuwerke SM, Kaza AK, Tribble CG, et al. Inhibition of compensatory lung growth in endothelial nitric oxide synthase-deficient mice. *Am J Physiol Lung Cell Mol Physiol*. 2002;282: L1272-L1278.
108. Han RN, Babaei S, Robb M, et al. Defective lung vascular development and fatal respiratory distress in endothelial NO synthase-deficient mice: a model of alveolar capillary dysplasia? *Circ Res*. 2004;94:1115-1123.
109. Burri PH, Hlushchuk R, Djonov V. Intussusceptive angiogenesis: its emergence, its characteristics, and its significance. *Dev Dynamics*. 2004;231:474-488.
110. deMello DE, Sawyer D, Galvin N, Reid LM. Early fetal development of lung vasculature. *Am J Respir Cell Mol Biol*. 1997;16:568-581.
111. deMello DE, Reid LM. Embryonic and early fetal development of human lung vasculature and its functional implications. *Pediatr Dev Pathol*. 2000;3:439-449.
112. Schachtner SK, Wang Y, Scott Baldwin H. Qualitative and quantitative analysis of embryonic pulmonary vessel formation. *Am J Respir Cell Mol Biol*. 2000;22:157-165.
113. Hall SM, Hislop AA, Haworth SG. Origin, differentiation, and maturation of human pulmonary veins. *Am J Respir Cell Mol Biol*. 2002;26:333-340.
114. Parera MC, van Dooren M, van Kempan M, et al. Distal angiogenesis: a new concept for lung vascular morphogenesis. *Am J Physiol Lung Cell Mol Physiol*. 2005;288:L141-L149.
115. Schwartz MA, Caldwell L, Cafasso D, Zheng H. Emerging pulmonary vasculature lacks fate specification. *Am J Physiol Lung Cell Mol Physiol*. 2009;296:L71-L81.
116. Greenberg JM, Thompson FY, Brooks SK, et al. Mesenchymal expression of vascular endothelial growth factors D and A defines vascular patterning in developing lung. *Dev Dyn*. 2002;224: 144-153.
117. Gebb SA, Shannon JM. Tissue interactions mediate early events in pulmonary vasculogenesis. *Dev Dyn*. 2000;217:159-169.
118. Carmeliet P, Ferreira V, Breier G, et al. Abnormal blood vessel development and lethality in embryos lacking a single VEGF allele. *Nature*. 1996;380:435-439.
119. Ferrara N, Gerber HP, LeCouter J. The biology of VEGF and its receptors. *Nat Med*. 2003;9: 669-676.
120. Fong GH, Rossant J, Gertsenstein M, Breitman ML. Role of the Flt-1 receptor tyrosine kinase in regulating the assembly of vascular endothelium. *Nature*. 1995;376:66-70.
121. Shalaby F, Rossant J, Yamaguchi TP, et al. Failure of blood-island formation and vasculogenesis in Flk-1-deficient mice. *Nature*. 1995;376:62-66.
122. Galambos C, Ng YS, Ali A, et al. Defective pulmonary development in the absence of heparin-binding vascular endothelial growth factor isoforms. *Am J Respir Cell Mol Biol*. 2002;27:194-203.
123. Akeson AL, Greenberg JM, Cameron JE, et al. Temporal and spatial regulation of VEGF-A controls vascular patterning in the embryonic lung. *Dev Biol*. 2003;264:443-455.
124. White AC, Lavine KJ, Ornitz DM. FGF9 and SHH regulate mesenchymal VEGFa expression and development of the pulmonary capillary network. *Development*. 2007;134:3743-3752.
125. Sato TN, Qin Y, Kozak CA, Audus KL. Tie-1 and Tie-2 define another class of putative receptor tyrosine kinase genes expressed in early embryonic vascular system. *Proc Natl Acad Sci USA*. 1993; 90:9355-9358.
126. Davis S, Aldrich TH, Jones PF, et al. Isolation of angiopoietin-1, a ligand for the TIE2 receptor, by secretion-trap expression cloning. *Cell*. 1996;87:1161-1169.
127. Augustin HG, Koh GY, Thurston G, Alitalo K. Control of vascular morphogenesis and homeostasis through the angiopoietin-tie system. *Nature Review/Mol Cell Biol*. 2009;6:165-177.
128. Iwama A, Hamaguchi I, Hashiyama M, et al. Molecular cloning and characterization of mouse TIE and TEK receptor tyrosine kinase genes and their expression in hematopoietic stem cells. *Biochem Biophys Res Commun*. 1993;195:301-309.

A

129. Maisonpierre PC, Suri C, Jones PF, et al. Angiopoietin-2, a natural antagonist for Tie2 that disrupts in vivo angiogenesis. *Science*. 1997;277:55-60.
130. Valenzuela DM, Griffiths JA, Rojas J, et al. Angiopoietins 3 and 4: diverging gene counterparts in mice and humans. *Proc Natl Acad Sci USA*. 1999;96:1904-1909.
131. Brindle NP, Saharinen P, Alitalo K. Signaling and functions of Angiopietin-1 in vascular protection. *Circ Res*. 2006;98:1014-1023.
132. Sato TN, Tozawa Y, Deutsch U, et al. Distinct roles of receptor tyrosin kinase Tie-1 and Tie-2 in blood vessel formation. *Nature*. 1995;376:70-74.
133. Suri C, Jones PF, Patan S, et al. Requisite role of angiopoietin-1, a ligand for tie2 receptor, during embryonic angiogenesis. *Cell*. 1996;87:1171-1180.
134. Dumont DJ, Gradwohl G, Fong GH, et al. Dominant-negative and targeted null mutations in the endothelial receptor tyrosin kinase, tek, reveal a critical role in vasculogenesis. *Genes Dev*. 1994;8:1897-1909.
135. Gale NW, Thurston G, Hackett SF, et al. Angiopoietin-2 is required for postnatal angiogenesis and lymphatic patterning, and only the latter role is rescued by Angiopoietin-1. *Dev Cell*. 2002;3: 411-423.
136. Hato T, Kimura Y, Morisada T, et al. Angiopoietins contribute to lung development by regulating pulmonary vascular network formation. *Biochem Biophys Res Commun*. 2009;381:218-223.
137. Rudge JS, Thurston G, Rancopoulos GD. Angiopoietin A and pulmonary hypertension: cause or cure? *Circ Res*. 2003;92:947-949.
138. Chu D, Sullivan CC, Du L, et al. A new animal model for pulmonary hypertension based on the overexpression of a single gene, angiopoietin-1. *Ann Thorac Surg*. 2004;77:449-456.
139. Zhao YD, Campbell AI, Robb M, et al. Protective role of angiopoietin-1 in experimental pulmonary hypertension. *Circ Res*. 2003;92:984-991.
140. Wang HU, Chen ZF, Aderson DJ. Molecular distinction and angiogenic interaction between embryonic arteries and veins revealed by ephrinB2 and its receptor EphB4. *Cell*. 1998;93:741-753.
141. Cheng N, Brantley DM, Chen J. The ephrins and Eph receptors in angiogenesis. *Cytokine Growth Factor Rev*. 2002;13:75-85.
142. Kuijper S, Turner CJ, Adams RH. Regulation of angiogenesis by Eph-Ephrin interactions. *Trands Cardiovasc Med*. 2007;17:145-151.
143. Gerety SS, Wang HU, Chen ZF, Aderson DJ. Symmetrical mutant phenotypes of the receptor EphB4 and its specific transmembrane ligands ephrin-B2 in cardiovascular development. *Mol Cell*. 1999;4: 403-414.
144. Adams RH, Wilkinson GA, Weiss C, et al. Roles of ephrinB ligands and EphB receptors in cardiovascular development: demarcation of arterial/venous domains, vascular morphogenesis, and sprouting angiogenesis. *Genes Dev*. 1999;13:295-306.
145. Wilkinson GA, Schittny JC, Reinhardt DP, Klein R. Role for ephrinB2 in postnatal lung alveolar development and elastic matrix integrity. *Dev Dyn*. 2008;237:2220-2234.
146. Taichman DB, Loomes KM, Schachtner SK, et al. Notch1 and Jagged1 expression by the developing pulmonary vasculature. *Dev Dyn*. 2002;225:166-175.
147. Kotecha S, Wangoo A, Silverman M, Shaw RJ. Increase in the concentration of transforming growth factor beta-1 in bronchoalveolar lavage fluid before development of chronic lung disease of prematurity. *J Pediatr*. 1996;128:464-469.
148. Ichiba H, Saito M, Yamano T. Amniotic fluid transforming growth factor-beta1 and the risk for the development of neonatal bronchopulmonary dysplasia. *Neonatology*. 2009;96:156-161.
149. Kunzmann S, Speer CP, Jobe AH, Kramer BW. Antenatal inflammation induced TGF-beta1 but suppressed CTGF in preterm lungs. *Am J Physiol Lung Cell Mol Physiol*. 2007;292: L223-L231.
150. Bland RD, Xu L, Ertsey R, et al. Dysregulation of pulmonary elastin synthesis and assembly in preterm lambs with chronic lung disease. *Am J Physiol Lung Cell Mol Physiol*. 2007;292: L1370-L1384.
151. Kumarasamy A, Schmitt I, Nave AH, et al. Lysyl oxidase activity is dysregulated during impaired alveolarization of mouse and human lungs. *Am J Respir Crit Care Med*. 2009;180:1239-1252.
152. Alejandre-Alcázar MA, Kwapiszewska G, Reiss I, et al. Hyperoxia modulates TGF-beta/BMP signaling in a mouse model of bronchopulmonary dysplasia. *Am J Physiol Lung Cell Mol Physiol*. 2007;292:L537-L549.
153. Zhou L, Dey CR, Wert SE, Whitsett JA. Arrested lung morphogenesis in transgenic mice bearing an SP-C-TGF-beta 1 chimeric gene. *Dev Biol*. 1996;175:227-238.
154. Vicencio AG, Lee CG, Cho SJ, et al. Conditional overexpression of bioactive transforming growth factor-beta1 in neonatal mouse lung: a new model for bronchopulmonary dysplasia? *Am J Respir Cell Mol Biol*. 2004;31:650-656.
155. Nakanishi H, Sugiura T, Streisand JB, et al. TGF-beta-neutralizing antibodies improve pulmonary alveologenesis and vasculogenesis in the injured newborn lung. *Am J Physiol Lung Cell Mol Physiol*. 2007;293:L151-L161.
156. Dasgupta C, Sakurai R, Wang Y, et al. Hyperoxia-induced neonatal rat lung injury involves activation of TGF-{beta} and Wnt signaling and is protected by rosiglitazone. *Am J Physiol Lung Cell Mol Physiol*. 2009;296:L1031-L1041.
157. Varga J, Pasche B. Transforming growth factor beta as a therapeutic target in systemic sclerosis. *Nat Rev Rheumatol*. 2009;5:200-206.
158. Leask A, Abraham DJ. All in the CCN family: essential matricellular signaling modulators emerge from the bunker. *J Cell Sci*. 2006;119:4803-4810.

A

159. Grotendorst GR. Connective tissue growth factor: a mediator of TGF-beta action on fibroblasts. *Cytokine Growth Factor Rev*. 1997;8:171-179.
160. Kothapalli D, Frazier KS, Welply A, et al. Transforming growth factor beta induces anchorage-independent growth of NRK fibroblasts via a connective tissue growth factor-dependent signaling pathway. *Cell Growth Differ*. 1997;8:61-68.
161. Grotendorst GR, Rahmanie H, Duncan MR. Combinatorial signaling pathways determine fibroblast proliferation and myofibroblast differentiation. *FASEB J*. 2004;18:469-479.
162. Duncan MR, Frazier KS, Abramson S, et al. Connective tissue growth factor mediates transforming growth factor beta-induced collagen synthesis: down-regulation by cAMP. *FASEB J*. 1999;13:1774-1786.
163. Che Z, Gao P, Shen W, et al. Angiotensin II-stimulated collagen synthesis in aortic adventitial fibroblasts is mediated by connective tissue growth factor. *Hypertension Res*. 2008;31:1233-1240.
164. Rodriguez-Vita J, Ruiz-Ortega M, Rupérez M, et al. Endothelin-1, via ETA receptor and independently of transforming growth factor-beta, increases the connective tissue growth factor in vascular smooth muscle cells. *Circ Res*. 2005;97:125-134.
165. Wu S, Capasso L, Lessa A, et al. High tidal volume ventilation up-regulates CTGF expression in the lung of newborn rats. *Pediatr Res*. 2008;63:245-250.
166. Chen, CM. Wang LF, Chou HC, et al. Up-regulation of connective tissue growth factor in hyperoxia-induced lung fibrosis. *Pediatr Res*. 2007;62:128-133.
167. Heng ECK, Huang Y, Black SA, Trackman PC. CCN2, connective tissue growth factor, stimulates collagen deposition by gingival fibroblasts via module 3 and alpha6- and beta1 integrins. *J Cell Biochem*. 2006;8:409-420.
168. Mercurio S, Latinkic B, Itasaki N, et al. Connective-tissue growth factor modulates WNT signalling and interacts with the WNT receptor complex. *Development*. 2004;131:2137-2147.
169. Abreu JG, Ketpura NI, Reversade B, De Robertis EM. Connective tissue growth factor (CTGF) modulates cell signaling by BMP and TGF-β. *Nature Cell Bio*. 2002;4:599-604.
170. Inoki I, Shiomi T, Hashimoto G, et al. Connective tissue growth factor binds vascular endothelial growth factor (VEGF) and inhibits VEGF-induced angiogenesis. *FASEB J*. 2002;16:219-221.
171. Kireeva ML, Latinkic BV, Kolesnikova TV, et al. Cyr61 and Fisp12 are both ECM-associated signaling molecules: activities, metabolism, and localization during development. *Experimental Cell Research*. 1997;233:63-77.
172. Wu S, Peng J, Duncan MR, et al. ALK-5 mediates endogenous and TGF-{beta}1-induced expression of CTGF in embryonic lung. *Am J Respir Cell Mol Biol*. 2007;36:552-561.
173. Ivkovic S, Yoon BS, Popoff SN, et al. Connective tissue growth factor coordinates chondrogenesis and angiogenesis during skeletal development. *Development*. 2003;130:2779-2791.
174. Baguma-Nibasheka M, Kablar B. Pulmonary hypoplasia in the connective tissue growth factor (CTGF) null mouse. *Dev Dyn*. 2008;237:485-493.
175. Kambas K, Chrysanthopoulou A, Kourtzelis I, et al. Endothelin-1 signaling promotes fibrosis in vitro in a bronchopulmonary dysplasia model by activating the extrinsic coagulation cascade. *J Immunol*. 2011;186(1):6568-6575.
176. Wallace MJ, Probyn ME, Zahra VA, et al. Early biomarkers and potential mediators of ventilation-induced lung injury in very preterm lambs. *Respir Res*. 2009;10:19.
177. Wu S, Platteau A, Chen S, et al. Conditional over-expression of connective tissue growth factor disrupts postnatal lung development. *Am J Respir Cell Mol Biol*. 2010;42:552-563.
178. Chen S, Rong M, Platteau A, et al. CTGF disrupts alveolarization and induces PH in neonatal mice: Implication in the pathogenesis of severe bronchopulmonary dysplasia. *Am J Physiol Lung Cell Mol Physiol*. 2011;300:L330-L340.
179. Alapati D, Rong M, Chen S, et al. CTGF antibody therapy attenuates hyperoxia-induced lung injury in neonatal rats. *Am J Respir Cell Mol Biol*. 2011;45(6):1169-1177.
180. Ponticos M, Holmes AM, Shi-wen X, et al. Pivotal role of connective tissue growth factor in lung fibrosis: MAPK-dependent transcriptional activation of type I collagen. *Arthritis Rheum*. 2009;60:2142-2155.
181. Huber PE, Bickelhaupt S, Peschke P, et al. Reversal of established fibrosis by treatment with the anti-CTGF monoclonal antibody FG-3019 in a murine model of radiation-induced pulmonary fibrosis. *Am J Respir Crit Care Med*. 2010;181:A1054.
182. Lassus P, Ristimäki A, Ylikorkala O, et al. Vascular endothelial growth factor in human preterm lung. *Am J Respir Crit Care Med*. 1999;159:1429-1433.
183. Bhatt AJ, Pryhuber GS, Huyck H, et al. Disrupted pulmonary vasculature and decreased vascular endothelial growth factor, Flt-1, and TIE-2 in human infants dying with bronchopulmonary dysplasia. *Am J Respir Crit Care Med*. 2001;164:1971-1980.
184. De Paepe ME, Mao Q, Powell J, et al. Growth of pulmonary microvasculature in ventilated preterm infants. *Am J Respir Crit Care Med*. 2006;173:204-211.
185. De Paepe ME, Patel C, Tsai A, et al. Endoglin (CD105) up-regulation in pulmonary microvasculature of ventilated preterm infants. *Am J Respir Crit Care Med*. 2008;178:180-187.
186. Maniscalco WM, Watkins RH, D'Angio CT, Ryan RM. Hyperoxic injury decreases alveolar epithelial cell expression of vascular endothelial growth factor (VEGF) in neonatal rabbit lung. *Am J Respir Cell Mol Biol*. 1997;16:557-567.
187. Hosford GE, Olson DM. Effects of hyperoxia on VEGF, its receptors, and HIF-2alpha in the newborn rat lung. *Am J Physiol Lung Cell Mol Physiol*. 2003;285:L161-L168.

188. Mokres LM, Parai K, Hilgendorff A, et al. Prolonged mechanical ventilation with air induces apoptosis and causes failure of alveolar septation and angiogenesis in lungs of newborn mice. *Am J Physiol Lung Cell Mol Physiol*. 2010;298:L23-L35.
189. Maniscalco WM, Watkins RH, Pryhuber GS, et al. Angiogenic factors and alveolar vasculature: development and alterations by injury in very premature baboons. *Am J Physiol Lung Cell Mol Physiol*. 2002;282:L811-L823.
190. Tambunting F, Beharry KD, Waltzman J, Modanlou HD. Impaired lung vascular endothelial growth factor in extremely premature baboons developing bronchopulmonary dysplasia/chronic lung disease. *J Investig Med*. 2005;53:253-262.
191. Cao L, Wang J, Tseu I, et al. Maternal exposure to endotoxin delays alveolarization during postnatal rat lung development. *Am J Physiol Lung Cell Mol Physiol*. 2009;296:L726-L737.
192. Kunig AM, Balasubramaniam V, Markham NE, et al. Recombinant human VEGF treatment enhances alveolarization after hyperoxic lung injury in neonatal rats. *Am J Physiol Lung Cell Mol Physiol*. 2005;289:L529-L535.
193. Kunig AM, Balasubramaniam V, Markham NE, et al. Recombinant human VEGF treatment transiently increases lung edema but enhances lung structure after neonatal hyperoxia. *Am J Physiol Lung Cell Mol Physiol*. 2006;291:L1068-L1078.
194. Thébaud B, Ladha F, Michelakis ED, et al. Vascular endothelial growth factor gene therapy increases survival, promotes lung angiogenesis, and prevents alveolar damage in hyperoxia-induced lung injury: evidence that angiogenesis participates in alveolarization. *Circulation*. 2005;112:2477-2486.
195. Le Cras TD, Spitzmiller RE, Albertine KH, et al. VEGF causes pulmonary hemorrhage, hemosiderosis, and air space enlargement in neonatal mice. *Am J Physiol Lung Cell Mol Physiol*. 2004;287: L134-L142.
196. Woessner JF. Matrix metalloproteinases and their inhibitors in connective tissue remodeling. *FASEB J*. 1991;5:2145-2154.
197. Murphy G, Willenbrock F. Tissue inhibitors of matrix metalloproteinases. *Methods Enzymol*. 1995;248:496-510.
198. Chakrabarti S, Patel KD. Matrix metalloproteinase-2 (MMP-2) and MMP-9 in pulmonary pathology. *Exp Lung Res*. 2005;31:599-621.
199. Tambunting F, Beharry KD, Hartleroad J, et al. Increased lung matrix metalloproteinase-9 levels in extremely premature baboons with bronchopulmonary dysplasia. *Pediatr Pulmonol*. 2005;39:5-14.
200. Chetty A, Cao GJ, Severgnini M, et al. Role of matrix metalloproteinase-9 in hyperoxic injury in developing lung. *Am J Physiol Lung Cell Mol Physiol*. 2008;295:L584-L592.
201. Cederqvist K, Sorsa T, Tervahartiala T, et al. Matrix metalopproteiase-2, -8 and -9 and TIMP-2 in tracheal aspirates from preterm infants with respiratory distress. *Pediatrics*. 2001;108:686-692.
202. Schulz CG, Sawicki G, Lemke RP, et al. MMP-2 and MMP-9 and their tissue inhibitors in the plasma of preterm and term neonates. *Pediatric Research*. 2004;55:794-801.
203. Ekekezie II, Thibeault DW, Simon SD, et al. Low levels of tissue inhibitors of metalloproteinases with a high matrix metalloproteinase-9/tissue inhibitor of metalloproteinase-1 ratio are present in tracheal aspirate fluids of infants who develop chronic lung disease. *Pediatrics*. 2004;113: 1709-1714.
204. Sweet DG, Curley AE, Chesshyre E, et al. The role of matrix metalloproteinases-9 and -2 in development of neonatal chronic lung disease. *Acta Paediatr*. 2004;93:791-796.

1

CHAPTER 2

Genetic Influences in Lung Development and Injury

Vineet Bhandari, MD, DM

2

- Genetic Influences in Lung Development: Animal Models
- Genetic Influences in Lung Development: Clinical Context of RDS
- Genetic Influences in Injury to the Developing Lung: Animal Models
- Genetic Influences in Injury to the Developing Lung: Clinical Context of BPD
- Conclusions

Normal lung development occurs in phases that correspond to the complexity of the lung architecture. In humans, the first phase, the embryonic (E) phase, occurs at 4 to 7 weeks postmenstrual age (embryonic day [E] 9.5 to E12 in mice). The pseudoglandular phase occurs next, from 5 to 17 weeks postmenstrual age (E12-E16.5 in mice). At 16 to 26 weeks postmenstrual age (E16.5-E17.5 in mice), the canalicular phase occurs. The saccular phase occurs at 24 to 38 weeks postmenstrual age (E17.5 to postnatal [PN] day 4 in mice). The last phase, the alveolar phase, occurs from about 32 weeks postmenstrual age until about 18 months after birth, with the majority of the alveolarization process occurring 5 to 6 months after birth (PN4-PN28, but mostly completed by PN14, in mice).[1] Intrinsic to the process of normal lung development is alveolarization, which incorporates the processes of vascular development with multiple cell-to-cell interactions between epithelial cells (type I and type II pneumocytes [TIPs, TIIPs, respectively), fibroblasts, interstitial cells, and endothelial cells.[2] A key aspect of lung maturation is the presence of functional pulmonary surfactant. Surfactant is composed mostly of a mixture of phospholipids and surfactant proteins (SPs), specifically, A, B, C, and D.

Because the majority of the preterm births occur in the late canalicular/early saccular phase of lung development, this chapter focuses on disruptions of lung development/maturation, and their impact on lung injury, that are due to alteration of specific genes that occur during these periods in animal models. Primarily, the effects on alveolar formation are discussed. In addition, the role of genetics in the most relevant clinical conditions in the premature newborn, respiratory distress syndrome (RDS) and bronchopulmonary dysplasia (BPD), respectively, are considered.

Genetic Influences in Lung Development: Animal Models

Adenosine Triphosphate–Binding Cassette Transporter A3

Mice lacking *ABCA3*, the gene for adenosine triphosphate–binding cassette transporter A3 (ABCA3), developed normally in utero; however, these mice died from respiratory failure within 1 hour after birth.[3] Histologic and ultrastructural analyses at E18.5 revealed a significant reduction in phosphatidylglycerol (PG) and failure to develop mature lamellar bodies in TIIP, leading to a lack of secreted surfactant.[3] No data was reported about SPs. These data suggest a crucial role for ABCA3 in surfactant secretion and postnatal adaptation at birth.

β-Catenin

Conditional deletion of the *β-catenin* gene in epithelial cells of the lung caused large, epithelium-lined bronchiolar tubules extending to the lung periphery, with few terminal alveolar saccules, at E18.5.[4] There was reduced expression of *SP-A, SP-C,* and vascular endothelial growth factor A (*VEGFA*), but *SP-B* was present.[4] Mice died of respiratory failure at birth if deletion of the *β-catenin* gene was activated at E0.5 with use of the SP-C promoter, but there was no alteration in lung structure or survival if deletion occurred from E14.5 to E15.5 with use of the Clara cell secretory protein (CCSP) promoter.[4]

Bone Morphogenetic Protein 4

Misexpression of human bone morphogenetic protein 4 (BMP4) gene (*Bmp4*) throughout the distal epithelium under the control of the SP-C promoter/enhancer was found to lead to lungs that had fewer terminal buds separated by abundant mesenchyme.[5] By 18.5 days in the mouse, the lung lobes contained huge epithelial sacs apparently separated by thickened mesenchyme.[5] Gremlin 1 (Grem1) is a protein that preferentially antagonizes BMP2 and BMP4.[6] Knockout of the *Grem1* gene leads to a murine phenotype of renal agenesis, limb defects, and abnormal alveolar septation.[6] The pulmonary phenotype noted in lung epithelium with conditionally deleted *BMP4*[7] was somewhat similar to that reported for BMP receptor type 1A (*BMPR-1A*) (see later).

Bone Morphogenetic Protein Receptor Type 1A

In one study, antenatal conditional knockout of the gene for alveolar epithelial cell–specific *BMPR-1A* (also known as *Alk3*) led to neonatal lethality in the mice, with lungs showing a thickened mesenchyme, lack of lamellar body formation, and decreased SP-C.[8] The decreased saccular formation could be a result of reduced cell proliferation as well as cell death.[8] Interestingly, if the *Alk3* conditional knockout was induced after birth (PN1), it did not affect neonatal survival or lung morphology.[8] No changes were noted in the fibroblast growth factor (FGF), Sonic hedgehog (Shh), and transforming growth factor β1 (TGF-β1) signaling pathways, whereas the Wnt pathway appeared to be activated in the mutant lungs.[8] Other investigators also reported on a conditional knockout of *Alk3* in lung epithelial cells using a different noninducible approach, and noted abnormally large fluid-filled sacs with reduced cell proliferation, increased cell death, and decreased SP-C.[7] Interestingly, this finding was accompanied by decreased messenger RNA (mRNA) expression of Forkhead box *a2* (Foxa2), *Nmyc*, and *Shh.*[7] Some of the discrepant findings in these murine models could potentially be due to the different background strains of the mice used.[8]

Coactivator-Associated Arginine Methyltransferase 1

Coactivator-associated arginine methyltransferase 1 (CARM1) is one of the members of the protein arginine methyltransferase family that regulate multiple cellular functions including transcription and translation. $Carm1^{-/-}$ null mutant mice die in utero or soon after birth.[9] Histologic examination of their lungs revealed small alveolar spaces that failed to inflate.[9] A more detailed analysis at E18.5 demonstrated hypercellularity of TIIP as a result of proliferation and blocked differentiation to TIP.[10] Although the mRNA expression of SP-A was decreased, no changes were noted for the other SPs. However, immunohistochemistry showed SP-C protein to be increased.[10] The researchers suggested that loss of CARM1 disrupts glucocorticoid receptor (GR) signaling.[10]

CCAAT Enhancer–Binding Protein α

In a study the conditional Cre/LoxP system, targeted to respiratory epithelial cells, deletion of the *Cebpa* gene, which encodes for CCAAT enhancer–binding protein α (C/EBPα), led to a pulmonary phenotype of impaired maturation. At E18.5, the lungs of mice lacking C/EBPα had diminished dilation of peripheral saccules with thickened mesenchyme, a lack of TIP, and absence of lamellar bodies in TIIPs.[11] There was a significant reduction of levels of SPsA, B, C, and D and of ABCA3 protein but increased *TGF-β2* mRNA expression in the lung. In addition, it was noted that normal expression of C/EBPα was dependent on *Foxa2* (codes for FOXA2 protein) and *Titf1* (codes for thyroid transcription factor 1 [TTF-1] protein) genes.[11] These data suggest a critical interactive role for these transcription factors in controlling lung maturation.

Cytidylyltransferase-α

The major phospholipid component of pulmonary surfactant is phosphatidylcholine (PC). The latter is produced by the cytidine-5-diphosphocholine (CDP-choline) pathway, in which cytidylyltransferase (CCT) regulates the rate-limiting step. The major isoform of CCT in the lung is CCTα, the activation of which is responsible for the induction of pulmonary surfactant in the fetal and neonatal lung.[12] Overexpression of full-length CCTα, that is, CCTα$^{1\text{-}367}$, in TIIPs was found to cause no embryonic or postnatal lethality.[13] At E18, lung liquid fluid of mice with this overexpression had increased PC content with no difference in SPs; however, CCTα overexpression led to increased glycogen content in TIIPs, a finding that contrasts with the normal decline in glycogen content and increased surfactant PC synthesis at late gestation.[13] Like full-length CCTα, CCTα$^{203\text{-}367}$ had higher glycogen content in the lungs of mice at E18, but there was no significant accumulation of glycogen in the CCTα$^{1\text{-}239}$ transgenic mice. The investigators in this study speculated that the P domain contained in the C-terminus of CCTα encompassing CCTα$^{203\text{-}367}$ is the most likely candidate contributing to the phenotype.[13]

Targeted deletion of CCTα in respiratory epithelial cells (at E6.5-E7.5 or E10.5-E12.5 till birth at E18.5-E19.5) led to a neonatal pulmonary phenotype characterized histologically by reduced peripheral saccules with thickened septa and clinically by severe respiratory distress and death within 10 minutes of delivery.[14] Loss of CCTα initiated at E16.5 led to normal lungs and only 10% mortality at term birth. Deletion of CCTα between E8.5 and E12.5 (deletion of CCTα in cells destined to form the gas exchange region of the lung) or between E12.5 and E16.5 (deletion of CCTα in cells destined to form TIPs and TIIPs) reduced PC content in the neonatal lungs.[14] The mRNA expression of *SP A, B, C,* or *D* was not affected, but values of SP-A, SP-C, and SP-D proteins were reduced and that of SP-B elevated, suggesting an impact on the translation or turnover of these proteins.[14] Hence, CCTα in respiratory epithelial cells is critical for postnatal adaptation at birth in mice.

Endothelial Nitric Oxide Synthase

Some investigators have reported that lungs of endothelial nitric oxide synthase null (*eNOS*$^{-/-}$ mice exhibited reduced saccular volume and marked septal thickening at E18.[15] Although there was no difference in SPs, levels of PC were decreased in the bronchoalveolar lavage fluid at birth in the *eNOS*$^{-/-}$ mice.[15] Others have reported normal lung development in *eNOS*$^{-/-}$ mice.[16]

Epidermal Growth Factor Receptor

Epidermal growth factor receptor (EGFR) belongs to a family of tyrosine kinase receptors and may be bound by various ligands, including epidermal growth factor (EGF), TGF-α, and regulate cellular processes. The pulmonary phenotype of *EGFR*$^{-/-}$ mice at E18.5 and at term (E21-E22) was found to consist of undifferentiated respiratory epithelium in the bronchioles and thickened cellular alveolar septa, suggesting an arrest in lung maturation.[17,18]

ErbB4

A transgenic mice model was used to study the impact of receptor tyrosine kinase receptor ErbB4, a member of the epidermal growth factor receptor subfamily, on fetal lung development.[19] Morphometric analyses revealed a delayed structural development with a significant decrease in saccular size at E17 to E18, keeping these lungs in the canalicular stage. Levels of SP-B mRNA and protein as well as surfactant phospholipid synthesis and secretion were decreased at E17 to E18, with SP-D protein significantly decreased at E18.[19]

Eyes Absent

Eyes absent (Eya) is a transcription factor/protein phosphatase that regulates cell lineage specification and proliferation. *Eya1*$^{-/-}$ embryos and newborn mice lungs exhibit defects in the smooth muscle of bronchi and major blood vessels, leading to pulmonary hemorrhage.[20] Genetic reduction of Shh partially rescues the pulmonary phenotype of *Eya1*$^{-/-}$, in addition to restoring fibroblast growth factor 10 (FGF10) expression.[20] These data support a role for Eya1 that is upstream of Shh-FGF10 signaling and that affects lung epithelial, mesenchymal, and vascular development.

Fibroblast Growth Factor 8

Lung development occurs normally through the embryonic and pseudoglandular stages in FGF8 conditional and hypomorphic mutants but is disrupted in the canalicular stage by excess proliferation, failure of TIP differentiation, and abnormal septal and vascular remodeling.[21] These changes result in postnatal respiratory failure and mortality.[21]

Fibroblast Growth Factor 18

At E18.5, lungs of *Fgf18*$^{-/-}$ mice were reported to have reduced alveolar spaces and thickened interstitial mesenchyme.[22] There were no differences in the expression of *CCSP*, TIP and TIIP markers, *BMP4*, and *Shh*. Interestingly, lungs of *Fgf18*$^{-/-}$ mice also showed transiently decreased proliferating activity in epithelial and mesenchymal cells during the terminal saccular phase.[22]

Forkhead Box f1

In one study, haploinsufficiency of the gene for Forkhead box f1 (*Foxf1*) had a neonatal lethality of 55% within a few hours of birth.[23] Mice exhibiting less than 50% levels of Foxf1 expression had diminished sacculation of the lung periphery and decreased SP-B.[23] However, the predominant phenotype was that of pulmonary hemorrhage, which was associated with loss of tight junctions between TIP and endothelial cells.[23]

Forkhead Box m1

Conditional deletion of the gene for Foxm1 in lung epithelial cells was found to cause respiratory failure and neonatal lethality at birth.[24] At E17.5 and E18.5, there was diminished size of the peripheral saccules, with thickened mesenchyme and decreased TIP and TIIP markers, suggesting delayed maturation.[24] One study has reported that transgenic lung cell–specific overexpression of Foxm1 resulted in epithelial hyperplasia, inhibition of lung sacculation, and absence of pro-SP-C at E18.5 or PN1.[25]

Gata6

Conditional loss of transcription factor Gata6 in lung epithelium has been observed to lead to increased airway dilation[26] and at E18.5 to demonstrate decreased expression of airway and alveolar epithelial cell markers in mice.[26] The Wnt–β-catenin signaling pathway was upregulated, with increased expression of *Nmyc* and *Bmp4*, in these lungs.[26] Re-expression of *Fzd2* (which encodes a Wnt receptor) or decreased β-catenin expression resulted in an incomplete rescue, because the neonatal mice still succumbed to respiratory failure at birth.[26]

Using a lung epithelial cell–targeted Gata6/Engrailed transgenic mice model, Yang and colleagues[27] noted that at E17.5 the distal airways were lined with thick, cuboidal TIIP. At E19.5, numbers of interalveolar septa were decreased with thickened mesenchyme, with a marked lack of TIP.[27] No differences were observed in *TTF-1* or *SP-A*, but there was a marked attenuation of endogenous *SP-C* expression. Furthermore, there were a reduced number of airways with *CCSP* and *Foxj1* expression. *Aqp5* is a TIP marker, the levels of which were reduced, but the level of *Foxp2* (expressed in distal airway epithelium) was increased.[27] These data suggest that Gata6 is important in differentiation to TIIPs and TIPs during the late canalicular/early saccular phase of lung development.

In another study, mouse lungs with elevated Gata6 values at E18.5 demonstrated abnormally shaped and sized distal alveoli, with thickened mesenchyme.[28] Molecular analyses suggested a block in the terminal differentiation to mature TIIPs and TIPs.[28]

2

Glucocorticoid Receptor

Mice with lung epithelial cell–specific knockout of the GR were found to have higher mortality at PN0.5 secondary to respiratory failure.[29] At E18.5, these mice had increased lung tissue cellularity and thickened septa, reduced mRNA expression of *SPs A, B, C,* and *D*, but no changes in *ABCA3*, *TTF-1*, or *FOXA2*.[29]

G Protein–Coupled Receptor 4

Some G-protein–coupled receptor 4 (GPR4) null mutant mice were reported to die on PN1 owing to respiratory distress. The bronchiolar epithelium had abnormal cells with enlarged clear cytoplasm.[30] These cells expanded to multiple layers extending to the respiratory and terminal bronchioles in the peripheral lung.[30] This lung epithelial metaplasia appeared to be transient and reversible because it was not seen in adult mice.[30]

Hepatocyte Nuclear Factor-3β

Hepatocyte nuclear factor-3β (HNF-3β), a member of the winged helix family, is a transcription factor. Lung epithelial cell–specific overexpression of *HNF-3β* was found to lead to a phenotype in which saccules were absent, the lung tubules were lined with columnar epithelial cells lacking lamellar bodies, but there were also areas of normal lung architecture, at E18.5 in transgenic mice.[31] In the affected areas of the lung, the expression of the SPs were variable, although SP-A, pro-SP-B, pro-SP-C, and CCSP were not detected by immunohistochemistry.[31] The expression of *VEGF* mRNA was decreased, but *Shh* mRNA was not altered in the abnormal epithelial cells of the transgenic lungs.[31] The data suggest that HNF-3β limits cellular diversity in the respiratory epithelial cells in the developing lung.

Homeobox a-5

The homeobox (Hox) genes are a family of transcription factors that are responsible for the positioning of body structures of an organism. Besides the laryngotracheal defects in *Hoxa-5* null mutant mice, the lungs at E18.5 have a thickening of the alveolar walls. By birth, the mice have poorly inflated alveoli, and a majority die from respiratory failure.[32] Expression of *TTF-1* and *HNF-3β* was decreased but that of *Nmyc* was increased in the mutant lungs.[32] Levels of *SP-A*, *Sp-B*, and *Sp-C* mRNA and of SP-B protein were decreased in the mutant lungs.[32]

Kruppel-Like Factor 5

Kruppel-like factor 5 (KLF5) is a zinc-finger transcription factor. Conditional deletion of *Klf5* in respiratory epithelial cells in mice was found to lead to a pulmonary phenotype consisting of thickened saccules with absence of lamellar bodies in TIIP and decreases in saturated PC, SP-B protein, and *Vegfa* at E18.5.[33] This combination resulted in perinatal respiratory failure and mortality at birth. Signaling pathways implicated were those of VEGF, PDGF, TGF-β2, and FGF.[33]

Lysophosphatidylcholine Acyltransferase 1

Formation of saturated PC occurs by deacylation of monounsaturated PC by phospholipase A_2 (PLA_2), followed by reacylation with lysophosphatidylcholine acyltransferase (LPCAT).[34] Saturated PC levels in the homozygous hypomorphic *Lpcat1* allele (decreased expression by ≈50%) newborn lungs were not that different in the dead and alive mice (46% vs. 60%, respectively).[34] Both pro-SP-C and mature SP-C levels were decreased in a majority of these mice.[34]

Macrophage Migration Inhibitory Factor

Increased mortality was observed in prematurely delivered mouse pups that were genetically deficient in migration inhibitory factor (MIF) at E18.[35] Histologic evaluation demonstrated that the lungs of $MIF^{-/-}$ pups were immature and had lower levels of VEGF and corticosterone, two factors that promote fetal lung maturation.[35] Interestingly, this phenotype could be rescued with exposure to maternal MIF.[35]

GlcNac *N*-Deacetylase/*N*-Sulfotranferase-1

GlcNac *N*-deacetylase/*N*-sulfotranferase-1 (NDST-1) is an enzyme catalyzing modifications of the glycosaminoglycan chains of heparin sulfate proteoglycans. Disruption of *Ndst-1* was found to lead to birth of mice who succumbed to respiratory failure soon after birth.[36] Histologic evaluation revealed atelectasis and thicker alveolar septa, reduced numbers of lamellar bodies, and decreased surfactant phospholipids.[36]

Nmyc

Nmyc is a member of a small family of proto-oncogenes that are involved in cell growth, differentiation, and death.[37] Lung epithelial cell–targeted overexpression of *Nmyc* has been observed to lead to a phenotype of distal epithelial tubules with abundant mesenchyme at E18.5, accompanied by hyperproliferation and cell death.[37] Conditional deletion of *Nymc* in the lung epithelium led to severely abnormal lungs characterized by numerous large fluid-filled sacs that contained cellular debris, were lined by highly attenuated epithelial cells, and were separated by a thin layer of mesoderm at E18.5.[37] These defects were accompanied by inhibition of cell proliferation and enhanced cell death.[37]

Platelet-Derived Growth Factor-A

Platelet-derived growth factors (PDGFs) bind to cell surface receptors and are involved in fibroblast proliferation and chemotaxis. In one study, overexpression of *PDGF-A* in lung epithelial cells led to an arrest in the canalicular stage at E18.5.[38] Lungs in transgenic mice were hypercellular with thickened mesenchyme and an increased rate of cellular proliferation.[38] In comparison with lungs of control mice, CCSP staining response was weaker, whereas SP-B staining response was increased in the lungs of transgenic mice.[38]

Platelet-Derived Growth Factor-C

Lung epithelial cell–targeted overexpression of *PDGF-C* was reported to lead to a phenotype consisting of lungs that were arrested in the canalicular stage, were hypercellular, and had tubular air spaces surrounded by thickened mesenchyme, at E18.5.[39] CCSP and SP-B staining responses were present in the lungs of transgenic mice, suggesting appropriate differentiation of small airway cells and TIIP but a delay in TIP differentiation.[39]

Prophet of Pit 1

Approximately half of mutant mice that were null for the gene prophet of Pit 1 (*Prop1*) died of respiratory failure in one study. Neonatal lungs were atelectatic, contained excess mesenchymal tissue and had decreased levels of the proteins SP-B and TTF-1.[40] The penetrance of the RDS phenotype was dependent on the strain of mice used. It was increased with the higher contribution of the 129S1 background and decreased with a higher contribution of the B6 background.[40] Investigators of the study speculated that multiple anterior pituitary hormone deficiencies in the *Prop1* null mutant mice could be responsible for the pulmonary phenotype.[40]

Pten

Pten is a multifunctional phosphatase whose major substrate is phosphotidylinosotol-3,4,5-triphosphate, a lipid second-messenger molecule. It has a major role as a tumor suppressor gene and is involved in the development of various tissues.[41] Using a lung targeted conditional knockout strategy, Yanagi and associates[41] observed that loss of *Pten* at E10 to E16 led to neonatal lethality secondary to respiratory failure. The lung phenotype was that of impaired differentiation of terminal sacs and alveolar epithelial cells. Thickened septa and reduced production of SPs were noted.[41] The investigators speculated that the activation of the Shh pathway in these mice may be due to enhanced P13K/Akt signaling.[41]

2

Retinoic Acid Receptor β

Histologic evaluation of lungs of retinoic acid receptor β (*RAR*β)$^{-/-}$mice revealed that alveolar saccules were larger at PN4 than those in wild-type mice, though the lung volumes did not differ.[42] The rate of formation of alveoli was twice as fast in lungs of *RAR*β$^{-/-}$ mice as in lungs of wild-type mice at PN4 and PN21.[42]

Sonic Hedgehog

Lung-targeted overexpression of *Shh* in mice was reported to lead to smaller newborn lungs characterized by thickened mesenchyme and lack of alveoli, leading to neonatal lethality.[43]

Surfactant Protein-B

Clark and associates[44] reported that lack of SP-B in mice lungs did not affect antenatal survival or development; however, it resulted in universal postnatal lethality with respiratory failure. Histologic evaluation found the lung morphology to be normal. Ultrastructure analysis, however, showed the lungs of absent SP-B mice to be characterized by absence of tubular myelin and lamellar bodies in the TIIP.[44] A separate study reported that mice with reduced amounts of SP-B (*SP-B*$^{+/-}$ mice) were found to abnormal pulmonary function,[45] and another that *SP-B*$^{-/-}$ mice could be rescued by selective restoration in the TIIP.[46] The critical requirement for SP-B in postnatal pulmonary adaptation is highlighted by these studies.

Thyroid Transcription Factor-1

One study found that the pulmonary phenotype of *TTF-1*$^{-/-}$ mice, which have tracheal and bronchial tubules with nearly complete loss of peripheral lung parenchyma, could not be rescued by SP-C–targeted overexpression of TTF-1, confirming that TTF-1 is upstream of SP-C.[47] In another study, at E18 to E18.5, *TTF-1*–homozygous mice bearing a mutant allele, in which seven serine phosphorylation sites were mutated, had hypoplastic lungs.[48] The pulmonary phenotype was characterized by impairment of terminal differentiation of TIIP and of vascularization. In addition, there was a significant reduction in proteins SP-B and SP-C.[48]

Transforming Growth Factor-β1

TGF-β1 has been implicated in fetal lung development. Using a targeted approach to respiratory cells (with SP-C), Zhou and coworkers[49] produced transgenic mice in which *TGF-β1* was selectively expressed. The lungs of these mice at E16 contained fewer acinar buds, whereas those at E18.5 were noted to be arrested at the late pseudoglandular phase. In addition, the researchers found decreased expression of *CCSP* and pro-*SP-C*, suggesting interference with epithelial cell differentiation.[49] This finding supports a critical role for TGF-β1 in murine lung morphogenesis.

Transforming Growth Factor-β3

TGF-β3$^{-/-}$ mice were reported to die soon after birth. Their lungs were characterized by atelectasis, pseudoglandular histology, lack of alveolar septa, mesenchymal thickening and hypercellularity, and a lack of staining for SP-C.[50] In addition, there was extensive intrapulmonary and pleural hemorrhage.[50]

Transforming Growth Factor-β Receptor II

Mice produced with epithelial cell–specific conditional deletion of TGF-β receptor II (*TGF-βRII*) had a normal lung phenotype at birth (PN1); however, by PN7 a significant maturational arrest of alveolarization was noted, and it persisted till adulthood.[51] Cell proliferation was decreased, but cell death was not increased in the lungs of these mice.[51]

Vascular Endothelial Growth Factor

In one study, activating the hypoxia-inducible transcription factors HIF-1α and HIF-2α, which bind the hypoxia-response element in the VEGF promoter, upregulated VEGF.[52] HIF-2α is expressed in fetal TIIP. This study found that loss of HIF-2α did not affect lung development during the pseudoglandular or canalicular phase. In the saccular phase, thinning of the alveolar septa at birth was impaired in *HIF-2α*$^{-/-}$ mice, and production of surfactant phospholipids and of SPs A, B, and D was decreased.[52] This phenotype of impaired lung maturation led to early neonatal death secondary to respiratory failure, which could be somewhat rescued by intra-amniotic and intratracheal administration of VEGF.[52]

Another study reported that at E17.5, conditional targeted deletion of *Vegf-A* in the murine lung alveolar epithelium led to fewer and more dilated terminal tubules.[53] At E18.5, the lungs showed an impairment of primary septa formation and dysregulated vasculature. The researchers in this study proposed that these findings suggest a role for endothelium-derived hepatocyte growth factor signaling pathway in normal septa formation.[53] Another study found that at PN0.5, lungs from mice deficient in the isoforms VEGF164 and VEGF188 had defective alveolar septa development, which resulted in distended and underdeveloped alveoli.[54]

Using a conditional, lung-targeted transgenic system, Bhandari and coworkers[55] found that overexpression of human *VEGF165* led to enhanced murine lung maturation, an effect that appeared to be restricted to a specific developmental window from after E18 up to PN7. Interestingly, although short-term VEGF administration does not lead to hemorrhage or angiogenesis,[52] longer exposure to VEGF does cause pulmonary hemorrhage,[55,56] which could be blocked by nitric oxide inhibition with no apparent deleterious effect on lung maturation.[55] These data show the therapeutic potential for VEGF in the clinical context; however, the timing and duration of exposure need to be carefully controlled.

Wingless-Int 7b

Mutant mice that were null for wingless-Int7b (*Wnt7b*) (with the *lacZ*-coding region replacing the coding region of the first exon) were reported to die in the perinatal period with respiratory failure. The distal airways of these mutant mice had large numbers of TIIPs (normal expression of *SP-C*), but no TIPs (with severe attenuation of aquaporin 5 [*Aqp5*] levels) at E18.5, suggesting a delay in epithelial cell differentiation.[57] The presence of pulmonary hemorrhage, secondary to defects in the vascular smooth muscle cells of the pulmonary vessels, was also an important feature.[57]

Summary

It is obvious from the studies just described that effects on the pulmonary developmental/maturational phenotype of modifications in specific genes depend on the mouse strain and are temporally regulated. This deduction suggests that additional genetic influences can affect the lung phenotype of a specific genetically altered murine lung and that their timing can play a significant role. In addition, data suggest that mice from different colonies with the same genotype may not have the same phenotype, because structural differences in alveolar size in inbred mouse strains have been observed.[58] This finding needs to be kept in mind when one is translating data to the clinical context, analyzing genetic associations in human neonates with RDS.

Genetic Influences in Lung Development: Clinical Context of RDS

RDS is a disease process resulting from absence or a diminished amount of surfactant in the newborn lung. Prematurity, therefore, plays a crucial role in the development of RDS. The incidence is inversely proportional to gestational age (GA) and birth weight (BW), with approximately 71% of neonates with BW between 501 and 750 grams affected, compared with 23% of those with BW between 1250 and 1500 grams.[59] In addition to prematurity, multiple additional factors have been implicated in the pathogenesis of RDS. These include maternal, intrapartum, and neonatal variables, such as advanced maternal age,[60] chorioamnionitis,[61,62] mode of delivery,[63] gender,[64,65] and birth order.[66-69] In preterm infants of the same GA, the clinical severity of RDS varies widely. Given the preceding descriptions of multiple genes affecting lung maturation, it is not surprising that genetic factors have been suggested to be implicated in predisposing premature neonates to RDS.

Twin Studies in RDS

Previous twin studies have evaluated the genetic contribution to RDS, with contradictory results.[68,70-72] The first two studies, published in 1971[70] and 2002,[71] showed that RDS had a significant genetic component. The 1971 study evaluated 31 twin pairs and suggested that RDS has a genetic component.[70] The second study, a retrospective review of all twins born during a 19-year period (1976 to 1995) in Amsterdam, suggested a strong genetic influence but included only 80 pairs with a GA of 30 to 34 weeks,[71] a population that has a fairly low risk for RDS.

Another study evaluating 100 same-gender twin pairs with RDS, found an insignificant genetic contribution.[72] In a different study, the same investigators concluded that environmental factors predominate over genetic factors, on the basis of a lack of difference in the concordance of RDS between same-gender and opposite-gender twins.[68] Although this study included a large number of twin pairs, the investigators inferred the zygosity by regarding all the gender-discordant pairs as dizygotic (DZ) and then estimating the number of monozygotic (MZ) twin pairs from the gender-concordant cohort.[68] Interpretation of the results of these four studies is limited by sample size, variability in the methods for confirmation of zygosity, and the exclusion of confounding variables known to contribute to the risk for RDS.[73] Using a large sample size, a standard method for ascertaining zygosity, and including and controlling for virtually all major known non-genetic (i.e., environmental) risk factors for RDS, Levit and colleagues[73] reported that a significant portion (49.7%) of the variance in liability to RDS was the result of genetic factors alone, suggesting a significant genetic susceptibility to RDS in preterm infants.

Candidate Genes and RDS

ABCA3

Karjalaeinen and associates[74] concluded that their findings suggest an association of rs13332514 alleles in the *Abca3* gene with a prolonged course of RDS in very premature infants (n = 155).[74] Another study reported that mutation E292V in the *Abca3* gene occurred on a unique haplotype derived from a combination of two common ABCA3 haplotypes and was over-represented in newborns with RDS (n = 420, total cohort).[75]

Table 2-1 GENETIC ALLELIC VARIANTS OF SURFACTANT PROTEINS (SPS) A AND B ASSOCIATED WITH RISK FOR RESPIRATORY DISTRESS SYNDROME (RDS)

Marker	Reference No. for Study	Polymorphism/ Haplotype	N	RDS Susceptibility
SP-A1	152	$6A^3/6A^3$ or $6A^3/*$	73	Decreased
	153	$6A^3$-$1A^1$ or $6A^4$-$1A^5$	107	Decreased
	154	$6A^2/6A^2$	921	Increased
		$6A^2$	921	Decreased
	155	(allele) $6A^2$	176	Increased
		(allele) $6A^3$	176	Decreased
	152	$6A^2/6A^2$	511	Increased
SP-A2	152	1A°/1A° or 1A°/*	511	Increased
SP-A2	156	$1A^0/1A^0$	241	Increased
		$1A^1/1\ A^1$	241	Decreased
SP-A1-A2	153	(haplotype) $6A^2$-$1A^0$	107	Increased
SP-B	156	Intron 4	241	Increased/Decreased
	157	SP-B Ile131 Thr	684	Determines the SP-A allele effect on RDS
	152	9306 A/G or del/*	511	Increased
		1580 T/T	73	Decreased
		Intron 4 ins variant	73	Increased
SP-B	136	Intron 4	198	Increased
	154	Exon 4 genotype Thr/Thr	921	Increased
		SP-B Ile/Thr	921	Decreased
SP-D/SP-A2	158	(haplotype) DA160-A/SP-A2 $1A^1$ Also DA11-T present in SP-A–containing haplotypes	132	Decreased

Endothelial Nitric Oxide Synthase

Sivasli and coworkers[76] found no association between Glu298Asp and T(−786)C polymorphisms in the *eNOS* gene and development of respiratory distress in premature neonates (n = 50)

Surfactant Proteins A, B, C, and D

The studies of *SP-A* and *SP-B* genes associated with RDS are summarized in Table 2-1. Logistic regression analysis, when gender was included as a confounding factor, revealed that SP-C alleles coding for 138 Asn or 186 Asn were independent risk factors for RDS.[77] In a later study, a variant of the *SP-D* gene (rs1923537; A-to-G substitution, 11208A>G) was found to be associated with a lower prevalence of RDS.[78]

G Protein–Coupled Receptor A (GPRA)

A case-control study has suggested an association between GPRA (also known as GPR154) and susceptibility to RDS.[79]

Miscellaneous

Capasso and associates[80] investigated polymorphisms in specific cytokines (interleukin-10 [IL-10]-1082 G>A; IL-10-592 A>C, IL-8-251 A>T, tumor necrosis factor [TNF]-α-308 G>A) and their association with RDS (n = 176, preterms; n = 164 full-term controls). The only significant differences were found in IL-10-1082, with the risk of RDS significantly lower in preterm infants with GG and GA genotypes than in those with the AA genotype.

In 62 preterm infants, Oretti and colleagues[81] analyzed the following polymorphisms and their association with RDS: C1236T, G2677T, and C3435T polymorphisms in the ABC, subfamily B, member 1 (*ABCB1*) gene; BclI, N363S, and ER22/23EK in the nuclear receptor subfamily 3, group C, member 1, GR (*NR3C1*) gene; I105V in the glutathione-S-transferase subclass P1 (*GST-P1*) gene; and GST-M1 and GST-T1 deletions. All of the infants had been born to mothers who had received a full course of antenatal betamethasone. Univariate analysis showed that the heterozygous and homozygous presence of the I105V variant in the *GST-P1* gene seemed to confer protection against the occurrence of RDS ($P = 0.032$) but no association for all the other polymorphisms.[81]

In another study, no association was found between BclI, N363S, and ER22/23EK polymorphisms of the *GR* gene and RDS, in infants (n = 125) with or without exposure to antenatal betamethasone.[82]

Conclusion

Despite the plethora of developmentally appropriate murine models of specific gene alterations that impact on lung development, it is surprising that most of the clinical studies on RDS have focused primarily on SPs. Although certain specific haplotypes of SPs and ABCA3 have shown promise, the results are not definitive. The major drawbacks are the small sample sizes, variation in race/ethnic backgrounds, lack of replication cohorts, and, most important, lack of functional correlation. It is critical to show that if a specific single-nucleotide polymorphism (SNP) or haplotype is identified as having a possible association with the phenotype of RDS, the SNP or haplotype must have a functional impact in developmentally appropriate premature infants.

Genetic Influences in Injury to the Developing Lung

Animal Models

Given the multitude of genes (as discussed earlier) and signaling pathways that are responsible for lung maturation and postnatal adaptation, injury to the immature lung can significantly impair these processes. In addition, depending on the degree and duration of injury, resolution can lead to a normal lung or repair can result in marked perturbations of the pulmonary phenotype, with long-term consequences. The developing lung of the premature newborn is commonly exposed to stretch, infectious agents/mediators, and high concentrations of oxygen, with deleterious effect. This section of the chapter focuses on the genetic influences on the developing lung, mostly in the late saccular and early alveolar phases, especially those due to the environmental insults noted previously. Ventilation-induced lung injury in very preterm lambs have identified *IL-1, IL-6, IL-8,* connective tissue growth factor (*CTGF*), cysteine-rich 61 (*CYR61*), and early growth response factor 1 (*EGR1*) mRNA upregulation.[83] Exposure to hyperoxia has been well-recognized mode of injury to the developing lung that leads to a phenotype resembling human BPD[84] and accompanied by alterations in gene expression.[85]

Angiopoietin 1

Angs signal through the Tie2 receptor and are involved with vascular remodeling, hyperoxia-induced lung injury, and BPD.[86,87] Transgenic mice generated with SP-C targeting and cartilage oligomeric matrix protein (COMP)–Ang1 resulted in neonatal mice, of which 50% died from respiratory failure.[88] The surviving mice had lung histology suggestive of human BPD.[88]

Connective Tissue Growth Factor

Conditional overexpression of *CTGF* from PN1 to PN14 led to thickened alveolar septa, decreased secondary septal formation, and decreased formation of alveolar capillary network.[89] These data demonstrate that overexpression of *CTGF* disrupts alveolarization and pulmonary vasculature and induces fibrosis during the critical period of lung development. This histology is probably more reminiscent of "old" rather than "new" BPD.[90]

A

Fas-Ligand

Hyperoxia-induced injury to the developing lung is characterized by an influx of inflammatory cells, increased pulmonary permeability, and endothelial and epithelial cell death.[91] The induction of cell death responses regulated by shared common mediators of apoptotic and necrotic pathways.[91] The Fas/Fas-ligand (Fas-L) receptor–mediated cell death–signaling pathway is one of those well characterized.[92] Targeted upregulation of *Fas-L* in respiratory epithelial cells in transgenic mice was found to disrupt alveolar development, decrease vascular density, and increase post-neonatal mortality[92] between E19 and PN7.

Fibroblast Growth Factors 3 and 4

A study found that double-null mutant mice lacking both *FGF3* and *FGF4* had normal lungs at PN2; however, by PN9, there was evidence of failure of secondary septation.[93] This defect in alveolar development was quite obvious by PN21. Elastin synthesis is normally shut off following the alveolar phase, the remodeling of the lung extracellular matrix then being carried out by metalloelastases. Histochemical staining suggested that there was a failure in this elastin "shutting off" process in the lungs of the double-mutant mice.[93]

Fibroblast Growth Factor Receptor 2

Conditional lung epithelial cell targeted transgenic overexpression of a soluble dominant-negative fibroblast growth factor receptor 2 (*FGFR2*)—designated as FGFR-HFc—led to a pulmonary phenotype of large, simplified alveoli, resembling emphysema in adults, when activated from E14.5 to birth.[94] These alterations in lung architecture persisted till adulthood. Lungs were normal if the FGFR2 inhibition occurred only in the PN period.[94]

Interferon-γ

Using a unique triple transgenic interferon-γ (IFNγ)–overexpressing, lung-targeted newborn mouse model, Harijith and colleagues[95] observed a lung phenotype of impaired alveolarization resembling human BPD.[95] IFNγ-mediated abnormal lung architecture was associated with increased cell death and upregulation of cell death pathway mediators caspases 3, 6, 8 and 9, and Ang2. There were also increases in cathepsins B, H, K, L, and S as well as matrix metalloproteinase (MMPs) 2, 9, 12, and 14.[95] Interestingly, the IFNγ-induced pulmonary phenotype could be rescued, and survival was prolonged in hyperoxia with concomitant partial deficiency of MMP9.[95] Also, as evidence of clinical relevance, the investigators showed increased levels of downstream targets of IFNγ (CXCL10 and CXCL11) in baboon and human lungs with BPD.[95] The preceding data are in accord with earlier work in newborn *MMP9*$^{-/-}$ mice in hyperoxia.[96]

Interleukin-1β

Backstrom and associates[97] reported that conditional overexpression of human *IL-1β* in the saccular stage caused arrest in alveolar development and airway remodeling in a murine model; however, activation in the late canalicular–early saccular stage did not adversely affect lung development, growth, or survival of the pups. Interestingly, earlier work by the same group of investigators reported that MMP9 deficiency worsened the lung injury in IL-1β–overexpressing transgenic mice.[98]

Interleukin-6

Lung-targeted IL-6 overexpression was reported to cause significantly increased mortality, DNA injury, and upregulation of caspases and cell death mediators (including Fas and Fas-L) upon exposure to hyperoxia in neonatal transgenic mice.[99] In addition, there was upregulation of Ang2 mRNA and protein,[99] an angiogenic factor that has been implicated in hyperoxia-induced lung injury and BPD.[86]

Interleukin-11

Using a regulated lung epithelial cell–targeted overexpression approach, Ray and coworkers[100] observed that IL-11, when activated in utero or in the immediate PN period (for 10-14 days), led to lungs with large, simplified alveoli.[100] This phenotype was not noted when IL-11 was "turned on" in mature adult (i.e. after 4 weeks of age) lungs. This finding suggests that IL-11–induced impairment of alveolarization is developmentally regulated.

2

Platelet-Derived Growth Factor-A

The lungs of *PDGF-A*$^{-/-}$ mice older than 2 weeks were found to have large air spaces, suggesting a lack of alveolarization.[101] This defect in alveolar development occurred after PN4 and was apparent by PN7, because at PN4, saccules were present in the lungs of heterozygous and null mutant mice.[101] This defect was progressive because airway spaces continued to expand and the process was accompanied by a significant deficiency of alveolar myofibroblasts.[101]

Stroma-Derived Factor 1

Stroma-derived factor 1 (SDF-1) (also known as CXCL2) is a cell-signaling cytokine and a chemoattractant. It is the only known ligand for CXCR4 and CXCR7. Using conditional mice, Chen and colleagues[102] induced SDF-1 disruption on PN7. At PN14, there were enlarged alveolar spaces. Expression of *FGF-7* and *FGF-10* mRNAs was significantly decreased. Because SDF-1 staining was localized to vascular endothelial cells, analysis of angiogenic factors revealed that mRNA expression of *Flk-1*, a receptor for VEGF, was also significantly decreased.[102] However, there was no significant changes in mRNA expression of *Tie-2, FGF-R2, TGF-β2, TGF-β1, VEGF164,* or *eNOS*.[102]

Thy-1 (CD90)

Thy-1 (also known as CD90) is a glycophosphatidylinositol (GPI)–linked outer membrane leaflet glycoprotein that is expressed predominantly on subsets of fibroblasts and lymphocytes. *Thy-1*$^{-/-}$ mice were found to have abnormal alveolarization by PN14, and inhibition of TGF-β signaling improved alveolar development and lung function.[103]

Tissue Inhibitor of Metalloproteinase 3

Tissue inhibitors of metalloproteinases (TIMPs) regulate the extracellular matrix degradation by MMPs. In *TIMP3*-null mutant mice, Gill and coworkers[104] described significant air space enlargement over the first 2 weeks of PN life; specifically, on PNs 1, 5, 9, and 14. The enlargement was accompanied by increased MMP2 activity. Maternal treatment with a synthetic metalloproteinase inhibitor from E16.5 was associated with a partial rescue of the lung phenotype on PN1.[104]

Transforming Growth Factor-α

Overexpression of *TGF-α* in a conditional lung-targeted transgenic murine model, when activated from E16.5 to E18.5, significantly decreased survival in the PN period.[105] On lung histology at E17.5, after 1 day of activation (with doxycycline), there was increased parenchymal cellularity. On E18.5, there was extensive thickening of the septa in saccules and mesenchyme of blood vessels and airways, along with abundant lipofibroblasts.[105] These changes were accompanied by upregulation of EGFR.[105] No severe defects in epithelial maturation or of surfactant deficiency were evident.[105] When TGF-α was activated in the alveolar phase (PN3-PN5), the lungs showed arrest of septation and enlarged air spaces with abnormal vasculature,[106] suggestive of human BPD.

Transforming Growth Factor-β1

Overexpression of human *TGF-β1* in a conditional, lung-targeted triple-transgenic mouse model in the alveolar phase (PN7-PN14) led to a phenotype of enlarged alveoli, thickened cellular septa, and dysregulated vasculature, reminiscent of human BPD.[107] A similar picture was also reported after transfer of human *TGF-β1* gene using an adenoviral vector in the lungs of rat pups.[108]

A

Thyroid Transcription Factor-1

Interestingly, SP-C–targeted increased expression of *TTF-1* in murine lungs led to impaired alveolarization, inflammation, TIIP hyperplasia, and increased SP-B by PN14.[47] These data suggest that enhanced TTF-1 may have a role in lung injury and repair in the developing lung.

Vascular Endothelial Growth Factor

Most developmentally appropriate animal and human data suggest that exposure to hyperoxia and/or ventilation-induced lung injury leads to an increase in VEGF levels, followed by a decrease in VEGF in animals or humans demonstrating BPD.[84] Such an early increase in VEGF could lead to pulmonary vascular leak and injury, followed by a later "protective" response if VEGF levels are increased (rather than decreased, as in BPD). Conforming to this notion, transgenic overexpression of lung-targeted VEGF in a neonatal murine model led to enhanced lung injury, but no difference in mortality, upon exposure to hyperoxia in the saccular/alveolar phase (PN1-PN7).[55]

Summary

These data suggest that the developmental stage at the time of lung injury is a critical factor in the development of the pulmonary phenotype of BPD.

Genetic Influences in Injury to the Developing Lung: Clinical Context of BPD

BPD, the most common chronic respiratory disease in infants, occurs from disruption of the developmental program of the immature lung.[109] BPD is a complex disorder with multiple factors involved in the pathogenesis of the pulmonary phenotype characterized by a dysmorphic microvascular network and fewer, larger, simplified alveoli.[109-112] Figure 2-1 illustrates a proposed pathogenesis of BPD. Factors such as ventilation, sepsis (which includes chorioamnionitis and localized and systemic infections), and hyperoxia act on an immature lung, leading to the production of multiple molecular mediators. The balance of inflammatory and anti-inflammatory effects propels the process of lung injury highlighted by cell death. This step is followed by either resolution of injury (normal lung) or repair (BPD). The actions of the molecular mediators involved in lung development and injury are influenced by allelic differences of genes that create differential results. The sequence of events is highlighted by the time frames suggesting developmental regulation of the response of the lung to the inciting factors. Differential interactions between genetic susceptibility and environmental factors would create intermediate phenotypes that would modify the degree of lung repair, manifested as mild to severe BPD. Mild BPD is defined as a need for supplemental oxygen (O_2) for at least 28 days but not at postmenstrual age (PMA) of 36 weeks or at discharge. Moderate BPD is defined as the need for O_2 for at least 28 days in addition to treatment with more than 30% O_2 at 36 weeks PMA. Severe BPD is defined as need for O_2 for at least 28 days in addition to more than 30% O_2 and/or positive-pressure ventilation at 36 weeks PMA.[113,114] In some of the studies discussed in the following sections, the older definitions of the need for supplemental O_2 for 28 days or more or at 36 weeks PMA are used.

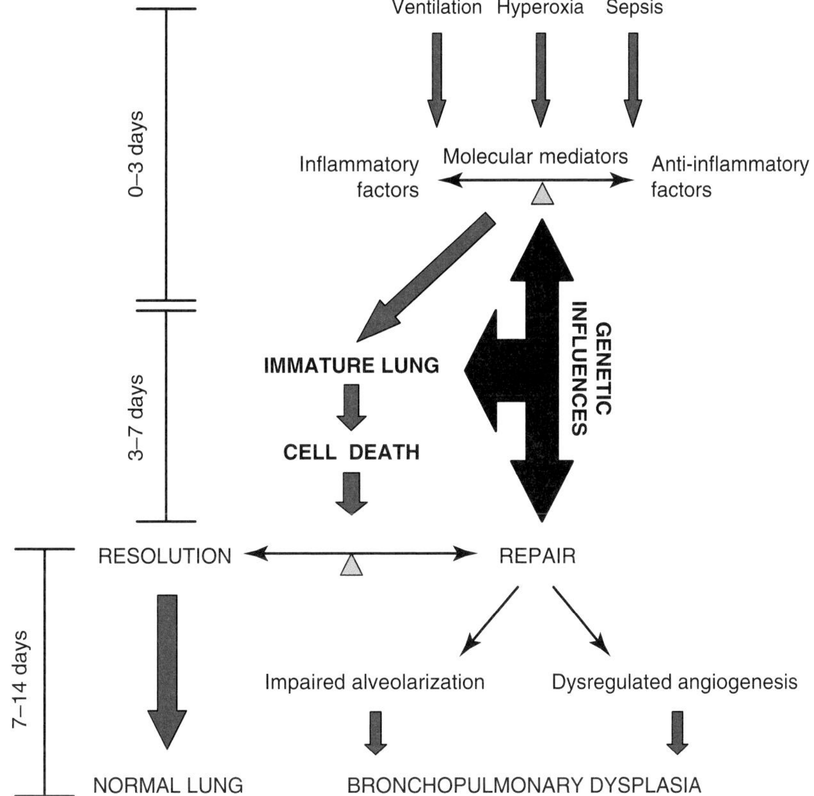

Figure 2-1 Genetic influences on lung development and injury modify the multiple processes that lead to the clinical pulmonary phenotypes of BPD.

2

Twin Studies in Bronchopulmonary Dysplasia

Studies have suggested a link between genetic susceptibility and risk for BPD when evaluated in twins.[69,115,116] In a study of premature twins (n = 108), after adjustment of data for BW, GA, gender, RDS, pneumothorax, and patent ductus arteriosus, BPD status in one twin was found to be a highly significant predictor of BPD in the other twin, irrespective of birth order, Apgar scores, and other factors.[117] These studies, however, had some significant limitations, including small sample sizes, lack of definitive zygosity analyses, and older definitions of BPD.

In a later study (n = 450 twin pairs), after data were controlled for the effects of the other significant risk factors, genetic modeling of twin data showed that 65.2% of the variance in liability for BPD could be accounted for by a combination of shared genetic and environmental factors.[112]

The contribution by genetic factors alone was further analyzed by comparison of 63 monozygotic and 189 dizygotic twin pairs. After data were controlled for covariates such as BW, GA, gender, RDS, Apgar scores, duration of ventilation, and birth order, genetic factors were found to account for 53% of the variance in liability for BPD.[112] The data proving that genetic factors are a significant component of BPD have been confirmed by an independent study using an even more stringent definition of BPD.[118]

Candidate Genes and Bronchopulmonary Dysplasia

Adhesion Molecules

Dystroglycan

The N494H homozygous genotype for DAG1 (codes for dystroglycan, an extracellular matrix receptor stabilizing the plasma membrane) was found more often in patients with BPD (n = 11, defined as O_2 requirement at 36 weeks PMA) than in those without BPD (n = 22).[119] No correction was performed for differences in GA, BW, or other known confounding variables.

L-Selectin

L-selectin is expressed on leukocytes. The pro213ser polymorphism causes an amino acid alteration in the short consensus repeat domain-1 of L-selectin and could potentially alter leukocyte-endothelial interactions.[120] In a cohort of low BW singleton infants, the 213ser allele of L-selectin was found to confer greater risk for BPD (28-day definition; n = 24) compared with 101 infants without BPD.[120]

A

Antioxidants

Glutathione-S-Transferase

GSTs provide an important line of cellular defense against reactive oxygen species (ROS). The *GST-P1* gene, which encodes the human class GST p, has an SNP at nucleotide 313 that causes a valine-to-isoleucine change at amino acid 105. The valine isoform is better at reducing oxidative toxins.[121] After data were controlled for race and gender, Manar and colleagues[122] found that patients with BPD (n = 35; controls = 98) were less likely to be homozygous for the valine/valine isoform and more likely to possess the less efficient isoleucine isoform.

Microsomal Epoxide Hydrolases

Microsomal enzymes metabolize ROS by catalyzing the hydrolysis of various epoxides and reactive epoxide intermediates. The alteration in the 113tyr isoform to histidine leads to slower catalysis of reduction of ROS metabolites. Manar and colleagues[122] found that their patients with BPD had an approximate six-fold increase (not statistically significant) in 113his homozygotes.

Inflammatory Mediators

Interleukin-4

Because IL-4 downregulates many of the inflammatory mediators that are elevated in tracheal aspirates from infants with BPD, it may have a protective effect. In a case-control study of IL-4 polymorphisms in infants with RDS requiring ventilation (n = 224), there were no significant differences in allelic frequencies of the IL-4 intron 3 or IL-4 promoter polymorphisms between those who did and did not have BPD.[123]

Interleukin 10

IL-10 inhibits mononuclear cell synthesis of a variety of pro-inflammatory cytokines, including TNF, IL-1α, IL-1β, IL-6, IL-8, IFN-γ, IL-12, IL-18, and chemokines. By inhibiting synthesis and promoting degradation of pro-inflammatory cytokines, IL-10 may diminish inflammation, cell injury and cell death known to occur in BPD. The A allele at position 1082 is associated with lower IL-10 production.[124] The frequency of this SNP in ventilated infants (n=294) had no significant effect on BPD.[125]

Interferonγ

IFNγ is considered a Th1 cytokine and has effects on regulation of cell growth and differentiation as well as activation of monocytes/macrophages, cytotoxic T cells, and natural killer cells. Infant carriers of the IFNγ+874T allele (n = 153) were found to be protected against BPD in comparison with the IFNγ+874AA genotype.[126]

Mannose-Binding Lectin 2

Mannose-binding lectin (MBL) (encoded by the *MBL2* gene), a collectin, activates the complement system in an antibody-independent manner and enhances phagocytosis.[127] Low serum levels of MBL and *MBL2* genetic variants have been associated with infection in premature newborns; however, genotype–MBL concentration correlations may not always be true in individuals.[127] In a study of premature infants (n = 75), the R52C mutation of *MBL2* was associated with an increased risk of BPD (36 weeks PMA definition) after data were corrected for GA and BW.[127]

Macrophage Migration Inhibitory Factor

A 2010 study reported that the MIF-173*C allele, which predisposes to higher MIF production, was associated with a lower incidence of BPD, independent from mechanical ventilation and oxygen exposure.[128] These data support the earlier finding that low levels of MIF in tracheal aspirates of neonates predispose them to development of BPD.[35]

Monocyte Chemoattractant Protein-1

Chemokines such as monocyte chemoattractant protein-1 (MCP-1) have chemotactic, homing, and activating effects on leukocytes. The A/G polymorphism at MCP-1-2518 was found not to be associated with BPD in ventilated infants (n = 178) or with differences in MCP-1 concentration in tracheal aspirates from the infants.[129]

2

Transforming Growth Factor-β1

As mentioned before, TGF-β1 has been implicated in fetal lung development and in animal models of BPD. In ventilated infants (n = 178) in one study the TGF-β1+915 noncoding C-to-G SNP, which is associated with decreased production of TGF-β1 in vitro (C allele), was found to have no effect on the development of BPD.[129] In another study (n = 192), no association was found between BPD and the TGF-β1 (915G/C) SNP.[130] In a third study (n =181), no association was found between BPD and the following SNPs of TGF-β1: −800G>A, −509C>T, 10T>C, 25G>C.[131]

Tumor Necrosis Factor

Because TNF is one of the principal mediators of the inflammatory cascade, high levels of TNFα may promote chronic inflammation by overwhelming counter-regulatory mechanisms, whereas low levels may decrease the risk for and severity of BPD.[132]

A-to-G substitutions at positions 308 and 238 for TNFα and position 250 for TNFβ have been studied. The A alleles of TNFα-308 and TNFβ-250 have been associated with increased levels of TNFα, whereas the A allele of TNFα-238 produces lower levels after stimulation. The inverse is true for the TNFα and TNFβ levels in the presence of the G allele at the positions specified above.

No difference in allele frequencies were found in one study of ventilated infants (n = 178) genotyped for the TNFα-308 A-to-G allele between those in whom BPD developed and those in whom it did not.[129] In another study, the allele frequencies of TNFα-308 and TNFβ-250 were comparable in BPD cases (n = 51; 36 weeks PMA definition) and controls (n = 69).[132] Although the investigators of the second study suggest that the A allele in TNFα-238 genotype is protective for BPD, the number of subjects is small, and the correlation was relatively weak.[132] In contrast, other investigators have reported no association with severity of BPD for the following TNFα SNPs: −1031, −863, −857, −308, and −238.[133] A meta-analysis (n = 804) of the TNFα-308 A-to-G SNP did not show any association with BPD.[134] The authors of the meta-analysis concluded that future research efforts to define genetic predisposition to BPD should focus on alternative candidate genes.[134]

Surfactant Proteins A, B, and D

The SP-A 6A[6] allele appears to be over-represented in infants with BPD.[135] More than 27 loss-of-function mutations resulting in lethal neonatal respiratory failure have been identified in the *SP-B* gene. Of the several known common variants, the most common is the frameshift in exon 4 (121ins2), which accounts for 60% to 70% of mutations. In one study that evaluated SP-B intron 4 polymorphisms, group 1 (n = 111, with the intron 4 wild type) and group 2 (n = 29, with intron 4 variations) were comparable for GA, BW, and gender. The incidence of BPD (28-day definition) was higher in infants in group 2. Use of the 36-week definition of BPD resulted in loss of that association.[136] In a study from Finland, the frequency of the SP-B intron

4 deletion variant allele was higher in infants with BPD (n = 67) than in controls (n = 178).[137]

In a family-based association study, in the *SP-B* gene, allele B-18_C was associated with susceptibility to BPD (36-week PMA definition; n = 19) and the microsatellite marker AAGG_6 was associated with susceptibility to BPD (28-day definition, n = 52′ 36-week PMA. n=19)/[138] Haplotype analysis showed ten susceptibility haplotypes, one protective haplotype for SP-B, and two protective haplotypes for SP-A–SP-D.[138]

In a later study, the variant of the *SP-D* gene (rs1923537; 11208A>G) (n = 284) which was associated with a lower prevalence of RDS, was also associated with decreased BPD (28-day definition).[78]

A

Miscellaneous

Adenosine Triphosphate–Binding Cassette Transporter A3

In one study (n = 368), an SNP (rs13332514) of *Abca3* was associated with BPD(28-day definition).[74]

Angiotensin-Converting Enzyme

Renin, secreted exclusively by the kidneys into the circulation, splits the decapeptide angiotensin I (AT-I) from the amino terminal end of angiotensinogen. Angiotensin-converting enzyme (ACE) converts the physiologically inactive AT-I to the active AT-II, which mostly occurs in endothelial cells in the lung. AT-II, a direct vasoconstrictor, stimulates the adrenal cortex to produce aldosterone, which causes sodium and hence water absorption in the distal collecting tubules of the kidneys. Therefore, it is postulated that the extracellular fluid retention via aldosterone resulting from ACE polymorphisms that increase AT-II may increase BPD susceptibility. The *ACE* gene contains a polymorphism consisting of either the presence (insertion, I) or absence (deletion, D) of a 287–base pair alu repeat in intron 16. The D allele is associated with greater ACE activity in both tissue and plasma. In a study reported by Yanamandra and colleagues,[139] ACE I and D alleles were genotyped in ventilated infants (n = 245); 88 (35.9%) infants were homozygous DD, 107 (43.7%) were heterozygous ID, and 50 (20.4%) were homozygous II. There were no significant differences between genotype groups with respect to ethnicity, GA, BW, or gender. The ACE ID polymorphism was found to have no effect on development of BPD for either the 28-day or the 36-week definition.[139] In another study comparing infants with BPD (n = 51) to controls (n = 60), it was reported that infants with DD or ID genotypes of ACE were more likely to have BPD than infants with the II genotype. However, more infants with DD or ID genotypes did not have BPD (51/97 = 53%) than did (46/97 = 47%), and the real difference in this study were the 23 infants with II, with the I allele not being "causative." The researchers further noted that the number of D alleles correlated with severity, but they had a small number of infants with mild (16/62) and moderate (46/62) BPD.[140]

Factor VII

The factor VII-323 del/ins (323 A1/A2) promoter polymorphism has been shown to result in an approximately 20% decrease in factor VII coagulant activity.[141] This polymorphism was found in one study to be a potential protective factor against BPD (n = 1004).[141] However, a smaller study (n = 192) did not confirm the finding.[130] The biochemical explanation for an effect in BPD remains unknown.

Factor-XIII

A study in Turkish infants (n = 192) did not reveal any association between BPD and the Val34Leu SNP.[130]

Human Leukocyte AntigenA2

Seventy-seven preterm infants were HLA genotyped in one of the earliest prospective blinded studies associating genes with BPD.[142] All infants with BPD (defined only by chest radiograph) had HLA-A2 antigens.[142]

Insulin-Like Growth Factor-I and its Receptor

Insulin-like growth factor-1 (IGF-1), with most effects mediated through its receptor, IGF-1R, is involved in both prenatal and postnatal lung growth. In one study, low serum IGF levels were associated with BPD (n = 22).[143] In contrast, expression of IGF-1 and IGF-1R, as detected by immunocytochemistry in human lung tissue obtained at autopsy, was found in another study to be low during fetal development (n = 6), acutely upregulated in RDS (n = 5), and further upregulated in BPD (n = 4).[144] In other studies, no association was found between CA repeats in the IGF-1 promoter and BPD (n = 181)[131] or between an IGF-1R non-coding G-to-A SNP at +3174 and development of BPD (n = 132).[145] In the second study, the SNP in the IGF-1R was used as a proxy for IGF-1 plasma levels. However, the ability of this SNP to predict IGF-1 levels is at best tenuous, with very wide standard errors (GG: 2.95 ± 2.61, AG: 2.34 ± 2.41, AA: 1.94 ± 2.17),[146] raising concern about the utility of the assay and the results of the preceding BPD study.[145]

Matrix Metalloproteinase-16

After data adjustment for BW and ethnic origin, Hadchouel and coworkers[147] found that the TT genotype of MMP16 C/T (rs2664352) and the GG genotype of MMP16 A/G (rs2664349) to be protective of BPD (n = 284).

5,10-Methylenetetrahydrofolate reductase

In individuals homozygous for the 677C>T polymorphism, specific,10-methylenetetrahydrofolate reductase (5,10-MTHFR) enzyme activity is reduced to approximately one third. In addition, the *5,10-MTHFR* enzyme is more unstable than the normal isoforms and can cause the plasma homocysteine level to almost double. Hence, one team of investigators chose the 5,10-MTHFR gene as a candidate gene for BPD, because numerous studies have demonstrated the correlation between hyperhomocysteinemia and increased production of ROS and oxidant stress, known to be involved in the pathogenesis of BPD. However, they found no association (n = 181).[131]

Vascular Endothelial Growth Factor

Investigators in the preceding study have also found that VEGF–460CC homozygotes have a lower risk than babies with –460TT or –460TC genotypes (n = 181), although VEGF serum concentrations were no different.[131] In addition, no association was found between the VEGF 405G>C SNP and BPD or the serum VEGF levels.[131]

Transporter Associated with Antigen Processing

Together, transporter associated with antigen processing 1 (TAP1) and TAP2 proteins translocate peptides from the cytosol to major histocompatibility complex (MHC) class I molecules in the endoplasmic reticulum. TAP1 polymorphisms may play a role in inflammation, specifically affecting IFNγ responsiveness and activation of adhesion molecules. In a study of infants (n = 224) in the Taiwanese population, no association was noted between BPD and the TAP1 DpnII polymorphism.[148]

Urokinase

Urokinase is an enzyme that catalyzes the conversion of plasminogen to plasmin, thus stimulating fibrinolysis and degradation of major basement membrane glycoproteins such as fibronectin and laminin.[149] In a study of preterm infants (n = 204) from Taiwan, the frequency of the urokinase 3′-UTR (untranslated region) polymorphism did not differ significantly between those in whom BPD did and did not develop.[150]

Summary

Genetic association studies of BPD have attempted to identify specific candidate genes involved in the biologic pathways regulating the processes noted in Figure 2-1. These have been summarized in Tables 2-2 to 2-6. These studies, however, mostly involve small sample sizes, and a majority of them have not been replicated

Table 2-2 GENETIC ALLELIC VARIANTS OF ADHESION MOLECULES ASSOCIATED WITH RISK FOR BRONCHOPULMONARY DYSPLASIA (BPD)

Marker*	Reference No. for Study	Polymorphism	N	BPD Susceptibility
DAG1	119	N449H	33	Increased in homozygotes
L-selectin	120	pro213ser	125	Increased

*See text for explanation of marker abbreviations.

A

Table 2-3 GENETIC ALLELIC VARIANTS OF ANTIOXIDANTS ASSOCIATED WITH RISK FOR BRONCHOPULMONARY DYSPLASIA (BPD)

Marker*	Polymorphism	N	BPD Susceptibility
GST	Valine/isoleucine	35	Increased (ile) Decreased (val)
mEPHx	tyr113his	35	None

*See text for explanation of marker abbreviations.
Data from Manar MH, Brown MR, Gauthier TW, et al. Association of glutathione-S-transferase-P1 (GST-P1) polymorphisms with bronchopulmonary dysplasia. *J Perinatol.* 2004;24:30-35.

Table 2-4 GENETIC ALLELIC VARIANTS OF INFLAMMATORY MEDIATORS ASSOCIATED WITH RISK FOR BRONCHOPULMONARY DYSPLASIA (BPD)

Marker*	Reference No. for Study	Polymorphism	N	BPD Susceptibility
IL-4	123	Intron 3	224	None
		590 Promoter	224	None
IL-10	125	1082 Adenine/guanine	294	None
IFNγ	126	+874T	153	Decreased
MBL2	127	R52C	75	Increased
MIF	128	−173*C	91	Decreased
MCP-1	129	2518 Adenine/guanine	178	None
TGF-β1	129	915 Guanine/cytosine	178	None
	130		192	None
	131	−800G>A, −509C>T, 10T>C, 25G>C	181	None
TNF-α 238	132	Adenine/guanine	100	Decreased
	133		105	None
TNF-α 308	132		100	None
	129		178	None
	133		105	None
	134		804[†]	None
TNF-α-857	133	Cytosine/thymidine	105	None
TNF-α-863	133	Cytosine/adenine	105	None
TNF-α-1031	133	Thymidine/cytosine	105	None
TNF-β-250	132	Adenine/guanine	100	None

*See text for explanation of marker abbreviations.
[†]Meta-analysis.

Table 2-5 GENETIC ALLELIC VARIANTS OF SURFACTANT PROTEINS (SPS) A, B, AND D ASSOCIATED WITH RISK FOR BRONCHOPULMONARY DYSPLASIA (BPD)

Marker	Reference No. for Study	Polymorphism	N	BPD Susceptibility
SP-A1	135	6A6	46	Increased
SP-B	136	Intron 4	140	None
	138	Allele_6 AAGG	71	Increased
		B-18 (A/C)	71	Increased with allele C
SP-D	78	11208A>G	284	Decreased

in additional cohorts. In some cases, the *P* value is not compelling— as reflected by wide confidence intervals—and the association would probably disappear with most statistical corrections for multiple testing.

Regardless, these studies represent a shift in the way physicians and scientists have traditionally thought about BPD, from a disease that is exclusively developmental to one that is the consequence of interactions between genetic and environmental factors (see Fig. 2-1). The studies previously described interrogated variations of candidate genes in a wide distribution of sample sizes. Eleven studies have reported an increased or decreased risk. It is striking to note that the findings of only two have been replicated: for TNFα 238 and ACE insertion/deletion polymorphisms. Both these associations with BPD have not held up in studies with larger cohorts. This fact is not surprising. The frequency that genetic association is replicated in follow-up studies has been looked at in a meta-analyses.[151] About half of initial genetic association studies, even those with strong effects (odds ratio

Table 2-6 MISCELLANEOUS GENETIC ALLELIC VARIANTS ASSOCIATED WITH RISK FOR BRONCHOPULMONARY DYSPLASIA (BPD)

Marker	Reference No. for Study	Polymorphism	N	BPD Susceptibility
ABCA3	74	rs13332514	368	Increased
ACE	139	Insertion/deletion	245	None
	140	Deletion	111	Increased
Factor VII	141	323 Deletion/insertion	1004	Decreased
	130		192	None
Factor XIII	130	Val 34 Leu	192	None
HLA	142	A2	77	Increased
IGF-1	131	CA repeats in promoter	181	None
IGF-1R	145	IGF-1R G+3174	132	None
MMP16	147	C/T	284	Decreased in TT
MMP16	147	A/G	284	Decreased in GG
MTHFR	131	677C>T	181	None
VEGF	131	460T>C	181	–460CC homozygotes were at a lower risk than babies with –460TT or –460TC
VEGF	131	405G>C	181	None
TAP1	148	DpnII Adenine/guanine	224	None
Urokinase	150	3′ UTR	204	None

[OR] > 2.0) or with low *P* values (< 0.001), are not replicated. The reasons include population admixture (unmatched cases and controls), phenotypic heterogeneity (inclusion of both genetic and nongenetic cases), and commonly, underpowered studies (not enough subjects). It is therefore likely that subsequent studies with larger cohorts will diminish the initially reported association with BPD identified in smaller sample sizes.

Conclusions

A significant amount of information has been gleaned about the genes governing the process of lung development at the limits of viability, through the use of elegant genetic loss- and gain-of-function approaches in murine models. However, little progress has been made in terms of the translational aspect of pulmonary maturity. A potential explanation could be that increased use of antenatal steroids and availability of surfactant resulting in enhanced survival of neonates have potentially diminished the intensity of research in this direction. The reverse is true of BPD, in which there has been an explosion of genetic association studies, with limited progress in understanding of the genetic determinants of this complex disorder in animal models. One would hope, given the long-term consequences of BPD, that research would be intensified because understanding of the developmental regulation of lung maturation and response to injury could go a long way in elucidating pulmonary disorders in children and adults, including asthma and chronic obstructive pulmonary disease (COPD).

It is critical, therefore, to undertake human studies with sample sizes that would be adequately powered for robust genetic associations with RDS and BPD. Finally, it is also important to remember that identification of molecular determinants associated with RDS and BPD in such genetic studies does not necessarily mean that they are amenable to specific therapeutic targeting. Once they are identified, the next logical step would involve their validation with the use of developmentally appropriate animal models of RDS and BPD, before confirmation in human neonates. Significant improvements in the outcome of premature neonates with RDS and/or at risk for BPD will likely depend on our ability to identify these genetic components and to specify therapeutic targets.

Acknowledgments

VB was supported by grants from NIH HL 074195, HL 085103, AHA 0755843T, ATS 07-005.

References

1. Copland I, Post M. Lung development and fetal lung growth. *Paediatr Respir Rev*. 2004;5(Suppl A):S259-S264.
2. Bourbon J, Boucherat O, Chailley-Heu B, et al. Control mechanisms of lung alveolar development and their disorders in bronchopulmonary dysplasia. *Ped Res*. 2005;57:38-46.
3. Fitzgerald ML, Xavier R, Haley KJ, et al. ABCA3 inactivation in mice causes respiratory failure, loss of pulmonary surfactant, and depletion of lung phosphatidylglycerol. *J Lipid Res*. 2007;48:621-632.
4. Mucenski ML, Wert SE, Nation JM, et al. beta-Catenin is required for specification of proximal/distal cell fate during lung morphogenesis. *J Biol Chem*. 2003;278:40231-40238.
5. Bellusci S, Henderson R, Winnier G, et al. Evidence from normal expression and targeted misexpression that bone morphogenetic protein (Bmp-4) plays a role in mouse embryonic lung morphogenesis. *Development*. 1996;122:1693-1702.
6. Michos O, Panman L, Vintersten K, et al. Gremlin-mediated BMP antagonism induces the epithelial-mesenchymal feedback signaling controlling metanephric kidney and limb organogenesis. *Development*. 2004;131:3401-3410.
7. Eblaghie MC, Reedy M, Oliver T, et al. Evidence that autocrine signaling through Bmpr1a regulates the proliferation, survival and morphogenetic behavior of distal lung epithelial cells. *Dev Biol*. 2006;291:67-82.
8. Sun J, Chen H, Chen C, et al. Prenatal lung epithelial cell-specific abrogation of Alk3-bone morphogenetic protein signaling causes neonatal respiratory distress by disrupting distal airway formation. *Am J Pathol*. 2008;172:571-582.
9. Yadav N, Lee J, Kim J, et al. Specific protein methylation defects and gene expression perturbations in coactivator-associated arginine methyltransferase 1-deficient mice. *Proc Natl Acad Sci U S A*. 2003;100:6464-6468.

10. O'Brien KB, Alberich-Jorda M, Yadav N, et al. CARM1 is required for proper control of proliferation and differentiation of pulmonary epithelial cells. *Development*. 2010;137:2147-2156.
11. Martis PC, Whitsett JA, Xu Y, et al. C/EBPalpha is required for lung maturation at birth. *Development*. 2006;133:1155-1164.
12. McCoy DM, Fisher K, Robichaud J, et al. Transcriptional regulation of lung cytidylyltransferase in developing transgenic mice. *Am J Respir Cell Mol Biol*. 2006;35:394-402.
13. Ridsdale R, Tseu I, Roth-Kleiner M, et al. Increased phosphatidylcholine production but disrupted glycogen metabolism in fetal type II cells of mice that overexpress CTP:phosphocholine cytidylyltransferase. *J Biol Chem*. 2004;279:55946-55957.
14. Tian Y, Zhou R, Rehg JE, et al. Role of phosphocholine cytidylyltransferase alpha in lung development. *Mol Cell Biol*. 2007;27:975-982.
15. Han RN, Babaei S, Robb M, et al. Defective lung vascular development and fatal respiratory distress in endothelial NO synthase-deficient mice: a model of alveolar capillary dysplasia? *Circ Res*. 2004;94:1115-1123.
16. Miller AA, Hislop AA, Vallance PJ, et al. Deletion of the eNOS gene has a greater impact on the pulmonary circulation of male than female mice. *Am J Physiol Lung Cell Mol Physiol*. 2005;289: L299-L306.
17. Sibilia M, Wagner EF. Strain-dependent epithelial defects in mice lacking the EGF receptor. *Science*. 1995;269:234-238.
18. Miettinen PJ, Warburton D, Bu D, et al. Impaired lung branching morphogenesis in the absence of functional EGF receptor. *Dev Biol*. 1997;186:224-236.
19. Liu W, Purevdorj E, Zscheppang K, et al. ErbB4 regulates the timely progression of late fetal lung development. *Biochim Biophys Acta*. 2010;1803:832-839.
20. El-Hashash AH, Al Alam D, Turcatel G, et al. Eyes absent 1 (Eya1) is a critical coordinator of epithelial, mesenchymal and vascular morphogenesis in the mammalian lung. *Dev Biol*. 2010.
21. Yu S, Poe B, Schwarz M, et al. Fetal and postnatal lung defects reveal a novel and required role for Fgf8 in lung development. *Dev Biol*. 2010;347:92-108.
22. Usui H, Shibayama M, Ohbayashi N, et al. Fgf18 is required for embryonic lung alveolar development. *Biochem Biophys Res Commun*. 2004;322:887-892.
23. Kalinichenko VV, Lim L, Stolz DB, et al. Defects in pulmonary vasculature and perinatal lung hemorrhage in mice heterozygous null for the Forkhead Box f1 transcription factor. *Dev Biol*. 2001;235:489-506.
24. Kalin TV, Wang IC, Meliton L, et al. Forkhead Box m1 transcription factor is required for perinatal lung function. *Proc Natl Acad Sci U S A*. 2008;105:19330-19335.
25. Wang IC, Zhang Y, Snyder J, et al. Increased expression of FoxM1 transcription factor in respiratory epithelium inhibits lung sacculation and causes Clara cell hyperplasia. *Dev Biol*. 2010;347: 301-314.
26. Zhang Y, Goss AM, Cohen ED, et al. A Gata6-Wnt pathway required for epithelial stem cell development and airway regeneration. *Nat Genet*. 2008;40:862-870.
27. Yang H, Lu MM, Zhang L, et al. GATA6 regulates differentiation of distal lung epithelium. *Development*. 2002;129:2233-2246.
28. Koutsourakis M, Keijzer R, Visser P, et al. Branching and differentiation defects in pulmonary epithelium with elevated Gata6 expression. *Mech Dev*. 2001;105:105-114.
29. Manwani N, Gagnon S, Post M, et al. Reduced viability of mice with lung epithelial-specific knockout of glucocorticoid receptor. *Am J Respir Cell Mol Biol*. 2010;43:599-606.
30. Yang LV, Radu CG, Roy M, et al. Vascular abnormalities in mice deficient for the G protein-coupled receptor GPR4 that functions as a pH sensor. *Mol Cell Biol*. 2007;27:1334-1347.
31. Zhou L, Dey CR, Wert SE, et al. Hepatocyte nuclear factor-3beta limits cellular diversity in the developing respiratory epithelium and alters lung morphogenesis in vivo. *Dev Dyn*. 1997;210: 305-314.
32. Aubin J, Lemieux M, Tremblay M, et al. Early postnatal lethality in Hoxa-5 mutant mice is attributable to respiratory tract defects. *Dev Biol*. 1997;192:432-445.
33. Wan H, Luo F, Wert SE, et al. Kruppel-like factor 5 is required for perinatal lung morphogenesis and function. *Development*. 2008;135:2563-2572.
34. Bridges JP, Ikegami M, Brilli LL, et al. LPCAT1 regulates surfactant phospholipid synthesis and is required for transitioning to air breathing in mice. *J Clin Invest*. 2010;120:1736-1748.
35. Kevill KA, Bhandari V, Kettunen M, et al. A role for macrophage migration inhibitory factor in the neonatal respiratory distress syndrome. *J Immunol*. 2008;180:601-608.
36. Fan G, Xiao L, Cheng L, et al. Targeted disruption of NDST-1 gene leads to pulmonary hypoplasia and neonatal respiratory distress in mice. *FEBS Lett*. 2000;467:7-11.
37. Okubo T, Knoepfler PS, Eisenman RN, et al. Nmyc plays an essential role during lung development as a dosage-sensitive regulator of progenitor cell proliferation and differentiation. *Development*. 2005;132:1363-1374.
38. Li J, Hoyle GW. Overexpression of PDGF-A in the lung epithelium of transgenic mice produces a lethal phenotype associated with hyperplasia of mesenchymal cells. *Dev Biol*. 2001;239:338-349.
39. Zhuo Y, Hoyle GW, Shan B, et al. Over-expression of PDGF-C using a lung specific promoter results in abnormal lung development. *Transgenic Res*. 2006;15:543-555.
40. Nasonkin IO, Ward RD, Raetzman LT, et al. Pituitary hypoplasia and respiratory distress syndrome in Prop1 knockout mice. *Hum Mol Genet*. 2004;13:2727-2735.
41. Yanagi S, Kishimoto H, Kawahara K, et al. Pten controls lung morphogenesis, bronchioalveolar stem cells, and onset of lung adenocarcinomas in mice. *J Clin Invest*. 2007;117:2929-2940.

42. Massaro GD, Massaro D, Chan WY, et al. Retinoic acid receptor-beta: an endogenous inhibitor of the perinatal formation of pulmonary alveoli. *Physiol Genomics*. 2000;4:51-57.
43. Bellusci S, Furuta Y, Rush MG, et al. Involvement of Sonic hedgehog (Shh) in mouse embryonic lung growth and morphogenesis. *Development*. 1997;124:53-63.
44. Clark JC, Wert SE, Bachurski CJ, et al. Targeted disruption of the surfactant protein B gene disrupts surfactant homeostasis, causing respiratory failure in newborn mice. *Proc Natl Acad Sci U S A*. 1995;92:7794-7798.
45. Tokieda K, Whitsett JA, Clark JC, et al. Pulmonary dysfunction in neonatal SP-B-deficient mice. *Am J Physiol*. 1997;273:L875-L882.
46. Lin S, Na CL, Akinbi HT, et al. Surfactant protein B (SP-B) –/– mice are rescued by restoration of SP-B expression in alveolar type II cells but not Clara cells. *J Biol Chem*. 1999;274: 19168-19174.
47. Wert SE, Dey CR, Blair PA, et al. Increased expression of thyroid transcription factor-1 (TTF-1) in respiratory epithelial cells inhibits alveolarization and causes pulmonary inflammation. *Dev Biol*. 2002;242:75-87.
48. DeFelice M, Silberschmidt D, DiLauro R, et al. TTF-1 phosphorylation is required for peripheral lung morphogenesis, perinatal survival, and tissue-specific gene expression. *J Biol Chem*. 2003;278: 35574-35583.
49. Zhou L, Dey CR, Wert SE, et al. Arrested lung morphogenesis in transgenic mice bearing an SP-C-TGF-beta 1 chimeric gene. *Dev Biol*. 1996;175:227-238.
50. Kaartinen V, Voncken JW, Shuler C, et al. Abnormal lung development and cleft palate in mice lacking TGF-beta 3 indicates defects of epithelial-mesenchymal interaction. *Nat Genet*. 1995;11: 415-421.
51. Chen H, Zhuang F, Liu YH, et al. TGF-beta receptor II in epithelia versus mesenchyme plays distinct roles in the developing lung. *Eur Respir J*. 2008;32:285-295.
52. Compernolle V, Brusselmans K, Acker T, et al. Loss of HIF-2alpha and inhibition of VEGF impair fetal lung maturation, whereas treatment with VEGF prevents fatal respiratory distress in premature mice. *Nat Med*. 2002;8:702-710.
53. Yamamoto H, Yun EJ, Gerber HP, et al. Epithelial-vascular cross talk mediated by VEGF-A and HGF signaling directs primary septae formation during distal lung morphogenesis. *Dev Biol*. 2007;308: 44-53.
54. Ng YS, Rohan R, Sunday ME, et al. Differential expression of VEGF isoforms in mouse during development and in the adult. *Dev Dyn*. 2001;220:112-121.
55. Bhandari V, Choo-Wing R, Lee CG, et al. Developmental regulation of NO-mediated VEGF-induced effects in the lung. *Am J Respir Cell Mol Biol*. 2008;39:420-430.
56. Le Cras TD, Spitzmiller RE, Albertine KH, et al. VEGF causes pulmonary hemorrhage, hemosiderosis, and air space enlargement in neonatal mice. *Am J Physiol Lung Cell Mol Physiol*. 2004;287: L134-L142.
57. Shu W, Jiang YQ, Lu MM, et al. Wnt7b regulates mesenchymal proliferation and vascular development in the lung. *Development*. 2002;129:4831-4842.
58. Soutiere SE, Tankersley CG, Mitzner W. Differences in alveolar size in inbred mouse strains. *Respir Physiol Neurobiol*. 2004;140:283-291.
59. Fanaroff AA, Stoll BJ, Wright LL, et al. Trends in neonatal morbidity and mortality for very low birthweight infants. *Am J Obstet Gynecol*. 2007;196:147 e141-e148.
60. Dani C, Reali MF, Bertini G, et al. Risk factors for the development of respiratory distress syndrome and transient tachypnoea in newborn infants. Italian Group of Neonatal Pneumology. *Eur Respir J*. 1999;14:155-159.
61. Dempsey E, Chen MF, Kokottis T, et al. Outcome of neonates less than 30 weeks gestation with histologic chorioamnionitis. *Am J Perinatol*. 2005;22:155-159.
62. Namavar Jahromi B, Ardekany MS, Poorarian S. Relationship between duration of preterm premature rupture of membranes and pulmonary maturation. *Int J Gynaecol Obstet*. 2000;68:119-122.
63. Ziadeh SM, Sunna E, Badria LF. The effect of mode of delivery on neonatal outcome of twins with birthweight under 1500 grams. *J Obstet Gynaecol*. 2000;20:389-391.
64. Klein JM, Nielsen HC. Androgen regulation of epidermal growth factor receptor binding activity during fetal rabbit lung development. *J Clin Invest*. 1993;91:425-431.
65. Luerti M, Parazzini F, Agarossi A, et al. Risk factors for respiratory distress syndrome in the newborn. A multicenter Italian survey. Study Group for Lung Maturity of the Italian Society of Perinatal Medicine. *Acta Obstet Gynecol Scand*. 1993;72:359-364.
66. Hacking D, Watkins A, Fraser S, et al. Respiratory distress syndrome and birth order in premature twins. *Arch Dis Child Fetal Neonatal Ed*. 2001;84:F117-F121.
67. Balchin I, Whittaker JC, Lamont RF, et al. Timing of planned cesarean delivery by racial group. *Obstet Gynecol*. 2008;111:659-666.
68. Marttila R, Kaprio J, Hallman M. Respiratory distress syndrome in twin infants compared with singletons. *Am J Obstet Gynecol*. 2004;191:271-276.
69. Shinwell ES, Blickstein I, Lusky A, et al. Effect of birth order on neonatal morbidity and mortality among very low birthweight twins: a population based study. *Arch Dis Child Fetal Neonatal Ed*. 2004;89:F145-F148.
70. Myrianthopoulos NC, Churchill JA, Baszynski AJ. Respiratory distress syndrome in twins. *Acta Genet Med Gemellol (Roma)*. 1971;20:199-204.
71. van Sonderen L, Halsema EF, Spiering EJ, et al. Genetic influences in respiratory distress syndrome: a twin study. *Semin Perinatol*. 2002;26:447-449.

A

72. Marttila R, Haataja R, Ramet M, et al. Surfactant protein B polymorphism and respiratory distress syndrome in premature twins. *Hum Genet*. 2003;112:18-23.
73. Levit O, Jiang Y, Bizzarro MJ, et al. The genetic susceptibility to respiratory distress syndrome. *Pediatr Res*. 2009;66:693-697.
74. Karjalainen MK, Haataja R, Hallman M. Haplotype analysis of ABCA3: association with respiratory distress in very premature infants. *Ann Med*. 2008;40:56-65.
75. Garmany TH, Wambach JA, Heins HB, et al. Population and disease-based prevalence of the common mutations associated with surfactant deficiency. *Pediatr Res*. 2008;63:645-649.
76. Sivasli E, Babaoglu M, Yasar U, et al. Association between the Glu298Asp and T(-786)C polymorphisms of the endothelial nitric oxide synthase gene and respiratory distress in preterm neonates. *Turk J Pediatr*. 2010;52:145-149.
77. Lahti M, Marttila R, Hallman M. Surfactant protein C gene variation in the Finnish population—association with perinatal respiratory disease. *Eur J Hum Genet*. 2004;12:312-320.
78. Hilgendorff A, Heidinger K, Bohnert A, et al. Association of polymorphisms in the human surfactant protein-D (SFTPD) gene and postnatal pulmonary adaptation in the preterm infant. *Acta Paediatr*. 2009;98:112-117.
79. Pulkkinen V, Haataja R, Hannelius U, et al. G protein-coupled receptor for asthma susceptibility associates with respiratory distress syndrome. *Ann Med*. 2006;38:357-366.
80. Capasso M, Avvisati RA, Piscopo C, et al. Cytokine gene polymorphisms in Italian preterm infants: association between interleukin-10-1082 G/A polymorphism and respiratory distress syndrome. *Pediatr Res*. 2007;61:313-317.
81. Oretti C, Marino S, Mosca F, et al. Glutathione-S-transferase-P1 I105V polymorphism and response to antenatal betamethasone in the prevention of respiratory distress syndrome. *Eur J Clin Pharmacol*. 2009;65:483-491.
82. Bertalan R, Patocs A, Vasarhelyi B, et al. Association between birth weight in preterm neonates and the BclI polymorphism of the glucocorticoid receptor gene. *J Steroid Biochem Mol Biol*. 2008;111: 91-94.
83. Wallace MJ, Probyn ME, Zahra VA, et al. Early biomarkers and potential mediators of ventilation-induced lung injury in very preterm lambs. *Respir Res*. 2009;10:19.
84. Bhandari V. Hyperoxia-derived lung damage in preterm infants. *Semin Fetal Neonatal Med*. 2010;15:223-229.
85. Wagenaar GT, ter Horst SA, van Gastelen MA, et al. Gene expression profile and histopathology of experimental bronchopulmonary dysplasia induced by prolonged oxidative stress. *Free Radic Biol Med*. 2004;36:782-801.
86. Bhandari V, Choo-Wing R, Lee CG, et al. Hyperoxia causes angiopoietin 2-mediated acute lung injury and necrotic cell death. *Nat Med*. 2006;12:1286-1293.
87. Aghai ZH, Faqiri S, Saslow JG, et al. Angiopoietin 2 concentrations in infants developing bronchopulmonary dysplasia: attenuation by dexamethasone. *J Perinatol*. 2008;28:149-155.
88. Hato T, Kimura Y, Morisada T, et al. Angiopoietins contribute to lung development by regulating pulmonary vascular network formation. *Biochem Biophys Res Commun*. 2009;381:218-223.
89. Wu S, Platteau A, Chen S, et al. Conditional overexpression of connective tissue growth factor disrupts postnatal lung development. *Am J Respir Cell Mol Biol*. 2010;42:552-563.
90. Bhandari A, Bhandari V. Pitfalls, problems, and progress in bronchopulmonary dysplasia. *Pediatrics*. 2009;123:1562-1573.
91. Bhandari V. Molecular mechanisms of hyperoxia-induced acute lung injury. *Front Biosci*. 2008;13: 6653-6661.
92. De Paepe ME, Gundavarapu S, Tantravahi U, et al. Fas-ligand-induced apoptosis of respiratory epithelial cells causes disruption of postcanalicular alveolar development. *Am J Pathol*. 2008;173: 42-56.
93. Weinstein M, Xu X, Ohyama K, et al. FGFR-3 and FGFR-4 function cooperatively to direct alveogenesis in the murine lung. *Development*. 1998;125:3615-3623.
94. Hokuto I, Perl AK, Whitsett JA. Prenatal, but not postnatal, inhibition of fibroblast growth factor receptor signaling causes emphysema. *J Biol Chem*. 2003;278:415-421.
95. Harijith A, Choo-Wing R, Cataltepe S, et al. A role for matrix 9 in IFNγ-mediated injury in developing lungs: Relevance to bronchopulmonary dysplasia. *Am J Respir Cell Mol Biol*. 2011;44: 621-630.
96. Chetty A, Cao GJ, Severgnini M, et al. Role of matrix metalloprotease-9 in hyperoxic injury in developing lung. *Am J Physiol Lung Cell Mol Physiol*. 2008;295:L584-L592.
97. Backstrom E, Hogmalm A, Lappalainen U, et al. developmental stage is a major determinant of lung injury in a murine model of bronchopulmonary dysplasia. *Pediatr Res*. 2011;69:312-318.
98. Lukkarinen H, Hogmalm A, Lappalainen U, et al. Matrix metalloproteinase-9 deficiency worsens lung injury in a model of bronchopulmonary dysplasia. *Am J Respir Cell Mol Biol*. 2009;41:59-68.
99. Choo-Wing R, Nedrelow JH, Homer RJ, et al. Developmental differences in the responses of IL-6 and IL-13 transgenic mice exposed to hyperoxia. *Am J Physiol Lung Cell Mol Physiol*. 2007;293: L142-L150.
100. Ray P, Tang W, Wang P, et al. Regulated overexpression of interleukin 11 in the lung. Use to dissociate development-dependent and -independent phenotypes. *J Clin Invest*. 1997;100:2501-2511.
101. Bostrom H, Willetts K, Pekny M, et al. PDGF-A signaling is a critical event in lung alveolar myofibroblast development and alveogenesis. *Cell*. 1996;85:863-873.
102. Chen WC, Tzeng YS, Li H, et al. Lung defects in neonatal and adult stromal-derived factor-1 conditional knockout mice. *Cell Tissue Res*. 2010;342:75-85.

2

103. Nicola T, Hagood JS, James ML, et al. Loss of Thy-1 inhibits alveolar development in the newborn mouse lung. *Am J Physiol Lung Cell Mol Physiol*. 2009;296:L738-L750.
104. Gill SE, Pape MC, Leco KJ. Absence of tissue inhibitor of metalloproteinases 3 disrupts alveologenesis in the mouse. *Dev Growth Differ*. 2009;51:17-24.
105. Kramer EL, Deutsch GH, Sartor MA, et al. Perinatal increases in TGF-{alpha} disrupt the saccular phase of lung morphogenesis and cause remodeling: microarray analysis. *Am J Physiol Lung Cell Mol Physiol*. 2007;293:L314-L327.
106. Le Cras TD, Hardie WD, Deutsch GH, et al. Transient induction of TGF-alpha disrupts lung morphogenesis, causing pulmonary disease in adulthood. *Am J Physiol Lung Cell Mol Physiol*. 2004;287:L718-L729.
107. Vicencio AG, Lee CG, Cho SJ, et al. Conditional overexpression of bioactive transforming growth factor-beta1 in neonatal mouse lung: a new model for bronchopulmonary dysplasia? *Am J Respir Cell Mol Biol*. 2004;31:650-656.
108. Gauldie J, Galt T, Bonniaud P, et al. Transfer of the active form of transforming growth factor-beta 1 gene to newborn rat lung induces changes consistent with bronchopulmonary dysplasia. *Am J Pathol*. 2003;163:2575-2584.
109. Baraldi E, Filippone M. Chronic lung disease after premature birth. *N Engl J Med*. 2007;357:1946-1955.
110. Bhandari A, Bhandari V. Pathogenesis, pathology and pathophysiology of pulmonary sequelae of bronchopulmonary dysplasia in premature infants. *Front Biosci*. 2003;8:e370-e380.
111. Bhandari A, Bhandari V. Bronchopulmonary dysplasia: an update. *Indian J Pediatr*. 2007;74:73-77.
112. Bhandari V, Bizzarro MJ, Shetty A, et al. Familial and genetic susceptibility to major neonatal morbidities in preterm twins. *Pediatrics*. 2006;117:1901-1906.
113. Jobe AH, Bancalari E. Bronchopulmonary dysplasia. *Am J Respir Crit Care Med*. 2001;163:1723-1729.
114. Ehrenkranz RA, Walsh MC, Vohr BR, et al. Validation of the National Institutes of Health consensus definition of bronchopulmonary dysplasia. *Pediatrics*. 2005;116:1353-1360.
115. Chen SJ, Vohr BR, Oh W. Effects of birth order, gender, and intrauterine growth retardation on the outcome of very low birth weight in twins. *J Pediatr*. 1993;123:132-136.
116. Nielsen HC, Harvey-Wilkes K, MacKinnon B, et al. Neonatal outcome of very premature infants from multiple and singleton gestations. *Am J Obstet Gynecol*. 1997;177:653-659.
117. Parker RA, Lindstrom DP, Cotton RB. Evidence from twin study implies possible genetic susceptibility to bronchopulmonary dysplasia. *Semin Perinatol*. 1996;20:206-209.
118. Lavoie PM, Pham C, Jang KL. Heritability of bronchopulmonary dysplasia, defined according to the consensus statement of the national institutes of health. *Pediatrics*. 2008;122:479-485.
119. Concolino P, Capoluongo E, Santonocito C, et al. Genetic analysis of the dystroglycan gene in bronchopulmonary dysplasia affected premature newborns. *Clin Chim Acta*. 2007;378:164-167.
120. Derzbach L, Bokodi G, Treszl A, et al. Selectin polymorphisms and perinatal morbidity in low-birthweight infants. *Acta Paediatr*. 2006;95:1213-1217.
121. Hayes JD, Strange RC. Glutathione S-transferase polymorphisms and their biological consequences. *Pharmacology*. 2000;61:154-166.
122. Manar MH, Brown MR, Gauthier TW, et al. Association of glutathione-S-transferase-P1 (GST-P1) polymorphisms with bronchopulmonary dysplasia. *J Perinatol*. 2004;24:30-35.
123. Lin HC, Su BH, Chang JS, et al. Nonassociation of interleukin 4 intron 3 and 590 promoter polymorphisms with bronchopulmonary dysplasia for ventilated preterm infants. *Biol Neonate*. 2005;87:181-186.
124. Turner DM, Williams DM, Sankaran D, et al. An investigation of polymorphism in the interleukin-10 gene promoter. *Eur J Immunogenet*. 1997;24:1-8.
125. Yanamandra K, Boggs P, Loggins J, et al. Interleukin-10-1082 G/A polymorphism and risk of death or bronchopulmonary dysplasia in ventilated very low birth weight infants. *Pediatr Pulmonol*. 2005;39:426-432.
126. Bokodi G, Derzbach L, Banyasz I, et al. Association of interferon gamma T+874A and interleukin 12 p40 promoter CTCTAA/GC polymorphism with the need for respiratory support and perinatal complications in low birthweight neonates. *Arch Dis Child Fetal Neonatal Ed*. 2007;92:F25-F29.
127. Capoluongo E, Vento G, Rocchetti S, et al. Mannose-binding lectin polymorphisms and pulmonary outcome in premature neonates: a pilot study. *Intensive Care Med*. 2007;33:1787-1794.
128. Prencipe G, Auriti C, Inglese R, et al. A polymorphism in the macrophage migration inhibitory factor promoter is associated with bronchopulmonary dysplasia. *Pediatr Res*. 2011;69:142-147.
129. Adcock K, Hedberg C, Loggins J, et al. The TNF-alpha-308, MCP-1-2518 and TGF-beta1+915 polymorphisms are not associated with the development of chronic lung disease in very low birth weight infants. *Genes Immun*. 2003;4:420-426.
130. Atac FB, Ince DA, Verdi H, et al. Lack of association between FXIII-Val34Leu, FVII-323 del/ins, and transforming growth factor beta1 (915G/T) gene polymorphisms and bronchopulmonary dysplasia: a single-center study. *DNA Cell Biol*. 2010;29:13-18.
131. Kwinta P, Bik-Multanowski M, Mitkowska Z, et al. Genetic risk factors of bronchopulmonary dysplasia. *Pediatr Res*. 2008;64:682-688.
132. Kazzi SN, Kim UO, Quasney MW, et al. Polymorphism of tumor necrosis factor-alpha and risk and severity of bronchopulmonary dysplasia among very low birth weight infants. *Pediatrics*. 2004;114:e243-e248.

A

133. Strassberg SS, Cristea IA, Qian D, et al. Single nucleotide polymorphisms of tumor necrosis factor-alpha and the susceptibility to bronchopulmonary dysplasia. *Pediatr Pulmonol.* 2007;42:29-36.
134. Chauhan M, Bombell S, McGuire W. Tumour necrosis factor (−308A) polymorphism in very preterm infants with bronchopulmonary dysplasia: a meta-analysis. *Arch Dis Child Fetal Neonatal Ed.* 2009; 94:F257-F259.
135. Weber B, Borkhardt A, Stoll-Becker S, et al. Polymorphisms of surfactant protein A genes and the risk of bronchopulmonary dysplasia in preterm infants. *Turk J Pediatr.* 2000;42:181-185.
136. Makri V, Hospes B, Stoll-Becker S, et al. Polymorphisms of surfactant protein B encoding gene: modifiers of the course of neonatal respiratory distress syndrome? *Eur J Pediatr.* 2002;161: 604-608.
137. Rova M, Haataja R, Marttila R, et al. Data mining and multiparameter analysis of lung surfactant protein genes in bronchopulmonary dysplasia. *Hum Mol Genet.* 2004;13:1095-1104.
138. Pavlovic J, Papagaroufalis C, Xanthou M, et al. Genetic variants of surfactant proteins A, B, C, and D in bronchopulmonary dysplasia. *Dis Markers.* 2006;22:277-291.
139. Yanamandra K, Loggins J, Baier RJ. The angiotensin converting enzyme insertion/deletion polymorphism is not associated with an increased risk of death or bronchopulmonary dysplasia in ventilated very low birth weight infants. *BMC Pediatr.* 2004;4:26.
140. Kazzi SN, Quasney MW. Deletion allele of angiotensin-converting enzyme is associated with increased risk and severity of bronchopulmonary dysplasia. *J Pediatr.* 2005;147:818-822.
141. Hartel C, Konig I, Koster S, et al. Genetic polymorphisms of hemostasis genes and primary outcome of very low birth weight infants. *Pediatrics.* 2006;118:683-689.
142. Clark DA, Pincus LG, Oliphant M, et al. HLA-A2 and chronic lung disease in neonates. *JAMA.* 1982;248:1868-1869.
143. Hellstrom A, Engstrom E, Hard AL, et al. Postnatal serum insulin-like growth factor I deficiency is associated with retinopathy of prematurity and other complications of premature birth. *Pediatrics.* 2003;112:1016-1020.
144. Chetty A, Andersson S, Lassus P, et al. Insulin-like growth factor-1 (IGF-1) and IGF-1 receptor (IGF-1R) expression in human lung in RDS and BPD. *Pediatr Pulmonol.* 2004;37:128-136.
145. Balogh A, Treszl A, Vannay A, et al. A prevalent functional polymorphism of insulin-like growth factor system is not associated with perinatal complications in preterm infants. *Pediatrics.* 2006;117: 591-592.
146. Bonafe M, Barbieri M, Marchegiani F, et al. Polymorphic variants of insulin-like growth factor I (IGF-I) receptor and phosphoinositide 3-kinase genes affect IGF-I plasma levels and human longevity: cues for an evolutionarily conserved mechanism of life span control. *J Clin Endocrinol Metab.* 2003;88:3299-3304.
147. Hadchouel A, Decobert F, Franco-Montoya ML, et al. Matrix metalloproteinase gene polymorphisms and bronchopulmonary dysplasia: identification of MMP16 as a new player in lung development. *PLoS One.* 2008;3:e3188.
148. Lin HC, Su BH, Hsu CM, et al. No association between TAP1 DpnII polymorphism and bronchopulmonary dysplasia. *Acta Paediatr Taiwan.* 2005;46:341-345.
149. Wu HC, Chang CH, Chen WC, et al. Urokinase gene 3′-UTR T/C polymorphism is not associated with bladder cancer. *Genet Mol Biol.* 2004;27:15-16.
150. Lin HC, Su BH, Lin TW, et al. No association of urokinase gene 3′-UTR polymorphism with bronchopulmonary dysplasia for ventilated preterm infants. *Acta Paediatr Taiwan.* 2004;45:315-319.
151. Trikalinos TA, Ntzani EE, Contopoulos-Ioannidis DG, et al. Establishment of genetic associations for complex diseases is independent of early study findings. *Eur J Hum Genet.* 2004;12:762-769.
152. Floros J, Fan R, Diangelo S, et al. Surfactant protein (SP) B associations and interactions with SP-A in white and black subjects with respiratory distress syndrome. *Pediatr Int.* 2001;43:567-576.
153. Haataja R, Marttila R, Uimari P, et al. Respiratory distress syndrome: evaluation of genetic susceptibility and protection by transmission disequilibrium test. *Hum Genet.* 2001;109:351-355.
154. Marttila R, Haataja R, Guttentag S, et al. Surfactant protein A and B genetic variants in respiratory distress syndrome in singletons and twins. *Am J Respir Crit Care Med.* 2003;168:1216-1222.
155. Ramet M, Haataja R, Marttila R, et al. Association between the surfactant protein A (SP-A) gene locus and respiratory-distress syndrome in the Finnish population. *Am J Hum Genet.* 2000;66: 1569-1579.
156. Kala P, Ten Have T, Nielsen H, et al. Association of pulmonary surfactant protein A (SP-A) gene and respiratory distress syndrome: interaction with SP-B. *Pediatr Res.* 1998;43:169-177.
157. Haataja R, Ramet M, Marttila R, et al. Surfactant proteins A and B as interactive genetic determinants of neonatal respiratory distress syndrome. *Hum Mol Genet.* 2000;9:2751-2760.
158. Thomas NJ, Fan R, Diangelo S, et al. Haplotypes of the surfactant protein genes A and D as susceptibility factors for the development of respiratory distress syndrome. *Acta Paediatr.* 2007;96: 985-989.

CHAPTER 3

Perinatal Events and Their Influence on Lung Development and Function

Alan H. Jobe, MD, PhD, Suhas G. Kallapur, MD, and
Boris W. Kramer, MD, PhD

3

- Overview of Lung Development and Perinatal Events
- Lung Development: The Substrate for Adverse Events
- Lung Maturation
- Antenatal Corticosteroids
- Antenatal Infection/Inflammation
- Summary

Overview of Lung Development and Perinatal Events

Lung growth and development are the substrate on which all lung outcomes ultimately depend. This chapter emphasizes four categories of events that can modulate fetal and subsequent postnatal lung development and thus alter lung outcomes for a lifetime (Fig. 3-1). McElrath and colleagues[1] propose that there are two pathologic pathways that result in deliveries as very early gestational age (GA): intrauterine inflammation that is often chronic and aberrations of placentation/vascular development. Other examples of clinically relevant modulators of lung development are small for gestational age/intrauterine growth restriction (SGA/IUGR) and environmental exposures such as maternal tobacco and alcohol use. Lung maturation is a late phase of lung development that can be accelerated by antenatal corticosteroids and by fetal exposure to inflammation. Although infection can induce lung maturation, fetal exposures to acute or chronic chorioamnionitis also can injure the lung. There are two "elephants in the room" for this discussion of events that influence lung development. The first is the concept of what is normal. Any discussion of premature lungs is complicated by the lack of a normal comparison group with which to evaluate the impact of the perinatal event of interest. Although the words *all* or *never* should be sparingly used in biology and medicine, all very low-birth-weight (VLBW) deliveries must be regarded as adverse pregnancy outcomes. The 24-week postmenstrual age newborn who does not have respiratory distress syndrome (RDS) is a true wonder of nature.

The second "elephant" is the complexity of the entangled pathways that regulate lung development, injury, and repair for any perinatal event that affects the lung. These three cellular and molecular response programs share signaling pathways that are superimposed simultaneously or sequentially on the immature lung. This complexity confounds simple interpretations about what mediator is causing which outcome. Finally, outcomes such as bronchopulmonary dysplasia (BPD) and asthma/airway disease in childhood and later life may be initiated by fetal events that then are modulated by postnatal responses of the lungs. An example is early life exposures to viral infections.[2] This biologic complexity generates inconsistencies in clinical data and more than enough questions and controversies. In this chapter, we simply provide our current understanding of how prenatal exposures can change postnatal lung function based on both clinical information and animal models.

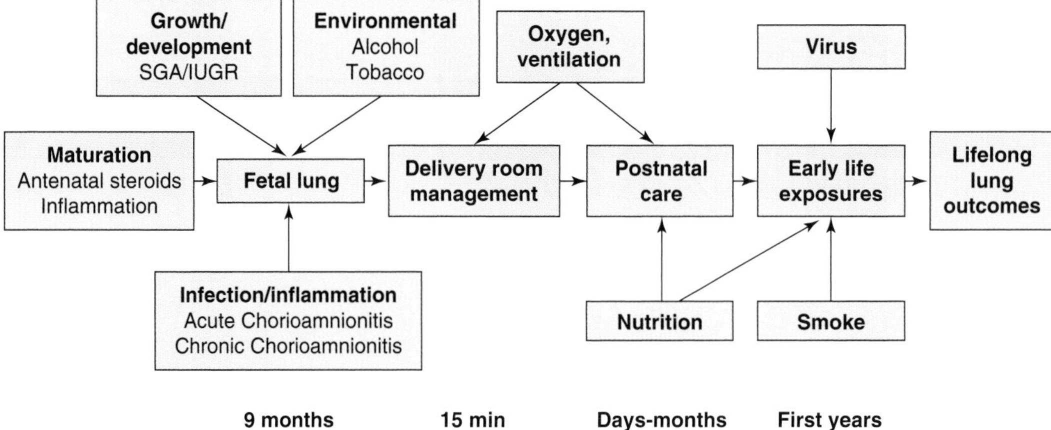

Figure 3-1 Sketch of factors that modulate the fetal lung development and function. Some effectors that alter lung development after delivery also are indicated. IUGR, intrauterine growth retardation; SGA, small for gestational age.

Lung Development: The Substrate for Adverse Events

Lung development is programmed by the fetus to be sufficiently mature to adapt rapidly to air breathing at birth. The timing of the structural development of the lung in Figure 3-2 is given as weeks from last menstrual period and from conception to emphasize the 2-week difference. Infants born by elective cesarean section as early term infants (38 weeks postmenstrual age) have more problems with pulmonary adaptation than infants born at 40 weeks postmenstrual age.[3,4] Late preterm infants have more lung adaptation problems and more RDS for each week of birth prior to 37 weeks.[5] Finally, lung adaptation abnormalities, RDS, and subsequently BPD become increasingly frequent as GA decreases into the early GA and very early GA categories of preterm infants.[6]

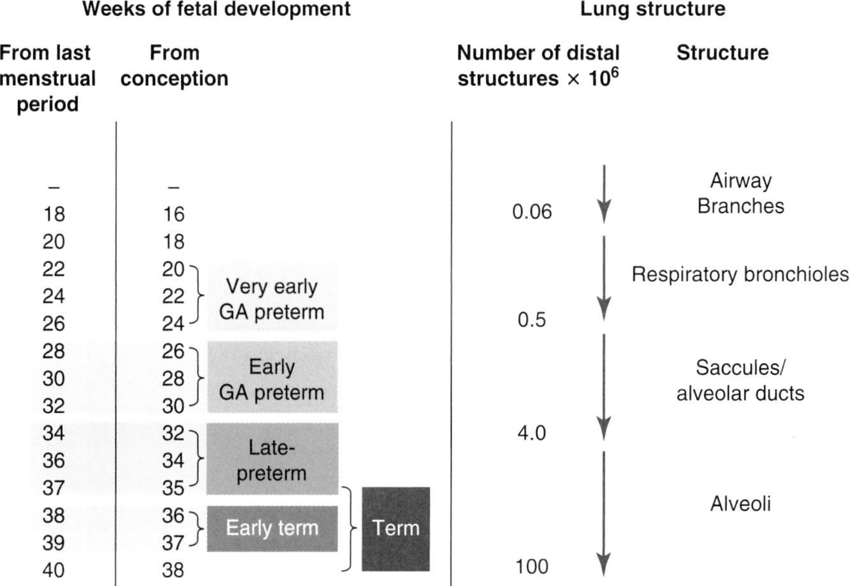

Figure 3-2 Timing of fetal lung development, emphasizing the 2-week difference in weeks between postmenstrual age and conceptional age. The lung progressively branches from airways to alveoli with a large increase in distal structures. The adult lung contains about 500 × 10^6 alveoli. GA, gestational age.[8]

Lung development includes development of the structural elements as well as functional maturation of fluid clearance pathways and the surfactant system. The major structural events are the completion of airway branching by about 18 weeks of gestation, followed by three generations of airway divisions to form respiratory bronchioles, and three more divisions to form alveolar ducts to about 32 to 36 weeks.[7] Subsequently, secondary septation or alveolarization occurs to term and for several years after birth. The changes in distal saccular numbers demonstrate the dynamic septation events that take the fetal lung from about 0.06×10^6 distal structures at 18 to 20 weeks to about 100×10^6 alveoli at term—a 1700-fold increase. Alveolar numbers increase only about fivefold from the term birth lung to the adult lung.[8] There is essentially no information about the variability of the timing of normal septation in the human lung. It is also not known whether very early lung maturation changes the timing of the later gestational septation events that generate respiratory bronchioles and alveolar ducts. Some forms of pulmonary hypoplasia may result from altered septation and airway development. The injury and repair associated with BPD do inhibit and delay alveolarization of the developing lung.[9]

Until recently, growth of new alveoli after early childhood was thought not to occur, but newer human anatomic and experimental data demonstrate that the healthy lung probably grows new alveoli and looses old alveoli continuously at a very slow rate.[10,11] Empirically, very preterm infants with a BPD-associated "arrest" in alveolar septation must be able to grow alveoli or they could not grow and survive. These lungs may not "catch up" to have lung volumes or alveolar numbers equivalent to normal lungs.[12] The questions for the future include how alveolar growth after very preterm birth and lung injury can be promoted.

Lung Maturation

From the clinical perspective, lung maturation has focused on RDS and the surfactant system since the seminal report from Avery and Mead[13] in 1959 that the lungs of infants who died of RDS had less surfactant. Lung maturation also includes epithelial development of ion/water regulation, thinning of the alveolar capillary barrier, and microvascular development. However, the disease RDS is the primary clinical indicator of lung immaturity. The first challenge is to define the timing of normal lung maturation, which is not an easy task if one assumes that most preterm infants are abnormal. In the 1970s, amniotic fluid was sampled from women with relatively normal gestations for the evaluation of surfactant components to test for lung maturation.[14] The lecithin/sphingomyelin (L/S) ratio was not greater than 2 until after 34 to 35 weeks of gestation, and phosphatidylglycerol was seldom detected prior to 34 weeks of gestation in normal pregnancies.[15] The true time course and the variability for the timing for normal lung maturation are not known with any precision for the human. However, lung maturity testing and inadvertent experiences with non-indicated cesarean sections prior to 37 weeks demonstrate that lung maturation, defined as absence of RDS, normally occurs after about 34 to 36 weeks in normal pregnancies

The diagnosis of RDS for very early GA preterm infants has been confounded in clinical series and epidemiologic studies by the common practice of intubation and ventilation with or without surfactant treatment shortly after birth. These intubated and ventilated infants likely carry the diagnosis RDS even if they are not receiving supplemental oxygen. Furthermore, if these infants have infection, transient tachypnea of the newborn, a degree of pulmonary hypoplasia, or apnea requiring ventilatory support, they likely will be said to have RDS or RDS plus another diagnosis. Attempts to minimize lung injury in very early GA infants using continuous positive airway pressure (CPAP) demonstrate that many very preterm infants do not have enough RDS to need surfactant or mechanical ventilation (Table 3-1).[16-18] Infants born at 24 weeks gestational age without RDS are surprisingly common.[19] These clinical experiences demonstrate that induced lung maturation is frequently sufficiently advanced to yield an infant without RDS. Because lung maturation (and RDS) is a continuum from severe immaturity to sufficient maturation to

Table 3-1 INCIDENCE OF RESPIRATORY DISTRESS SYNDROME IN VERY PRETERM INFANTS

Study	Number of Infants	Characteristics	% Treated with Surfactant
Verder et al[16]	397	27 ± 2 wk GA	42
Morley et al[17]; CPAP arm	307	964 ± 212 g	38
Finer et al[18]; CPAP arm	663	24-27 wk	67

CPAP, continuous positive airway pressure; GA, gestational age.

avoid RDS, we think that most very preterm infants have some degree of induced lung maturation. We suspect that the infant born at 24 to 26 weeks of gestation with severe lung immaturity and a poor response to surfactant and who dies of RDS/respiratory failure soon after birth is the infant with "normal" 25-week lungs or the infant with RDS-plus (RDS plus infection or pulmonary hypoplasia, for example).

At the margin of lung maturity in preterm sheep, a surfactant pool size of about 4 mg/kg is sufficient to support normal gas exchange with CPAP,[20] demonstrating that a small amount of surfactant is sufficient to protect the preterm lung from RDS. We have no good tests to quantify the degree of lung maturation prior to or soon after delivery. The L/S ratio or phosphatidylglycerol measurements in amniotic fluid are no longer commonly available, and other tests such as lamellar body number in amniotic fluid are imprecise. Samples of fetal lung fluid (intubated infants) or gastric aspirates soon after birth could provide information about surfactant and inflammation, but they are not used routinely. A clinical controversy is: Which very preterm infant should receive surfactant/ventilation or CPAP after birth? The controversy is based on the perceived risk for RDS and the ability of these infants to transition if treated by CPAP. The clinical trials demonstrate that the two approaches yield similar outcomes that marginally favor an initial trial of CPAP.[17,18] However, individualized treatments could be given if there were accurate assessments of the functional potential of the very preterm lung prior to delivery. Clearly, very preterm delivery is an event that profoundly changes the developing lung. However, there is no good information about how the preterm delivery and breathing, independent of oxygen exposure and injury, change the trajectory of subsequent lung development. We assume that preterm delivery does modify lung development because of the lung stretch from breathing and the striking changes in hormone milieu alter lung development in experimental models.[21,22] The implication is that independent of injury, lung structure at 40 weeks and throughout life will be different for infants born at 25 weeks or 35 weeks from those for infants born at 40 weeks.

Antenatal Corticosteroids

There is no controversy about the use of antenatal administration of corticosteroids for women at risk for preterm delivery at 24 to 34 weeks of gestation. This therapy was developed to reduce the risk of RDS, but it also decreases incidences of intraventricular hemorrhage and death. The therapy is supported by two National Institutes of Health Consensus Conferences,[23,24] an extensive meta-analysis,[25] and the endorsements of obstetric societies worldwide. Nevertheless, there are controversies about repeated treatments,[23] the drug and dose to be used,[26] and the responses of selected populations of patients.[5,27] We briefly review the effects of antenatal corticosteroids on fetal lungs and identify some of the remaining questions.

Maternal corticosteroid treatments have pleiotropic effects on the lung and other fetal organ systems. Corticosteroids upregulate families of genes and downregulate other genes. The net response in an organ such as the lung changes anatomy, physiology, and clinical outcomes (Table 3-2). The fetal primate lung responds to a

Table 3-2 EFFECTS OF ANTENATAL CORTICOSTEROIDS ON FETAL LUNGS

Anatomy/biochemistry	Thin mesenchyme of alveolar-capillary structures Increased saccular/alveolar gas volumes Decreased alveolar septation Increased antioxidant enzymes Increased surfactant
Physiology	Increased compliance Improved gas exchange Decreased epithelial permeability Protection of preterm lung from injury during resuscitation
Interactions with exogenous surfactant	Improvement in surfactant treatment responses Improvement in surfactant dose-response curve Decreased inactivation of surfactant
Clinical	Decreased incidence of respiratory distress syndrome No effect on incidence of bronchopulmonary dysplasia Decreased mortality

3-day maternal corticosteroid treatment, beginning at 63 days of gestation with a thinning of the mesenchyme and enlargement of air spaces[28] (Fig. 3-3). The functional effect is to increase lung gas volume. Treatments of primates or sheep at later gestational ages also increase lung gas volumes.[29] This increase in lung gas volume reflects two events, mesenchymal thinning and an interruption in alveolar septation such that saccular/alveolar numbers decrease and the sizes increase.[30] These anatomic changes in the lung to increase lung gas volumes occur within 15 hours and prior to an increase in alveolar surfactant in fetal sheep.[31] Although this effect is not reported in preterm infants, antenatal steroids increase the risk for pneumothorax for about 24 hours after treatment in preterm sheep and rabbits by reducing the rupture pressures of the lung, presumably by thinning the mesenchyme without increasing support structures.[32,33]

The physiologic changes that accompany the changes in lung structure and surfactant are an increase in lung compliance, improved gas exchange, and a decrease in the permeability of the air space epithelium. The corticosteroid effects on the fetal lung also change the interaction of the lung with both the endogenous surfactant and surfactant treatments. Surfactant treatment responses are better in animal models and in infants exposed to antenatal corticosteroids than in those not exposed.[34,35] The dose-response curves for endogenous surfactant or surfactant treatments are improved,[36,37] and the surfactant composition is altered to make it less susceptible to inactivation by proteinaceous pulmonary edema.[38] The decreased epithelial permeability also protects surfactant function. Lung injury during resuscitation with high tidal volumes was found to be decreased by fetal exposure to corticosteroids in preterm surfactant-deficient sheep.[39] The surfactant lipids and proteins do not increase in fetal sheep until 4 to 7 days after corticosteroid treatment.[40] Therefore, the early responses to antenatal corticosteroids result primarily from anatomic and other associated effects. The clinical correlates are a decrease in RDS and improved surfactant treatment responses. There was no consistent decrease in BPD in the placebo-controlled trials of antenatal corticosteroids conducted before 1990 or in clinical series since that era.[25] Two factors contribute to a lack of a BPD benefit: First, antenatal corticosteroids decrease mortality and salvage a population of infants that are at high risk of BPD, and second, currently, the great majority of infants at the highest risk for BPD are exposed to maternal corticosteroids. For example, Laughon and associates[41] found no relationship between antenatal corticosteroids and BPD, but with 90% of the infants exposed to this treatment in their study, the ability to detect an interaction was minimal (Table 3-3).

There remain a number of questions about the appropriate use and benefits of antenatal corticosteroids. Current practice is to treat with either 12 mg betamethasone acetate plus betamethasone phosphate given as a 2-dose treatment separated

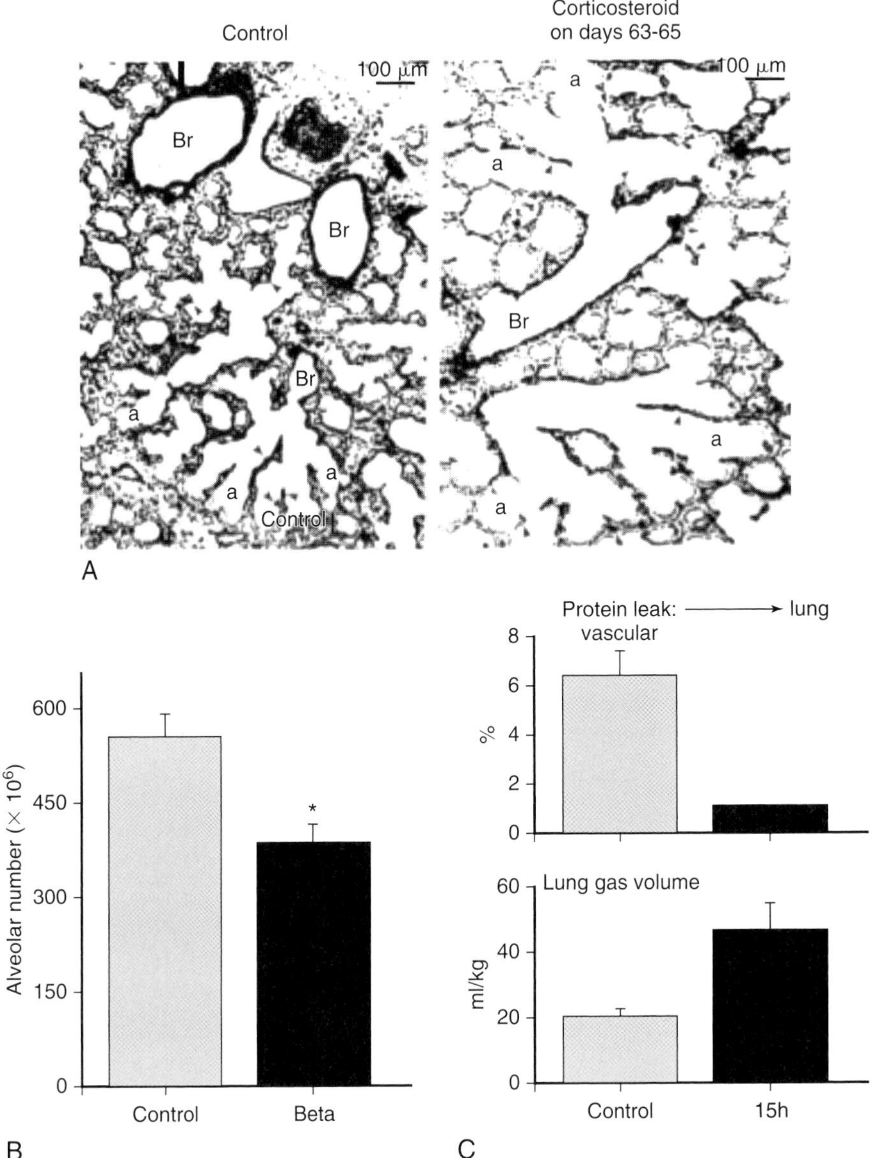

Figure 3-3 Examples of fetal corticosteroid responses. **A,** Corticosteroid responses of the very immature fetal monkey lung. Maternal triamcinolone (10 mg) treatment on days 63-65 of pregnancy cause mesenchymal loss and air space enlargement at 90 days of gestation. **B,** Alveolar numbers in fetal sheep lung were decreased 7 days following maternal treatments with 0.5 mg/kg betamethasone. **C,** An interval between fetal betamethasone treatment and delivery of 15 hours was sufficient to decrease vascular to alveolar leaks and increase lung gas volumes in betamethasone-exposed preterm and ventilated lambs. a, distal saccule; Br, bronchiole. (**A** from Bunton TE, Plopper CG: Triamcinolone-induced structural alterations in the development of the lung of the fetal rhesus macaque. *Am J Obstet Gynecol.* 1984;148:203-215; **B** from Willet KE, Jobe AH, Ikegami M, et al: Lung morphometry after repetitive antenatal glucocorticoid treatment in preterm sheep. *Am J Respir Crit Care Med.* 2001;163:1437-1443; **C** from Ikegami M, Polk D, Jobe A: Minimum interval from fetal betamethasone treatment to postnatal lung responses in preterm lambs. *Am J Obstet Gynecol.* 1996;174:1408-1413.)

by 24 hours or a 4-dose 12-hour interval treatment with dexamethasone phosphate.[26] These drugs are not equivalent, having different and complex pharmacokinetics in the mother and the fetus. In animal models, fetal lung maturation is induced with low and prolonged fetal exposures to betamethasone, but not with single high-dose exposures to dexamethasone.[42] The presently recommended drug doses and treatment intervals may not be optimal, but there are insufficient clinical

Table 3-3 PERINATAL ASSOCIATIONS WITH PATTERNS OF OXYGEN USE FOR RESPIRATORY DISEASE*

	Percentage of Population			
Perinatal Association	**Initial Low FIO_2**	**Increasing FIO_2**	**Persistent Lung Disease**	**$P < 0.05$**
Antenatal steroids	92	91	88	—
Prolonged rupture of membranes	27	21	20	—
Chorioamnionitis	55	54	53	—
Funisitis	40	33	32	—
Any organism – placenta	20	35	45	—
Surfactant treatment	78	89	97	+
Growth restriction	9	20	26	+
Bronchopulmonary dysplasia	17	51	67	+

*In 1340 infants of 23-27 weeks gestational age. Respiratory disease group by low FIO_2 for first 14 days and for more than 14 days, and by persistent high oxygen use and lung disease for more than 14 days.
Data from Laughon M, Allred EN, Bose C, et al: Patterns of respiratory disease during the first 2 postnatal weeks in extremely premature infants. *Pediatrics.* 2009;123:1124-1131.

data to recommend betamethasone or dexamethasone or to suggest other treatment strategies.

Trials with antenatal corticosteroids were completed by about 1990, and few infants who were delivered prior to 28 weeks gestational age were included in those trials. However, in clinical practice, the use of corticosteroids is routine for infants who are to be offered intensive care of gestational ages as low as 22 to 23 weeks (Table 3-4).[43] Because most of these extremely preterm infants have a diagnosis of RDS (appropriate or not), a decrease in RDS may not be a good indicator of benefit. For example, Garite and coworkers[44] found no decrease in RDS but did document decreased severity of RDS in early gestational age infants. As demonstrated in Figure 3-3, the primate lung can respond to antenatal corticosteroids at very early (pre-viable human equivalent) gestational ages, as do explants of human fetal lung at less than 20 weeks of gestation. There is no biologic reason to limit the use of antenatal corticosteroids to infants of a particular early gestational age. The decision should be based on the goals for care for each very preterm fetus.

Table 3-4 CHARACTERISTICS OF INFANTS OF 22 TO 28 WEEKS GESTATIONAL AGE CARED FOR IN NICHD NEONATAL RESEARCH NETWORK CENTERS*

Characteristic	**Percentage of Population Affected**
Antenatal corticosteroids	80
Antenatal antibiotics	67
Rupture of membranes >24 hr	25
Histologic chorioamnionitis[†]	48
Intrauterine growth restriction	8
Multiple births	25

*9575 infants receiving care from 2003 to 2007 at National Institute of Child Health and Human Development centers.
[†]82% of the entire population was evaluated.
Data from Stoll BJ, Hansen NI, Bell EF, et al: Neonatal outcomes of extremely preterm infants from the NICHD Neonatal Research Network. *Pediatrics.* 2010;126:443-456.

Repeated courses of antenatal corticosteroids are conceptually attractive because many early gestational age fetuses are not delivered within 7 days of maternal treatment and the benefits of therapy seem to decrease with time after treatment.[25] In animal models, second courses of corticosteroids progressively raise the indicators of fetal lung maturation.[29,45] The risks are adverse effects of repeated fetal exposures on fetal somatic and brain growth, effects that occur in animal models.[45] A meta-analysis of more than 2000 randomized pregnancies in trials published prior to 2008 reported a modest benefit in RDS and severe lung disease with no adverse effects for repeated courses of treatment.[46] A subsequent trial of 1858 women randomly assigned to a 14-day retreatment interval versus no retreatment found no benefit for RDS, mortality, or other outcomes, but a small decrease in birth weights and head circumferences.[47] Later reports of 2-year neurodevelopment outcomes are reassuring for infants exposed to fewer than four courses of antenatal corticosteroids.[48,49] Another option is a rescue treatment when a woman has received an initial treatment and again has a high risk of delivery prior to 34 weeks. There are no recommendations from learned societies about the use of repeated corticosteroid treatments.

Although the neonatal community is primarily concerned about the lung outcomes of very preterm infants, large populations of term infants delivered by elective cesarean section and late preterm infants delivered for multiple indications require respiratory care after birth. Sinclair[50] pointed out in 1995 that the early clinical trials demonstrated lung benefits for infants exposed to antenatal corticosteroids who were delivered after 32 to 34 weeks of gestation. The relative benefit of an approximate 50% decrease in RDS was similar for infants of all gestations, but the attack rate was low after 34 weeks of gestation, such that 100 women would need to be treated to prevent one case of RDS. However, the current obstetric practice of frequent obstetrical interventions for late-preterm and early-term pregnancies may now result in more infants with respiratory morbidities including RDS. There are no recent randomized controlled trial data for the use of antenatal corticosteroids for late-preterm deliveries,[5] but the Eunice Kennedy Shriver National Institute of Child Health and Human Development (NICHD) has launched a trial to evaluate antenatal steroids for this population. A provocative randomized trial of antenatal corticosteroids for 998 women scheduled for elective cesarean delivery demonstrated that respiratory distress decreased with use of corticosteroids for deliveries at 37 weeks from 11.4% to 5.4% and for deliveries at 39 weeks from 1.5% to 0.6% (Table 3-5).[51] The potential benefits of antenatal steroids in the developing world may be substantial, because in this environment, where neonatal intensive care is not always available, late-preterm infants with RDS can die. Antenatal corticosteroid therapy is one of the great successes in improving pulmonary and overall outcomes, but many questions remain.

Table 3-5 A RANDOMIZED CONTROLLED TRIAL OF ANTENATAL BETAMETHASONE FOR ELECTIVE CESAREAN DELIVERY

Feature	Control Group	Betamethasone Group	*P* Value or Risk Ratio (95% Confidence Interval)
ICU admission for respiratory distress (number)	24	11	0.02
Incidence if ICU admissions (%)	5.1	2.4	0.46 (0.23-0.93)
Transient tachypnea of newborn (%)	4	2	0.54 (0.26-1.12)
RDS (%)	1.1	0.2	0.21 (0.03-1.32)

ICU, intensive care unit; RDS, respiratory distress syndrome.
Data from Stutchfield P, Whitaker R, Russell I: Antenatal betamethasone and incidence of neonatal respiratory distress after elective caesarean section: Pragmatic randomised trial. *BMJ*. 2005;331:662.

Antenatal Infection/Inflammation

Overview of Fetal Inflammation

The human fetus is normally considered to be in an environment protected from infection. However, the human fetus can be exposed to a variety of pathogens, which may initiate an inflammatory process in the placenta, chorioamnion, or fetus. For example, human fetuses are exposed to viral pathogens as a consequence of maternal viremia. The patterns of injury to agents such as varicella and cytomegalovirus depend on the period of gestation during which the infection occurs. Similarly, the fetus can acquire a spirochete infection with syphilis or a parasitic infection with toxoplasmosis secondary to maternal infection, and each causes characteristic syndromes depending on the gestational timing of exposure. These infections are not generally viewed as predominantly inflammatory, although the fetal injury and immune responses have inflammatory characteristics. Asphyxia with injury to fetal tissue also causes inflammation as part of the injury and the repair process. Similarly, normal labor is associated with an increase in proinflammatory mediators.[52] Both innate and acquired inflammatory responses of the fetus are generally considered to be less effective than those in the child or adult because the response systems in the fetus are immature and pregnancy is an immune-suppressive environment.[53] For example, fetal inflammatory responses to pathogens such as group B streptococcus and *Listeria monocytogenes* are blunted, resulting in severe infection and often death of the fetus or newborn. The most common fetal infectious exposure is to chorioamnionitis, which is associated with preterm labor and delivery.[54] In this section, we present the questions and controversies about the associations of chorioamnionitis with a range of effects on the fetal and newborn lung.

Diagnosis of Chorioamnionitis

Chorioamnionitis can be either a clinical syndrome or a silent, indolent process. The clinical diagnosis of chorioamnionitis is made when a pregnant woman has a constellation of findings that include fever, a tender uterus, an elevated blood granulocyte count, and bacteria and/or inflammatory cells in amniotic fluid and often preterm or prolonged rupture of membranes.[55] The diagnosis of clinical chorioamnionitis is frequently made for near-term or term labors, and the infection can be caused by highly virulent organisms. Before 30 weeks of gestation, *clinical chorioamnionitis* is most often diagnosed after attempts to delay preterm delivery or with preterm prolonged rupture of membranes. Another method to diagnose chorioamnionitis is by histopathology of the chorioamnion with inflammation, indicating *histologic chorioamnionitis*. The amount of infiltration of the chorioamnion by inflammatory cells and the intensity of secondary changes are used to grade the severity of the fetal exposure to inflammation.[56] Inflammation of the cord, called *funisitis*, is generally considered to indicate a more advanced inflammatory process that involves the fetus.[57] Another diagnostic approach is to culture amniotic fluid or fetal membranes for organisms or to assay amniotic fluid for the presence of proinflammatory mediators such as tumor necrosis factor α (TNFα) and interleukin-1 (IL-1) and IL-6.[58] With the recognition that only a minority of organisms in the human biome can be cultured, polymerase chain reaction (PCR) and DNA sequencing techniques are being used to demonstrate that chorioamnionitis is often polymicrobial with organisms that cannot be cultured.[59] Technologies to identify multiple proteins in biologic fluids also are being adapted to develop proteomic biomarkers for chorioamnionitis in amniotic fluid.[60] These technologies have the potential to rapidly diagnose inflammation and to identify specific organisms. Such approaches will change the understanding of fetal exposures to inflammation and specific organisms.

The chorioamnion is fetal tissue, and the amniotic fluid surrounding the fetus is in direct contact with the fetal gut, skin, and lung.[57] Therefore, the fetus will be exposed to inflammation if there is histologic chorioamnionitis or if the amniotic fluid contains mediators of inflammation. The Venn diagram in Figure 3-4 illustrates the diagnostic conundrum. Clinical chorioamnionitis does not correlate well with

3

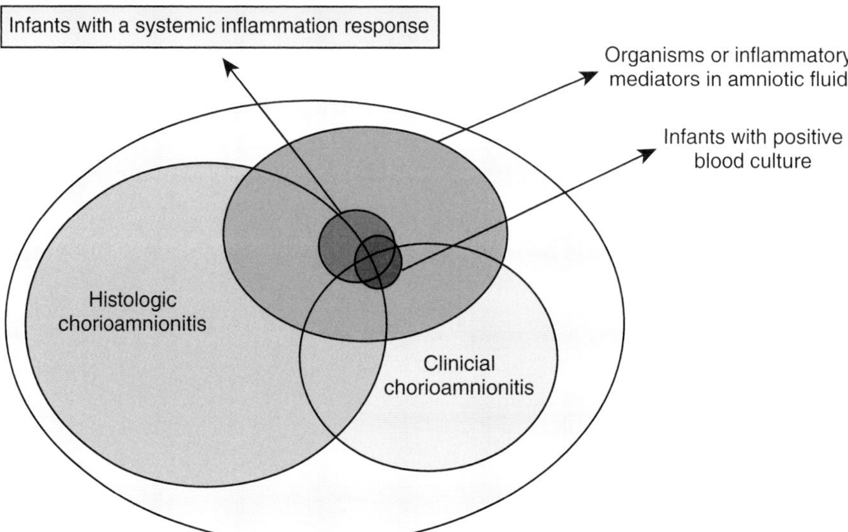

Figure 3-4 Venn diagram illustrating the overlapping relationships among different ways to diagnose chorioamnionitis and the outcomes of sepsis and systemic inflammatory syndromes. The *outer circle* represents preterm deliveries prior to 30 weeks of gestation.

the subsequent diagnosis of histologic chorioamnionitis, and an amniotic fluid diagnosis of infection may or may not predict chorioamnionitis associated with preterm delivery. PCR-based analyses of amniotic fluid call into question the assumption that fetal colonization with organisms is abnormal and will cause preterm delivery. Gerber and associates[61] demonstrated that 11% of 254 presumably normal amniotic fluid samples collected at 15 to 19 weeks of gestation for genetic analysis were PCR-positive for *Ureaplasma urealyticum*. Although 17 of the 29 *Ureaplasma*-positive pregnancies in their study had preterm labor, only 2 fetuses were delivered before 34 weeks of gestation. Perni and colleagues[62] analyzed 179 amniotic fluid samples, finding 13% positive for *Ureaplasma* and 6% positive for *Mycoplasma hominis*; also, 28 of the 33 pregnancies with positive amniotic fluid samples did not deliver preterm. Later attempts to extensively culture the placenta/chorioamnion have recovered multiple organisms of low virulence that include vaginal flora.[63] The severity of the chorioamnionitis does not correlate well with the organisms but tends to be more severe with *Ureaplasma* and *Mycoplasma* species.[64,65] Furthermore, in many preterm deliveries, polymicrobial organisms are recovered by culture or PCR from the amniotic fluid. The unknowns are the association of organisms with pregnancies that do not deliver preterm and the variety of organisms that might be identified by PCR. For example, Steel and coworkers[66] used a fluorescent probe for a common 16s ribosomal RNA bacterial sequence and identified organisms deep within the membranes of all preterm deliveries and many term deliveries. These results suggest that the human pregnancy can tolerate colonization/infection with low-pathogenicity organisms.

There is no clear answer to the question "What is chorioamnionitis?" The multiple ways to make the diagnosis are not necessarily congruent. Furthermore, if one accepts that chorioamnionitis results from colonization/infection, then the diagnosis is imprecise in the extreme in relation to how infectious diseases are generally diagnosed. The diagnosis of an infection includes the identity of the organism, an estimate of the duration of infection, its intensity, and specific sites of involvement. The diagnosis of chorioamnionitis contains none of these elements. Research is now linking genetically determined inflammatory response characteristics of the mother and fetus with prematurity.[67] The chronic indolent chorioamnionitis associated with prematurity may result from the interaction of the environment and the genetically determined immunomodulatory characteristics of the mother and fetus. Challenges for the future are how to better diagnose and to understand what makes patients susceptible to chorioamnionitis, and how to quantify the severity potential for fetal injury from the chorioamnionitis.

Clinical Pulmonary Outcomes of Fetal Exposure to Inflammation/Infection

A decreased incidence of RDS was associated with preterm prolonged rupture of the membranes, a surrogate marker for chorioamnionitis, as early as 1974.[68] Watterberg and associates[69] reported in 1996 that ventilated preterm infants exposed to histologic chorioamnionitis had a lower incidence of RDS but a higher incidence of BPD than infants not exposed to chorioamnionitis. Furthermore, the initial tracheal aspirates from infants exposed to chorioamnionitis contained proinflammatory mediators such as IL-1, IL-6, and IL-8, indicating that the lung inflammation was of antenatal origin.[70,71] Other reports support that association. Clinical chorioamnionitis was associated with decreased death in all infants born at or before 26 weeks of gestation in the United Kingdom and Ireland in 1995.[72] Hannaford and colleagues[73] identified *U. urealyticum* as an organism of fetal origin that was associated with a decreased risk of RDS. Lahra and coworkers[74] noted, in a population of 724 preterm infants, that RDS was decreased for infants exposed to histologic chorioamnionitis (odds ratio [OR] 0.49, 95% confidence interval [95%CI] 0.31-0.78) or chorioamnionitis plus funisitis (OR 0.23, 95% CI 0.15-0.35) relative to no chorioamnionitis. This group also reported their 13-year experience that histologic chorioamnionitis (with or without funisitis) was associated with a decreased risk of BPD (OR 0.58, 95% CI 0.51-0.67).[75]

In contrast, there are other reports associating chorioamnionitis with poor pulmonary and other outcomes. Hitti and associates,[76] for example, reported that high levels of TNFα in amniotic fluid predicted prolonged postnatal ventilation, suggesting early and persistent lung injury from chorioamnionitis. Ramsey and colleagues[77] also demonstrated that chorioamnionitis increased neonatal morbidities. Laughon and coworkers,[41] after extensively evaluating and culturing the placentas of 1340 infants born before 28 weeks of gestation, found no association between histologic chorioamnionitis, funisitis, or specific organisms and the initial oxygen requirements of the infants or BPD (see Table 3-3). The Canadian Neonatal Network also reported that clinical chorioamnionitis was not predictive of RDS or BPD.[78]

These discrepant reports need to be understood within the complexities of the diagnosis of chorioamnionitis as well as the factors contributing to the diagnosis of RDS or BPD. Van Marter and associates[79] evaluated the outcomes of ventilated and VLBW infants and found that chorioamnionitis was associated with a decreased incidence of BPD (OR 0.2). However, BPD was increased if the infant had been exposed to chorioamnionitis and either underwent mechanical ventilation for more than 7 days (OR 3.2) or had postnatal sepsis (OR 2.9). Lahra and coworkers[75] noted the same associations in an unselected population of 761 infants with gestation less than 30 weeks. BPD was lower in infants exposed to histologic chorioamnionitis than in infants without chorioamnionitis, as noted previously. However, the combination of histologic chorioamnionitis and postnatal sepsis increased the risk for BPD (OR 1.98 95% CI 1.15-3.39). These reports demonstrate that antenatal and postnatal exposures interact to change outcomes such as BPD. Been and colleagues[80,81] reported that newborns exposed to chorioamnionitis with fetal involvement had more severe RDS and impaired surfactant treatment responses. In contrast, infants exposed to chorioamnionitis without fetal involvement had minimal lung disease. The severity of the chorioamnionitis and postnatal interventions confound simple correlations between chorioamnionitis and outcomes such as RDS and BPD.

Other studies to explore the associations of antenatal inflammation with postnatal lung outcomes are the measurements of proinflammatory cytokines in cord plasma and tracheal aspirates collected shortly after birth. In general, cord plasma from early gestational deliveries had higher proinflammatory cytokine levels than cord plasma from term deliveries, but the median values were not greatly different,[82] suggesting little useful resolution between the preterm and term populations. Although Ambalavanam and coworkers[83] could detect differences in blood cytokines collected within 4 hours of birth for infants in whom BPD developed from those without BPD, the resolution between the populations was not clinically useful for the prediction of risk of BPD. Similarly, Paananen and associates[84] found higher selected cord plasma cytokine levels in infants exposed to severe chorioamnionitis. The cord cytokine levels decreased with age for infants at lower risk for BPD, but cord cytokine levels were not reliable predictors of BPD. Because histologic chorioamnionitis is a retrospective diagnosis, De Dooy and colleagues[71] could predict chorioamnionitis from IL-8 levels in tracheal aspirates collected soon after birth, but the clinical utility of that information also is unclear. Been and colleagues[85] did find that vascular endothelial growth factor levels in initial tracheal aspirates were predictive of BPD. However, there is no compelling evidence that measurements of proinflammatory mediators in cord plasma or tracheal aspirates will identify high-resolution biomarkers for either chorioamnionitis or the pulmonary outcomes RDS and BPD.

The inconsistent clinical correlates most likely result from the imprecise nature of the diagnosis of chorioamnionitis and its association with different populations of infants. An example of the inconsistency is the diagnosis of fetal exposures by histologic chorioamnionitis or by blood culture for *Ureaplasma* collected from the cord at delivery and the outcomes of RDS and BPD for the same cohort of consecutive patients (Table 3-6).[86,87] The associations with histologic chorioamnionitis and culture positivity for *Ureaplasma* for BPD are the *opposite* of those for RDS in the same cohort of patients. The diagram in Figure 3-5 may help show the findings. A progressive chorioamnionitis caused by virulent organisms may cause severe postnatal lung and systemic inflammation with the outcomes of more severe RDS, BPD, or sepsis/death. Such outcomes are relatively infrequent in VLBW infants who are not stillborn. Fewer than 2% of VLBW infants have positive blood culture results at birth.[88] Chronic, indolent chorioamnionitis caused by organisms such as *Ureaplasma* can induce lung maturation (less RDS), but that maturation may be associated with more BPD.[69] These associations may depend on how the diagnosis of chorioamnionitis is made (clinical, histopathologic, other), and the population of infants studied (ventilated only, all VLBW infants, other selected populations). In an attempt to better establish a cause-and-effect relationship, Viscardi and associates[89] correlated

Table 3-6 PULMONARY AND SYSTEMIC OUTCOMES FOR CONSECUTIVELY TREATED INFANTS BORN BEFORE 30 WEEKS OF GESTATION AND EXPOSED TO INFECTION*

Outcome	Percentage of Population: Yes	Percentage of Population: No	P Value
Histologically Diagnosed Chorioamnionitis			
Respiratory distress syndrome	61	73	0.008
Bronchopulmonary dysplasia	17	17	NS
Fetal inflammatory response syndrome	44	18	<0.001
Positive Result of Cord Blood Culture			
Respiratory distress syndrome	66	65	NS
Bronchopulmonary dysplasia	27	10	0.001
Fetal inflammatory response syndrome	41	26	0.007

*A comparison of fetal exposures diagnosed by histologic chorioamnionitis or positive results of cord blood cultures for *Ureaplasma* or *Mycoplasma*.

Data from Andrews WW, Goldenberg RL, Faye-Petersen O, et al: The Alabama Preterm Birth study: Polymorphonuclear and mononuclear cell placental infiltrations, other markers of inflammation, and outcomes in 23- to 32-week preterm newborn infants. *Am J Obstet Gynecol.* 2006;195:803-808; and Goldenberg RL, Andrews WW, Goepfert AR, et al: The Alabama Preterm Birth Study: umbilical cord blood *Ureaplasma urealyticum* and *Mycoplasma hominis* cultures in very preterm newborn infants. *Am J Obstet Gynecol.* 2008;198:43 e41-e45.

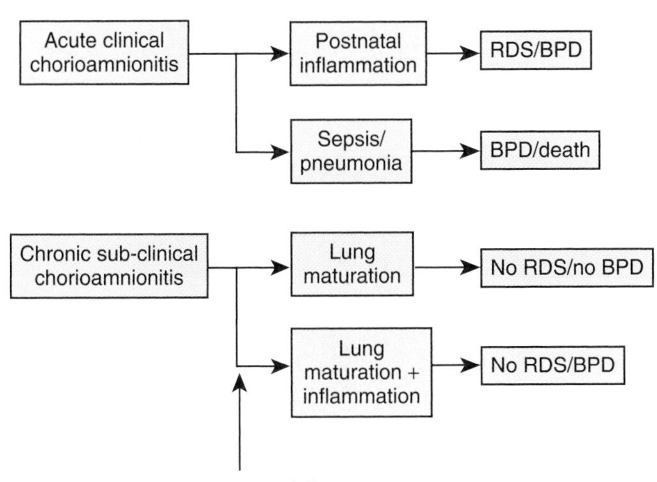

Figure 3-5 Overview of outcomes of acute clinical or chronic subclinical chorioamnionitis. Acute chorioamnionitis with virulent organisms is likely to cause severe lung disease or death. In contrast, chronic chorioamnionitis may improve lung outcomes by inducing lung maturation. However, bronchopulmonary dysplasia (BPD) may occur if the inflammation in the fetal lung is increased by postnatal exposures to oxygen, ventilation or postnatal sepsis. RDS, respiratory distress syndrome.

3

the intensity of the inflammatory response to chorioamnionitis in the fetal membranes with the clinical outcome of BPD (Fig. 3-6). More severe chorioamnionitis at delivery predicted a higher incidence and greater severity of BPD. However, clinicians do not know for how long the chorioamnionitis was present or what organisms were responsible. The fetus will have a graded response to chorioamnionitis that is based on currently poorly defined variables, such as the organism and the duration of fetal exposure.

Experimental Results: The Link between Fetal Exposure to Inflammation and Lung Maturation

The inconsistencies of the associations between chorioamnionitis/fetal inflammation and lung outcomes relate to the imprecision in diagnosis of fetal exposures, postnatal management, and the imprecision of the diagnoses RDS and BPD. Clinical associations also provide no information about mechanisms of the effects. Animal models

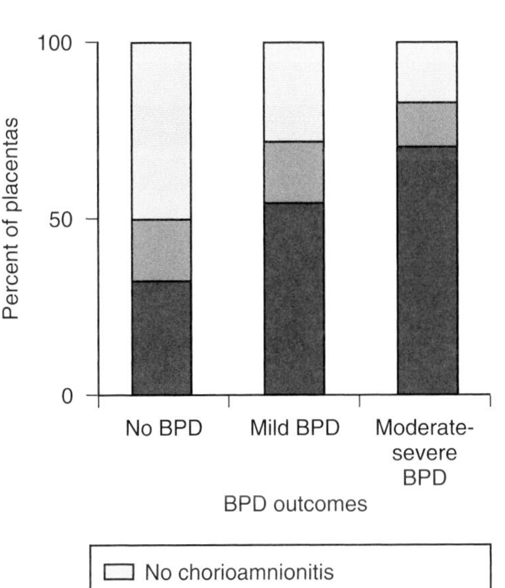

Figure 3-6 Relationship of severity of chorioamnionitis by histologic grading with the severity of bronchopulmonary dysplasia (BPD). Infants with moderate to severe BPD were more likely to have been exposed to more severe histologic chorioamnionitis. (Data from Viscardi RM, Muhumuza CK, Rodriguez A, et al: Inflammatory markers in intrauterine and fetal blood and cerebrospinal fluid compartments are associated with adverse pulmonary and neurologic outcomes in preterm infants. *Pediatr Res.* 2004;55:1009-1017.)

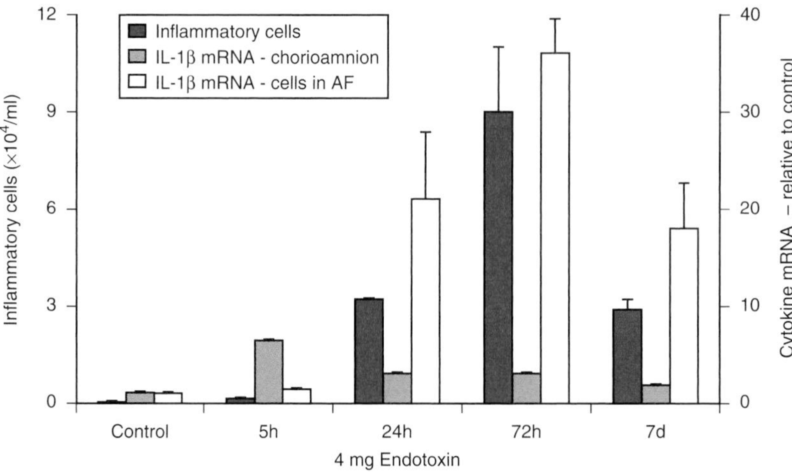

Figure 3-7 Intra-amniotic injection of endotoxin caused chorioamnionitis in fetal sheep. The intra-amniotic injection of endotoxin increased inflammatory cells in amniotic fluid (AF) and interleukin-1β (IL-1β) messenger RNA (mRNA) in both the chorioamnion and the cells in the amniotic fluid. (Data from Kramer BW, Moss TJ, Willet K, et al: Dose and time response after intra-amniotic endotoxin in preterm lambs. *Am J Respir Crit Care Med.* 2001;164:982-988.)

have consistently demonstrated that fetal exposure to inflammation causes lung injury and induces lung maturation. The first experiment demonstrating that inflammation induced lung maturation was reported in 1997 by Bry and colleagues.[90] In studies to evaluate the effects of the proinflammatory cytokines on preterm labor in rabbits, intra-amniotic injection of IL-1α caused increases in the surfactant proteins SP-A and SP-B and increased lung compliance. Our group found that intra-amniotic injection of the proinflammatory mediator endotoxin from *Escherichia coli* in sheep caused chorioamnionitis (inflammatory cells and increased IL-1β and IL-6 messenger RNA (mRNA) expression in the chorioamnion), inflammatory cells in amniotic fluid, and increased IL-8 protein levels in amniotic fluid (Fig. 3-7).[91,92] The chorioamnionitis was accompanied by inflammation of the fetal lung, as demonstrated by recruitment of granulocytes to the fetal lung tissue and air spaces within 24 hours and expression of multiple proinflammatory mediators (Fig. 3-8).[93,94] Apoptosis of lung cells increased at 24 hours, and proliferation increased at 3 days. This lung inflammation/injury sequence included multiple indicators of lung microvascular injury—epithelial nitric oxide synthase and vascular endothelial growth factor decreased, and medial smooth muscle hypertrophied.[94] Thus, intra-amniotic endotoxin caused lung inflammation and an injury sequence.

Inflammation was associated with the induction of the mRNAs for the surfactant proteins within 12 to 24 hours, persistent elevation of those mRNAs for weeks, and an increase in alveolar surfactant proteins and lipids with improved lung function within 5 to 7 days.[91,95] The improvement in lung function was accompanied by a decrease in mesenchymal tissue and an increase in potential gas volume in the fetal lung. The residual effects of the injury at 7 days were greater thickness of the pulmonary microvessels and a reduction in secondary septation of the alveoli.[94,96] However, the net effect was a lung that was easier to ventilate because of improved compliance and that had better gas exchange (Fig. 3-9). Of note, the lung injury followed by maturation sequence did not result from "fetal stress," because fetal blood cortisol levels did not increase. Lung inflammation resulted in accelerated lung maturation.

Intra-amniotic endotoxin in sheep was found to induce a cascade of inflammatory mediators in the chorioamnion and amniotic fluid. The fetal lung could be signaled by a systemic inflammatory response or by direct contact with endotoxin or mediators from the amniotic fluid. There was a modest fetal systemic response

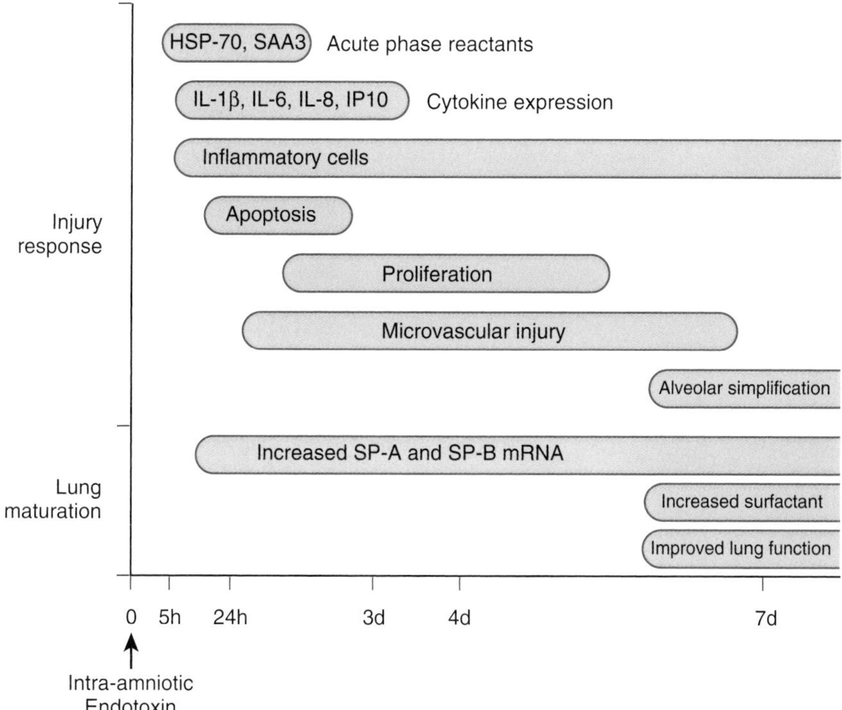

Figure 3-8 Time course of lung injury and lung maturation responses in fetal sheep to an intra-amniotic injection of endotoxin. The lung initially has an inflammation and injury response, which are followed by lung maturation. d, day(s); h, hour(s); HSP-70, heat shock protein 70; IL, interleukin; IP10, Interferon gamma – inducing protein 10; mRNA, messenger RNA; SP, surfactant protein.

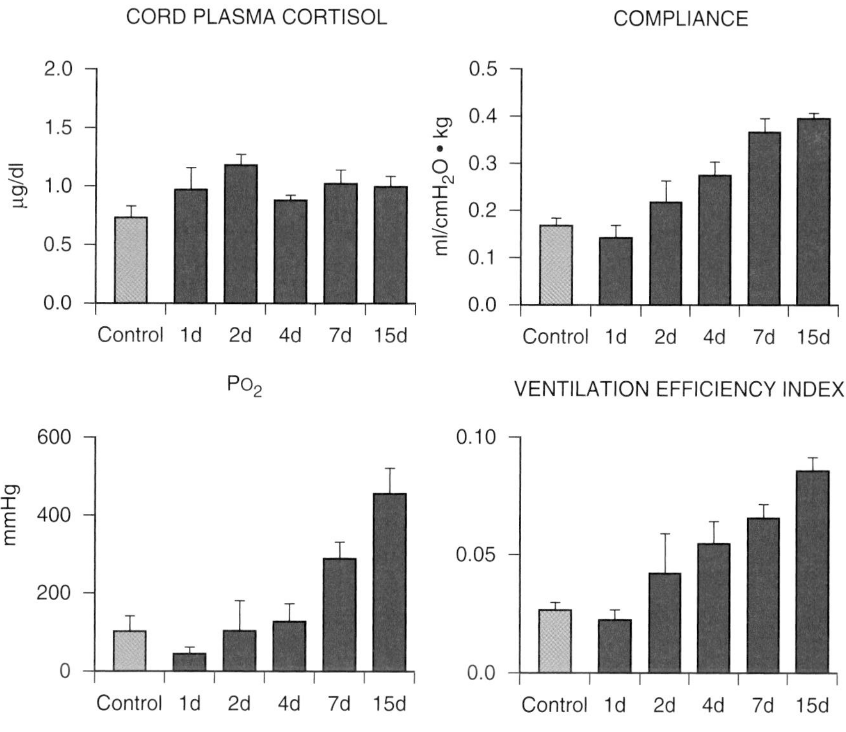

Figure 3-9 Cord plasma cortisol values and lung function following intra-amniotic injections of endotoxin for intervals from 1 day to 15 days before preterm delivery and mechanical ventilation of lambs. Plasma cortisol values did not increase from the low fetal values. Lung function increased progressively following the intra-amniotic injection of endotoxin. (Redrawn from Jobe AH, Newnham JP, Willet KE, et al: Endotoxin induced lung maturation in preterm lambs is not mediated by cortisol. *Am J Respir Crit Care Med.* 2000;162:1656-1661.)

to intra-amniotic endotoxin that included increased expression of the acute-phase reactant serum amyloid A3 and inflammation in the fetal liver.[93,97-99] Blood granulocytes decreased at 2 days, and granulocytes and platelets increased at 7 days. To test for systemic signaling to the fetal lung, Moss and colleagues[100] isolated the lung from the amniotic fluid surgically with collection of the fetal lung fluid in a bag placed in the amniotic cavity. Intra-amniotic endotoxin induced chorioamnionitis but not lung inflammation or lung maturation. In contrast, a 24-hour tracheal infusion of endotoxin induced both lung inflammation and lung maturation. This same result was achieved in another study with a fetal tracheal infusion of IL-1 as the proinflammatory agonist.[101] Therefore, the sequence from fetal lung inflammation to maturation did not result from a lung response to a systemic fetal inflammatory response. Also, new mediators resulting from the chorioamnionitis were not required for the response. Rather, direct contact of the fetal lung—presumably the airway epithelium—with endotoxin or IL-1 given by intra-amniotic injection or tracheal infusion induced the lung maturation. The initial inflammation is thought to result from responses to the mediators by the airway epithelium, because the airways express the acute-phase reactants heat shock protein 70 (Hsp70) and serum amyloid A3 (SAA3), and there are very few monocytes/macrophages present in the fetal lung to initiate an inflammatory response. However, in chronic chorioamnionitis, the inflammatory products of the chorioamnionitis or organisms in the amniotic fluid probably are mediating the responses of the fetal lungs.

A

Mediators that Induce Fetal Lung Responses

Innate immune responses are signaled by a family of pattern recognition molecules called the Toll-like receptors (TLRs). TLR4 recognizes endotoxin from gram-negative organisms, TLR2 signals gram-positive organisms, and TLR3 recognizes double-stranded RNA from viral pathogens, for example. The chorioamnion has TLRs, but there is very little information about the pattern of responses or the expression of the TLRs in the human fetus.[102] The inflammatory cells in the chorioamnion may be of maternal origin when organisms localized between the endometrium and chorioamnion initiate the inflammation.[103] The fetal rabbit lung expresses low levels of TLR2 and TLR4, and mRNA levels of TLRs 2, 3, and 4 remain unchanged for the last third of gestation in the fetal mice and sheep.[104,105] Empirically, *E. coli* endotoxin induces a rapid inflammatory response in the fetal sheep lung, as does IL-1, a cytokine that signals inflammation through a receptor that shares receptor elements and the signaling pathways with endotoxin. A high dose of a TLR2 agonist given by intra-amniotic injection in sheep induced less inflammation than did endotoxin and had inconsistent effects on lung maturation. Blood monocytes from preterm sheep also do not respond as well as monocytes from adult sheep to challenge with TLR agonists.[106] The fetus may not respond uniformly to different TLR agonists.

Ureaplasma given by intra-amniotic injection in sheep can colonize the amniotic fluid and fetal lung as early as 50 days of gestation (term is 150 days) and cause low-grade chronic lung inflammation and lung maturation (Table 3-7).[107] In fetal sheep, the innate inflammatory response to *Ureaplasma* is modest, with an increase in neutrophils by 3 days and persistent changes in lymphocyte populations in the lung.[108] The organism is not cleared from the fetal lungs. Colonization with *Ureaplasma* also does not cause fetal death or injury, a result similar to the outcomes of human pregnancies in which amniotic fluid samples were PC-positive for *Ureaplasma* at 15 to 19 weeks of gestation.[61,62] However, the fetal lungs have increased surfactant and persistent elevations in mRNAs for surfactant proteins. This model of chronic colonization/infection of the fetal lung with *Ureaplasma* may closely resemble the clinical effects of *Ureaplasma* associated with preterm deliveries in humans.

These experiments demonstrate that fetal sheep can respond to a variety of proinflammatory agonists and can be colonized with *Ureaplasma*, the organisms most frequently associated with preterm delivery in the human. However, fetal responses do not simply replicate responses in the adult. For example, fetal sheep do not respond to intra-amniotic or intravascular injections of sheep recombinant

Table 3-7 MEASUREMENTS AFTER INTRA-AMNIOTIC INJECTION OF *Ureaplasma parvum* IN SHEEP FETUSES*

	Controls	*Ureaplasma* Group
Result of culture for *Ureaplasma*	Negative	Positive
Plasma cortisol (mg/dL)	0.43 +/− 0.05	0.54 +/− 0.06
Measurements in bronchiolar lavage fluid†:		
Inflammatory cells ($\times 10^6$/kg)	0.1 +/− 0.06	6.7 +/− 1.2
Protein (mg/kg)	85 +/− 21	34 +/− 3
Saturated phosphatidylcholine (mmol/kg)	6.7 +/− 3.0	0.2 +/− 0.1
Lung gas volume (mL/kg)	11.2 +/− 1.5	28.5 +/− 2.8

*Intra-amniotic injection of 2×10^7 colony-forming units of *Ureaplasma parvum* at 67 days gestational age (GA) for sheep fetuses; measurements made at 124 days GA.

†Values per kg are expressed per kg body weight; all values for the *Ureaplasma* animals are different from those in controls except plasma cortisol.

Data from Moss TJ, Nitsos I, Kramer BW, et al: Intra-amniotic endotoxin induces lung maturation by direct effects on the developing respiratory tract in preterm sheep. *Am J Obstet Gynecol.* 2002;187:1059-1065.

TNFα,[109] and as noted previously, responses to TLR2 agonist were insufficient to consistently induce lung maturation. The spectrum of the response potential of the fetus and the fetal lung to the multiple mediators of innate immune responses remains to be studied. Clinical responses also may reflect the polymicrobial nature of the chorioamnionitis. Questions that remain relate to receptor expression, the cell localization of that expression, the response potential of the signaling pathways, and the maturity of the integration of innate and acquired immune responses.

Early Gestational Fetal Lung Responses to Inflammation

The interval from fetal exposure to chorioamnionitis and lung inflammation or lung maturation is not known in the human, primarily because of the lack of precision about the diagnosis of chorioamnionitis. In fetal sheep, significant lung maturation is not detected until 4 to 7 days after an intra-amniotic injection of endotoxin.[95] Lung maturation is striking if the interval between intra-amniotic endotoxin injection and preterm delivery is 15 days. Intra-amniotic *Ureaplasma* did not induce lung maturation within 7 days but did induce lung maturation when given 14 to 45 days before preterm delivery.[107] Intra-amniotic endotoxin given at 60 days of gestation (40% of gestation) to fetal sheep resulted in a doubling of lung-saturated phosphatidylcholine, increased SP-A, SP-B, and SP-C mRNA, and improved in lung function 65 days later, with preterm delivery at 125 days of gestation.[110] The fetal sheep lung can respond to intra-amniotic endotoxin/chorioamnionitis across a wide range of gestational ages. The question how early in gestation an inflammatory stimulus can modulate fetal lung development remains unanswered in the clinical context. However, the frequent occurrence of early lung maturation and chorioamnionitis suggests to us that inflammation is the major mediator of lung maturation in the very preterm infant.

Mechanisms of Inflammation-Mediated Lung Maturation

The mechanisms responsible for inflammation-induced lung maturation are not well understood. In the human, chorioamnionitis is associated with an increase in cortisol in cord blood collected at delivery,[111] and of course, glucocorticoids induce lung maturation. The clinical samples were from infants who had been exposed to chorioamnionitis and who were delivered as a result of preterm labor, which may represent a selected population—because some women with chronic chorioamnionitis may not deliver prematurely. In fetal sheep, endotoxin-, IL-1–, or *Ureaplasma*-induced chorioamnionitis *does not* induce preterm labor, preterm delivery, or increases in fetal blood cortisol levels sufficient to induce lung maturation.

The minimal amount of *E. coli* endotoxin given by intra-amniotic injection that will induce lung maturation in the fetal sheep is 1 to 4 mg, and doses as high as 100 mg induce lung maturation without increasing the amount of lung inflammation or causing fetal injury or preterm delivery.[92,95] Doses of intra-amniotic endotoxin smaller than 1 mg cause less inflammation and no lung maturation. In general, the amount of lung inflammation induced by chorioamnionitis correlated with the amount of lung maturation. These results indicate that low amounts of lung inflammation do not induce lung maturation and that above some minimal level there is a dose-response relationship between lung inflammation and lung maturation. Our group used a monoclonal antibody to the integrin CD18 to block endotoxin-induced lung inflammation, which also prevented lung maturation (Fig. 3-10).[112] In contrast,

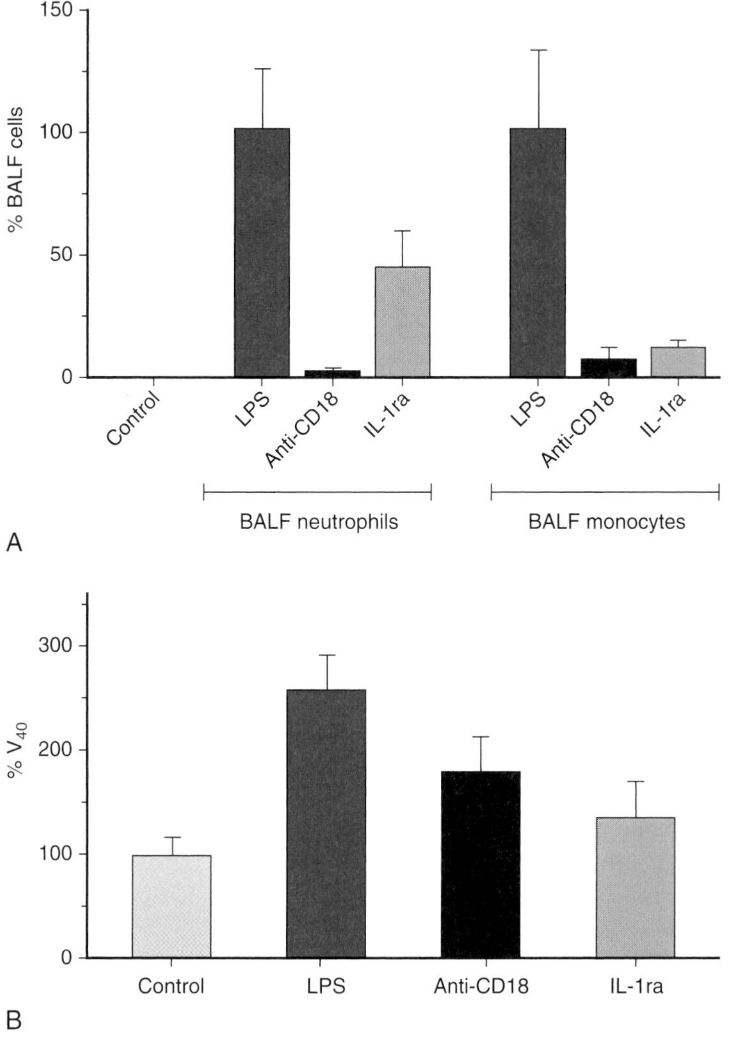

Figure 3-10 Anti–CD18 antibody and IL-1 receptor antagonist (IL-1ra) block lung inflammation and maturation in fetal sheep. **A,** Fetal sheep were given an anti–CD18 antibody by intramuscular injection or IL-1ra into the amniotic fluid 3 hours before intra-amniotic (IA) lipopolysaccharide (LPS). Both treatments decreased the numbers of neutrophils and monocytes in bronchoalveolar lavage fluid (BALF), indicating almost complete blockade of the endotoxin-induced lung inflammation at 2 days. **B,** The treatments also decreased lung gas volumes, measured at 40 cm H_2O pressure (V_{40}) relative to LPS, indicating decreased lung maturation. (Data from Kallapur SG, Moss JTM, Newnham JP, et al: Recruited inflammatory cells mediate endotoxin-induced lung maturation in preterm fetal lambs. *Am J Respir Crit Care Med.* 2005;172:1315-1321; and Kallapur SG, Nitsos I, Moss TJ, et al: IL-1 mediates pulmonary and systemic inflammatory responses to chorioamnionitis induced by lipopolysaccharide. *Am J Respir Crit Care Med.* 2009;179:955-961.)

inflammation and lung maturation induced by IL-I was not blocked by this anti-CD18 antibody. This experiment links inflammation to lung maturation and further demonstrates that different proinflammatory agonists can recruit inflammatory cells to the fetal lungs by different mechanisms.

This inflammation-maturation relationship was further examined with use of an IL-1 receptor blocker.[113] IL-1α is a potent inducer of chorioamnionitis, lung inflammation, and lung maturation. IL-1α also induces the expression of IL-1β in the chorioamnion, and cells in amniotic fluid and the fetal lung. When the IL-1 receptor antagonist IL-1ra was given into the amniotic fluid, about 80% of the lung inflammatory response to intra-amniotic endotoxin was blocked, and lung maturation was decreased. These experiments demonstrate that inflammation is essential to the lung maturation response. There currently is no information about what products of lung inflammation signal lung maturation. Presumably, mediators produced locally in the distal lung parenchyma, possibly by granulocytes and/or monocytes, induce a signaling cascade resulting in the mesenchymal and type II cell changes that result in lung maturation. Insight into this signaling sequence may provide clues for the development of clinically practical strategies to induce lung maturation.

3

Experimental Chronic Chorioamnionitis

Although the majority of VLBW infants may be exposed to chronic chorioamnionitis, the duration and the intensity of the inflammatory exposure to the fetus remain undefined. A single proinflammatory fetal exposure from intra-amniotic injections of mediators caused acute lung inflammation followed by mild microvascular injury and an arrest in alveolar septation by 7 days.[94,96] Low-grade inflammation (increased inflammatory cells) persisted for weeks. Live *Ureaplasma* caused mild inflammation despite prolonged persistence in the fetal lung.[107] The clinically relevant question is how the fetal lung copes with prolonged exposures to inflammatory agonists such as endotoxin. Surprisingly, few VLBW infants seem to have severe pneumonia after preterm birth despite exposure to infection/inflammation. Although a single intrauterine exposure to endotoxin caused histologic changes consistent with a mild BPD phenotype in experimental animals, infants are not born with BPD. A possible exception is the rapid development of the BPD variant described by radiologic changes as the Wilson-Mikity syndrome, which has been associated with chorioamnionitis.[114] However, in general, severe lung injury and pneumonia are infrequent after the histologic chorioamnionitis associated with preterm birth.

Our group has modeled chronic endotoxin-induced chorioamnionitis with repeated weekly intra-amniotic injections of endotoxin and with osmotic pumps that deliver endotoxin continuously over 28 days to the amniotic fluid. A prolonged fetal exposure resulting from a 28-day intra-amniotic infusion of endotoxin from 53% to 72% of gestation caused striking lung maturation and increases in surfactant with decreased alveolar septation at 125 days (83% of gestation).[110] When the lungs of the fetal sheep were examined at 138 days of gestation, low-grade inflammation persisted 30 days after the end of endotoxin administration and surfactant was increased as a residual effect of the induced lung maturation (Fig. 3-11).[115] Remarkably, all anatomic indicators of the arrest of alveolar septation seen at 125 days of gestation had disappeared by 138 days of gestation. There also were no biochemical or histologic indicators of microvascular injury.

Weekly intra-amniotic injections with 10 mg endotoxin given at 100 days, 107 days, 114 days, and 121 days of gestation resulted in the recovery of 3.3×10^7 inflammatory cells per kg body weight by bronchoalveolar lavage at 145 days of gestation, just prior to term.[115] In contrast, control lungs had less than 10^4 inflammatory cells in bronchoalveolar lavage fluid. At 145 days of gestation and 24 days after repeated intra-amniotic endotoxin injections, the mRNA for the proinflammatory cytokine IL-1β in lung tissue was higher than in control, as was the amount of surfactant, but there were no changes in the lung architecture or microvasculature (Fig. 3-12). These results demonstrate that the fetal lung can adapt to chronic inflammation and that despite a brief interference with alveolar septation and

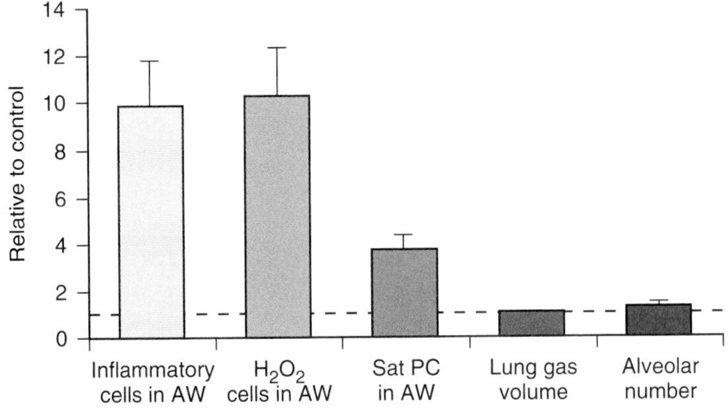

A

Figure 3-11 Residual effects at 138 days of gestation of the intra-amniotic infusion of 1 mg/day of endotoxin for 28 days of gestation, from day 80 to day 108 days, in fetal sheep. All measurements are expressed relative to the control group, which was normalized to 1.0 (*dashed line*). Residual indicators of inflammation were the number of inflammatory cells in bronchoalveolar lavage (BAL) and their ability to produce hydrogen peroxide (H_2O_2). Although the amount of saturated phosphatidylcholine (Sat PC) in alveolar wash (AW) was increased, lung structure was not altered. (Data from Kallapur SG, Nitsos I, Moss TJM, et al: Chronic endotoxin exposure does not cause sustained structural abnormalities in the fetal sheep lungs. *Am J Physiol Lung Cell Mol Physiol.* 2005;288:L966-L974.)

microvascular development, the fetal lung corrects the deficits and can continue to develop. *Ureaplasma* also causes subtle alterations in lung structure after a 14-day exposure, but the changes do not persist with more chronic exposures.[108,116]

Immune Modulation from Fetal Exposures to Inflammation

The fetus is presumed to have naïve and immature immune responses, but a fetal challenge or priming of innate immunity may be contributing to postnatal lung and other organ diseases in preterm infants. Fetal sheep exposed to intra-amniotic

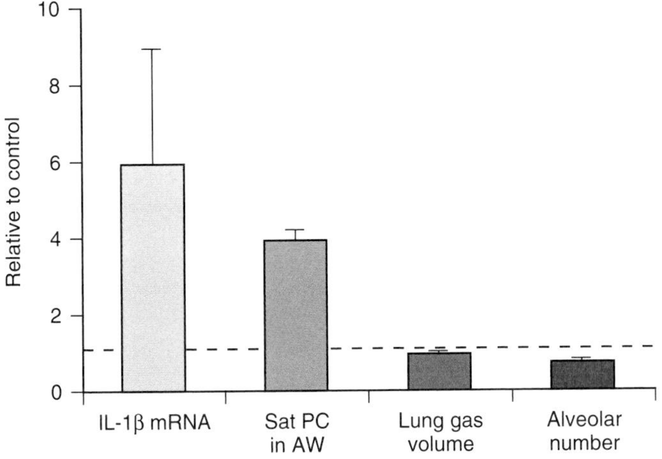

Figure 3-12 Residual effects of weekly intra-amniotic injections of endotoxin on fetal sheep lungs at term. Fetal sheep were exposed to four intra-amniotic injections of 10 mg endotoxin at weekly intervals beginning at 100 days gestation. At delivery 24 days after the final injection, expression of interleukin 1β (IL-1β) messenger RNA (mRNA) in lung tissue was increased, the amount of saturated phosphatidylcholine (Sat PC) in alveolar wash (AW) was increased, but lung gas volumes and alveolar numbers were similar to control values. The control values were normalized to 1.0 and are indicated by the *dashed line*. (Data from Kallapur SG, Nitsos I, Moss TJM, et al: Chronic endotoxin exposure does not cause sustained structural abnormalities in the fetal sheep lungs. *Am J Physiol Lung Cell Mol Physiol.* 2005;288:L966-L974.)

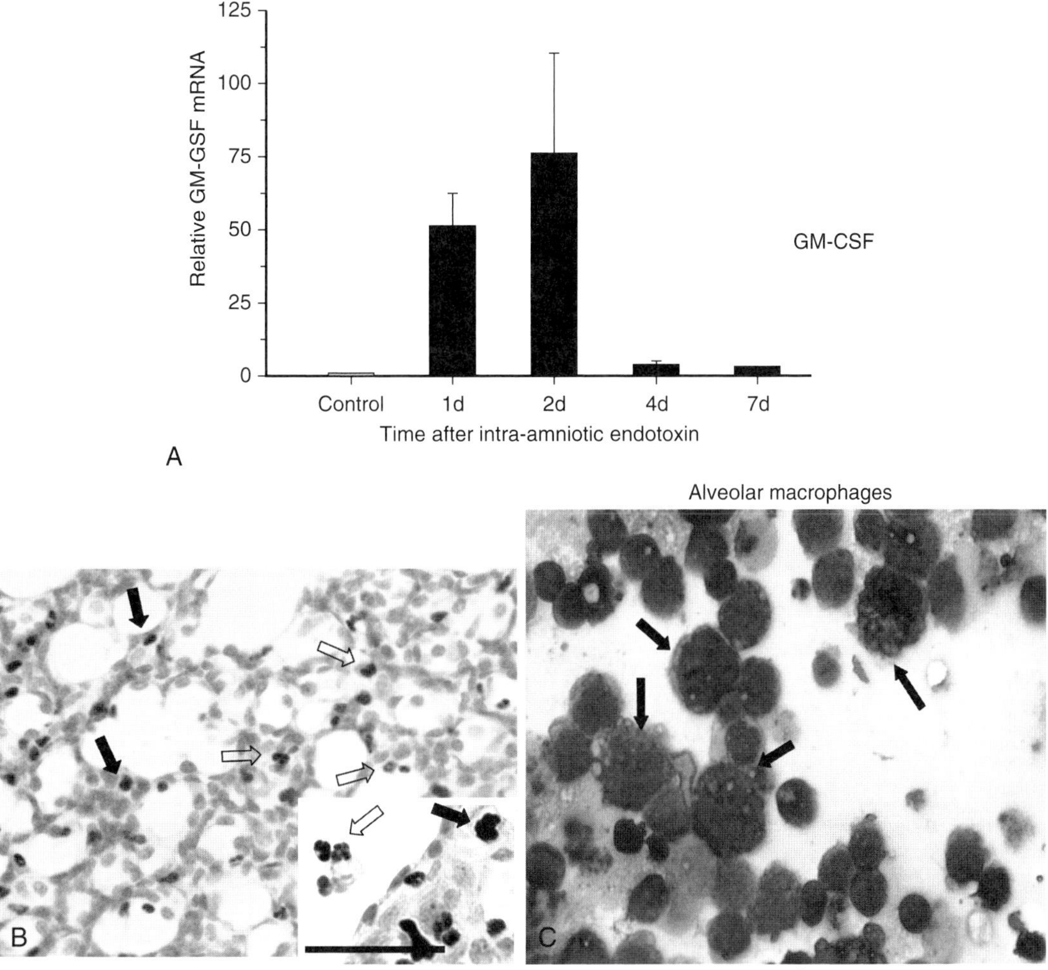

Figure 3-13 Intra-amniotic administration of lipopolysaccharide (LPS) matures alveolar macrophages in the fetal lungs. **A,** Following the intra-amniotic injection (IA) of 10 mg LPS, granulocyte-monocyte colony-stimulating factor (GM-CSF) is induced in the fetal lung and (B) PU.1-positive cells appear in the lung, indicating maturation from monocytes to macrophages. Expression is localized to nuclei of monocyte cells (filled arrows) and neutrophils (open arrows). **C,** By 7 days (d), mature-appearing alveolar macrophages (arrows) are in high numbers in alveolar washes. mRNA, messenger RNA. (Data from Kramer BW, Joshi SN, Moss TJ, et al: Endotoxin-induced maturation of monocytes in preterm fetal sheep lung. *Am J Physiol Lung Cell Mol Physiol.* 2007;293:L345-L353.)

lipopolysaccharide (LPS) have more lymphocytes and monocytes in the air spaces after delivery and ventilation.[117] Of note, the normal fetal lung contains few mature macrophages, but lungs exposed to endotoxin contain large numbers of histologically mature macrophages. Exposure to endotoxin recruits immature monocytes into the fetal lung and induces maturation via granulocyte-monocyte colony-stimulating factor and induction of the transcription factor PU.1 within 7 days (Fig. 3-13).[118] A fetal exposure to LPS also matures the function of blood monocytes and increases regulatory lymphocytes (CD4/CD25 and gamma/delta T cells) in the posterior mediastinal node draining the lungs and in the fetal thymus.[119] Fetal inflammatory cells that do not make or respond to TNFα can respond after fetal exposure to endotoxin. A second exposure to intra-amniotic endotoxin after an initial exposure renders the fetal lung and blood monocytes unresponsive to challenge with endotoxin—a state of *endotoxin tolerance*.[120] The single fetal exposure to endotoxin also increases immune cell responses to the other TLR agonists, and a second endotoxin exposure blunts cell responses to other TLR agonists—a condition called *cross-tolerance*.[121] Long-term fetal exposure to live *Ureaplasma* also induces a tolerance response to intra-amniotic endotoxin. These results demonstrate complex immune modulations by the fetus that could modify the postnatal responses to mechanical ventilation, oxygen, nutrition, or secondary sepsis that would change short-term clinical outcomes such as later-onset sepsis, BPD, and necrotizing enterocolitis. These possible relationships between fetal exposures and subsequent postnatal immune responses are just another layer of complexity challenging the understanding of clinical outcomes. A large literature is being developed about how fetal exposures to inflammation may promote airway disease and asthma,[122] which is beyond the scope of this review.

Antenatal Corticosteroid Treatments and Chorioamnionitis

Corticosteroids are given antenatally to more than 80% of the women at risk for preterm delivery before 30 weeks of gestation, and the majority of these women have undiagnosed (histologic) chorioamnionitis.[41,55] The majority of women with preterm rupture of membranes have histologic chorioamnionitis. Thus, preterm rupture of membranes is a surrogate marker for chorioamnionitis. The current recommendation is to give antenatal corticosteroids with preterm rupture of membranes, because the treatment reduces the incidences of RDS, intraventricular hemorrhage, and death.[123] In clinical series, antenatal corticosteroids are of benefit for preterm deliveries that in retrospect had associated histologic chorioamnionitis.[124] A 2011 meta-analysis of observational studies identified benefit of corticosteroid treatment in women with chorioamnionitis (Table 3-8).[125] Antenatal corticosteroids also decrease the fetal inflammatory response syndrome in preterm infants exposed to histologic chorioamnionitis.[124]

Although there is no specific clinical information available about how corticosteroids influence chorioamnionitis, the corticosteroids might suppress inflammation—a potential benefit—or increase the risk of progressive inflammation—a potential risk. Both outcomes seem possible on the basis of the small amount of information available from experimental studies: Maternal treatment with betamethasone suppressed the inflammation caused by intra-amniotic endotoxin in the chorioamnion and lungs of fetal sheep (Fig. 3-14).[98,126] Inflammatory cells and proinflammatory cytokine expression were suppressed for about 2 days after the betamethasone treatment, but subsequently inflammation was *increased* in the lungs of lambs exposed to both maternal betamethasone and intra-amniotic endotoxin in comparison with lambs exposed to endotoxin alone 5 and 15 days after the exposures (Fig. 3-15). Lung maturation was greater in lambs exposed to

Table 3-8 META-ANALYSIS OF OBSERVATIONAL STUDIES OF ANTENATAL CORTICOSTEROID TREATMENTS FOR WOMEN WITH CHORIOAMNIONITIS

	Odds Ratio	95% Confidence Interval
Histologic Diagnosis of Chorioamnionitis (5 studies)		
Mortality of newborn	0.45	0.30-0.68
Respiratory distress syndrome	0.53	0.40-0.71
Bronchopulmonary dysplasia	0.79	0.35-1.83
Severe intraventricular hemorrhage	0.39	0.19-0.82
Clinical Diagnosis of Chorioamnionitis (4 studies)		
Mortality of newborn	0.77	0.36-1.65
Respiratory distress syndrome	0.73	0.48-1.12
Bronchopulmonary dysplasia	0.80	0.37-1.74
Severe intraventricular hemorrhage	0.29	0.10-0.89

Data from Been JV, Degraeuwe PL, Kramer BW, Zimmermann LJ: Antenatal steroids and neonatal outcome after chorioamnionitis: a meta-analysis. *BJOG.* 2011;118:113-122.

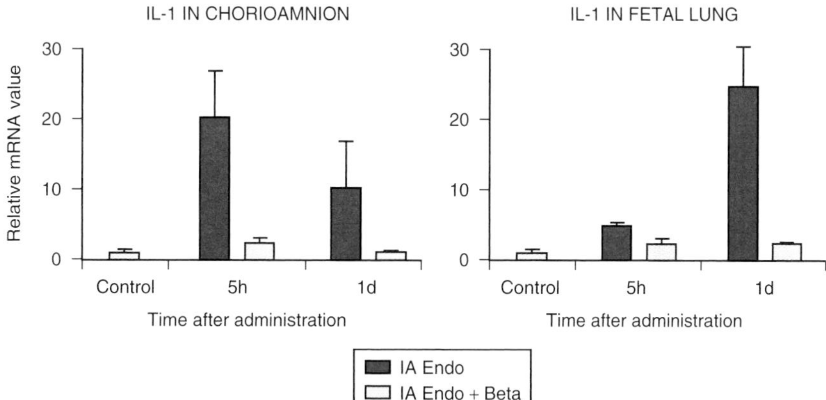

Figure 3-14 Maternal betamethasone suppressed the inflammation induced by intra-amniotic (IA) administration of endotoxin in the chorioamnion and fetal lung. The expression of interleukin-1β (IL-1β) messenger RNA (mRNA) was decreased to control values by maternal betamethasone given to sheep 3 hours (h) before IA endotoxin. (Data from Newnham J, Kallapur SG, Kramer BW, et al: Betamethasone effects on chorioamnionitis induced by intra-amniotic endotoxin in sheep. *Am J Obstet Gynecol.* 2003;189:1458-1466; and Kallapur SG, Kramer BW, Moss TJ, et al: Maternal glucocorticoids increase endotoxin-induced lung inflammation in preterm lambs. *Am J Physiol Lung Cell Mol Physiol.* 2003;284:L633-L642.)

both betamethasone and endotoxin than to either treatment alone (Fig. 3-16).[127] A surprising result was that growth restriction induced by betamethasone did not occur with concurrent endotoxin exposure. These results in fetal sheep support the clinical observations that betamethasone can further decrease RDS in the presence of histologic chorioamnionitis.[124] In fetal sheep the lung maturational response to endotoxin was larger and more uniform than the response to betamethasone. A distinct difference in the responses is the rapid improvement in lung function within 15 hours after betamethasone and the delay for an improvement in lung function of at least 4 days following intra-amniotic endotoxin.[31,95] Betamethasone also seems to augment the lung maturation induced by chronic fetal *Ureaplasma* colonization.[128]

The increased inflammation in the fetal sheep lungs that occurs 5 to 15 days after combined betamethasone and endotoxin exposures is a potential concern. Such effects have not been apparent clinically, but they have not been evaluated. A

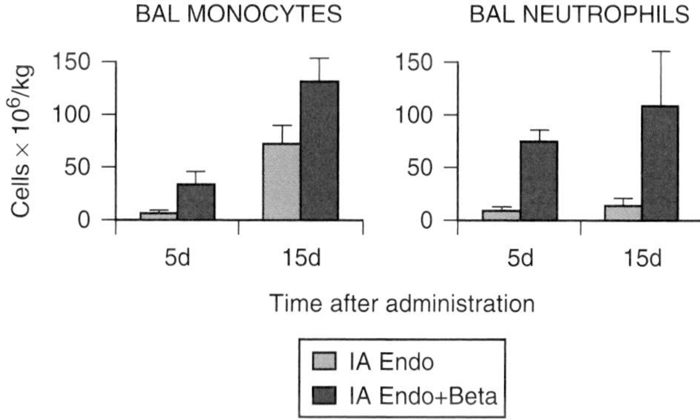

Figure 3-15 Inflammation is increased in the fetal lung by maternal betamethasone 5 days (d) and 15 days after intra-amniotic (IA) administration of endotoxin. The monocytes and neutrophils recovered by bronchoalveolar lavage (BAL) were higher if fetuses were exposed to maternal betamethasone prior to intra-amniotic endotoxin than if they were exposed to the endotoxin alone. (Data from Kallapur SG, Kramer BW, Moss TJ, et al: Maternal glucocorticoids increase endotoxin-induced lung inflammation in preterm lambs. *Am J Physiol Lung Cell Mol Physiol.* 2003;284:L633-L642.)

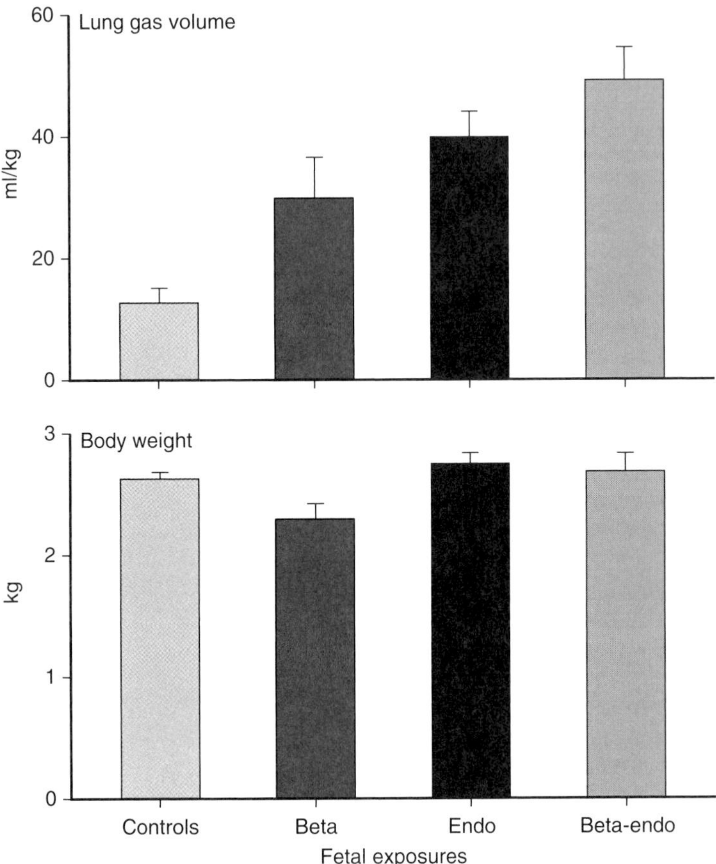

Figure 3-16 Lung gas volumes and body weights of fetal sheep 7 days after exposure to maternal betamethasone (Beta), intra-amniotic endotoxin (Endo), or both (Beta-endo). Maximal lung gas volume measured at an airway pressure of 40 cm H_2O, increased with either treatment but was largest with both treatments. Only maternal betamethasone decreased fetal weight, and this effect was prevented by concurrent endotoxin exposure. (Redrawn from Newnham JP, Moss TJ, Padbury JF, et al: The interactive effects of endotoxin with prenatal glucocorticoids on short-term lung function in sheep. *Am J Obstet Gynecol.* 2001;185:190-197.)

potential mechanism to explain the increased inflammation is that both betamethasone and the endotoxin "mature" an immature inflammatory system. Blood monocytes from fetal sheep have decreased responses in vitro to endotoxin stimulation in comparison with monocytes from adult sheep (Fig. 3-17).[129] However, 7 days after the fetal exposures, the monocytes respond to endotoxin in vitro similarly to monocytes from adult sheep. Maternal betamethasone also initially suppresses the fetal monocyte, but function is increased 7 days after the maternal treatment.[130] These results illustrate just how clinically complex interactions between exposures may be.

These experiments in fetal sheep describe simultaneous exposures to betamethasone and chorioamnionitis. The more likely clinical scenarios are the superposition of maternal betamethasone treatments on chronic, subclinical chorioamnionitis or maternal betamethasone treatments followed by the acute onset of chorioamnionitis. There is just no information about how timing of exposures may alter clinical outcomes. Repetitive courses of betamethasone treatments may be a concern, particularly when chorioamnionitis is present. The clinical dilemma is that histologic chorioamnionitis is a retrospective diagnosis of a clinically silent process.

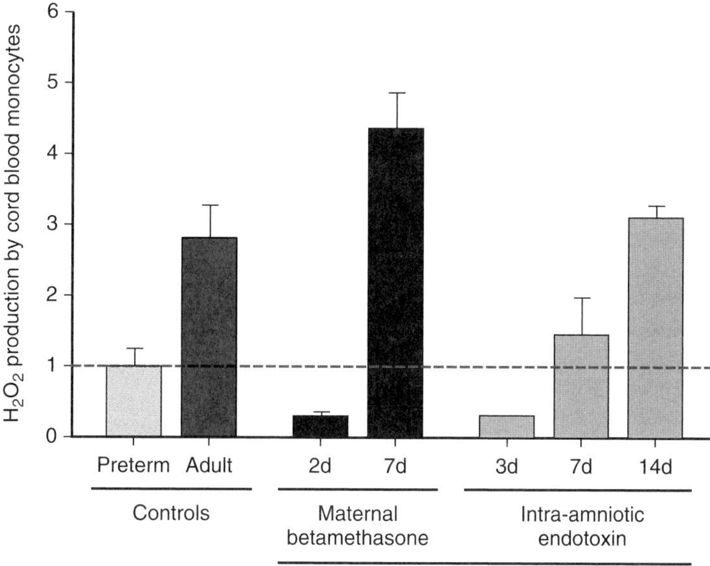

Figure 3-17 Production of hydrogen peroxide (H_2O_2) by cord blood monocytes from preterm lambs and blood monocytes from adult sheep on challenge in vitro with endotoxin. The monocytes from the preterm sheep produce less H_2O_2 than the monocytes from adult sheep. Maternal betamethasone suppressed monocyte function at 2 days (d) but enhanced monocyte function at 7 days. Intra-amniotic endotoxin also initially suppressed then enhanced monocyte function. (Data from Kramer BW, Ikegami M, Moss TJ, et al: Endotoxin-induced chorioamnionitis modulates innate immunity of monocytes in preterm sheep. *Am J Respir Crit Care Med.* 2005;171:73-77; and Kramer BW, Ikegami M, Moss TJ, et al: Antenatal betamethasone changes cord blood monocyte responses to endotoxin in preterm lambs. *Pediatr Res.* 2004;55: 764-768.)

Intrauterine Growth Restriction/Small for Gestational Age

Fetuses identified to have IUGR on the basis of estimates of fetal size and Doppler flow patterns of the fetal circulation and infants born SGA according to standardized growth charts are overlapping populations with varied causes for the inadequate growth. For the preterm segment of this population, the majority of infants result from pregnancies with associated hypertension or preeclampsia,[131] excluding genetic and chromosomal abnormalities. Lung disease after term or near-term delivery has not been well studied but is not appreciated as a clinical problem. In contrast, preterm delivery of growth-restricted infants and infants of preeclamptic pregnancies are associated with an increased risk for RDS, despite the severe chronic stress experienced by the fetuses (Fig. 3-18).[132,133] Jelin and associates[134] also reported that preeclampsia with onset early in pregnancy increased the risk for SGA infants (OR 3.9, 59% CI 2.5-6.2) and for RDS (OR 1.5, 95% CI 1.1-2.2). The concept has been that fetal stress will increase fetal cortisol levels and induce lung maturation, but the stresses causing fetal growth restriction and preeclampsia do not decrease RDS relative to the comparison populations of preterm infants at comparable gestational ages. We suspect that the comparison group simply illustrates one "elephant in the room," in that the comparison population is enriched for infants exposed to chorioamnionitis, which is less frequent in IUGR/SGA infants. This interpretation suggests decreased RDS in both populations relative to a theoretical population of "normal" preterm infants. A reasonable conclusion is that preeclampsia/IUGR/SGA preterm infants are not protected from respiratory problems soon after birth, as captured by the diagnosis of RDS.

These small infants are at increased risk for mortality and BPD. In one study, IUGR or SGA status at birth raised mortality for infants at all gestations, and increased the need for respiratory support at 28 days of age primarily for infants

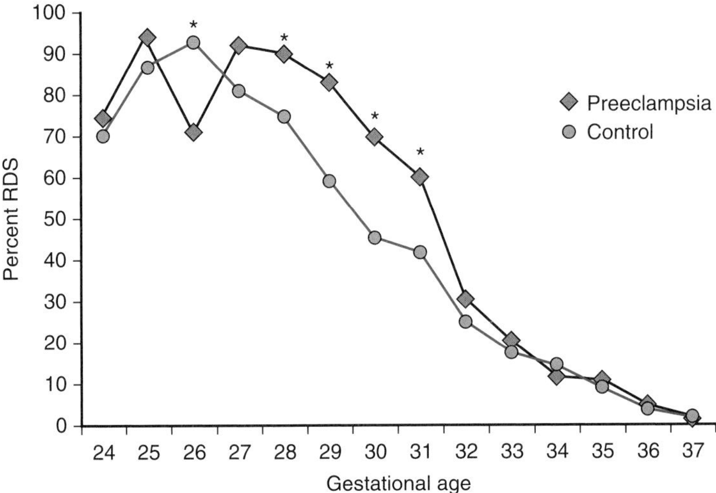

Figure 3-18 Epidemiologic data for incidences of respiratory distress syndrome (RDS) relative to gestational age. RDS incidence was higher for fetuses exposed to pre-eclampsia. (Data from Chang EY, Menard MK, Vermillion ST, et al: The association between hyaline membrane disease and preeclampsia. *Am J Obstet Gynecol.* 2004;191:1414-1417.)

born at 26 to 29 weeks gestational age.[135] Reiss and colleagues[136] reported an increased risk in BPD for infants with birth weights below the 10th percentile (OR 3.8, 95% CI 2.1-6.8). This relationship of increased BPD with low birth weight for gestational age is a continuum that includes less BPD at high birth weights for gestational age (Fig. 3-19).[131] Bose and coworkers[137] also demonstrated an increased risk of BPD through the use logistic regression models for 1241 infants who were born prior to 28 weeks of gestation and survived to 36 weeks gestational age. The predictors of BPD were gestational age and birth weights for gestational age below −1 Z score (OR 3.2, 95% CI 2.1-5.0), or −2 Z scores (OR 4.4, 95% CI 2.2-8.2). There are several possible explanations for the increased risk of BPD in infants born

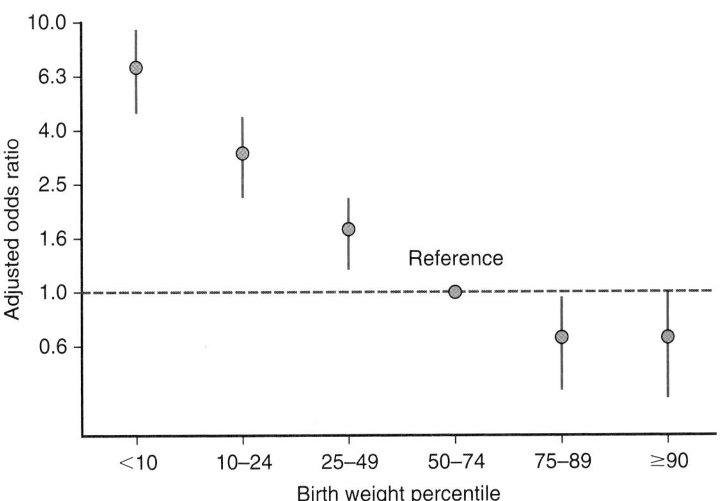

Figure 3-19 Odds ratios (circles) and 95% confidence intervals (*lines*) for bronchopulmonary dysplasia (BPD) for infants grouped by birth weight percentiles adjusted for gestational ages. The risk for BPD increases as birth weight percentile decreases from the reference group for the 50 to 74 percentiles. The risk of BPD is lower for the larger infants. (Data from Zeitlin J, El Ayoubi M, Jarreau PH, et al: Impact of fetal growth restriction on mortality and morbidity in a very preterm birth cohort. *J Pediatr.* 2010;157:733-739 e731.)

SGA. The somewhat trivial explanation is that the respiratory and nutritional care of smaller infants is more difficult technically than that for larger infants. For example, the 600-g 27-week infant may be kept on a ventilator because of perceived fragility longer than the 1000-g 27-week infant, with the consequence being increased BPD. However, biologic explanations likely contribute to this association. McElrath and associates[1] hypothesize that most severe prematurity results from either inflammation/infection or vascular developmental abnormalities that may progress from implantation. These vascular abnormalities (preeclampsia) are highly associated with fetal growth failure and an increased risk for BPD.[138] Therefore, the clinical data are consistent with the likelihood that small infants may have abnormal lung vascular development.

Antenatal corticosteroids decrease fetal growth in animal models and may decrease fetal growth with repetitive treatments in humans.[47] Thus, the combined effects of antenatal corticosteroid treatments on growth-restricted fetuses could be adverse. There are no targeted randomized trials of antenatal corticosteroids for these at-risk pregnancies, although antenatal corticosteroids are routinely used for pregnancies with preeclampsia and at risk for preterm delivery.[135] Data from the early randomized trials show no adverse effects of corticosteroid use with maternal hypertension or for SGA infants.[25] The available data from clinical series do not suggest that antenatal corticosteroids are of benefit for growth-restricted fetuses.[139] Thus, there remain questions about the benefit of antenatal corticosteroids for the growth-restricted fetus.

Experimental models demonstrate clear effects of decreased fetal growth on lung development. Fetal sheep become growth restricted if placental implantation sites are decreased prior to pregnancy. Lipsett and colleagues[140] reported that fetal growth restriction caused a reduction in the gas exchange surface density of the fetal lung with smaller alveoli. Growth-restricted preterm fetal sheep had reduced surfactant protein levels, indicating delayed lung maturation despite high fetal cortisol levels.[141] Similarly, fetal growth restriction caused by an hypoxic environment in mice decreased mRNA expression of the surfactant proteins.[142] Exposure of growth-restricted fetal sheep to corticosteroids altered cardiovascular responses and increased indicators of brain injury relative to normally grown comparison groups.[143,144] Although the causes of fetal growth restriction in humans differ from those in the animal models, the lungs may have abnormal structure and maturation. Fetal growth restriction has now been recognized as a major predictor of BPD, and multiple questions remain about the mechanisms that promote BPD in these at-risk fetuses.

Environmental Factors and Lung Disease

Multiple environmental factors could modulate lung development in the fetus and have consequences after birth. The field of fetal and early neonatal exposures that may increase risks for asthma in children and chronic lung diseases in adults is captured in the research fields into the early origins of adult diseases and the hygiene hypothesis. Studies have focused primarily on term infant populations, and these subjects are beyond the scope of this review. However, we briefly explore two fetal exposures that may be underappreciated modulators of fetal lung development and that have not been adequately explored in relation to lung diseases in preterms. In a perspective written in 2001, Pierce and Nguyen[145] itemized the multiple effects of maternal cigarette smoking on fetal and newborn lung growth and function in animal models. These include decreased lung size and volume, changes in lung collagen and elastin, greater alveolar size, and increased type II cell numbers. Maternal smoking induced airway remodeling in fetal mice,[146] the presumed substrate for the airway disease reported in infants exposed to environmental smoke.[147] Maternal smoking was associated with increases in L/S ratio and cortisol in amniotic fluid in humans,[148] and nicotine altered developmental programs in the fetal lungs of rats.[149] Infants who were exposed to maternal smoking and who died of sudden infant death syndrome had fewer alveolar attachment points on airways.[150] These observations are consistent with the hypothesis that maternal smoking may alter lung structural and maturational development in very preterm infants, an effect that will be reflected in disease incidences such as RDS, BPD, and more frequent airway reactivity. Populations of very preterm infants have not been evaluated for such effects.

A less studied exposure with possible effects on the preterm lung is maternal alcohol use. The fetal alcohol syndrome that includes fetal growth restriction and impaired neurodevelopment is well described. Exposure of fetal sheep to alcohol for the last third of gestation decreased surfactant protein mRNA expression but increased extracellular matrix deposition.[151] Changes in cytokine levels in the fetal lungs could result in altered immune status. Alcohol abuse alters the redox state of the adult lung, in which adult respiratory distress syndrome is more likely to develop with an injury.[152] The effects of maternal alcohol abuse on lung function and injury in preterm infants remain unexplored.

Summary: The Complexities

Premature delivery is an abnormal event, and the preterm infant must have sufficiently developed lungs to survive, often with the help of multiple interventions such as antenatal corticosteroids, surfactant, and mechanical ventilation. The experimental literature relating to lung development and maturity is vast and informative, but the story becomes quite messy when clinical experiences are considered. There are just too many variables that influence the status of the preterm lung at delivery. Gestational age and birth weight are the overriding predictors of outcomes. Maternal/fetal diseases such as preeclampsia and chorioamnionitis have potent effects on the fetal lung, but both have a spectrum of effects, from decreased risks to increased risks of RDS or BPD. Antenatal corticosteroids clearly benefit preterm infants overall, but how they further modulate the pregnancy abnormalities resulting in preterm delivery probably differ for each abnormality and with the timing of the fetal exposures. Environmental exposures such as smoke and alcohol are seldom considered relative to lung disease in the preterm. Other factors, such as genetic background, race, and fetal sex, are not discussed in this chapter. Finally, the diagnoses of RDS and BPD are imprecise and also represent spectrums of severity. The pathophysiology that accompanies RDS or BPD results in large part from how the preterm is managed clinically. As clinicians, we can understand populations of infants, but we are poor at predicting the outcomes for individual very preterm infants. Our failures result from a lack of a basic understanding of how lung developmental programs interact with injury programs and repair programs that are superimposed during the fetal period on the abnormalities that result in preterm delivery. The fetus then is assaulted by postnatal events—oxygen, mechanical ventilation, infection. It is a wonder of nature that very low-birth-weight infants can survive and that most of the survivors have relatively normal lung function in childhood.

References

1. McElrath TF, Hecht JL, Dammann O, et al. Pregnancy disorders that lead to delivery before the 28th week of gestation: an epidemiologic approach to classification. *Am J Epidemiol*. 2008;168: 980-989.
2. Martinez FD. Respiratory syncytial virus bronchiolitis and the pathogenesis of childhood asthma. *Pediatr Infect Dis J*. 2003;22:S76-S82.
3. Tita AT, Landon MB, Spong CY, et al. Timing of elective repeat cesarean delivery at term and neonatal outcomes. *N Engl J Med*. 2009;360:111-120.
4. Cheng YW, Nicholson JM, Nakagawa S, et al. Perinatal outcomes in low-risk term pregnancies: do they differ by week of gestation? *Am J Obstet Gynecol*. 2008;199:370 e371-e377.
5. Joseph KS, Nette F, Scott H, Vincer MJ. Prenatal corticosteroid prophylaxis for women delivering at late preterm gestation. *Pediatrics*. 2009;124:e835-e843.
6. Stoll BJ, Hansen NI, Bell EF, et al. Neonatal outcomes of extremely preterm infants from the NICHD Neonatal Research Network. *Pediatrics*. 2010;126:443-456.
7. Burri PH. Structural aspects of prenatal and postnatal development and growth of the lung. In: McDonald JA, ed. *Lung Growth and Development*. New York: Marcel Dekker, Inc.; 1997:1-35.
8. Ochs M, Nyengaard JR, Jung A, et al. The number of alveoli in the human lung. *Am J Respir Crit Care Med*. 2004;169:120-124.
9. Coalson JJ, Winter V, deLemos RA. Decreased alveolarization in baboon survivors with bronchopulmonary dysplasia. *Am J Respir Crit Care Med*. 1995;152:640-646.
10. Burri PH. Structural aspects of postnatal lung development—alveolar formation and growth. *Biol Neonate*. 2006;89:313-322.

11. Schittny JC, Mund SI, Stampanoni M. Evidence and structural mechanism for late lung alveolarization. *Am J Physiol Lung Cell Mol Physiol*. 2008;294:L246-L254.
12. Balinotti JE, Chakr VC, Tiller C, et al. Growth of lung parenchyma in infants and toddlers with chronic lung disease of infancy. *Am J Respir Crit Care Med*. 2010;181:1093-1097.
13. Avery ME, Mead J. Surface properties in relation to atelectasis and hyaline membrane disease. *Am J Dis Child*. 1959;97:517-523.
14. Gluck L, Kulovich M, Borer RC, et al. Diagnosis of the respiratory distress syndrome by amniocentesis. *Am J Obstet Gynecol*. 1971;109:440-445.
15. Hallman M, Kulovich M, Kirkpatrick E, et al. Phosphatidylinositol and phosphatidylglycerol in amniotic fluid: indices of lung maturity. *Am J Obstet Gynecol*. 1976;125:613-617.
16. Verder H, Albertsen P, Ebbesen F, et al. Nasal continuous positive airway pressure and early surfactant therapy for respiratory distress syndrome in newborns of less than 30 weeks' gestation. *Pediatrics*. 1999;103:E24.
17. Morley CJ, Davis PG, Doyle LW, et al. Nasal CPAP or intubation at birth for very preterm infants. *N Engl J Med*. 2008;358:700-708.
18. Finer NN, Carlo WA, Walsh MC, et al. Early CPAP versus surfactant in extremely preterm infants. *N Engl J Med*. 2010;362:1970-1979.
19. Ammari A, Suri MS, Milisavljevic V, et al. Variables associated with the early failure of nasal CPAP in very low birth weight infants. *J Pediatr*. 2005;147:341-347.
20. Mulrooney N, Champion Z, Moss TJ, et al. Surfactant and physiological responses of preterm lambs to continuous positive airway pressure. *Am J Respir Crit Care Med*. 2005;171:1-6.
21. Bland RD, Ertsey R, Mokres LM, et al. Mechanical ventilation uncouples synthesis and assembly of elastin and increases apoptosis in lungs of newborn mice: Prelude to defective alveolar septation during lung development? *Am J Physiol Lung Cell Mol Physiol*. 2008;294:L3-L14.
22. Mokres LM, Parai K, Hilgendorff A, et al. Prolonged mechanical ventilation with air induces apoptosis and causes failure of alveolar septation and angiogenesis in lungs of newborn mice. *Am J Physiol Lung Cell Mol Physiol*. 2010;298:L23-L35.
23. Antenatal Corticosteroids Revisited: Repeat Courses. NIH Consens Statement Online. 2000;17: 1-10.
24. Consensus development panel on the effect of corticosteroids for fetal maturation on perinatal outcomes. *JAMA*. 1995;273:413-418.
25. Roberts D, Dalziel S. Antenatal corticosteroids for accelerating fetal lung maturation for women at risk of preterm birth. *Cochrane Database Syst Rev*. 2006;(3):CD004454.
26. Brownfoot FC, Crowther CA, Middleton P. Different corticosteroids and regimens for accelerating fetal lung maturation for women at risk of preterm birth. *Cochrane Database Syst Rev*. 2008;(4): CD006764.
27. Hayes EJ, Paul DA, Stahl GE, et al. Effect of antenatal corticosteroids on survival for neonates born at 23 weeks of gestation. *Obstet Gynecol*. 2008;111:921-926.
28. Bunton TE, Plopper CG. Triamcinolone-induced structural alterations in the development of the lung of the fetal rhesus macaque. *Am J Obstet Gynecol*. 1984;148:203-215.
29. Jobe AH, Newnham J, Willet K, et al. Fetal versus maternal and gestational age effects of repetitive antenatal glucocorticoids. *Pediatrics*. 1998;102:1116-1125.
30. Willet KE, Jobe AH, Ikegami M, et al. Lung morphometry after repetitive antenatal glucocorticoid treatment in preterm sheep. *American Journal Respiratory and Critical Care Medicine*. 2001;163: 1437-1443.
31. Ikegami M, Polk D, Jobe A. Minimum interval from fetal betamethasone treatment to postnatal lung responses in preterm lambs. *Am J Obstet Gynecol*. 1996;174:1408-1413.
32. Elkady T, Jobe AH. Corticosteroids and surfactant increase lung volumes and decrease rupture pressures of preterm rabbit lungs. *J Appl Physiol*. 1987;63:1616-1621.
33. Willet KE, Jobe AH, Ikegami M, et al. Pulmonary interstitial emphysema following intrauterine exposure to glucocorticoids in preterm sheep. *Am J Respir Crit Care Med*. 2000;162:1087-1094.
34. Jobe AH, Mitchell BR, Gunkel JH. Beneficial effects of the combined use of prenatal corticosteroids and postnatal surfactant on preterm infants. *Am J Obstet Gynecol*. 1993;168:508-513.
35. Ikegami M, Polk D, Tabor B, et al. Corticosteroid and thyrotropin-releasing hormone effects on preterm sheep lung function. *J Appl Physiol*. 1991;70:2268-2278.
36. Ikegami M, Jobe AH, Yamada T, Seidner S. Relationship between alveolar saturated phosphatidylcholine pool sizes and compliance of preterm rabbit lungs: The effect of maternal corticosteroid treatment. *Am Rev Respir Dis*. 1989;139:367-369.
37. Seidner S, Pettenazzo A, Ikegami M, Jobe A. Corticosteroid potentiation of surfactant dose response in preterm rabbits. *J Appl Physiol*. 1988;64:2366-2371.
38. Ueda T, Ikegami M, Jobe AH. Developmental changes of sheep surfactant: in vivo function and in vitro subtype conversion. *J Appl Physiol*. 1994;76:2701-2706.
39. Hillman NH, Pillow JJ, Ball MK, et al. Antenatal and postnatal corticosteroid and resuscitation induced lung injury in preterm sheep. *Respir Res*. 2009;10:124.
40. Bachurski CJ, Ross GF, Ikegami M, et al. Intra-amniotic endotoxin increases pulmonary surfactant components and induces SP-B processing in fetal sheep. *Am J Physiol Lung Cell Mol Physiol*. 2001;280:L279-L285.
41. Laughon M, Allred EN, Bose C, et al. Patterns of respiratory disease during the first 2 postnatal weeks in extremely premature infants. *Pediatrics*. 2009;123:1124-1131.
42. Jobe AH, Nitsos I, Pillow JJ, et al. Betamethasone dose and formulation for induced lung maturation in fetal sheep. *American Journal of Obstetrics and Gynecology*. 2009;201:611 e611-617.

43. Onland W, de Laat M, Mol BW, Offringa M. Effects of antenatal corticosteroids given prior to 26 weeks' gestation: a systematic review of randomized controlled trials. *Am J Perinatol*. 2010.
44. Garite TJ, Rumney PJ, Briggs GG, et al. A randomized, placebo-controlled trial of betamethasone for the prevention of respiratory distress syndrome at 24 to 28 weeks' gestation. *Am J Obstet Gynecol*. 1992;166:646-651.
45. Ikegami M, Jobe AH, Newnham J, et al. Repetitive prenatal glucocorticoids improve lung function and decrease growth in preterm lambs. *Am J Respir Crit Care Med*. 1997;156:178-184.
46. Crowther CA, Harding JE. Repeat doses of prenatal corticosteroids for women at risk of preterm birth for preventing neonatal respiratory disease. *Cochrane Database Syst Rev*. 2007;(3):CD003935.
47. Murphy KE, Hannah ME, Willan AR, et al. Multiple courses of antenatal corticosteroids for preterm birth (MACS): a randomised controlled trial. *Lancet*. 2009;372:2143-2151.
48. Wapner RJ, Sorokin Y, Mele L, et al. Long-term outcomes after repeat doses of antenatal corticosteroids. *N Engl J Med*. 2007;357:1190-1198.
49. Crowther CA, Doyle LW, Haslam RR, et al. Outcomes at 2 years of age after repeat doses of antenatal corticosteroids. *N Engl J Med*. 2007;357:1179-1189.
50. Sinclair JC. Meta-analysis of randomized controlled trials of antenatal corticosteroid for the prevention of respiratory distress syndrome: discussion. *Am J Obstet Gynecol*. 1995;173:335-344.
51. Stutchfield P, Whitaker R, Russell I. Antenatal betamethasone and incidence of neonatal respiratory distress after elective caesarean section: pragmatic randomised trial. *BMJ*. 2005;331:662.
52. Stjernholm-Vladic Y, Stygar D, Mansson C, et al. Factors involved in the inflammatory events of cervical ripening in humans. *Reprod Biol Endocrinol*. 2004;2:74.
53. Marshall-Clarke S, Reen D, Tasker L, Hassan J. Neonatal immunity: how well has it grown up? *Immunol Today*. 2000;21:35-41.
54. Goldenberg RL, Culhane JF, Iams JD, Romero R. Epidemiology and causes of preterm birth. *Lancet*. 2008;371:75-84.
55. Goldenberg RL, Hauth JC, Andrews WW. Intrauterine infection and preterm delivery. *N Engl J Med*. 2000;342:1500-1507.
56. Redline RW, Wilson-Costello D, Borawski E, et al. Placental lesions associated with neurologic impairment and cerebral palsy in very low-birth-weight infants. *Arch Pathol Lab Med*. 1998;122: 1091-1098.
57. Romero R, Espinoza J, Chaiworapongsa T, Kalache K. Infection and prematurity and the role of preventive strategies. *Semin Neonatol*. 2002;7:259-274.
58. Yoon BH, Romero R, Jun JK, et al. Amniotic fluid cytokines (interleukin-6, tumor necrosis factor-alpha, interleukin-1 beta, and interleukin-8) and the risk for the development of bronchopulmonary dysplasia. *Am J Obstet Gynecol*. 1997;177:825-830.
59. DiGiulio DB, Romero R, Amogan HP, et al. Microbial prevalence, diversity and abundance in amniotic fluid during preterm labor: a molecular and culture-based investigation. *PLoS ONE*. 2008;3:e3056.
60. Buhimschi IA, Christner R, Buhimschi CS. Proteomic biomarker analysis of amniotic fluid for identification of intra-amniotic inflammation. *BJOG*. 2005;112:173-181.
61. Gerber S, Vial Y, Hohlfeld P, Witkin SS. Detection of *Ureaplasma urealyticum* in second-trimester amniotic fluid by polymerase chain reaction correlates with subsequent preterm labor and delivery. *J Infect Dis*. 2003;187:518-521.
62. Perni SC, Vardhana S, Korneeva I, et al. *Mycoplasma hominis* and *Ureaplasma urealyticum* in midtrimester amniotic fluid: association with amniotic fluid cytokine levels and pregnancy outcome. *Am J Obstet Gynecol*. 2004;191:1382-1386.
63. Onderdonk AB, Delaney ML, DuBois AM, et al. Detection of bacteria in placental tissues obtained from extremely low gestational age neonates. *Am J Obstet Gynecol*. 2008;198:110 e111-e117.
64. Hecht JL, Onderdonk A, Delaney M, et al. Characterization of chorioamnionitis in 2nd-trimester C-section placentas and correlation with microorganism recovery from subamniotic tissues. *Pediatr Dev Pathol*. 2008;11:15-22.
65. Oh KJ, Lee KA, Sohn YK, et al. Intraamniotic infection with genital mycoplasmas exhibits a more intense inflammatory response than intraamniotic infection with other microorganisms in patients with preterm premature rupture of membranes. *Am J Obstet Gynecol*. 2010;203:211 e211-e218.
66. Steel JH, Malatos S, Kennea N, et al. Bacteria and inflammatory cells in fetal membranes do not always cause preterm labor. *Pediatr Res*. 2005;57:404-411.
67. Reiman M, Kujari H, Ekholm E, et al. Interleukin-6 polymorphism is associated with chorioamnionitis and neonatal infections in preterm infants. *J Pediatr*. 2008;153:19-24.
68. Richardson CJ, Pomerance JJ, Cunningham MD, Gluck L. Acceleration of fetal lung maturation following prolonged rupture of the membranes. *Am J Obstet Gynecol*. 1974;118:1115-1118.
69. Watterberg KL, Demers LM, Scott SM, Murphy S. Chorioamnionitis and early lung inflammation in infants in whom bronchopulmonary dysplasia develops. *Pediatrics*. 1996;97:210-215.
70. Groneck P, Goetze-Speer B, Speer CP. Inflammatory bronchopulmonary response of preterm infants with microbial colonization of the airways at birth. *Arch Dis Child*. 1996;74:F51-F55.
71. De Dooy J, Colpaert C, Schuerwegh A, et al. Relationship between histologic chorioamnionitis and early inflammatory variables in blood, tracheal aspirates, and endotracheal colonization in preterm infants. *Pediatr Res*. 2003;54:113-119.
72. Costeloe K, Hennessy E, Gibson AT, et al. The EPICure study: outcomes to discharge from hospital for infants born at the threshold of viability. *Pediatrics*. 2000;106:659-671.
73. Hannaford K, Todd DA, Jeffery H, et al. Role of *Ureaplasma urealyticum* in lung disease of prematurity. *Arch Dis Child Fetal Neonatal Ed*. 1999;81:F162-F167.

A

74. Lahra MM, Beeby PJ, Jeffery HE. Maternal versus fetal inflammation and respiratory distress syndrome: a 10-year hospital cohort study. *Arch Dis Child Fetal Neonatal Ed*. 2009;94:F13-F16.
75. Lahra MM, Beeby PJ, Jeffery HE. Intrauterine inflammation, neonatal sepsis, and chronic lung disease: a 13-year hospital cohort study. *Pediatrics*. 2009;123:1314-1319.
76. Hitti J, Krohn MA, Patton DL, et al. Amniotic fluid tumor necrosis factor-alpha and the risk of respiratory distress syndrome among preterm infants. *Am J Obstet Gynecol*. 1997;177:50-56.
77. Ramsey PS, Lieman JM, Brumfield CG, Carlo W. Chorioamnionitis increases neonatal morbidity in pregnancies complicated by preterm premature rupture of membranes. *Am J Obstet Gynecol*. 2005;192:1162-1166.
78. Soraisham AS, Singhal N, McMillan DD, et al. A multicenter study on the clinical outcome of chorioamnionitis in preterm infants. *American Journal of Obstetrics and Gynecology*. 2009;200:372 e371-e376.
79. Van Marter LJ, Dammann O, Allred EN, et al. Chorioamnionitis, mechanical ventilation, and postnatal sepsis as modulators of chronic lung disease in preterm infants. *J Pediatr*. 2002; 140:171-176.
80. Been JV, Rours IG, Kornelisse RF, et al. Chorioamnionitis alters the response to surfactant in preterm infants. *Journal of Pediatrics*. 2010;156:10-15 e11.
81. Been JV, Rours IG, Kornelisse RF, et al. Histologic chorioamnionitis, fetal involvement, and antenatal steroids: effects on neonatal outcome in preterm infants. *Am J Obstet Gynecol*. 2009;201: 587 e1-e8.
82. Matoba N, Yu Y, Mestan K, et al. Differential patterns of 27 cord blood immune biomarkers across gestational age. *Pediatrics*. 2009;123:1320-1328.
83. Ambalavanan N, Carlo WA, D'Angio CT, et al. Cytokines associated with bronchopulmonary dysplasia or death in extremely low birth weight infants. *Pediatrics*. 2009;123:1132-1141.
84. Paananen R, Husa AK, Vuolteenaho R, et al. Blood cytokines during the perinatal period in very preterm infants: relationship of inflammatory response and bronchopulmonary dysplasia. *J Pediatr*. 2009;154:39-43 e33.
85. Been JV, Debeer A, van Iwaarden JF, et al. Early alterations of growth factor patterns in bronchoalveolar lavage fluid from preterm infants developing bronchopulmonary dysplasia. *Pediatr Res*. 2010;67:83-89.
86. Andrews WW, Goldenberg RL, Faye-Petersen O, et al. The Alabama Preterm Birth study: polymorphonuclear and mononuclear cell placental infiltrations, other markers of inflammation, and outcomes in 23- to 32-week preterm newborn infants. *Am J Obstet Gynecol*. 2006;195:803-808.
87. Goldenberg RL, Andrews WW, Goepfert AR, et al. The Alabama Preterm Birth Study: umbilical cord blood *Ureaplasma urealyticum* and *Mycoplasma hominis* cultures in very preterm newborn infants. *Am J Obstet Gynecol*. 2008;198:43 e41-e45.
88. Stoll BJ, Hansen N, Fanaroff AA, et al. Changes in pathogens causing early-onset sepsis in very-low-birth-weight infants. *N Engl J Med*. 2002;347:240-247.
89. Viscardi RM, Muhumuza CK, Rodriguez A, et al. Inflammatory markers in intrauterine and fetal blood and cerebrospinal fluid compartments are associated with adverse pulmonary and neurologic outcomes in preterm infants. *Pediatr Res*. 2004;55:1009-1017.
90. Bry K, Lappalainen U, Hallman M. Intraamniotic interleukin-1 accelerates surfactant protein synthesis in fetal rabbits and improves lung stability after premature birth. *J Clin Invest*. 1997;99: 2992-2999.
91. Kallapur SG, Willet KE, Jobe AH, et al. Intra-amniotic endotoxin: Chorioamnionitis precedes lung maturation in preterm lambs. *Am J Physiol*. 2001;280:L527-L536.
92. Kramer BW, Moss TJ, Willet K, et al. Dose and time response after intra-amniotic endotoxin in preterm lambs. *American Journal of Respiratory and Critical Care Medicine*. 2001;164:982-988.
93. Kramer BW, Kramer S, Ikegami M, Jobe A. Injury, inflammation and remodeling in fetal sheep lung after intra-amniotic endotoxin. *American Journal of Physiology Lung Cellular & Molecular Physiology*. 2002;283:L452-L459.
94. Kallapur SG, Bachurski CJ, Le Cras TD, et al. Vascular changes following intra-amniotic endotoxin in preterm lamb lungs. *Am J Physiol Lung Cell Mol Physiol*. 2004;287:L1178-L1185.
95. Jobe AH, Newnham JP, Willet KE, et al. Endotoxin induced lung maturation in preterm lambs is not mediated by cortisol. *Am J Respir Crit Care Med*. 2000;162:1656-1661.
96. Willet K, Jobe A, Ikegami M, et al. Antenatal endotoxin and glucocorticoid effects on lung morphometry in preterm lambs. *Pediatric Research*. 2000;48:782-788.
97. Bieghs V, Vlassaks E, Custers A, et al. Chorioamnionitis induced hepatic inflammation and disturbed lipid metabolism in fetal sheep. *Pediatric Research*. 2010;68:466-472.
98. Kallapur SG, Kramer BW, Moss TJ, et al. Maternal glucocorticoids increase endotoxin-induced lung inflammation in preterm lambs. *Am J Physiol Lung Cell Mol Physiol*. 2003;284:L633-L642.
99. Kramer BW, Ikegami M, Moss TJ, et al. Antenatal betamethasone changes cord blood monocyte responses to endotoxin in preterm lambs. *Pediatric Research*. 2004;55:764-768.
100. Moss TJ, Nitsos I, Kramer BW, et al. Intra-amniotic endotoxin induces lung maturation by direct effects on the developing respiratory tract in preterm sheep. *American Journal of Obstetrics and Gynecology*. 2002;187:1059-1065.
101. Sosenko IR, Jobe AH. Intra-amniotic endotoxin increases lung antioxidant enzyme activity in preterm lambs. *Pediatric Research*. 2003;53:679-683.
102. Kim YM, Romero R, Chaiworapongsa T, et al. Toll-like receptor-2 and -4 in the chorioamniotic membranes in spontaneous labor at term and in preterm parturition that are associated with chorioamnionitis. *Am J Obstet Gynecol*. 2004;191:1346-1355.

3

103. Steel JH, O'Donoghue K, Kennea NL, et al. Maternal origin of inflammatory leukocytes in preterm fetal membranes, shown by fluorescence in situ hybridisation. *Placenta*. 2005;26:672-677.
104. Harju K, Glumoff V, Hallman M. Ontogeny of Toll-like receptors Tlr2 and Tlr4 in mice. *Pediatr Res*. 2001;49:81-83.
105. Hillman NH, Moss TJ, Nitsos I, et al. Toll-like receptors and agonist responses in the developing fetal sheep lung. *Pediatric Research*. 2008;63:388-393.
106. Kramer BW, Jobe AH. The clever fetus: responding to inflammation to minimize lung injury. *Biol Neonate*. 2005;88:202-207.
107. Moss TJ, Nitsos I, Ikegami M, et al. Experimental intra-uterine Ureaplasma infection in sheep. *American Journal of Obstetrics and Gynecology*. 2005;192:1179-1186.
108. Collins JJ, Kallapur SG, Knox CL, et al. Inflammation in fetal sheep from intra-amniotic injection of *Ureaplasma parvum*. *Am J Physiol Lung Cell Mol Physiol*. 2010;299:L852-L860.
109. Ikegami M, Moss TJ, Kallapur SG, et al. Minimal lung and systemic responses to TNFα in preterm sheep. *American Journal of Physiology*. 2003;285:L121-L129.
110. Moss TM, Newnham J, Willet K, et al. Early gestational Intra-amniotic endotoxin: Lung function, surfactant and morphometry. *American Journal of Respiratory and Critical Care Medicine*. 2002;165: 805-811.
111. Watterberg KL, Scott SM, Naeye RL. Chorioamnionitis, cortisol, and acute lung disease in very low birth weight infants. *Pediatrics*. 1997;99:E6.
112. Kallapur SG, Moss TJ, Newnham JP, et al. Recruited inflammatory cells mediate endotoxin-induced lung maturation in preterm fetal lambs. *American Journal of Respiratory and Critical Care Medicine*. 2005;172:1315-1321.
113. Kallapur SG, Nitsos I, Moss TJ, et al. IL-1 mediates pulmonary and systemic inflammatory responses to chorioamnionitis induced by lipopolysaccharide. *American Journal of Respiratory and Critical Care Medicine*. 2009;179:955-961.
114. Hodgman JE. Relationship between Wilson-Mikity syndrome and the new bronchopulmonary dysplasia. *Pediatrics*. 2003;112:1414-1415.
115. Kallapur SG, Nitsos I, Moss TJ, et al. Chronic endotoxin exposure does not cause sustained structural abnormalities in the fetal sheep lungs. *American Journal of Physiology Lung Cellular & Molecular Physiology*. 2005;288:L966-L974.
116. Polglase GR, Hillman NH, Pillow JJ, et al. Ventilation mediated injury following preterm delivery of Ureaplasma colonized fetal lambs. *Pediatr Res*. 2010;67:630-635.
117. Ikegami M, Jobe A. Postnatal lung inflammation increased by ventilation of preterm lambs exposed antenatally to *E. coli* endotoxin. *Pediatric Research*. 2002;52:356-362.
118. Kramer BW, Joshi SN, Moss TJ, et al. Endotoxin-induced maturation of monocytes in preterm fetal sheep lung. *Am J Physiol Lung Çell Mol Physiol*. 2007;293:L345-L353.
119. Kramer BW, Kallapur SG, Moss TJ, et al. Modulation of fetal inflammatory response on exposure to lipopolysaccharide by chorioamnion, lung, or gut in sheep. *American Journal of Obstetrics and Gynecology*. 2009;202:77 e71-e79.
120. Kallapur SG, Jobe AH, Ball MK, et al. Pulmonary and systemic endotoxin tolerance in preterm fetal sheep exposed to chorioamnionitis. *J Immunol*. 2007;179:8491-8499.
121. Kramer BW, Kallapur SG, Moss TJ, et al. Intra-amniotic LPS modulation of TLR signaling in lung and blood monocytes of fetal sheep. *Innate Immun*. 2009;15:101-107.
122. Lee AJ, Lambertmont VA, Pillow JJ, et al. Fetal responses to lipopolysaccharide-induced chorioamnionitis alter immune and airway responses in 7-week-old sheep. *American Journal of Obstetrics and Gynecology*. 2011;204:364 e17-e24.
123. Harding JE, Pang J, Knight DB, Liggins GC. Do antenatal corticosteroids help in the setting of preterm rupture of membranes? *Am J Obstet Gynecol*. 2001;184:131-139.
124. Goldenberg RL, Andrews WW, Faye-Petersen OM, et al. The Alabama preterm birth study: corticosteroids and neonatal outcomes in 23- to 32-week newborns with various markers of intrauterine infection. *Am J Obstet Gynecol*. 2006;195:1020-1024.
125. Been JV, Degraeuwe PL, Kramer BW, Zimmermann LJ. Antenatal steroids and neonatal outcome after chorioamnionitis: a meta-analysis. *BJOG*. 2011;118:113-122.
126. Newnham J, Kallapur SG, Kramer BW, et al. Betamethasone effects on chorioamnionitis induced by intra-amniotic endotoxin in sheep. *American Journal of Obstetrics and Gynecology*. 2003;189: 1458-1466.
127. Newnham JP, Moss TJ, Padbury JF, et al. The interactive effects of endotoxin with prenatal glucocorticoids on short-term lung function in sheep. *Am J Obstet Gynecol*. 2001;185:190-197.
128. Moss TJM, Nitsos I, Knox CL, et al. Ureaplasma colonization of amniotic fluid and efficacy of antenatal corticosteroids for preterm lung maturation in sheep. *American Journal of Obstetrics and Gynecology*. 2009;200:96 e1-e6.
129. Kramer BW, Ikegami M, Moss TJ, et al. Endotoxin-induced chorioamnionitis modulates innate immunity of monocytes in preterm sheep. *Am J Respir Crit Care Med*. 2005;171:73-77.
130. Kramer BW, Ikegami M, Moss TJ, et al. Antenatal betamethasone changes cord blood monocyte responses to endotoxin in preterm lambs. *Pediatr Res*. 2004;55:764-768.
131. Zeitlin J, El Ayoubi M, Jarreau PH, et al. Impact of fetal growth restriction on mortality and morbidity in a very preterm birth cohort. *J Pediatr*. 2010;157:733-739 e1.
132. Tyson JE, Kennedy K, Broyles S, Rosenfeld CR. The small for gestational age infant: Accelerated or delayed pulmonary maturation? Increased or decreased survival? *Pediatrics*. 1995;95:534-538.
133. Chang EY, Menard MK, Vermillion ST, et al. The association between hyaline membrane disease and preeclampsia. *Am J Obstet Gynecol*. 2004;191:1414-1417.

A

134. Jelin AC, Cheng YW, Shaffer BL, et al. Early-onset preeclampsia and neonatal outcomes. *J Matern Fetal Neonatal Med*. 2010;23:389-392.
135. Garite TJ, Clark R, Thorp JA. Intrauterine growth restriction increases morbidity and mortality among premature neonates. *Am J Obstet Gynecol*. 2004;191:481-487.
136. Reiss I, Landmann E, Heckmann M, et al. Increased risk of bronchopulmonary dysplasia and increased mortality in very preterm infants being small for gestational age. *Arch Gynecol Obstet*. 2003;269:40-44.
137. Bose C, Van Marter LJ, Laughon M, et al. Fetal growth restriction and chronic lung disease among infants born before the 28th week of gestation. *Pediatrics*. 2009;124:e450-e458.
138. Hansen AR, Barnes CM, Folkman J, McElrath TF. Maternal preeclampsia predicts the development of bronchopulmonary dysplasia. *Journal of Pediatrics*. 2009;156:532-536.
139. Torrance HL, Derks JB, Scherjon SA, et al. Is antenatal steroid treatment effective in preterm IUGR fetuses? *Acta Obstet Gynecol Scand*. 2009;88:1068-1073.
140. Lipsett J, Tamblyn M, Madigan K, et al. Restricted fetal growth and lung development: a morphometric analysis of pulmonary structure. *Pediatr Pulmonol*. 2006;41:1138-1145.
141. Orgeig S, Crittenden TA, Marchant C, et al. Intrauterine growth restriction delays surfactant protein maturation in the sheep fetus. *Am J Physiol Lung Cell Mol Physiol*. 2010;298:L575-L583.
142. Gortner L, Hilgendorff A, Bahner T, et al. Hypoxia-induced intrauterine growth retardation: effects on pulmonary development and surfactant protein transcription. *Biol Neonate*. 2005;88:129-135.
143. Miller SL, Supramaniam VG, Jenkin G, et al. Cardiovascular responses to maternal betamethasone administration in the intrauterine growth-restricted ovine fetus. *Am J Obstet Gynecol*. 2009;201:613 e1-e8.
144. Miller SL, Chai M, Loose J, et al. The effects of maternal betamethasone administration on the intrauterine growth-restricted fetus. *Endocrinology*. 2007;148:1288-1295.
145. Pierce RA, Nguyen NM. Prenatal nicotine exposure and abnormal lung function. *Am J Respir Cell Mol Biol*. 2002;26:10-13.
146. Blacquiere MJ, Timens W, Melgert BN, et al. Maternal smoking during pregnancy induces airway remodelling in mice offspring. *Eur Respir J*. 2009;33:1133-1140.
147. Hylkema MN, Blacquiere MJ. Intrauterine effects of maternal smoking on sensitization, asthma, and chronic obstructive pulmonary disease. *Proc Am Thorac Soc*. 2009;6:660-662.
148. Lieberman E, Torday J, Barbieri R, et al. Association of intrauterine cigarette smoke exposure with indices of fetal lung maturation. *Obstet Gynecol*. 1992;79:564-570.
149. Rehan VK, Wang Y, Sugano S, et al. In utero nicotine exposure alters fetal rat lung alveolar type II cell proliferation, differentiation, and metabolism. *Am J Physiol Lung Cell Mol Physiol*. 2007;292: L323-L333.
150. Elliot JG, Carroll NG, James AL, Robinson PJ. Airway alveolar attachment points and exposure to cigarette smoke in utero. *Am J Respir Crit Care Med*. 2003;167:45-49.
151. Sozo F, O'Day L, Maritz G, et al. Repeated ethanol exposure during late gestation alters the maturation and innate immune status of the ovine fetal lung. *Am J Physiol Lung Cell Mol Physiol*. 2009;296:L510-L518.
152. Joshi PC, Guidot DM. The alcoholic lung: epidemiology, pathophysiology, and potential therapies. *Am J Physiol Lung Cell Mol Physiol*. 2007;292:L813-L823.

3

CHAPTER 4

Hypoxia and Hyperoxia: Effects on the Newborn Pulmonary Circulation

Stephen Wedgwood, PhD, Paul T. Schumacker, PhD, and
Robin H. Steinhorn, MD

4

- **Overview of Reactive Oxygen Species**
- **Hypoxia and the Pulmonary Circulation**
- **Hyperoxia and the Pulmonary Circulation**
- **Therapeutic Implications**

Oxygen is one of the most abundant elements on the earth and in the known universe. The lung is the human organ that is exposed to the highest concentrations of atmospheric oxygen, and as such, it has developed an intricate array of responses to alterations in oxygen concentrations. Neonatal life is particularly interesting in this regard, because the fetus must survive and grow in a relatively hypoxic environment and then adapt within minutes to an oxygen-rich atmosphere. This chapter discusses how the pulmonary vasculature responds to acute and chronic hypoxia and hyperoxia, focusing especially on the role of reactive oxygen species as mediators of these responses.

Overview of Reactive Oxygen Species

The vascular effects of both hypoxia and hyperoxia are mediated largely through the formation of reactive oxygen species (ROS). ROS are small molecules derived from molecular oxygen that serve as important vascular signaling molecules, as regulators of vascular tone and function, and as a potential source of vascular injury through their interaction with proteins, DNA, RNA, and lipids.[1,2] Multiple enzymatic oxidase systems can contribute to generation of ROS in vessel walls, and each system has specific roles in vascular physiology and pathophysiology. Antioxidant systems also regulate vascular signaling pathways by scavenging ROS. In the endothelium, mitochondria, xanthine oxidase, cytochrome P-450, and cyclooxygenase can generate ROS that influence vascular function, whereas under stress conditions, an uncoupling of endothelial nitric oxide synthase (eNOS) can also contribute (Fig. 4-1).[3,4] In vascular smooth muscle, nicotinamide adenine dinucleotide phosphate (reduced form) (NADPH) oxidases (Noxs) and mitochondria can function as significant sources of ROS generation.[5-9]

ROS-generating systems donate an electron to molecular oxygen to generate superoxide anion (O_2^-), the precursor for hydrogen peroxide and other reactive species. Superoxide dismutases (SODs) generate hydrogen peroxide (H_2O_2) through dismutation of superoxide, although spontaneous dismutation can occur at low pH even in the absence of SOD. H_2O_2 induces vasoconstriction, which is blocked by scavengers such as catalase and glutathione peroxidase. In the presence of SOD, superoxide is relatively short-lived, and its negative charge renders it relatively impermeable to biologic membranes. By contrast, H_2O_2 has a longer half-life, is uncharged, and is freely diffusible through aquaporins in membranes. As such, H_2O_2 is an important intracellular and extracellular signaling molecule. Superoxide can also react with other radicals, such as nitric oxide (NO^-) to form peroxynitrite

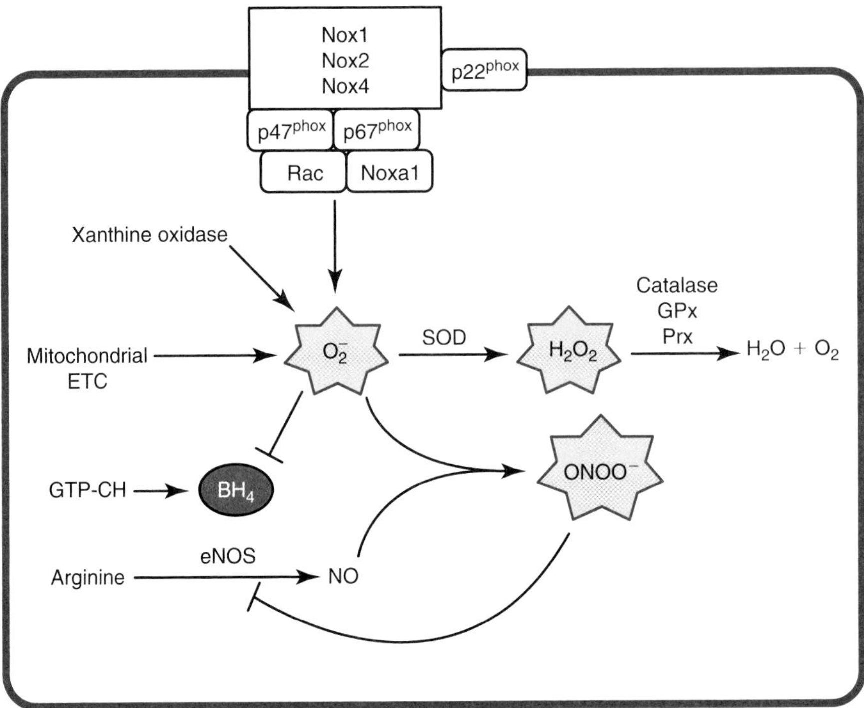

Figure 4-1 Schematic of cellular sources of reactive oxygen species as outlined in the first part of this chapter. BH_4, tetrahydrobiopterin; eNOS, endothelial nitric oxide synthase; ETC, electron transport chain; GPx, glutathione peroxidase; GTP-CH_1, guanosine triphosphate–cyclohydrolase; H_2O_2, hydrogen peroxide; NO, nitric oxide; Nox, nicotinamide adenine dinucleotide phosphate (reduced form) (NADPH) oxidase; $ONOO^-$, peroxynitrite; Prx, peroxiredoxin; SOD, superoxide dismutase. Other abbreviations in figure are names of protein subunits; see text for details.

($ONOO^-$), an exceptionally reactive oxidant that can promote vascular dysfunction by nonspecific nitration of proteins, with significant consequences for their functions. In the presence of iron, H_2O_2 can generate hydroxyl radicals through the Fenton reaction. However, these highly reactive radicals are unlikely to participate in signaling pathways and are therefore exclusively involved in cell damage responses.

Cellular Sources of Reactive Oxygen Species

Mitochondrial Electron Transport Chain

Mitochondria were the first described cellular source of ROS.[10] During normal oxidative phosphorylation, most of the electrons traveling down the mitochondrial electron transport chain (ETC) are transferred to molecular oxygen at the terminal cytochrome oxidase, generating H_2O. However, a small fraction of these electrons are captured by O_2 at more proximal sites, resulting in the formation of superoxide radical. Superoxide generated at complex I, II or III of the ETC can result in oxidant stress in the mitochondrial matrix or intermembrane space, depending on the site of formation.[11] In some conditions, such as atherosclerosis, the mitochondria appear to become dysfunctional and the leak of electrons is enhanced.[12] Angiotensin II is believed to increase ROS generation via mechanisms involving Nox isoforms in the endothelium,[13] whereas mitochondrial ROS appear to trigger increased Nox activity in hypoxic pulmonary arteries,[14] suggesting an important interplay between these sources of ROS. A full understanding of the mechanisms by which ligand-receptor interactions at the plasma membrane trigger ROS production, and the targets of those signals, has not yet been established. Nevertheless, receptor-mediated ROS signaling appears to be critical for initiating the physiologic cellular responses to vasoactive agonists.

NADPH Oxidases

Noxs were first discovered in phagocytes as the enzymes responsible for the respiratory burst. Seven Nox enzymatic subtypes have since been identified in a wide range of cell types, which include vascular cell expression of the Nox1, Nox2, and Nox4 homologs. Nox enzymes transfer electrons from NADPH to molecular oxygen, producing superoxide intracellularly or extracellularly, depending on the isoforms and the subcellular location of the enzyme. Each of these Nox family members is regulated by specific physiologic mechanisms, and dysregulation of expression or activity may transition oxidant signaling into oxidant stress in vascular cells in the lung, thereby contributing to pulmonary vascular dysfunction. However, major questions remain regarding how Nox systems are regulated by interaction with other proteins and posttranslational modifications.

4

Nox1 is expressed in vascular smooth muscle, endothelium, and adventitia[15,16] and has been localized to membranes, including plasma membranes,[17] caveolae,[6] and endosomes.[18] Nox1 activity requires the association with other protein subunits, including $p22^{phox}$, $p47^{phox}$, Noxa1, and Rac.[16,19] Because superoxide neutralizes the vasodilatory effects of NO, Nox1 would be expected to induce vasoconstriction, and its role in vascular signaling has been studied primarily in systemic hypertension. In vascular smooth muscle, stretch, various growth factors, and inflammatory mediators (e.g., interleukin 1β [IL-1β]) induce Nox1 expression, but other agonists, such as angiotensin II, appear to stimulate upstream signaling cascades that lead to enzyme activation.[20] Studies using several animal models have strongly implicated Nox1 in vascular dysfunction due to vascular inflammation and angiotensin II–induced hypertension.[21,22] Nox1 stimulates vascular smooth muscle proliferation,[15] suggesting that it may also play a role in vascular remodeling associated with hypertension. Together these findings have identified Nox1 as an attractive target for the treatment of vascular disease.

The Nox2 isoform is expressed in phagocytic cells as well as in cells constituting the vascular wall and is activated by pathways very similar to those for Nox1. It requires assembly of protein subunits, including $p22^{phox}$, $p47^{phox}$, $p67^{phox}$ and Rac, for activation. Nox2 is perhaps the best characterized system in terms of its regulation, in which phosphorylation of the p47 subunit by protein kinase C triggers assembly of the complex.[23] When assembled in the plasma membrane, Nox2 secretes superoxide into the extracellular space, but when endocytotic vesicles arising from the plasma membrane are formed, the superoxide is secreted into the lysosome.[24,25] Like Nox 1, Nox2 produces superoxide that is associated with vasoconstriction. Nox2 expression correlates inversely with endothelium-dependent relaxation in aorta,[26,27] whereas increased Nox2 subunit expression was found to raise superoxide levels and impair pulmonary vasorelaxation in both lamb and piglet models of neonatal pulmonary hypertension.[28,29] Studies in transgenic mice have implicated Nox2 in hypertension induced by hypoxia,[30] deoxycorticosterone acetate (DOCA)–salt,[31] and renal artery clipping,[32] but Nox2 knockout had no effect on hypertension induced by angiotensin II.[33]

Nox4 is much more abundantly expressed in vascular cells than are Nox1 and Nox2.[34-36] Nox4 was initially thought to require only $p22^{phox}$ for activity and to be constitutively active,[37] although newer data indicate that polymerase delta interacting protein 2 (Poldip2) may interact with Nox4 to enhance its activity.[38] Nox4 activity appears to be regulated primarily by expression, and its expression is upregulated by stimuli such as shear stress and transforming growth factor β (TGF-β) in vascular cells.[19,22] Nox4 has been shown to generate both superoxide and H_2O_2, depending on the stimulus and the cell type,[39] and Nox4 has been implicated in the regulation of several cellular processes including migration, growth, and differentiation.[20] Nox4 may also contribute to hypoxia-induced pulmonary hypertension,[40] although data from genetic models with altered Nox4 expression are just emerging, and the question of whether Nox4 participates in hypoxia-induced pulmonary vascular remodeling is not yet established.

All of these Nox enzymes contribute to normal vascular function through their modulation of intracellular signaling pathways, and their expression in different cellular subcompartments likely indicates that each plays a distinct role. Abnormal regulation of the expression and activities of these isoenzymes alone or in combination can result in the development of vascular disease. Furthermore, ROS can activate Nox expression and activity, resulting in further ROS generation and creating a positive feedback loop.[15,41-43] Additional studies are needed to identify targets associated with the deleterious mechanisms of Nox-induced ROS that also leave intact those pathways that are required for normal vascular function.

A

Nitric Oxide Synthase

Endothelial NOS converts L-arginine and molecular oxygen to L-citrulline and the vasodilator NO using O_2 as well as electrons from NADPH, and is thus an important regulator of vascular tone. The activity of eNOS is normally regulated by cytosolic calcium levels, which bind to a calmodulin subunit of the complex. In addition, phosphoinositide 3-kinase (PI3K) signaling leads to activation of eNOS in response to its phosphorylation by the protein kinase Akt. NO derived from eNOS activates soluble guanylate cyclase in vascular smooth muscle, leading to generation of cyclic guanosine monophosphate (cGMP) and vasodilation. Mechanisms that inhibit eNOS activity or attenuate downstream NO signaling can induce vasoconstriction. Newer data indicate that vasoconstriction is not only due to reduced production or bioavailability of NO, but that eNOS is also a potential source of ROS when the enzyme becomes "uncoupled," resulting in incomplete reduction of molecular oxygen with the formation of superoxide. eNOS uncoupling can occur via several mechanisms including degradation or oxidation of cofactors, such as tetrahydrobiopterin (BH_4) and heat shock protein 90 (Hsp90), or by inactivation of the enzyme through increased peroxynitrite levels.[42,44] Increased Nox activity may be an important trigger for eNOS uncoupling,[45,46] suggesting that abnormal regulation of ROS can promote oxidant production from additional sources, thus sustaining or amplifying a pathologic state.

Xanthine Oxidase

The endothelium-bound enzyme xanthine oxidase (XO) is another cellular source of superoxide, and increased XO activity was demonstrated in patients with idiopathic pulmonary arterial hypertension.[47] In endothelial cells, shear stress was found to activate XO in a Nox-dependent fashion.[13] These data suggest that crosstalk between different cellular sources of ROS contributes to the pathogenesis of vascular disease and hypertension. Increased superoxide generation by Nox and XO decreases bioavailable NO and attenuates vasodilation. The subsequent formation of peroxynitrite induces uncoupling of eNOS and mitochondria, resulting in a further increase in ROS generation and Nox expression.[20] A better characterization of the dysregulated pathways involved may lead to the identification of therapeutic targets for the treatment of diseases arising from increased vascular ROS generation.

Peroxynitrite

Vascular superoxide anions react with NO in a diffusion-limited reaction to form the highly reactive intermediate peroxynitrite, which has multiple nonspecific cellular targets, including protein tyrosine residues. Peroxynitrite is believed to contribute to various forms of cardiovascular, inflammatory, aging, and neurodegenerative diseases as well as to loss of vascular endothelium-dependent responses and impairment of myocardial contractility in some conditions. Its concentrations can be regulated by limiting superoxide generation or by enhancing superoxide scavenging by superoxide dismutases as described later. Peroxynitrite is highly reactive, and its lifetime is measured in nanoseconds. Like hydroxyl radicals, peroxynitrite is unlikely to participate in cell signaling pathways because it tends to react nonspecifically with virtually all biologic molecules. This lack of specificity limits its usefulness as a signaling molecule, although it likely contributes to nonspecific oxidant stress in disease states.

ROS Scavengers

Cells also regulate ROS levels through a wide variety of enzymatic scavengers that are developmentally regulated.[48,49] In general, the expression of these ROS scavengers is specific to certain subcellular compartments, so alterations in expression of an enzyme may affect oxidant stress in one compartment but not in another. Moreover, most antioxidant enzymes are selective for a single type of ROS molecule. For example, SOD degrades superoxide to H_2O_2 but is ineffective in degrading other species. By shortening the lifetime of superoxide, one might predict that SOD would also increase H_2O_2 in the cell, but this is not the case. The lifetime of H_2O_2 produced by SOD is regulated by the rate of degradation by enzymes such as glutathione peroxidase and peroxiredoxins.[50]

4

All mammalian tissues contain three forms of superoxide dismutase: Cu/ZnSOD (SOD1), MnSOD (SOD2), and extracellular superoxide dismutase (ecSOD or SOD3). Cu/ZnSOD is expressed in the cytosol and intermembrane space of the mitochondria, MnSOD is expressed in the matrix of mitochondria, and ecSOD is secreted to the extracellular space, where it binds to the extracellular matrix. The ecSOD activity is particularly worthy of additional discussion because it accounts for a significant component of the total SOD activity in blood vessel walls.[51] Extracellular SOD is a secretory Cu,Zn-containing protein with an SOD domain, a secretory signal, and a positively charged domain that mediates its attachment to the extracellular matrix. It is synthesized predominantly by the vascular smooth muscle cells. It is more highly expressed in the lung than in most other tissues,[52,53] and genetic deletion of ecSOD augments the lethality of hyperoxia in the mouse. Because ecSOD is believed to partition between cell surfaces and extracellular fluids, there may be a unique role for ecSOD in protecting against superoxide produced in extracellular spaces of the lung. Vascular ecSOD is present in high concentrations between the endothelium and smooth muscle surrounding blood vessels, the same domain that NO must pass through to stimulate smooth muscle relaxation. This finding suggests that high concentrations of ecSOD in this region are especially important in maintaining low superoxide concentrations and preserving NO function.[54] Finally, ecSOD can potentially permit paracrine oxidant signaling, by converting extracellular superoxide (secreted by Nox2-type systems) into H_2O_2, which can diffuse into nearby cells. MnSOD is localized to the mitochondria and is responsible for protecting against generation of excessive mitochondrial superoxide. Mice with homozygous deletion of the MnSOD gene die from oxidative stress shortly after birth.[55] Mice lacking one allele of MnSOD demonstrate hypertension with aging and in response to a high-salt diet,[56] whereas mice overexpressing MnSOD demonstrate attenuated angiotensin II–induced hypertension and Nox activity.[57]

Catalase, which is found in nearly every living organism, functions to catalyze the decomposition of H_2O_2 to water and oxygen. However, mice deficient in catalase develop normally, indicating that other, complementary antioxidant systems must be present.[58] The glutathione peroxidase (GPx) and peroxiredoxin systems utilize reduced glutathione to scavenge H_2O_2 and are therefore critical for minimizing oxidant stress and for regulating redox signaling pathways. GPx levels were found to be decreased in the lungs of patients with IPAH,[59] although genetic deletion of GPx-1 did not affect the rise in aortic pressure or vascular hypertrophy induced by angiotensin II.[60] By contrast, deletion of peroxiredoxin 1 (Prx-1) induces hemolytic anemia and a significant reduction in lifespan,[61] whereas deletion of Prx-3 leads to oxidant-mediated lung inflammation and an enhanced susceptibility to lipopolysaccharide challenge.[62]

Taken together, these data suggest that impaired endogenous antioxidant activity might contribute to ROS-induced vascular dysfunction and pulmonary hypertension. Furthermore, the targeting of exogenous antioxidants to specific subcellular locations may be more effective in treating vascular diseases than global antioxidants, which may also interfere with essential cellular signaling pathways.

A

Hypoxia and the Pulmonary Circulation

Acute Hypoxic Vasoconstriction

During placental respiration, the most highly oxygenated blood enters the fetus from the umbilical vein and must be efficiently directed to the systemic circulation after its return to the inferior vena cava and the right heart. In addition, in utero the lungs are filled with hypoxic amniotic fluid, so oxygen would be lost from the fetus if the pulmonary alveolar vessels were perfused with oxygenated blood. For efficient direction of oxygenated blood to the systemic circulation and minimizing of oxygen loss, almost 90% of fetal blood flow is diverted past the lungs through anatomic shunts through the foramen ovale and the ductus arteriosus. Blood flow in the pulmonary circulation is further restricted by hypoxia-induced constriction of small pulmonary arteries. This *hypoxic pulmonary vasoconstrictor response* is reversed at birth by the sudden increase in lung oxygenation when the newborn takes the first breath. However, the responsiveness to hypoxia is retained into adulthood, and pulmonary hypertension can be triggered by travel to high altitude, by hypoxic lung disease, or by intermittent obstructive sleep apnea.

Pulmonary arterial smooth muscle cells undergo calcium-dependent contraction in response to acute hypoxia, indicating that the O_2 responsiveness is intrinsic to vascular cells. The role of oxidant signaling in triggering this response has been controversial, with earlier work suggesting that decreases in ROS production may lead to redox-dependent closure of voltage-dependent potassium channels, plasma membrane depolarization, and entry of Ca^{2+} through voltage-dependent L-type channels.[63,64] However, later work has shown that hypoxia increases ROS production in pulmonary arterial smooth muscle cells, primarily from the mitochondria[65,66] but also from Nox4 in the cytosol.[67] These ROS signals trigger the release of intracellular calcium from the endoplasmic reticulum, which in turn triggers relocation of stromal interaction molecule 1 (STIM1, the endoplasmic reticulum Ca^{2+} sensor), to the plasma membrane, where it facilitates the assembly of calcium release–activated calcium (CRAC) channels.[68] In support of this model, one study showed that antioxidants abrogate the acute vasoconstriction response to hypoxia in the intact lung.[65] Moreover, increases in oxidant signaling are detected in pulmonary artery smooth muscle cells during acute hypoxia.[69,70] Interventions that augment the scavenging of ROS signals also attenuate the hypoxia-induced increases in cytosolic calcium in these cells.[71] Collectively, these observations suggest that oxidant signals are generated in pulmonary vascular cells during hypoxia and that these signals trigger the acute vasoconstriction response.

Chronic Hypoxia–Induced Pulmonary Hypertension

During chronic hypoxia, sustained constriction of pulmonary arteries causes pulmonary arterial hypertension, leading to right ventricular hypertrophy. If this condition persists for more than a few weeks, the walls of pulmonary arteries remodel through a process that involves hypertrophy and hyperplasia of smooth muscle cells and in some cases the endothelium.[30] After the vessels have remodeled, the pulmonary hypertension can become refractory to vasodilating drugs and the restoration of normoxia, most likely because reorganization of the extracellular matrix restricts the ability of the vessel to dilate. Although we tend to think of these events as a consequence of neonatal hypoxia due to lung disease or apnea, the fetus may also be subjected to chronic intrauterine hypoxia during gestation because of maternal or placental factors, and fetal lambs born after pregnancy at high altitude exhibit vascular remodeling and enhanced pulmonary constrictor responses that can persist despite return to sea level and even until adulthood.[72,73]

The role of oxidant signaling and oxidant stress in the hypoxia-induced remodeling process is not yet fully understood. A substantial number of studies tend to implicate oxidant stress as a causative or amplifying factor in the remodeling of pulmonary arteries in chronic hypoxia, but a clear identification of the systems contributing to the generation and clearance of ROS has not been established. Superoxide levels have been shown to be increased in the pulmonary arteries of mice exposed to 10% oxygen for 3 weeks.[30] Furthermore these increases, along with increases in right ventricular hypertrophy and pulmonary vascular remodeling, were found to be absent in mice lacking Nox2.[30] Increased Nox4 expression was also demonstrated in the pulmonary arteries of hypoxic mice and in the lungs of patients with idiopathic pulmonary arterial hypertension (IPAH),[40] although it is important to note that IPAH represents an entirely different class of pulmonary arterial hypertension from the form induced by chronic or intermittent hypoxia. In a mouse model of obstructive sleep apnea induced by long-term intermittent hypoxia, hypertension and vascular remodeling was associated with increased lung expression of $p22^{phox}$ and Nox4,[74] although these changes were attenuated in Nox2 knockout mice, indicating that more than one Nox isoform may be required for remodeling. Resolution of the role of the various Nox isoforms has been complicated by the absence of highly selective inhibitors of the Nox isoforms and by the possible involvement, interdependence, or redundancy among various Nox isoforms.

4

Other sources of ROS may also contribute to vascular remodeling responses. In hypoxia-exposed rats, lung XO activity was increased and treatment with the antioxidant *N*-acetylcysteine or with the XO inhibitor allopurinol attenuated hypoxia-induced vascular remodeling and hypertension.[75] Allopurinol also decreased both hypoxia-induced serum and lung XO activity and vascular superoxide and vascular remodeling, and partially restored endothelium-dependent arterial relaxation in rats.[76]

Activity of critical ROS scavengers may also be adversely affected by hypoxia. SOD1 expression was decreased in the pulmonary arteries of newborn piglets exposed to hypoxia.[77] Conversely, transgenic mice overexpressing ecSOD displayed attenuated chronic hypoxia-induced pulmonary hypertension, vascular remodeling, and redox-sensitive gene expression.[78]

If the generation of ROS is important, how might they contribute to the remodeling process? Hypoxia-induced mitochondrial ROS stabilize hypoxia-inducible factor 1α (HIF-1α),[79] a key transcription factor that can initiate or potentiate vascular remodeling via the upregulation of growth factors including vascular endothelial growth factor (VEGF).[80,81] $HIF\text{-}1\alpha^{+/-}$ heterozygous mice demonstrated less hypoxia-induced pulmonary hypertension and vascular remodeling than wild-type littermates.[82] Similarly, $HIF\text{-}2\alpha^{+/-}$ heterozygous mice displayed less vascular remodeling along with greater vasoconstrictor levels than wild-type mice.[83] Hypoxia failed to induce pulmonary hypertension and pulmonary arterial medial thickening in knockout mice lacking VEGF-B,[84] suggesting that this growth factor also plays a prominent role in hypoxia-induced vascular remodeling. However, a full analysis of the cell-specific roles of ROS signaling and HIF-1/HIF-2 in pulmonary hypertension has not yet emerged.

There has also been interest in how dysregulation of NOS function may contribute to pulmonary vascular disease induced by hypoxia. Overexpression of eNOS in transgenic mice has been reported to attenuate hypoxia-induced pulmonary hypertension and pulmonary arterial remodeling.[85] Moreover, augmentation of cGMP concentrations induced by the phosphodiesterase type 5 (PDE5) inhibitor sildenafil also blunt pulmonary vascular dysfunction and remodeling after exposure to hypoxia.[86] These findings have sparked interest in whether greater superoxide generation may also contribute to hypoxia-induced hypertension through impairment of NO signaling. In hypoxia-exposed rats, decreased eNOS activity was found to be associated with an abnormal interaction with its regulatory proteins.[87] Furthermore, augmenting synthesis of the eNOS cofactor tetrahydrobiopterin attenuated both the acute constrictor response to hypoxia and hypoxia-induced pulmonary hypertension.[88] In newborn piglets exposed to hypoxia, supplementation with L-citrulline to raise L-arginine levels was reported to attenuate pulmonary hypertension and increase NO production.[89] It appears that augmentation of NO-mediated vasodilation at multiple points within its signaling pathway may be helpful in blunting hypoxia-induced pulmonary hypertension.

Collectively, these studies indicate that increased ROS, arising from multiple sources, stimulate hypoxia-induced pulmonary hypertension by several mechanisms, including impaired NO-mediated vasodilation and increased growth factor–mediated vascular remodeling. Animal models of hypoxia may help identify additional strategies that can be used to augment the efficacy of therapies currently used to treat and/or prevent pulmonary hypertension.

A

Hyperoxia and the Pulmonary Circulation

Short-Term Effects of Hyperoxia

The fetus thrives in utero under relative hypoxic conditions, supported by the placenta. At birth, pulmonary vascular resistance (PVR) must rapidly drop to allow right ventricular output to be directed to the pulmonary circulation. The increase in oxygen tension that occurs at birth is one of the most important stimuli to facilitate this rapid transition. In approximately 10% of all deliveries, these transitional changes do not occur normally, leading to respiratory distress, hypoxemia, and pulmonary hypertension. As a result, it is not surprising that one of the first therapeutic uses of oxygen was for resuscitation of a newborn by Francoise Chaussier in 1780. Currently, high oxygen concentrations, up to 100% oxygen, are routinely used to treat hypoxemia and reverse pulmonary vasoconstriction in infants with neonatal pulmonary hypertension.[90] Until very recently, hyperoxic gas mixtures were also recommended whenever an infant required resuscitative measures. Although the use of hyperoxic gas mixtures may provide short-term benefits, there is an emerging understanding that hyperoxia may also greatly exaggerate oxidative stress in multiple cellular compartments of the normal and diseased pulmonary vasculature.

In order to better understand the acute effects of hyperoxia on the early transitional pulmonary vasculature, Lakshminrusimha and colleagues[91] ventilated healthy newborn lambs with 21%, 50%, or 100% oxygen for the first 30 minutes of life and found that initial ventilation with 100% oxygen decreased PVR more rapidly and to a greater degree than ventilation with 21% oxygen. All three groups were weaned to 21% oxygen and studied approximately 4 hours later to determine whether these early brief exposures to hyperoxia affected subsequent pulmonary vascular reactivity. Although pulmonary constrictor responses to hypoxia and thromboxane were similar in all the groups, a significant impairment of pulmonary dilator response to inhaled NO and endogenous NO (stimulated by acetylcholine) was selectively observed in the 100% oxygen group (Fig. 4-2). Additional groups of lambs were briefly ventilated with 100% or 21% oxygen at birth and recovered in 21% oxygen for a 24-hour period, followed by isolation of resistance pulmonary arteries for in vitro reactivity studies. Brief exposures to 100% oxygen resulted in significantly exaggerated contractile responses by the pulmonary arteries to norepinephrine and potassium chloride in comparison with responses of vessels from animals ventilated with 21% oxygen.[92] These studies indicate that the short-term pulmonary vascular benefits of hyperoxia need to be weighed against longer-lasting effects that increase contractility and diminish the vasodilator responses that are critical for the normal pulmonary vascular transition.

Many practitioners might be concerned that an infant born with pulmonary vascular remodeling will require resuscitation with hyperoxic gas mixtures to achieve sufficient early improvement in oxygenation and/or pulmonary vasodilation. Parallel studies performed in models of pulmonary hypertension have helped clarify the potential benefits for this population. In lambs with persistent pulmonary hypertension (PPHN), brief resuscitation with 21% and 50% oxygen did not significantly increase PaO_2 from fetal levels but did significantly decrease PVR, probably secondary to exposure to ventilation and a severalfold increase in alveolar oxygen levels.[95] Although 100% oxygen led to a greater rise in PaO_2, mean levels increased only to 40 ± 5 mm Hg. Surprisingly, and unlike in control lambs, ventilation with 100% O_2 did not enhance the decrease in pulmonary artery (PA) pressure or PVR or increase pulmonary blood flow more than 21% or 50% O_2. In addition, similar to what was

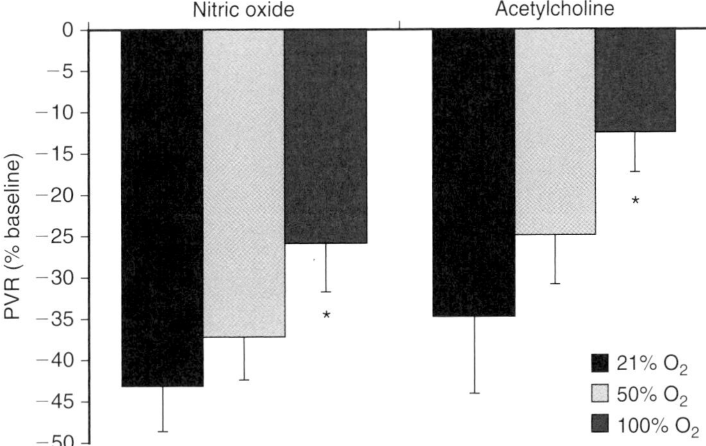

Figure 4-2 Healthy early newborn lambs were exposed to brief, 30-minute ventilations with 21%, 50%, or 100% oxygen immediately upon delivery. After return to room air for 2-3 hours, pulmonary hypertension was induced by a thromboxane analog. Pulmonary vascular relaxations to endogenous nitric oxide (NO) (as stimulated by acetylcholine) or inhaled NO were significantly blunted in the lambs that were initially resuscitated with 100% oxygen. (Adapted from Lakshminrusimha S, Russell JA, Steinhorn RH, et al. Pulmonary hemodynamics in neonatal lambs resuscitated with 21%, 50%, and 100% oxygen. *Pediatr Res.* 2007;62: 313-318.)

observed in healthy lambs, prior exposure to 100% oxygen significantly blunted the magnitude of response to inhaled NO.[95]

Because of the lack of obvious benefit and the potential for harm, the routine use of high oxygen concentrations for initial delivery room resuscitation is no longer recommended.[93] However, the optimal concentration of oxygen to treat hypoxemic respiratory failure and/or pulmonary hypertension in the neonatal intensive care unit (NICU) setting remains controversial and poorly studied. In clinical practice, only limited information (i.e., calculated alveolar PO_2 and measured arterial PO_2) is typically available to evaluate the relative effect of higher oxygen mixtures on pulmonary vasodilation. Rudolph and Yuan,[94] who first reported the relationship between PaO_2 and PVR in young, healthy calves in 1966, found that PVR rose steeply when the PaO_2 fell below 50 mm Hg but decreased minimally when the PaO_2 was more than 50 mm Hg. Equivalent studies in neonatal lambs ventilated with 10%, 21%, 50%, or 100% oxygen found striking similarity in the relationship between PaO_2 and PVR in both healthy lambs and lambs with PPHN (Fig. 4-3). Although both the normal and remodeled vasculature constricted vigorously in response to hypoxia, raising FIO_2 to greater than 50% or PaO_2 to more than 50 to 60 mm Hg produced little additional reduction of PVR in both groups.[91,95] These findings suggest that the vasodilatory effects of supplemental oxygen reach a plateau at about 50% oxygen or a PaO_2 of 50 to 60 mm Hg and are similar to previous clinical observations in children with bronchopulmonary dysplasia and pulmonary hypertension.[96]

If hyperoxia diminishes the vasodilator response to endogenous and exogenous NO, ROS generated during exposure to hyperoxia could affect multiple targets within the NO-cGMP signaling pathway. As the primary enzyme responsible for regulating cGMP concentrations in the vasculature, the cGMP-specific phosphodiesterase (PDE5) is a crucial regulator of NO-mediated vascular relaxation in the normal pulmonary vascular transition after birth.[97] A significant increase in pulmonary vascular PDE5 expression and activity was noted after ventilation with hyperoxia in both healthy and PPHN lambs, raising the possibility that PDE5 activity may serve as an important mediator in the vascular reactivity changes induced by oxygen and hyperoxia.[98,99]

Farrow and associates[98] extended these in vivo findings with more mechanistically oriented in vitro studies conducted in pulmonary artery smooth muscle cells

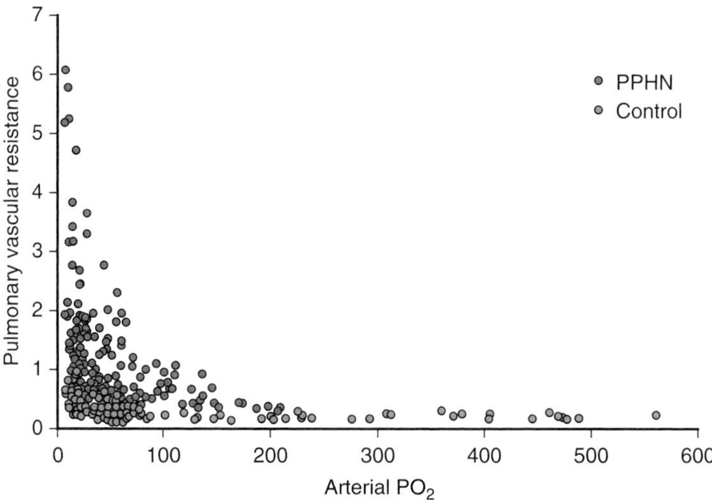

Figure 4-3 Changes in pulmonary vascular resistance (PVR) in 2- to 3-hour-old control lambs and lambs with persistent pulmonary hypertension (PPHN) in response to changes in inspired oxygen concentration. PVR in control and PPHN lambs significantly decreases when the oxygen concentration increases from 10 to 21 to 50% oxygen. Severe hypoxic vasoconstriction is observed in the PPHN lambs. However, PVR does not decrease further when oxygen is increased from 50% to 100% O_2 in either control or PPHN lambs. (Data replotted from Lakshminrusimha S, Swartz DD, Gugino SF, et al. Oxygen concentration and pulmonary hemodynamics in newborn lambs with pulmonary hypertension. *Pediatr Res.* 2009;66: 539-544.)

(PASMCs) isolated from healthy late-gestation fetal lambs. As might be expected, exposure to hyperoxia for 24 hours increased oxidative stress within fetal PASMCs. Furthermore, hyperoxia significantly blunted the expected rise in cGMP after exposure to exogenous NO. In addition, exposure of fetal pulmonary vascular cells to hyperoxia increased PDE5 mRNA and protein expression as well as phosphorylation and activity.[98] Like the findings in ventilated lambs, a dose-response effect of hyperoxia was noted, with a stepwise increase in PDE5 activity as oxygen levels rose from 21% to 50% to 95%. These results led to speculation that ROS may serve as critical mediators in crosstalk between oxygen and PDE5. In support of that hypothesis, a single dose of hydrogen peroxide (H_2O_2) was sufficient to induce changes in PDE5 expression, phosphorylation, and activity that mirrored those seen after exposure to hyperoxia. Because the effects of exogenously administered H_2O_2 would be expected to be transient, these last experiments are similar to the brief in vivo exposures to hyperoxia. Furthermore, the hyperoxia-induced changes in cGMP response and PDE5 expression and activity were reversed by pretreatment with a chemical antioxidant (*N*-acetylcysteine). Inhibition of PDE5 activity with sildenafil also partially rescued the cGMP response to exogenous NO, further confirming that hyperoxia affects cGMP signaling through increases in PDE5 activity.[98] 'The findings reported by Farrow and associates[98] confirm that ROS, in general, and H_2O_2, in particular, are sufficient to induce significant increases in PDE5 expression and activity in the PASMC that may promote vasoconstriction, poor NO response, and vascular remodeling.

Further experiments in pulmonary smooth muscle from lambs with PPHN found basal elevations in oxidant stress associated with depressed activity of extracellular SOD and elevated PDE5 activity relative to control pulmonary artery smooth muscle cells.[100,101] Hyperoxia exposure amplified these abnormalities in PPHN cells by increasing ROS, depressing ecSOD activity, and increasing PDE5 activity. Extracellular SOD facilitates NO-mediated vasodilation by removing extracellular superoxide and preventing the formation of peroxynitrite, so the inactivation of ecSOD may provide an additional explanation for the abnormalities in NO-cGMP signaling observed after ventilation of lambs with 100% oxygen. Interestingly, the changes in PDE5 activity were reversed with mitochondria-targeted catalase, indicating that targeting antioxidants to specific abnormalities in cellular subcompartmental production or clearance of ROS may eventually be possible.[100]

Chronic Hyperoxia

There is growing recognition that in preterm infants chronic lung disease is frequently associated with significant pulmonary hypertension and that abnormal vascular development can adversely affect parenchymal lung growth.[102] Although the studies previously described demonstrate that brief exposures to hyperoxia can induce vascular dysfunction in the newborn lung, long-term oxygen therapy is often required in preterm infants, and its relative benefits and risks for vascular function and development remain poorly understood.

In the first description of bronchopulmonary dysplasia (BPD), in 1967, Northway and coworkers[103] speculated that the condition might be partially due to oxygen toxicity. The development of surfactant improved survival for preterm infants but did not have a major affect on the overall incidence of BPD. The reason is likely that extremely preterm infants, born prior to 28 weeks of gestation, now routinely survive and must complete lung development from the late canalicular or saccular stage despite the presence of abnormal stimuli and stressors. Because the preterm lung is meant to grow in a low-oxygen intrauterine environment, it is ill-equipped to handle oxygen administration, and exposure even to normal ambient levels of oxygen represents relative hyperoxia at this critical developmental juncture. The "new BPD" is thus believed to be a form of arrested lung development that occurs when the preterm lung attempts to adapt to air breathing during this developmentally sensitive period. Later studies of BPD have also highlighted the interdependence of pulmonary vascular development and epithelial lung development—when one is damaged, the other appears likely to follow suit.

Several investigators have found evidence for early elevations in oxidant stress, in the form of elevated lipid or protein oxidation products, in infants who subsequently experience BPD.[104,105]

The alterations in pulmonary vascular signaling induced by hyperoxia, oxygen-dependent transcription factors, and ROS are therefore a subject of particularly intense investigation. Long-term exposure of neonatal rodents to high oxygen concentrations does not produce the early lethality noted in adult models. However, hyperoxia predictably causes structural changes that closely resemble those seen in human BPD, including alveolar simplification, abnormal pulmonary vascular development, and increased pulmonary vascular contractility[106,107]; these models have been used to explore potential mechanisms of oxidant-induced lung injury. Long-term oxygen exposure inhibits ecSOD activity, probably through peroxynitrite-mediated protein nitration,[101,108] and this inhibition would be expected to exacerbate elevations in ROS levels, diminish NO-mediated effects, and promote vascular dysfunction. Nox1 expression was found to be increased in mouse lung cell lines exposed to 72 hours of hyperoxia, whereas hyperoxia-induced ROS generation and lung injury was attenuated in Nox1-deficient mice.[109] Although most studies suggest that Nox2 and Nox4 are upregulated by hypoxia, later studies have shown that hyperoxia increases both Nox2 and Nox4 expression in human pulmonary artery endothelial cells studied in vitro.[110] It is possible that targeted Nox inhibition may attenuate ROS generation and improve NO signaling during hyperoxic exposure, although in one study, knockdown of one Nox isoform led to simultaneous upregulation of the other, suggesting the existence of compensatory mechanisms.[110] Also, Yang and colleagues[111] showed that hyperoxia activated the transcription factor nuclear factor κB (NF-κB) in the lungs of neonatal but not adult mice. Surprisingly, these researchers found that NF-κB activation reduced lung inflammation and increased neonatal tolerance of hyperoxia. Although the survival effect is counterintuitive, NF-κB can also activate pro-inflammatory genes such as tumor necrosis factor TN-α and interleukin-1β, which may contribute to abnormal lung development later in life.

A

Oxygen exposure also disrupts expression of other key transcriptional regulators of normal fetal development, such as HIF. Genetic inactivation of HIF-1 or HIF-2 is lethal in embryonic mice, and inhibition of HIF by oxygen administration may promote abnormal lung development in extremely premature neonates. The oxygen-dependent loss of VEGF is another probable contributor to these events, and the effects of HIF inhibition may be mediated in part by suppression of VEGF.[112] Later studies of genetic mouse models have provided evidence of a critical role for VEGF and its receptors during vascular development.[102] Loss of a single VEGF allele results in early embryonic lethality, and targeted disruption of the VEGF gene causes defective lung angiogenesis and early embryonic death. During fetal development, low oxygen tension and its mediators (including HIF) maintain VEGF expression, and exposure to oxygen suppresses these normal developmental patterns of expression. In support of this theory, decreased VEGF and VEGF receptor expression is found in animal models of BPD as well as in the lungs of premature infants who died with BPD.[113,114] Interestingly, NO production, which is also disrupted by preterm birth, not only mediates downstream effects of VEGF during lung development but also may upregulate VEGF expression.

Even later studies have explored whether neonatal hyperoxic exposure leads to long-term, or even permanent, alterations of vascular development and function. In one study, neonatal rat pups were exposed to 80% oxygen between postnatal days 3 and 10, followed by recovery in room air. At 6 months of age, the oxygen-exposed rats displayed higher blood pressure and systemic vascular dysfunction, associated with a trend toward elevations of vascular superoxide.[115] Yee and colleagues[116] exposed neonatal mice to 100% oxygen or room air between postnatal days 1 and 4, and then allowed them to return to room air. The investigators reported that at 67 weeks of age, the oxygen-exposed mice had right ventricular hypertrophy, pruning of the distal lung microvasculature, and nearly 50% mortality.[116] These studies raise the important concern that oxygen-induced pulmonary vascular remodeling and pulmonary hypertension in very low birth weight babies may persist well beyond infancy. Understanding the mechanisms that produce these potentially permanent alterations will be critical to learning how to prevent and/or reverse them.

In the consideration of how best to titrate supplemental oxygen therapy in the clinical setting, the optimal oxygen saturation value for extremely low-birth-weight infants during the first weeks of life remains highly controversial. Random assignment of infants who required oxygen supplementation after 32 weeks to lower oxygen saturation ranges (91%-94% versus 95%-98%) reduced the incidence of BPD.[117] However, much still needs to be learned about optimal saturation limits during the earlier phases of critical illness. In a large trial of extremely low birth weight infants, early randomization to even lower oxygen saturation limits (85%-89%) significantly reduced the incidence of BPD and of retinopathy of prematurity in comparison with a group treated with oxygen saturation limits of 91% to 94%.[118] However, predischarge mortality was unexpectedly 27% higher (19.9% overall) in the "'low' saturation" group. No obvious or single cause for mortality has yet been elucidated, but as the sensitivity and accuracy of oximeters continue to improve, the survival advantage of higher saturation limits appears to be even stronger than originally estimated.[119] This finding indicates that although lower oxygen tensions clearly benefit lung development, other organs may require higher oxygen delivery, and the therapeutic window for oxygen administration to extremely preterm babies appears to be exceptionally narrow.

Therapeutic Implications

NO/cGMP Modulation

Because normal vascular endothelial function depends so heavily on sufficient NO production by NOS, restoring NOS activity is an especially attractive therapeutic target. NO production correlates closely with intracellular concentrations of its essential cofactor tetrahydrobiopterin (BH_4), and when NO levels are insufficient,

NOS becomes "uncoupled," contributing to oxidant stress.[120] The rate-determining step for BH_4 is its synthesis by guanosine triphosphate–cyclohydrolase (GTP-CH1). Mice with impaired GTP-CH1 activity exhibit reduced lung BH_4 levels and spontaneous development of vascular remodeling and pulmonary hypertension.[88] Conversely, congenital overexpression of GTP-CH1 in vascular endothelium protects mice from hypoxic pulmonary hypertension. In piglets with pulmonary hypertension induced by chronic hypoxia, combined therapy with BH_4 and a superoxide dismutase mimetic restores endothelial function.[121] Evidence from one study also indicates that GTP-CH1 is a redox-sensitive enzyme and that antioxidant treatment may restore NOS activity in part by restoring GTP-CH1 expression and BH_4 synthesis.[122] Other investigators have proposed that oxidative stress may reduce BH_4 activity through its conversion to dihydrobiopterin.[123] The approval by the U.S. Food and Drug Administration and the European Commission of sapropterin hydrochloride, a synthetic form of BH_4 for treatment of patients with phenylketonuria could pave the way to clinical testing of this agent in children with pulmonary hypertension.

4

Sufficient availability of the substrate L-arginine is also important for eNOS activity, and data from human infants suggest that sufficient synthesis of L-arginine is necessary for optimal NOS function during the neonatal period.[124] Exogenous L-arginine supplementation enhances NOS activity in vitro but has been less successful in vivo. However, L-arginine can be endogenously synthesized from L-citrulline by a recycling pathway consisting of two enzymes, argininosuccinate synthase (AS) and argininosuccinate lyase (AL). Studies indicate that exogenous L-citrulline may reverse NOS dysfunction in neonatal piglets exposed to chronic hypoxia.[125] L-Citrulline has also been used in clinical populations with some success. For example, in children undergoing cardiopulmonary bypass who are at risk for development of postoperative pulmonary hypertension, oral supplementation with L-citrulline increased plasma levels of both citrulline and arginine, and plasma citrulline levels greater than 37 μM/L appeared to protect against pulmonary hypertension.[126] Intravenous L-citrulline has been shown to be safe and well tolerated in children undergoing cardiopulmonary bypass,[127] and clinical trials of its use are under way.

Augmenting cGMP concentrations through other routes may also prevent or reverse pulmonary vascular remodeling due to oxidant stress. Experimental evidence suggests that NO suppresses hypoxic vasoconstriction,[128] and of course, clinical treatment of neonatal pulmonary hypertension with inhaled NO represents one of the most significant advances in neonatal intensive care in the last 20 years. New "activators" such as cinaciguat (BAY 58-2667) may increase soluble guanylate cyclase activity even in its oxidized, NO-resistant state.[129,130] Phosphodiesterase inhibitors are widely used for adult pulmonary hypertension, and if hyperoxia and/or oxidant stress increases PDE5 activity in the neonatal vasculature, these inhibitors may be especially useful treatment adjuncts. Treatment of neonatal rats with sildenafil during 2 weeks of hyperoxia was found to preserve alveolar growth and lung angiogenesis and to decrease pulmonary vascular resistance, right ventricular hypertrophy, and medial wall thickness of pulmonary arteries (Fig. 4-4).[131] These findings suggest that augmenting the NO/cGMP pathway partially restores the disruptions in alveolar development induced by hyperoxia. A later study in a similar neonatal rat model extended these findings and demonstrated that prophylactic sildenafil (prior to hyperoxia) decreased lung inflammation and improved lung cGMP, alveolarization, angiogenesis, and survival. Interestingly, rescue treatment with sildenafil (6 days after initiation of hyperoxia) significantly decreased pulmonary vessel medial wall thickness and reduced right ventricular hypertrophy, suggesting that the agent may be particularly useful in reversing pulmonary vascular dysfunction after hyperoxia.[132]

Antioxidants

If ROS produced during episodes of hypoxia or hyperoxia promote vasoconstriction, ROS scavengers such as SOD and catalase may augment responsiveness to inhaled NO and restore pulmonary vasodilation. In lambs with pulmonary hypertension, initial studies suggested that scavenging ROS with SOD with or without catalase

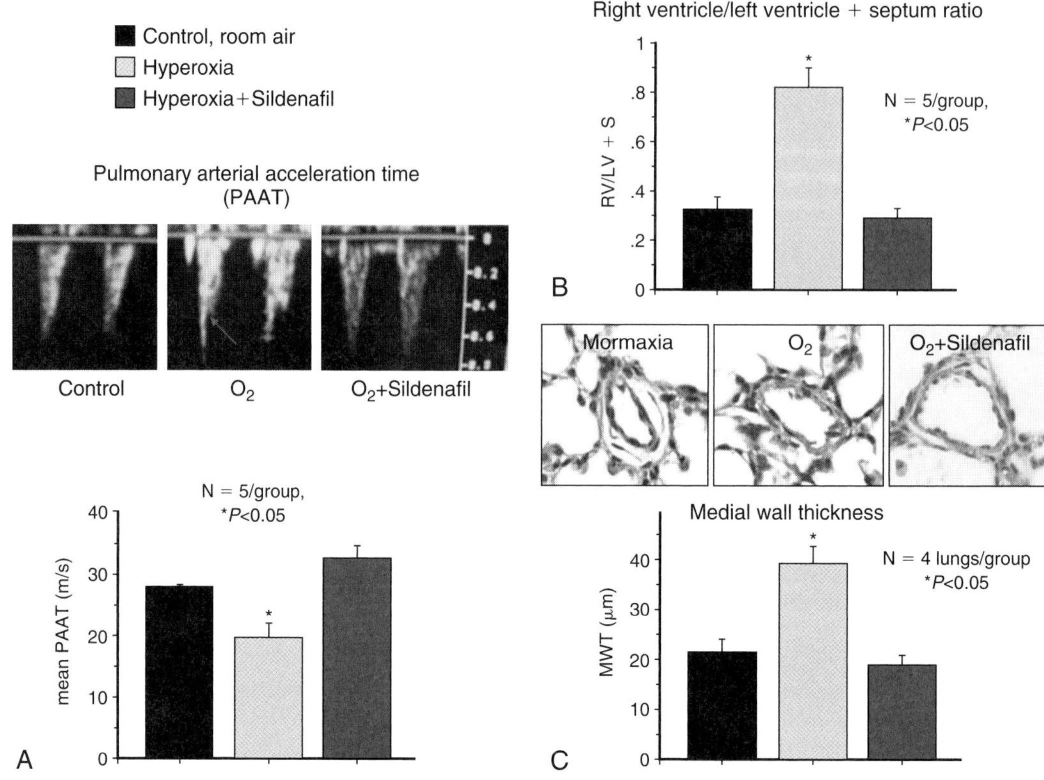

Figure 4-4 Long-term exposure to hyperoxia induces significant right ventricular (RV) hypertrophy and pulmonary vascular remodeling in neonatal rats in comparison with normoxic controls. Sildenafil treatment significantly reduced RV hypertrophy and medial wall thickness. LV, left ventricle/ventricular; S, septum. (Adapted from Ladha F, Bonnet S, Eaton F, et al. Sildenafil improves alveolar growth and pulmonary hypertension in hyperoxia-induced lung injury. *Am J Respir Crit Care Med.* 2005;172:750-756.)

enhanced pulmonary vascular relaxations to NO both in vitro and in vivo.[28,133] These studies were followed by preclinical studies in which a single intratracheal dose of recombinant human SOD (rhSOD) was found to dilate the pulmonary circulation[133] as well as improve oxygenation over a 24-hour period to a degree that was similar to that achieved with inhaled NO.[44] Furthermore, rhSOD blocked formation of oxidants such as peroxynitrite and isoprostanes and restored normal postnatal patterns of endogenous NOS and PDE expression and activity.[99,122] Thus, use of antioxidants may have multiple beneficial effects: Scavenging superoxide may increase the availability of both endogenous and inhaled NO and may also reduce oxidative stress, restore normal patterns of enzyme expression, and limit lung injury.

H_2O_2 levels are also increased in the pulmonary arteries of hypertensive lambs; catalase treatment was found to augment NO-mediated vasodilation in pulmonary arteries isolated from hypertensive lambs.[134] In lambs with PPHN that were ventilated with 100% oxygen, administration of intratracheal catalase improved oxygenation, increased ecSOD activity, and decreased vascular oxidative stress.[101] Intratracheal catalase also decreased PDE5 activity and increased pulmonary artery cGMP levels,[100] changes that may account for the improvements in oxygenation that were observed.[101]

Against the idea that antioxidant treatment might be useful for treating pulmonary hypertension is the very limited success in clinical trials of antioxidant treatments for a wide range of diseases, including prevention of BPD.[135] One explanation for the apparent lack of efficacy is that antioxidants may be ineffective in reversing disease pathology that has already progressed to the stage of vascular remodeling. Another consideration is that many antioxidant compounds attenuate oxidant stress but may also suppress normal ROS signaling pathways nonspecifically in multiple cell types, including those responsible for bacterial killing. A well-known example of this effect is the increase in rates of sepsis and necrotizing enterocolitis observed in preterm babies who were treated with pharmacologic doses of vitamin E.[136] In addition, we now understand that ROS signals are regulated in a cell-specific manner that is also highly localized to specific subcellular compartments or domains. By analogy, calcium plays a critical role in regulating diverse events in cells, and it, too, is tightly regulated in specific subcellular locations. Therapeutic agents such as L-type calcium channel inhibitors are effective because they specifically target a subset of calcium responses. To understand why systemic antioxidants have been ineffective, one should imagine the consequences of treating a disease like hypertension with a cell-permeable chelator of calcium ions! Fortunately, important progress is being made with novel antioxidant compounds that target specific locations such as mitochondria,[137] and small-molecule inhibitors of Nox isoforms are also beginning to appear. The possibility of being able to modify these systems more selectively represents an exciting prospect for future therapy.

Acknowledgments

This review was supported by grants HL54705 (RHS) and HL35440 (PTS) from the National Institutes of Health.

References

1. Rhoades R, Packer C, Roepke D, et al. Reactive oxygen species alter contractile properties of pulmonary arterial smooth muscle. *Can J Physiol Pharmacol*. 1990;68:1581-1589.
2. Demiryürek A, Wadsworth R. Superoxide in the pulmonary circulation. *Pharmacol Ther*. 1999;84:355-365.
3. Kukreja RC, Kontos HA, Hess ML, et al. PGH synthase and lipoxygenase generate superoxide in the presence of NADH or NADPH. *Circ Res*. 1986;59:612-619.
4. Mueller CF, Laude K, McNally JS, et al. ATVB in focus: redox mechanisms in blood vessels. *Arterioscler Thromb Vasc Biol*. 2005;25:274-278.
5. Archer SL, Gomberg-Maitland M, Maitland ML, et al. Mitochondrial metabolism, redox signaling, and fusion: a mitochondria-ROS-HIF-1alpha-Kv1.5 O2-sensing pathway at the intersection of pulmonary hypertension and cancer. *Am J Physiol Heart Circ Physiol*. 2008;294:H570-H578.
6. Hilenski LL, Clempus RE, Quinn MT, et al. Distinct subcellular localizations of Nox1 and Nox4 in vascular smooth muscle cells. *Arterioscler Thromb Vasc Biol*. 2004;24:677-683.
7. Lyle AN, Griendling KK. Modulation of vascular smooth muscle signaling by reactive oxygen species. *Physiol Bethesda*. 2006;21:269-280.
8. Waypa GB, Schumacker PT. Oxygen sensing in hypoxic pulmonary vasoconstriction: using new tools to answer an age-old question. *Exp Physiol*. 2008;93:133-138.
9. Wolin MS, Ahmad M, Gupte SA. Oxidant and redox signaling in vascular oxygen sensing mechanisms: basic concepts, current controversies, and potential importance of cytosolic NADPH. *Am J Physiol Lung Cell Mol Physiol*. 2005;289:L159-L173.
10. Jensen PK. Antimycin-insensitive oxidation of succinate and reduced nicotinamide-adenine dinucleotide in electron-transport particles. I. pH dependency and hydrogen peroxide formation. *Biochim Biophys Acta*. 1966;122:157-166.
11. Guzy RD, Schumacker PT. Oxygen sensing by mitochondria at complex III: the paradox of increased reactive oxygen species during hypoxia. *Exp Physiol*. 2006;91:807-819.
12. Madamanchi NR, Runge MS. Mitochondrial dysfunction in atherosclerosis. *Circ Res*. 2007;100:460-473.
13. Doughan AK, Harrison DG, Dikalov SI. Molecular mechanisms of angiotensin II-mediated mitochondrial dysfunction: linking mitochondrial oxidative damage and vascular endothelial dysfunction. *Circ Res*. 2008;102:488-496.
14. Rathore R, Zheng YM, Niu CF, et al. Hypoxia activates NADPH oxidase to increase ROS.i and Ca2+.i through the mitochondrial ROS-PKCepsilon signaling axis in pulmonary artery smooth muscle cells. *Free Radic Biol Med*. 2008;45:1223-1231.
15. Lassegue B, Clempus RE. Vascular NADPH oxidases: specific features, expression, and regulation. *Am J Physiol Regul Integr Comp Physiol*. 2003;285:R277-R297.
16. Csanyi G, Taylor WR, Pagano PJ. NOX and inflammation in the vascular adventitia. *Free Radic Biol Med*. 2009;47:1254-1266.
17. Zhang G, Zhang F, Muh R, et al. Autocrine/paracrine pattern of superoxide production through NADPH oxidase in coronary arterial myocytes. *Am J Physiol Heart Circ Physiol*. 2007;292:H483-H495.
18. Miller FJ Jr, Filali M, Huss GJ, et al. Cytokine activation of nuclear factor kappa B in vascular smooth muscle cells requires signaling endosomes containing Nox1 and ClC-3. *Circ Res*. 2007;101:663-671.

A

19. Brown DI, Griendling KK. Nox proteins in signal transduction. *Free Radic Biol Med*. 2009;47:1239-1253.
20. Lassegue B, Griendling KK. NADPH oxidases: Functions and pathologies in the vasculature. *Arterioscler Thromb Vasc Biol*. 2009;30:653-661.
21. Dikalova A, Clempus R, Lassegue B, et al. Nox1 overexpression potentiates angiotensin II-induced hypertension and vascular smooth muscle hypertrophy in transgenic mice. *Circulation*. 2005;112:2668-2676.
22. Bedard K, Krause KH. The NOX family of ROS-generating NADPH oxidases: physiology and pathophysiology. *Physiol Rev*. 2007;87:245-313.
23. Johnson JL, Park JW, Benna JE, et al. Activation of p47PHOX., a cytosolic subunit of the leukocyte NADPH oxidase. Phosphorylation of ser-359 or ser-370 precedes phosphorylation at other sites and is required for activity. *J Biol Chem*. 1998;273:35147-35152.
24. Chamseddine AH, Miller FJ Jr. Gp91phox contributes to NADPH oxidase activity in aortic fibroblasts but not smooth muscle cells. *Am J Physiol Heart Circ Physiol*. 2003;285:H2284-H2289.
25. Petry A, Djordjevic T, Weitnauer M, et al. NOX2 and NOX4 mediate proliferative response in endothelial cells. *Antioxid Redox Signal*. 2006;8:1473-1484.
26. Takenouchi Y, Kobayashi T, Matsumoto T, et al. Gender differences in age-related endothelial function in the murine aorta. *Atherosclerosis*. 2009;206:397-404.
27. Zemse SM, Hilgers RH, Webb RC. Interleukin-10 counteracts impaired endothelium-dependent relaxation induced by ANG II in murine aortic rings. *Am J Physiol Heart Circ Physiol*. 2007;292:H3103-H3108.
28. Brennan LA, Steinhorn RH, Wedgwood S, et al. Increased superoxide generation is associated with pulmonary hypertension in fetal lambs: a role for NADPH oxidase. *Circ Res*. 2003;92:683-691.
29. Fike CD, Slaughter JC, Kaplowitz MR, et al. Reactive oxygen species from NADPH oxidase contribute to altered pulmonary vascular responses in piglets with chronic hypoxia-induced pulmonary hypertension. *Am J Physiol Lung Cell Mol Physiol*. 2008;295:L881-L888.
30. Liu J, Zelko I, Erbynn E, et al. Hypoxic pulmonary hypertension: role of superoxide and NADPH oxidase gp91phox.. *Am J Physiol Lung Cell Mol Physiol*. 2006;290:L2-L10.
31. Fujii A, Nakano D, Katsuragi M, et al. Role of gp91phox-containing NADPH oxidase in the deoxycorticosterone acetate-salt-induced hypertension. *Eur J Pharmacol*. 2006;552:131-134.
32. Jung O, Schreiber J, Geiger H, et al. gp91phox-containing NADPH oxidase mediates endothelial dysfunction in renovascular hypertension. *Circulation*. 2004;109:1795-1801.
33. Touyz RM, Mercure C, He Y, et al. Angiotensin II-dependent chronic hypertension and cardiac hypertrophy are unaffected by gp91phox-containing NADPH oxidase. *Hypertension*. 2005;45:530-537.
34. Chen K, Kirber MT, Xiao H, et al. Regulation of ROS signal transduction by NADPH oxidase 4 localization. *J Cell Biol*. 2008;181:1129-1139.
35. Van Buul JD, Fernandez-Borja M, Anthony EC, et al. Expression and localization of NOX2 and NOX4 in primary human endothelial cells. *Antioxid Redox Signal*. 2005;7:308-317.
36. Kuroda J, Nakagawa K, Yamasaki T, et al. The superoxide-producing NADP.H oxidase Nox4 in the nucleus of human vascular endothelial cells. *Genes Cells*. 2005;10:1139-1151.
37. Serrander L, Cartier L, Bedard K, et al. NOX4 activity is determined by mRNA levels and reveals a unique pattern of ROS generation. *Biochem J*. 2007;406:105-114.
38. Lyle AN, Deshpande NN, Taniyama Y, et al. Poldip2, a novel regulator of Nox4 and cytoskeletal integrity in vascular smooth muscle cells. *Circ Res*. 2009;105:249-259.
39. Dikalov S, Dikalova A, Bikineyeva A, et al. Distinct roles of Nox1 and Nox4 in basal and angiotensin II-stimulated superoxide and hydrogen peroxide production. *Free Radic Biol Med*. 2008;45:1340-1351.
40. Mittal M, Roth M, Konig P, et al. Hypoxia-dependent regulation of nonphagocytic NADPH oxidase subunit NOX4 in the pulmonary vasculature. *Circ Res*. 2007;101:258-267.
41. DeMarco VG, Habibi J, Whaley-Connell AT, et al. Oxidative stress contributes to pulmonary hypertension in the transgenic mRen2.27 rat. *Am J Physiol Heart Circ Physiol*. 2008;294:H2659-H2668.
42. Lassegue B, Griendling KK. Reactive oxygen species in hypertension; An update. *Am J Hypertens*. 2004;17:852-860.
43. Li W, Miller FJ, Zhang H, et al. H(2)2.-induced O(2) production by a non-phagocytic NADP.H oxidase causes oxidant injury. *J Biol Chem*. 2001;276:29251-29256.
44. Lakshminrusimha S, Russell J, Wedgwood S, et al. Superoxide dismutase improves oxygenation and reduces oxidation in neonatal pulmonary hypertension. *Am J Respir Crit Care Med*. 2006;174:1370-1377.
45. Dikalova AE, Gongora MC, Harrison DG, et al. Upregulation of Nox1 in vascular smooth muscle leads to impaired endothelium-dependent relaxation via eNOS uncoupling. *Am J Physiol Heart Circ Physiol*. 2010;299:H673-H679.
46. Landmesser U, Dikalov S, Price SR, et al. Oxidation of tetrahydrobiopterin leads to uncoupling of endothelial cell nitric oxide synthase in hypertension. *J Clin Invest*. 2003;111:1201-1209..
47. Spiekermann S, Schenk K, Hoeper MM. Increased xanthine oxidase activity in idiopathic pulmonary arterial hypertension. *Eur Respir J*. 2009;34:276.
48. Asikainen TM, White CW. Pulmonary antioxidant defenses in the preterm newborn with respiratory distress and bronchopulmonary dysplasia in evolution: implications for antioxidant therapy. *Antioxid Redox Signal*. 2004;6:155-167.
49. Clerch LB, Massaro D. Rat lung antioxidant enzymes: differences in perinatal gene expression and regulation. *Am J Physiol*. 1992;263:L466-L470.

50. Rhee SG, Chae HZ, Kim K. Peroxiredoxins: a historical overview and speculative preview of novel mechanisms and emerging concepts in cell signaling. *Free Radic Biol Med*. 2005;38: 1543-1552.
51. Fukai T, Folz RJ, Landmesser U, et al. Extracellular superoxide dismutase and cardiovascular disease. *Cardiovasc Res*. 2002;55:239-249.
52. Oury TD, Chang L, Marklund S, et al. Immunocytochemical localization of extracellular superoxide dismutase in human lung. *Lab Invest*. 1994;70:889-898.
53. Oury TD, Day BJ, Crapo JD. Extracellular superoxide dismutase in vessels and airways of humans and baboons. *Free Radic Biol Med*. 1996;20:957-965.
54. Qin Z, Reszka KJ, Fukai T, et al. Extracellular superoxide dismutase ecSOD. in vascular biology: an update on exogenous gene transfer and endogenous regulators of ecSOD. *Transl Res*. 2008;151:68-78.
55. Li Y, Huang TT, Carlson EJ, et al. Dilated cardiomyopathy and neonatal lethality in mutant mice lacking manganese superoxide dismutase. *Nat Genet*. 1995;11:376-381.
56. Rodriguez-Iturbe B, Sepassi L, Quiroz Y, et al. Association of mitochondrial SOD deficiency with salt-sensitive hypertension and accelerated renal senescence. *J Appl Physiol*. 2007;102: 255-260.
57. Dikalova AE, Bikineyeva AT, Budzyn K, et al. Therapeutic targeting of mitochondrial superoxide in hypertension. *Circ Res*. 2010;107:106-116.
58. Ho YS, Xiong Y, Ma W, et al. Mice lacking catalase develop normally but show differential sensitivity to oxidant tissue injury. *J Biol Chem*. 2004;279:32804-32812.
59. Masri F, Comhair S, Dostanic-Larson I, et al. Deficiency of lung antioxidants in idiopathic pulmonary arterial hypertension. *Clin Transl Sci*. 2008;1:99-106.
60. Ardanaz N, Yang XP, Cifuentes ME, et al. Lack of glutathione peroxidase 1 accelerates cardiac-specific hypertrophy and dysfunction in angiotensin II hypertension. *Hypertension*. 2010;55: 116-123.
61. Neumann CA, Krause DS, Carman CV, et al. Essential role for the peroxiredoxin Prdx1 in erythrocyte antioxidant defence and tumour suppression. *Nature*. 2003;424:561-565.
62. Li L, Shoji W, Takano H, et al. Increased susceptibility of MER5 peroxiredoxin III knockout mice to LPS-induced oxidative stress. *Biochem Biophys Res Commun*. 2007;355:715-721.
63. Michelakis ED, Hampl V, Nsair A, et al. Diversity in mitochondrial function explains differences in vascular oxygen sensing. *Circ Res*. 2002;90:1307-1315.
64. Michelakis ED, Thebaud B, Weir EK, et al. Hypoxic pulmonary vasoconstriction: redox regulation of O2-sensitive K+ channels by a mitochondrial O2-sensor in resistance artery smooth muscle cells. *J Mol Cell Cardiol*. 2004;37:1119-1136.
65. Waypa GB, Chandel NS, Schumacker PT. Model for hypoxic pulmonary vasoconstriction involving mitochondrial oxygen sensing. *Circ Res*. 2001;88:1259-1266.
66. Waypa GB, Marks JD, Mack MM, et al. Mitochondrial reactive oxygen species trigger calcium increases during hypoxia in pulmonary arterial myocytes. *Circ Res*. 2002;91:719-726.
67. Li S, Tabar SS, Malec V, et al. NOX4 regulates ROS levels under normoxic and hypoxic conditions, triggers proliferation, and inhibits apoptosis in pulmonary artery adventitial fibroblasts. *Antioxid Redox Signal*. 2008;10:1687-1698.
68. Mungai P, Waypa G, Jairaman A, et al. Hypoxia triggers AMPK activation through ROS-mediated activation of CRAC channels. *Mol Cell Biol*. 2011;31:3531-3545.
69. Desireddi JR, Farrow KN, Marks JD, et al. Hypoxia increases ROS signaling and cytosolic Ca(2+) in pulmonary artery smooth muscle cells of mouse lungs slices. *Antioxid Redox Signal*. 2010; 12:595-602.
70. Waypa GB, Marks JD, Guzy R, et al. Hypoxia triggers subcellular compartmental redox signaling in vascular smooth muscle cells. *Circ Res*. 2010;106:526-535.
71. Waypa GB, Guzy R, Mungai PT, et al. Increases in mitochondrial reactive oxygen species trigger hypoxia-induced calcium responses in pulmonary artery smooth muscle cells. *Circ Res*. 2006; 99:970-978.
72. Herrera E, Riquelme R, Ebensperger G, et al. Long-term exposure to high-altitude chronic hypoxia during gestation induces neonatal pulmonary hypertension at sea level. *Am J Physiol Regul Integr Comp Physiol*. 2010;299:R1676-R1784.
73. Liu J, Gao Y, Negash S, et al. Long-term effects of prenatal hypoxia on endothelium-dependent relaxation responses in pulmonary arteries of adult sheep. *Am J Physiol Lung Cell Mol Physiol*. 2009;296:L547-L554.
74. Nisbet R, Graves A, Kleinhenz D, et al. The role of NADPH oxidase in chronic intermittent hypoxia-induced pulmonary hypertension in mice. *Am J Respir Cell Mol Biol*. 2009;40:601-609.
75. Hoshikawa Y, Ono S, Suzuki S, et al. Generation of oxidative stress contributes to the development of pulmonary hypertension induced by hypoxia. *J Appl Physiol*. 2001;90:1299-1306.
76. Jankov R, Kantores C, Pan J, et al. Contribution of xanthine oxidase-derived superoxide to chronic hypoxic pulmonary hypertension in neonatal rats. *Am J Physiol Lung Cell Mol Physiol*. 2008;294:L233-L245.
77. Dennis KE, Aschner JL, Milatovic D, et al. NADPH oxidases and reactive oxygen species at different stages of chronic hypoxia-induced pulmonary hypertension in newborn piglets. *Am J Physiol Lung Cell Mol Physiol*. 2009;297:L596-L607.
78. Nozik-Grayck E, Suliman H, Majka S, et al. Lung EC-SOD overexpression attenuates hypoxic induction of Egr-1 and chronic hypoxic pulmonary vascular remodeling. *Am J Physiol Lung Cell Mol Physiol*. 2008;295:L422-L430.

4

79. Guzy R, Hoyos B, Robin E, et al. Mitochondrial complex III is required for hypoxia-induced ROS production and cellular oxygen sensing. *Cell Metab.* 2005:401-408.
80. Forsythe JA, Jiang BH, Iyer NV, et al. Activation of vascular endothelial growth factor gene transcription by hypoxia-inducible factor 1. *Mol Cell Biol.* 1996;16:4604-4613.
81. Liu Y, Cox SR, Morita T, et al. Hypoxia regulates vascular endothelial growth factor gene expression in endothelial cells. Identification of a 5′ enhancer. *Circ Res.* 1995;77:638-643.
82. Yu AY, Shimoda LA, Iyer NV, et al. Impaired physiological responses to chronic hypoxia in mice partially deficient for hypoxia-inducible factor 1alpha. *J Clin Invest.* 1999;103:691-696.
83. Brusselmans K, Compernolle V, Tjwa M, et al. Heterozygous deficiency of hypoxia-inducible factor-2alpha protects mice against pulmonary hypertension and right ventricular dysfunction during prolonged hypoxia. *J Clin Invest.* 2003;111:1519-1527.
84. Wanstall JC, Gambino A, Jeffery TK, et al. Vascular endothelial growth factor-B-deficient mice show impaired development of hypoxic pulmonary hypertension. *Cardiovasc Res.* 2002;55:361-368.
85. Ozaki M, Kawashima S, Yamashita T, et al. Reduced hypoxic pulmonary vascular remodeling by nitric oxide from the endothelium. *Hypertension.* 2001;37:322-327.
86. Sebkhi A, Strange JW, Phillips SC, et al. Phosphodiesterase type 5 as a target for the treatment of hypoxia-induced pulmonary hypertension. *Circulation.* 2003;107:3230-3235.
87. Murata T, Sato K, Hori M, et al. Decreased endothelial nitric-oxide synthase eNOS activity resulting from abnormal interaction between eNOS and its regulatory proteins in hypoxia-induced pulmonary hypertension. *J Biol Chem.* 2002;277:44085-44092.
88. Khoo JP, Zhao L, Alp NJ, et al. Pivotal role for endothelial tetrahydrobiopterin in pulmonary hypertension. *Circulation.* 2005;111:2126-2133.
89. Ananthakrishnan M, Barr FE, Summar ML, et al. L-Citrulline ameliorates chronic hypoxia-induced pulmonary hypertension in newborn piglets. *Am J Physiol Lung Cell Mol Physiol.* 2009;297:L506-L511.
90. Farrow KN, Fliman P, Steinhorn RH. The diseases treated with ECMO: focus on PPHN. *Semin Perinatol.* 2005;29:8-14.
91. Lakshminrusimha S, Russell JA, Steinhorn RH, et al. Pulmonary hemodynamics in neonatal lambs resuscitated with 21%, 50%, and 100% oxygen. *Pediatr Res.* 2007;62:313-318.
92. Lakshminrusimha S, Russell JA, Steinhorn RH, et al. Pulmonary arterial contractility in neonatal lambs increases with 100% oxygen resuscitation. *Pediatr Res.* 2006;59:137-141.
93. Kattwinkel J, Perlman JM, Aziz K, et al. Part 15: Neonatal resuscitation: 2010 American Heart Association Guidelines for Cardiopulmonary Resuscitation and Emergency Cardiovascular Care. *Circulation.* 2010;122:S909-S919.
94. Rudolph AM, Yuan S. Response of the pulmonary vasculature to hypoxia and H+ ion concentration changes. *J Clin Invest.* 1966;45:399-411.
95. Lakshminrusimha S, Swartz DD, Gugino SF, et al. Oxygen concentration and pulmonary hemodynamics in newborn lambs with pulmonary hypertension. *Pediatr Res.* 2009;66:539-544.
96. Mourani PM, Ivy DD, Gao D, et al. Pulmonary vascular effects of inhaled nitric oxide and oxygen tension in bronchopulmonary dysplasia. *Am J Respir Crit Care Med.* 2004;170:1006-1013.
97. Lakshminrusimha S, Steinhorn RH. Pulmonary vascular biology during neonatal transition. *Clin Perinatol.* 1999;26:601-619.
98. Farrow KN, Groh BS, Schumacker PT, et al. Hyperoxia increases phosphodiesterase 5 expression and activity in ovine fetal pulmonary artery smooth muscle cells. *Circ Res.* 2008;102:226-233.
99. Farrow KN, Lakshminrusimha S, Czech L, et al. Superoxide dismutase and inhaled nitric oxide normalize phosphodiesterase 5 expression and activity in neonatal lambs with persistent pulmonary hypertension. *Am J Physiol Lung Cell Mol Physiol.* 2010;299:L109-L116.
100. Farrow K, Wedgwood S, Lee K, et al. Mitochondrial oxidant stress increases PDE5 activity in persistent pulmonary hypertension of the newborn. *Respir Physiol Neurobiol.* 2010;174:272-281.
101. Wedgwood S, Lakshminrusimha S, Fukai T, et al. Hydrogen peroxide regulates extracellular superoxide dismutase activity and expression in neonatal pulmonary hypertension. *Antioxid Redox Signal.* 2011;15(6):1497-1506.
102. Thebaud B, Abman SH. Bronchopulmonary dysplasia: where have all the vessels gone? Roles of angiogenic growth factors in chronic lung disease. *Am J Respir Crit Care Med.* 2007;175:978-985.
103. Northway WH Jr, Rosan RC, Porter DY. Pulmonary disease following respirator therapy of hyaline-membrane disease. Bronchopulmonary dysplasia. *N Engl J Med.* 1967;276:357-368.
104. Saugstad O. Oxygen and oxidative stress in bronchopulmonary dysplasia. *J Perinat Med.* 2010;38:571-577.
105. Ballard PL, Truog WE, Merrill JD, et al. Plasma biomarkers of oxidative stress: relationship to lung disease and inhaled nitric oxide therapy in premature infants. *Pediatrics.* 2008;121:555-561.
106. Warner BB, Stuart LA, Papes RA, et al. Functional and pathological effects of prolonged hyperoxia in neonatal mice. *Am J Physiol.* 1998;275:L110-L117.
107. Belik J, Jankov RP, Pan J, et al. Chronic O2 exposure enhances vascular and airway smooth muscle contraction in the newborn but not adult rat. *J Appl Physiol.* 2003;94:2303-2312.
108. Mamo LB, Suliman HB, Giles BL, et al. Discordant extracellular superoxide dismutase expression and activity in neonatal hyperoxic lung. *Am J Respir Crit Care Med.* 2004;170:313-318.
109. Carnesecchi S, Deffert C, Pagano A, et al. NADPH oxidase-1 plays a crucial role in hyperoxia-induced acute lung injury in mice. *Am J Respir Crit Care Med.* 2009;180:972-981.
110. Pendyala S, Gorshkova IA, Usatyuk PV, et al. Role of Nox4 and Nox2 in hyperoxia-induced reactive oxygen species generation and migration of human lung endothelial cells. *Antioxid Redox Signal.* 2009;11:747-764.

A

111. Yang G, Abate A, George AG, et al. Maturational differences in lung NF-kappaB activation and their role in tolerance to hyperoxia. *J Clin Invest*. 2004;114:669-678.
112. Maltepe E, Saugstad OD. Oxygen in health and disease: regulation of oxygen homeostasis—clinical implications. *Pediatr Res*. 2009;65:261-268.
113. Bhatt AJ, Pryhuber GS, Huyck H, et al. Disrupted pulmonary vasculature and decreased vascular endothelial growth factor, Flt-1, and TIE-2 in human infants dying with bronchopulmonary dysplasia. *Am J Respir Crit Care Med*. 2001;164:1971-1980.
114. Abman SH. Impaired vascular endothelial growth factor signaling in the pathogenesis of neonatal pulmonary vascular disease. *Adv Exp Med Biol*. 2010;661:323-335.
115. Yzydorczyk C, Comte B, Cambonie G, et al. Neonatal oxygen exposure in rats leads to cardiovascular and renal alterations in adulthood. *Hypertension*. 2008;52:889-895.
116. Yee M, White RJ, Awad HA, et al. Neonatal Hyperoxia Causes Pulmonary Vascular Disease and Shortens Life Span in Aging Mice. *Am J Pathol*. 178:2601-2610, 2011,.
117. Askie LM, Henderson-Smart DJ, Irwig L, et al. Oxygen-saturation targets and outcomes in extremely preterm infants. *N Engl J Med*. 2003;349:959-967.
118. Carlo WA, Finer NN, Walsh MC, et al. Target ranges of oxygen saturation in extremely preterm infants. *N Engl J Med*. 2010;362:1959-1969.
119. Stenson B, Brocklehurst P, Tarnow-Mordi W. Increased 36-week survival with high oxygen saturation target in extremely preterm infants. *N Engl J Med*. 2011;364:1680-1682.
120. Forstermann U. Nitric oxide and oxidative stress in vascular disease. *Pflugers Arch*. 2010;459: 923-939.
121. Nandi M, Leiper J, Arrigoni F, et al. Developmental regulation of GTP-CH1 in the porcine lung and its relationship to pulmonary vascular relaxation. *Pediatr Res*. 59:767-772. 2006;
122. Farrow KN, Lakshminrusimha S, Reda WJ, et al. Superoxide dismutase restores eNOS expression and function in resistance pulmonary arteries from neonatal lambs with persistent pulmonary hypertension. *Am J Physiol Lung Cell Mol Physiol*. 2008;295:L979-L987.
123. Mata-Greenwood E, Jenkins C, Farrow KN, et al. eNOS function is developmentally regulated: uncoupling of eNOS occurs postnatally. *Am J Physiol Lung Cell Mol Physiol*. 2006;290: L232-L241.
124. Pearson DL, Dawling S, Walsh WF, et al. Neonatal pulmonary hypertension—urea-cycle intermediates, nitric oxide production, and carbamoyl-phosphate synthetase function. *N Engl J Med*. 2001;344:1832-1838.
125. Ananthakrishnan M, Barr FE, Summar ML, et al. L-Citrulline ameliorates chronic hypoxia-induced pulmonary hypertension in newborn piglets. *Am J Physiol Lung Cell Mol Physiol*. 2009;297: L506-L511.
126. Smith HA, Canter JA, Christian KG, et al. Nitric oxide precursors and congenital heart surgery: a randomized controlled trial of oral citrulline. *J Thorac Cardiovasc Surg*. 2006;132:56-65.
127. Barr FE, Tirona RG, Taylor MB, et al. Pharmacokinetics and safety of intravenously administered citrulline in children undergoing congenital heart surgery: potential therapy for postoperative pulmonary hypertension. *J Thorac Cardiovasc Surg*. 134:319-326. 2007;
128. Wolin MS, Gupte SA, Neo BH, et al. Oxidant-redox regulation of pulmonary vascular responses to hypoxia and nitric oxide-cGMP signaling. *Cardiol Rev*. 2010;18:89-93.
129. Coggins MP, Bloch KD. Nitric oxide in the pulmonary vasculature. *Arterioscler Thromb Vasc Biol*. 2007;27:1877-1885.
130. Chester M, Tourneux P, Seedorf G, et al. Cinaciguat, a soluble guanylate cyclase activator, causes potent and sustained pulmonary vasodilation in the ovine fetus. *Am J Physiol Lung Cell Mol Physiol*. 2009;297:L318-L325.
131. Ladha F, Bonnet S, Eaton F, et al. Sildenafil improves alveolar growth and pulmonary hypertension in hyperoxia-induced lung injury. *Am J Respir Crit Care Med*. 2005;172:750-756.
132. de Visser YP, Walther FJ, Laghmani el H, et al. Sildenafil attenuates pulmonary inflammation and fibrin deposition, mortality and right ventricular hypertrophy in neonatal hyperoxic lung injury. *Respir Res*. 2009;10:30.
133. Steinhorn RH, Albert G, Swartz DD, et al. Recombinant human superoxide dismutase enhances the effect of inhaled nitric oxide in persistent pulmonary hypertension. *Am J Respir Crit Care Med*. 2001;164:834-839.
134. Wedgwood S, Steinhorn RH, Bunderson M, et al. Increased hydrogen peroxide downregulates soluble guanylate cyclase in the lungs of lambs with persistent pulmonary hypertension of the newborn. *Am J Physiol Lung Cell Mol Physiol*. 2005;289:L660-L666.
135. Davis JM, Parad RB, Michele T, et al. Pulmonary outcome at 1 year corrected age in premature infants treated at birth with recombinant human CuZn superoxide dismutase. *Pediatrics*. 2003;111:469-476.
136. Johnson L, Bowen FW Jr, Abbasi S, et al. Relationship of prolonged pharmacologic serum levels of vitamin E to incidence of sepsis and necrotizing enterocolitis in infants with birth weight 1,500 grams or less. *Pediatrics*. 1985;75:619-638.
137. Coulter CV, Kelso GF, Lin TK, et al. Mitochondrially targeted antioxidants and thiol reagents. *Free Radic Biol Med*. 2000;28:1547-1554.

4

CHAPTER 5

The Role of Nitric Oxide in Lung Growth and Function

Girija G. Konduri, MD

5

- Fetal Lung Development
- Angiogenic Factors and Their Receptors
- Nitric Oxide and Lung Development
- Role of Nitric Oxide in Lung Repair
- Regulation of NOS Activity through L-Arginine Availability
- Interaction of Antioxidant Enzyme Systems with Endogenous Nitric Oxide
- Relationship of Oxygen Tension with NOS Function and Lung Growth during Fetal Life
- Physiologic Role of Nitric Oxide in the Gas Exchange Function of the Lung
- Altered Lung Architecture in BPD and its Relation to NOS Signaling
- Application of Inhaled Nitric Oxide to Restore Lung Growth in Premature Neonates
- Summary

The lung is a highly complex specialized organ that is optimally prepared to take over the gas exchange function at birth. Development of the intricate air-blood interface in the lung, which brings capillary blood to within 0.1 μ of the gas phase in the alveolus, requires a series of highly coordinated steps during fetal life. This process involves synchronized development of the lung epithelial, vascular, and lymphatic systems. Although the structural changes in these compartments during gestation have been well characterized for a number of years, the molecular mechanisms involved remain unclear and are the focus of current studies. Emerging evidence suggests that nitric oxide (NO) is a key signal involved in the crosstalk between the developing epithelial and vascular compartments. This review focuses on the role of NO in normal lung development, repair of lung from injury, and the gas exchange function of lung. NO also plays a major role in the continuous repair and remodeling that occur in the lung throughout postnatal life. The importance of maintaining normal lung growth to the prevention of chronic lung disease in premature infants has been well recognized and covered extensively in the other chapters in this book.

Fetal Lung Development

This brief review outlines the major events that occur during fetal lung development as they relate to epithelial-vascular communications and the appropriate growth signals. A more detailed review of lung structural development is provided in the first chapter of this book. The lung buds arise as a pair of invaginations from primitive foregut endoderm during 4th embryonic week in the human fetus. Branching and differentiation of these endodermal buds occur within the surrounding mesoderm, leading to the growth of both parenchymal and vascular compartments within the lung. Interaction of the airway epithelium, derived from foregut endoderm with the surrounding mesoderm, is required for lung branching morphogenesis and development of vascular network.[1] This requirement for the interaction is a two-way process, as the epithelium requires mesenchymal cells for successful branching and the mesenchyme-derived vascular network requires growth factors from epithelial cells.[1] The developing capillary network surrounds the branching airways from early in gestation.[2] The vascular compartment follows the branching airways as a template as it develops in the lung mesenchyme and is most active around the terminal buds of branching airways. The central and peripheral components of the pulmonary arterial tree probably arise by distinct mechanisms.[2] The main pulmonary artery (PA) itself arises from truncus arteriosus at 8 weeks of human gestation. The pulmonary trunk connects with the arch pulmonary arteries, which are derived from the sixth branchial arteries coming from the dorsal aorta, to form the right and left pulmonary arteries. The precise mechanism of origin of the intrapulmonary vascular network remains unclear. Current evidence points to angioblasts derived from the mesenchyme surrounding lung buds as the major source of these vessels. The formation of this vascular network potentially occurs by two processes: *vasculogenesis,* which is the de novo formation of blood vessels from angioblasts within the mesoderm, and *angiogenesis,* which is a sprouting of blood vessels from the existing ones. The larger, proximal pulmonary arteries probably arise by angiogenesis from central arteries, whereas more distal vessels probably develop by de novo vasculogenesis from angioblasts in the lung mesenchyme. Fusion of these two vascular beds probably occurs at mid-gestation.

This model for pulmonary vascular growth is supported by studies using vascular casts and electron microscopy in the early gestation mouse lungs[2] and by findings in serial sections of human fetal lungs from early gestation.[2-3a] An alternate model proposed by Parera and colleagues[4] suggests that lung vascular growth occurs primarily by angiogenesis from the preexisting central vessels as a continuous process. In support of this hypothesis, they demonstrated that in early gestation mouse lung (embryonic day E9.5 (E9.5) to E13.5, corresponding to 6-14 weeks of human gestation), vascular networks that form around lung terminal buds are already connected to central vessels. It remains unclear whether species differences exist in the mechanism of formation of this vascular bed. Evidence also suggests that lung vascular growth occurs at all stages of lung development and continues postnatally during alveolar stage into adult life.[4,5] Regardless of the specific source of the vessels, epithelial-endothelial interactions are necessary for the proper development of vascular network around the branching airways and potential air spaces (Fig. 5-1). The guidance of vascular growth by epithelial cells in the airway and terminal buds involves a number of paracrine factors, including several that are angiogenic.[5] The mechanisms that govern the epithelial-endothelial crosstalk have lately been the subject of intense investigation (see Fig. 5-1). Available evidence suggests that the epithelial cells, particularly those around the terminal buds, release angiogenic factors, which interact with angioblasts in the surrounding mesenchyme. The important angiogenic signals include the family of fibroblast growth factors (FGFs), vascular endothelial growth factor (VEGF) and angiopoietins Ang1 and Ang2 (Table 5-1). NO appears to be at the center of this crosstalk, being released from both epithelial and endothelial cells to guide their mutually dependent growth to form the gas exchange unit.[6] NO, which is highly diffusible, serves as both an upstream and a downstream mediator for these signals (see Fig. 5-1).[6] The growing vascular network in turn modulates the growth and organization of epithelial cells into functional alveolar sacs.[5,6]

The interdependence of epithelial and vascular compartments in lung growth has been suggested by a number of previous studies. Prenatal constriction of the ductus arteriosus leads to in utero pulmonary hypertension and remodeling of vasculature in fetal lambs.[7-9] The decreased growth of vascular network in this model is also associated with hypoplasia of lungs due to impaired alveolar growth.[10] The

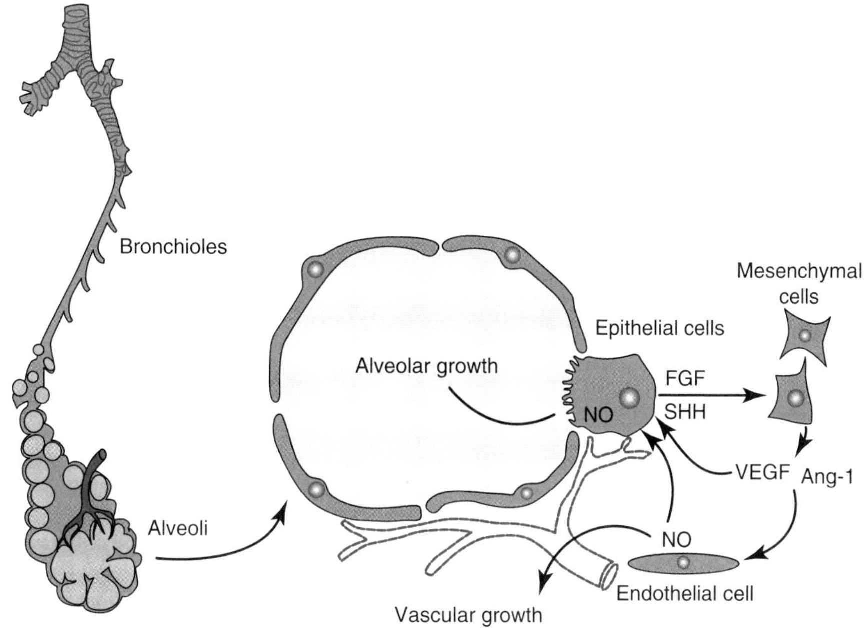

Figure 5-1 Proposed model for the coordinated growth of epithelial and vascularcompartments during fetal life. Release of growth signals, such as, fibroblastic growth factor-9 (FGF-9) and Sonic hedgehog factor (SHH), induces differentiation of mesenchymal cells to endothelial precursor cells, which release vascular endothelial growth factor (VEGF) and angiopoietin-1 (Ang1). These growth signals in turn promote release of nitric oxide (NO) from both epithelial and endothelial cells. NO, a diffusible signal, coordinates the growth of both units through upstream and downstream effects on growth factors and endothelial cell proliferation and migration.

impaired growth of the alveolar-vascular unit is accompanied by decreased expression of VEGF. This observation strongly supports the mutual requirement of vascular growth and alveolar formation.[10] Inhibition of angiogenesis in neonatal rats with drugs that inhibit endothelial cell proliferation, thalidomide or fumagilin, also leads to inhibition of alveolar growth.[11] Inhibition of endothelial cell migration alone through the use of a platelet endothelial cell adhesion molecule-1 (PECAM-1) antibody, without alteration of endothelial proliferation, decreases alveolar septation in neonatal rats.[12] These studies demonstrate the trophic effect that endothelial cells

Table 5-1 KEY ANGIOGENIC FACTORS THAT FUNCTION THROUGH NITRIC OXIDE (NO) SIGNALING AND THEIR EFFECTS ON LUNG GROWTH

Angiogenic Factor	Source	Target Cell	Receptor(s)	Downstream Mediator	Biologic Effect
Fibroblast growth factor (FGF) 9	Epithelial cells	Mesoderm cells	FGF receptor	VEGF	Differentiation to angioblasts and VEGF release
Vascular endothelial growth factor (VEGF)	Epithelial cells, angioblasts	Endothelial cells and their precursors	Flt-1 (VEGFR1) Flk-1 (VEGFR2)	NO	Cell proliferation, cell migration, and tube formation
angiopoietin-1	Epithelial cells	Endothelial cells	Tyrosine Kinase receptor Tie2 Tie1	NO	Stabilization of the vessel structure
angiopoietin-2	Epithelial cells	Endothelial cells	Tie2 Tie1	Unknown	Establishment of vascular connections

have on epithelial cell growth and organization of air spaces. Similarly, inhibition of alveolar growth during the exposure of neonatal rats to hypoxia or hyperoxia is associated with a reciprocal impairment of vascular growth.[13,14]

Angiogenic Factors and Their Receptors

A brief review of angiogenic factors released in the lung is necessary because NO is an integral part of their signaling pathways in the lung. VEGF is critical for early fetal lung growth and for maintaining the homeostasis of air-blood interface during postnatal life.[5] VEGF is a family of growth factors, of which VEGF-A is the most important member and the predominant form expressed in the fetal lung.[5] Its biologic effects are mediated by tyrosine kinase receptors Flt-1 (VEGFR1) and Flk-1 (VEGFR2). Among the other VEGF family members, VEGFB appears to be involved in the homeostatic mechanisms in established vascular beds and in neurons.[15,16] VEGFC and VEGFD, which interact with VEGFR3, appear predominantly in the lymphatic system in the lung[5] and are not discussed further in this review. VEGFA is referred to as *VEGF* in this review of lung development. VEGF is expressed in both pulmonary epithelium and mesenchyme from an early gestation and interacts with the receptor tyrosine kinases VEGFR1 and VEGFR2 on the angioblasts in mesenchyme, which are precursors of endothelial cells.[5] VEGFR2, is the active functional receptor for VEGF and mediates the proangiogenic effects, including stimulation of NO release.[17] The function of VEGFR1 is not clear, although it may sequester VEGF and help modulate the responses of VEGFR2.[17] VEGF is required for both angiogenesis and vasculogenesis in the lung.[5] The critical requirement of VEGF for lung development is demonstrated by the embryonic lethality of deletion of even a single copy of VEGF, which results in disruption of endothelial differentiation and capillary development in the lung buds.[18] Similarly, deletion of either of the VEGF receptors is also lethal to the embryo, with observation of disordered vascular development in the lung.[19,20] VEGF has several isoforms that result from alternate splicing of the eight-exon VEGF gene (VEGF121, VEGF145, VEGF165 VEGF189 and VEGF206 in humans).[17] These isoforms differ in their ability to bind heparin sulfate proteoglycans in the extra-cellular matrix. The smaller VEGF isoform (VEGF121) is more diffusible from lack of heparin binding and probably plays an important role as the signal from epithelial to mesenchymal cells for angiogenesis. The larger isoforms (VEGF189 and VEGF206) bind heparin sulfate and are localized to the extracellular matrix, where they remain biologically active.[21] The importance of each of these isoforms to lung development was shown in mice that express only VEGF120 (the mouse ortholog of human VEGF121).[22] These mice showed decreased development of the air-blood barrier and fewer air spaces in the parenchyma in comparison with their wild-type littermates.

The downstream effects of the activation of VEGFR2 are mediated by NO in the vascular endothelial cells (see Fig. 5-1).[17] VEGF facilitates crosstalk between epithelial and mesenchymal compartments in the developing lung.[5] Thus, VEGF signal is strongly expressed in the airway epithelium whereas VEGFR2, the functional target for VEGF, is expressed on angioblasts in the lung mesenchyme.[23] Similarly, NO released from endothelial cell precursor cells can stimulate VEGF release from epithelial cells (see Fig. 5-1).[6] This crosstalk with diffusion of the signals from epithelial/endothelial precursor cells coordinates the growth of vascular and airway compartments (see Fig. 5-1).[6] Inhibition of VEGF receptors during the neonatal period leads to impairment of alveolar and vascular growth in rats, suggesting the importance of this signal for lung development.[11] The role of NO in promoting lung growth is closely tied to its interaction with VEGF both upstream and downstream in the epithelial and vascular compartments, as described fully later.

VEGF effects are coordinated with the release of other important angiogenic factors, such as angiopoietins. Angiopoietins 1 through 4 are protein growth factors that are involved in angiogenesis. Ang1 and Ang2 are expressed in the embryonic phase of lung development in mice.[24] Their effects are signaled through their receptors, Tie1 and Tie2 (tyrosine kinases with immunoglobulin and EGF-like domains).

Ang1 promotes vascular stability through interaction with its receptor, Tie2, which is specifically expressed on endothelial cells.[24] Whereas VEGF induces formation of new capillaries, which are leaky, Ang1 stabilizes the vascular structure by promoting formation of endothelial tight junctions with adjacent cells and with matrix.[5] This cooperative function of VEGF and Ang1 is important to the formation of vascular network in the growing lung. Ang2 antagonizes the effect of Ang1 on Tie2. Ang1's interaction with Tie2 leads to the activation of protein kinases phosphoinositide-3 (PI3) kinase and akt, which signal downstream to activate release of NO synthase (NOS) and NO.[24] Although Ang2 decreases the proliferation of epithelial cells, it may play an important role in establishing vascular connections during angiogenesis. Both Ang1 and Ang 2 and their receptors, Tie1 and Tie2, are required for normal lung growth.[25-28] Null mutations in the genes for the angiopoietins and their receptors lead to disordered vascular development.[25,26] The loss of either Ang1 or Tie1/Tie2 receptors is lethal to the embryo.[26,27] The temporal and spatial coordination of angiopoietin and VEGF expression and their specific roles in promoting vascular growth in the lung require further investigation. Among the other angiogenic signals, FGF is a family of proteins that induce the differentiation of mesenchymal cells to angioblast lineage.[29] FGF-9, along with Sonic hedgehog factor (Shh), induces VEGF expression by the mesenchymal cells in the embryonic lung and is required for vascular growth in the lung (see Fig. 5-1).[29] Expression of FGF proteins and their downstream effects may precede the active release of VEGF to prepare the mesenchymal cells for commitment to vascular lineage.[29] A number of FGF proteins involved in angiogenesis in the lung signal through NO release from target cells.[30,31] NO in turn regulates FGF expression upstream.[6] The temporal sequence of the induction of NOS by FGF and VEGF in the mesenchymal cells probably plays specific roles in the organization of the vascular network during early branching morphogenesis.[32,33] This intriguing possibility requires further investigation.

Nitric Oxide and Lung Development

As mentioned previously, NO is the key molecule involved in the signaling pathway of several important angiogenic factors in the lung. NO is an upstream and downstream mediator for several angiogenic factors, including VEGF, FGF, and Ang1 (see Fig. 5-1).[6] NO is highly diffusible in the biologic systems and reacts with a number of targets, which include metal-containing enzymes such as guanylate cyclase (Fig. 5-2), thiol-containing proteins to form *S*-nitroso thiols, and other free radicals, such as superoxide.[34] These unique properties of NO facilitate its role in the crosstalk between parenchymal and vascular compartments in the lung. NO is the catalytic by-product (see Fig. 5-2) of the oxidation of terminal guanidino nitrogen of L-arginine to generate L-citrulline by the enzyme NO synthase (NOS). The three isoforms of NOS are designated NOS-1 (neuronal; nNOS), NOS-2 (inducible; iNOS) and NOS-3 (endothelial; eNOS) in the order of their discovery. Although they are homologous, they are coded by distinct genes and differ in the regulation of their activities and specific roles in cell biology. Their expression is also not restricted to the tissues suggested by the nomenclature. All three isoforms of NOS are expressed in the fetal lung.[35] Although the Ca^{++}-dependent NOS-1 and NOS-3 are expressed in the airway epithelial and endothelial cells,[35] NOS-2 expression is variable. NOS-2 expression has been described in the epithelial cells of the upper airway, in bronchial smooth muscle, and in macrophages.[36] Pulmonary vascular endothelial cells primarily express eNOS, whereas both eNOS and nNOS are expressed in the airway epithelial cells.[5] Studies in nonhuman primates suggest that nNOS is the major source of NO in the developing fetal lung.[35] The expression of both eNOS and nNOS increase by three-3 fold from 18 to 20 days of gestation in fetal rats[37] (80%-90% of term gestation, which is 22 days). Developmental studies in baboons demonstrated a marked increase in the expression and activity of all three NOS isoforms from 125 to 140 days (67%-75% of term) gestation.[35] The relative contributions of nNOS and eNOS to the epithelial-mesenchymal interactions remain unclear, partly because of a lack of selective inhibitors for these isoforms. However, studies done in eNOS knockout

A

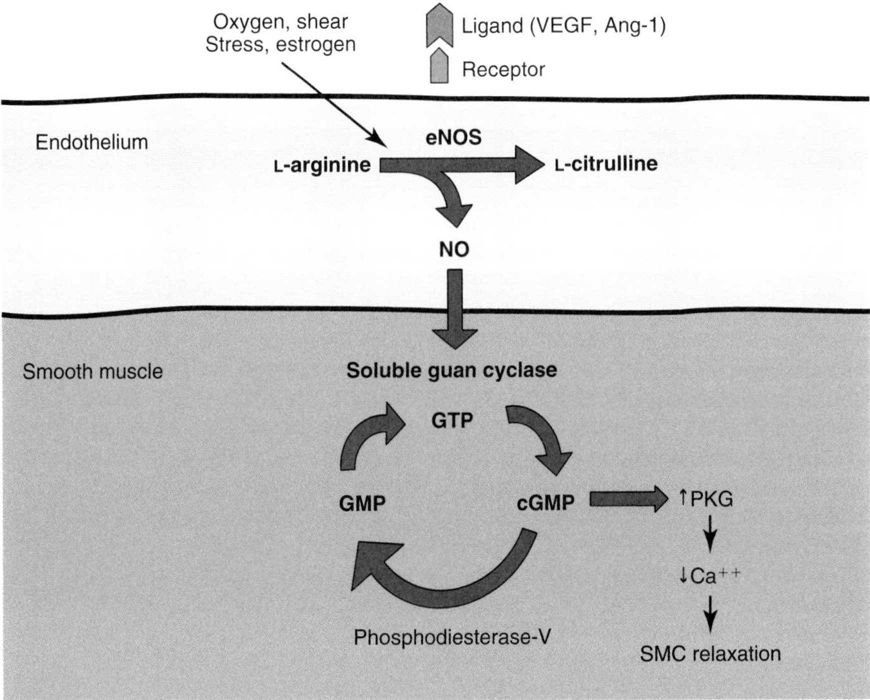

Figure 5-2 Biology of nitric oxide–cyclic guanosine monophosphate (NO-cGMP) system in the pulmonary artery. Several physiologic signals, including oxygen, shear stress, and vascular endothelial growth factor (VEGF), activate endothelial nitric oxide synthase (eNOS) to generate NO from substrates L-arginine and oxygen. NO diffuses to target cells such as vascular smooth muscle to stimulate the heme-containing protein, soluble guanylate cyclase. This stimulation results in the conversion of guanosine triphosphate (GTP) to cGMP, activation of protein kinase G (PKG), and smooth muscle cell (SMC) relaxation. Levels of cGMP are regulated by phosphodiesterase-V, which hydrolyzes cGMP and limits the duration of NO-mediated effects, such as vasodilation. Downstream effects of NO in epithelial cells are also mediated by cGMP.[41] (Adapted from Konduri GG: New approaches for persistent pulmonary hypertension of newborn. *Clin Perinatol.* 2004; 31:591-611.)

($eNOS^{-/-}$) mice demonstrate the importance of eNOS to the coordinated development of lung epithelial and vascular compartments, as described later.[38] Similar studies have not been done in $nNOS^{-/-}$ mice. Functional studies in mice demonstrated that nNOS knockout does not alter the basal PA pressure or the pressor response to hypoxia, although a deletion of even one allele for eNOS accentuates hypoxia-induced pulmonary hypertension.[39] Knockout of iNOS appears to increase the basal PA pressure slightly, probably in relation to a decrease in NO inhaled from the upper airway, which is largely contributed by iNOS.[40]

In contrast to our current understanding of NOS maturation and function in the fetal lung, the specific roles of the downstream mediator of NO (see Fig. 5-2), soluble guanylate cyclase (sGC), and the catalyst for cyclic guanosine monophosphate (cGMP) degradation, phosphodiesterase-V (PDE-V), in fetal lung growth are less clear. Studies done in fetal and neonatal rats demonstrated maturational increases in both sGC and PDE-5 at term gestation and in the neonatal pulmonary circulation.[41] The increase in PDE-V expression in the neonatal rat lung appears to parallel the changes in eNOS and sGC expression.[42] Expression of both sGC and PDE-V is also found in alveolar epithelium in the late-gestation fetal rat lung.[42] These data suggest the presence of the nitric oxide receptor sGC in developing epithelial and endothelial cells.[41] The potential modulation of lung growth by differential expression of sGC and PDE-5 during fetal life is tempting to consider but remains unexplored. In addition, although some studies were performed on the levels of sGC and PDE-V in the vascular smooth muscle (see Fig. 5-2), changes in the epithelial expression of sGC and PDE-V during early development remain unexplored. These studies are necessary for a comprehensive understanding of the role of the NO-cGMP system in both vascular and parenchymal lung growth.

The importance of NO to lung development was clearly demonstrated by studies in the genetic models of eNOS eNOS$^{-/-}$ mice.[38] Such mice have increased mortality in the neonatal period and suffer from respiratory distress. Autopsy studies show altered lung development with decreased alveolar septation, marked pruning of the pulmonary vascular tree, and enlargement and simplification of air spaces (Fig. 5-3). The lung histology of eNOS$^{-/-}$mice shows a decrease in air-blood interface and misalignment of pulmonary veins. The pulmonary veins in these lungs localize to bronchovascular bundle, sharing the adventitia with adjacent PA (see Fig. 5-3), in contrast to the normal location of pulmonary veins at the periphery of the acinus or the lobule of the lung.[5] These features found in eNOS$^{-/-}$ mice simulate the characteristic lung histology of alveolar capillary dysplasia (ACD), a lethal cause of respiratory failure in neonates.[5] The expression of several angiogenic factors, including VEGF/Flk1, angl/TIE2, and FGF2/FGFR, is decreased in the lungs of eNOS$^{-/-}$ mice.[38] These data provide strong evidence that NO is an important upstream regulator of these angiogenic factors. A potential mechanism by which NO regulates the expression of these factors is its effect on expression of HIF-1α. HIF-1α increases VEGF expression and angiogenesis in the lung.[43] Expression of both HIF-1α and VEGF is decreased in premature lambs and baboons with bronchopulmonary dysplasia (BPD), and increasing HIF-1α expression restores lung growth and VEGF expression.[44,45] VEGF is a potent agonist for NO release, which in turn mediates vascular growth by promoting tube formation and epithelial cell proliferation and migration (see Fig. 5-1). The VEGF-NO-VEGF pathway provides a mechanism for the crosstalk between epithelial and vascular compartments. In support of this concept, inhaled NO (INO) has been found to restore lung alveolar and vascular growth in rat pups following inhibition of VEGF signaling.[46] Studies in cultured fetal rat lung explants showed that NO donors promote airway branching morphogenesis (Fig. 5-4).[47] In contrast, inhibition of NO synthesis in lung explants using the arginine analog *N*-nitro-L-arginine methyl ester (L-NAME) leads to a failure of branching morphogenesis and vascular growth in the explants.[47] These data provide further evidence of the direct role of NO in lung development.

Role of Nitric Oxide in Lung Repair

Lung injury and the disordered lung growth that occurs in response are a well-recognized component of BPD in premature infants.[48] There is abundant evidence that alteration in normal growth signals leads to the abnormal lung architecture found in BPD.[5,49] Postmortem studies of lungs from babies with severe BPD demonstrate alveolar simplification with a lack of septation and decreased lung vascular growth.[49] These changes are similar to the observations made in neonatal animals exposed to hyperoxia or inhibition of VEGF receptors.[11,13] As a critical upstream and downstream mediator of angiogenic signals, NO plays an important role in the repair of lung after injury. The normal epithelial-mesenchymal interactions are disturbed in lung injury and BPD. Transition of epithelial to mesenchymal cells and their subsequent differentiation to myofibroblasts contribute to greater formation of collagen and fibrosis in the injured lung.[50] Increase in the transition of epithelial cells to myofibroblasts occurs under the influence of transforming growth factor-β (TGF-β).[51] NO attenuates the effects of TGF-β on the alveolar epithelial cells, preventing their transition to myofibroblasts.[52] The essential role of NO in modulating recovery from lung injury has been demonstrated by the response of eNOS knockout mice to hypoxia. Balasubramaniam and coworkers[53] investigated the effect of mild alveolar hypoxia (16% O_2) on lung development in wild-type mice, heterozygous mice missing one eNOS allele (eNOS$^{+/-}$), and homozygous knockout mice (eNOS$^{-/-}$).[53] Even this mild degree of hypoxia markedly inhibited the alveolar growth and led to alveolar simplification in eNOS$^{-/-}$ mice (Fig. 5-5). This impaired growth persisted in spite of the subsequent recovery of these mice in normoxia for 10 days. Exposure to iNO during recovery in normoxia largely restored lung growth in eNOS knockout

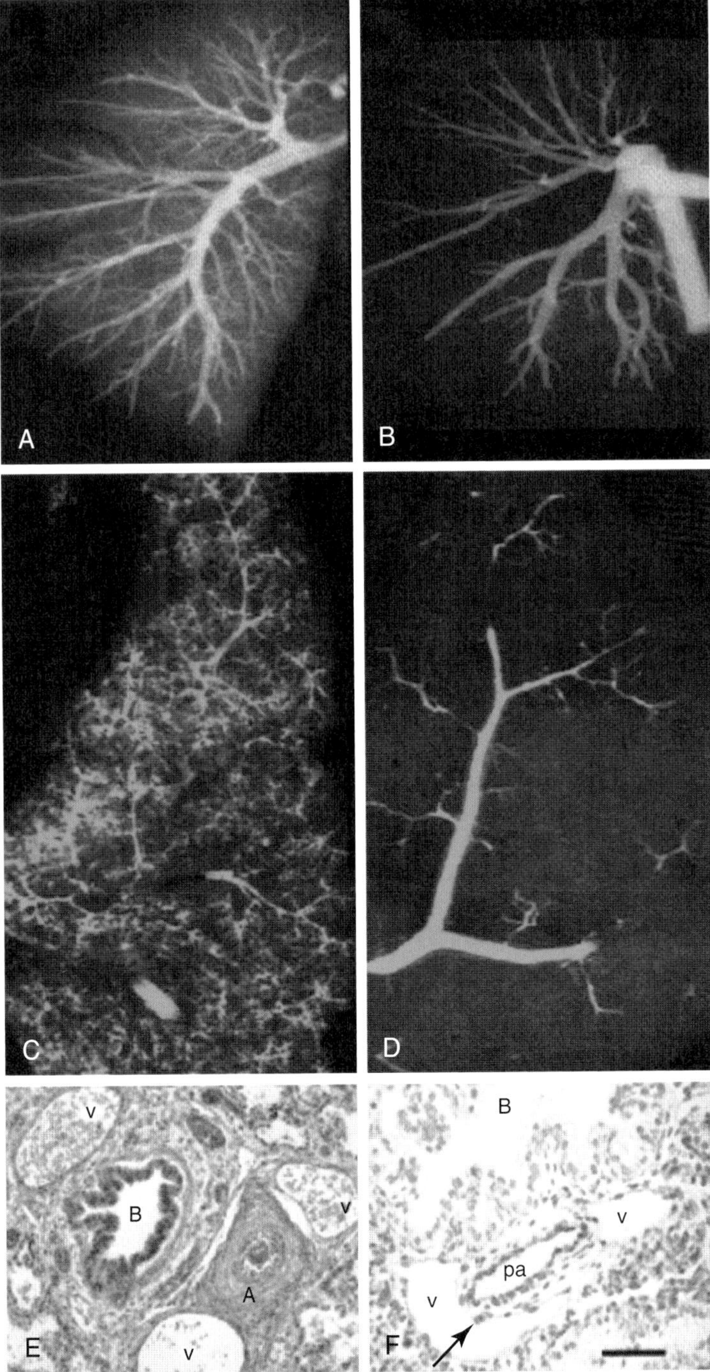

Figure 5-3 Effect of deletion of the endothelial nitric oxide synthase (eNOS) gene on fetal lung development in mice. Barium angiogram of normal human lung (**A**) and fluorescent microangiography of wild-type mouse lung (**C**) show uniform and diffuse filling of intra-acinar arterioles and distal vasculature. In contrast, barium angiogram of a human neonate who died of alveolar capillary dysplasia (ACD) (**B**) and microangiograph of an $eNOS^{-/-}$ mouse fetal lung (**D**) show marked pruning of the vascular tree due to lack of intra-acinar vasculature. Misalignment of pulmonary veins, with vein (V) sharing the same adventitia as the pulmonary artery (pa) (A) and bronchus (B), occurs in a human neonate with ACD (**E**) and an $eNOS^{-/-}$ mouse (**F**). (Figure 5- adapted from Han RNN, Stewart DJ. Defective lung vascular development in endothelial nitric oxide synthase-deficient mice. *Trends Cardiovasc Med.* 2006;16:29-34; ***A*** and ***B*** from DeMello DE. Pulmonary pathology. *Semin Neonatol.* 2004;9:311-329; ***E*** from Vick RN, Owens T, Moise KJ, Chescheir N, Bukowski TP. Urethral atresia in a neonate with alveolar capillary dysplasia and pulmonary venous misalignment. *Urology.* 2000;55:774.)

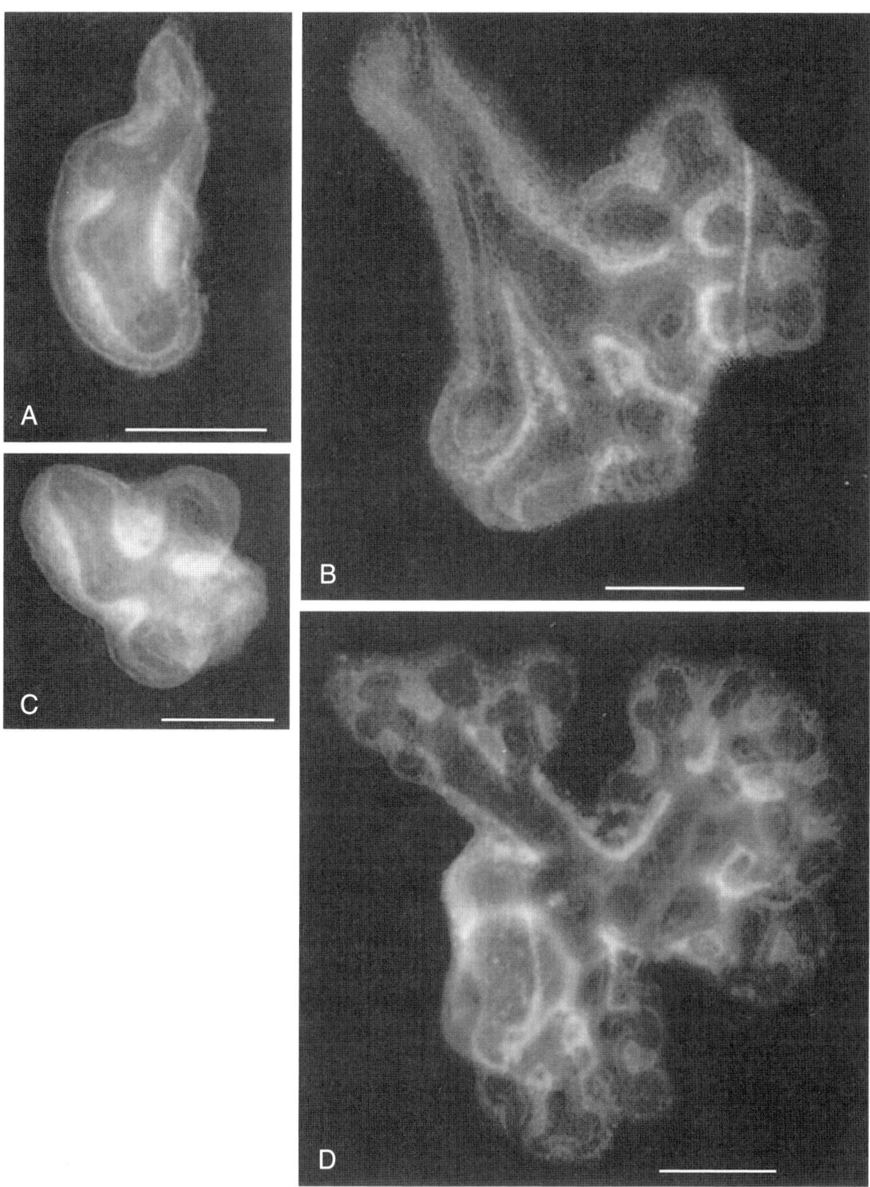

Figure 5-4 Branching morphogenesis of fetal rat lung explants taken at gestational day 13 and cultured for 72 hours. **A** and **B** show controls with fetal lung explant at 0 hours (**A**) and at 72 hours (**B**) in culture without added nitric oxide (NO) donor. When a nitric oxide donor, DETA-NO was added to the culture media at a concentration of 100 μM (**D**), branching of lung explants was greater than in the fetal lung explant at 0 hour (**C**). These data show that NO augments airway branching morphogenesis. (Adapted from Young SL, Evans K, Eu JP. Nitric oxide modulates branching morphogenesis in fetal rat lung explants. *Am J Physiol Lung Cell Mol Physiol.* 2002;282:L379-L385.)

5

mice, suggesting that NO was the critical missing piece for lung growth during early postnatal life in these mice (see Fig. 5-5).[53] VEGF expression was higher during room air recovery in both eNOS$^{+/-}$ and eNOS$^{-/-}$ mice than in wild type controls; whereas, VEGFR-2 expression increased in eNOS$^{+/-}$ mice.[53] These data suggest that VEGF signaling is increased, perhaps in an attempt to compensate for partial or complete loss of eNOS in the lung, during recovery from lung injury in knockout mice. The recovery of lung growth during NO exposure is associated with an increase in VEGFR2 expression in the eNOS$^{-/-}$ mice, although VEGF levels did not change significantly. These studies suggest that NO also has important downstream

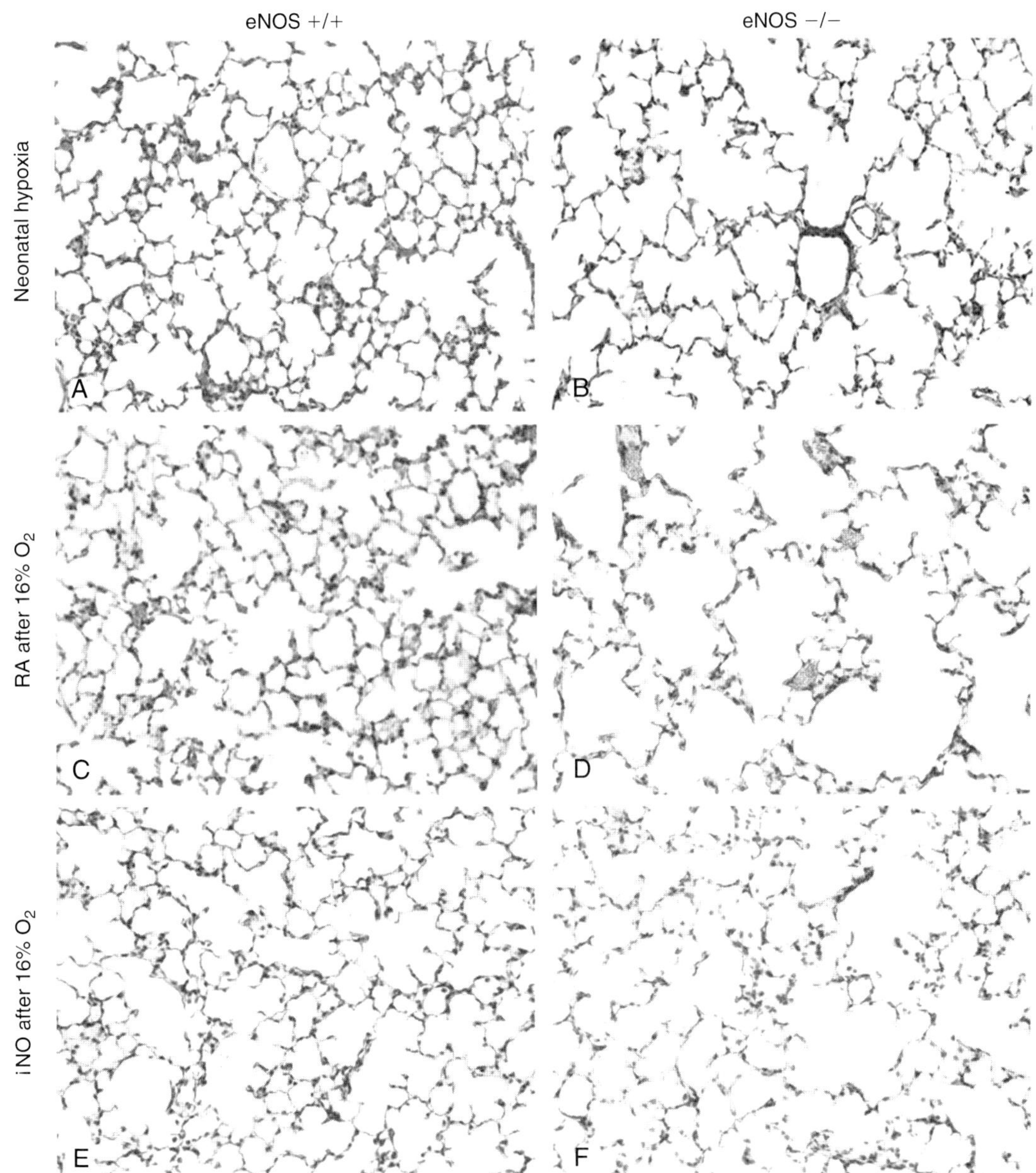

Figure 5-5 Inhaled nitric oxide (iNO) restores lung structure in the eNOS$^{-/-}$ mouse after brief postnatal exposure to mild hypoxia (16% O_2). Lung structure is abnormal with enlarged air spaces and a lack of alveolar septation in the eNOS$^{-/-}$ mice (**B**) in comparison with that in wild-type mice (**A**) after 10 days of neonatal exposure to mild hypoxia. The simplified air space structure persists in eNOS$^{-/-}$ mice exposed to neonatal hypoxia despite recovery in room air (**D**), whereas the lungs in wild-type mice show normal structure (**C**). The eNOS$^{-/-}$ mice that received iNO (10 ppm) during room air (RA) recovery (**F**) show restoration of lung alveolar structure, which is indistinguishable from that in lungs of wild-type mice (**E**). (Adapted from Balasubramaniam V, Maxey AM, Morgan DB, et al. Inhaled NO restores lung structure in eNOS-deficient mice recovering from neonatal hypoxia. *Am J Physiol Lung Cell Mol Physiol*. 2006;291:L119-L127.)

effects on VEGFR2, which mediates the angiogenic effects of VEGF in the lung. Compensatory lung growth, which normally occurs in the right lung after left pneumonectomy in mice, is also severely impaired in eNOS$^{-/-}$-mice.[54] This impaired growth is associated with decreased proliferation of alveolar epithelial cells and respiratory gas exchange area in the remaining right lung. In contrast, wild-type mice show marked increases in the proliferation rates of epithelial cells and gas exchange area of right lung after left pneumonectomy. This growth in wild-type mice is accompanied by increases in eNOS activity and expression and the expression of

NOS co-factor calmodulin in the remaining lung. The NOS antagonist, L-NAME, was found to inhibit this compensatory lung growth in pneumonectomized wild-type mice.[54] These data strongly suggest that NO is required for alveolar growth, which occurs as a component of lung repair. Hyperoxia exposure results in decreases in VEGF, VEGFR2, and eNOS expression in association with impaired alveolar and vascular growth in neonatal rat pups.[13] INO also improves impaired alveolarization in the hyperoxic rat pups.[13] These data support the concept that eNOS modulates both alveolar and vascular growth in the developing lung after injury. In contrast to the well-defined role of eNOS, the contributions of nNOS and iNOS to lung repair remain unclear. Further studies are needed in nNOS and iNOS knockout mice to define their specific roles in fetal lung development and the repair of postnatal lung after injury.

The critical role of NO in modulating lung injury was also demonstrated in primate and sheep models of respiratory distress syndrome. Afshar and colleagues[35] reported a decrease in the expression and activity of all three isoforms of NOS in a baboon model of BPD, which was initiated by premature delivery and support on mechanical ventilation.[35] Alveolar structure was disrupted in these baboon pups following 2 weeks of positive-pressure ventilation. Exposure to 5 ppm of INO therapy during mechanical ventilation preserved the alveolar structure, with normalization of lung growth, evidenced by DNA content and cell proliferation, elastin deposition, and stimulation of secondary crest formation.[55] These improvements occurred despite ongoing injury from mechanical ventilation to the lung structure. Expression of eNOS is also decreased in premature lambs undergoing long-term ventilation for respiratory distress syndrome (RDS).[56] INO administered to ventilated premature lambs decreases neutrophil influx and lung edema, suggesting modulation of the early inflammatory response to injury by NO.[57]

Role of Nitric Oxide in Maintaining the Lung Structure during Postnatal Life

Studies in rodent models demonstrated that both VEGF and NO play integral roles in maintaining the homeostasis of the air-blood barrier during postnatal life. Inhibition of VEGF receptors leads to changes similar to those of emphysema in adult rats with decreased expression of eNOS.[58] Decrease in VEGF expression leads to apoptosis of both endothelial and alveolar epithelial cells and makes the epithelial cells more vulnerable to oxidative stress and protease-mediated injury in chronic obstructive pulmonary disease (COPD).[58] NO protects the alveolar epithelial cells from superoxide-mediated injury, and INO decreases injury from hyperoxia in adult rats.[59] These studies suggest that NO plays a trophic role in maintaining the air-blood interface in the mature lung.

Regulation of NOS Catalytic Function and Its Alteration in Lung Injury

A proper understanding of NOS catalytic function is essential to a delineation of its role in lung development and the response to lung injury (Fig. 5-6). NOS is an oxidoreductase, and its catalytic function is among the most tightly regulated in the cell.[34] The carboxy terminal of the enzyme consists of the nicotinamide adenine dinucleotide phosphate (NADPH) reductase domain, and the amino terminal contains the heme-oxygenase domain with both heme and BH4 prosthetic groups.[34] The reductase and oxygenase domains are linked by a binding protein for calmodulin, which binds Ca^{++} and functions as a molecular switch for electron flow (see Fig. 5-6). BH4, an essential cofactor, activates heme-bound O_2 and stimulates efficient production of NO.[60] The catalytic activity of NOS also requires the presence of a substrate, L-arginine, and the chaperone, heat shock protein 90 (Hsp90), as a cofactor.[61] NOS functions as a homodimer and its activity is regulated by phosphorylation at several sites, which modulates electron flow through the reductase domain.[34] Hsp90 helps stabilize the NOS homodimer and facilitates phosphorylation and

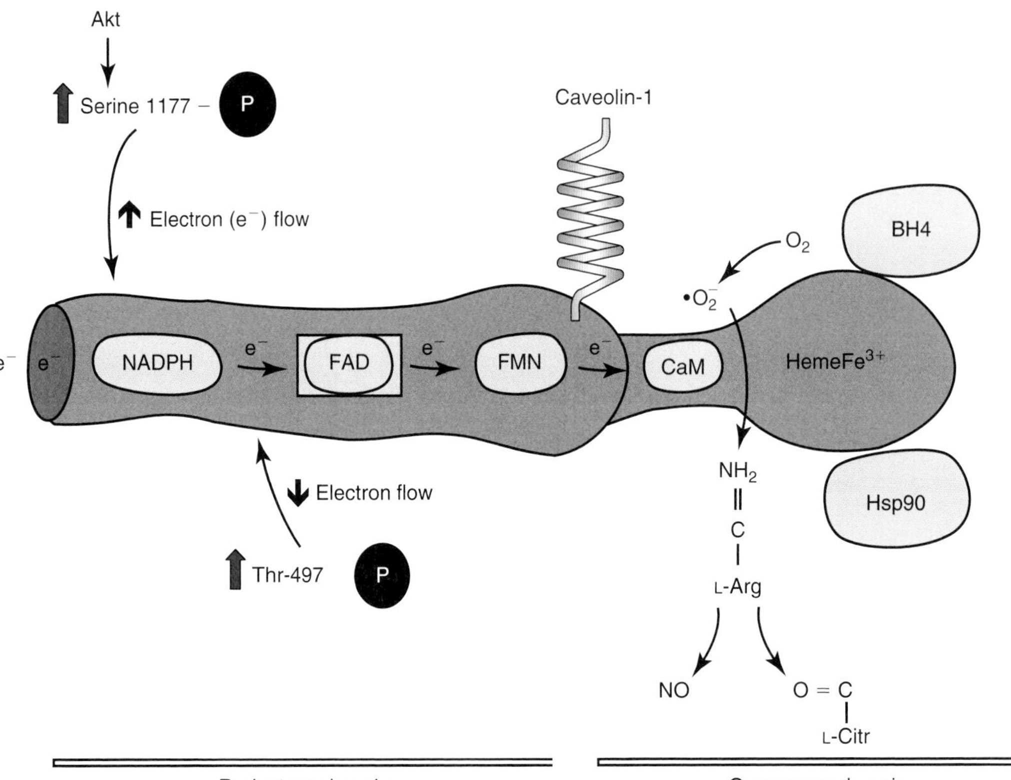

Figure 5-6 Regulation of endothelial nitric oxide synthase (eNOS) catalytic activity by phosphorylation and by cofactors. Several protein kinases modify NOS activity by phosphorylation at different serine and threonine residues. For example, serine-1177 phosphorylation by the kinase Akt increases and threonine-497 (Thr-497) phosphorylation decreases electron flow through the reductase domain of NOS. Caveolin-1 decreases and calmodulin promotes the electron flow to O_2. Interaction of cofactor BH4 and heat shock protein 90 (hsp90) with the heme oxygenase domain (HemeFe3$^+$) is required for oxidation of L-arginine (L-Arg) to generate NO. Decreases in BH4 or hsp90 association with NOS result in release of O_2^- instead of NO as the end product when NOS is stimulated. Although represented here as a monomer, NOS functions as a homodimer under physiologic conditions inside the cell. CaM, calmodulin; L-Citr, L-citrulline; FAD, flavine adenine dinucleotide; FMN, flavine mononucleotide; NADPH, nicotinamide adenine dinucleotide phosphate; P, phosphorylation.

coupling of electron flow to oxidation of arginine bound to the heme-oxygenase domain.[61] During normal catalytic function, oxidation of terminal guanidino nitrogen of arginine generates NO (see Fig. 5-6). Uncoupling of NOS activity can occur with the depletion of substrate, L-arginine, decreased availability of Hsp90, and depletion or oxidation of BH4.[62,63] Stimulation of uncoupled NOS leads to release of superoxide (O_2^- instead of nitric oxide as the catalytic end product. Increase in levels of O_2^- from NOS has been identified as a major contributor to injury in pulmonary hypertension[64,65] and in ventilator- or oxygen-induced lung injury.[66] Recoupling of NOS has been shown to ameliorate lung injury secondary to hyperoxia in neonatal rats.[67] The effect of increased superoxide from uncoupled NOS on lung growth is unclear. However, improved lung growth in response to L-citrulline supplementation in the hyperoxic neonatal rat model suggests that oxidative stress from eNOS contributes to impaired lung growth.[67] Oxidative stress also contributes to impaired angiogenesis of fetal PA endothelial cells.[68] Recoupling of NOS and scavenging of oxidative stress restore angiogenesis in these cells.[68] Impaired angiogenesis is an important cause of defective lung growth in BPD.[11] The possible reversal of impaired lung growth with the use of antioxidants remains unclear; the use of exogenous SOD in small clinical trials did not show a decrease in the incidence of BPD.[69] Exogenous recombinant SOD increases eNOS expression in neonatal lambs ventilated for persistent pulmonary hypertension of the newborn (PPHN).[70] Strategies to recouple endogenous NOS activity offer promise for repair of lung damage and restoration of lung growth in premature infants.

Role of BH4 in the Regulation of NOS Activity

As previously described, BH4 is an essential cofactor for NOS activity and overall redox balance in the cells.[60] BH4 facilitates NOS dimerization and oxidation of L-arginine to generate NO.[60] BH4 also facilitates the optimum interaction of NOS with its chaperone, Hsp90. Oxidation of BH4 leads to accumulation of BH2, which competes for the heme-binding site but is ineffective in stabilizing NOS.[60] Depletion of BH4 by oxidative stress leads to decreased NO availability in a variety of vascular diseases, including hypertension and diabetes.[63] BH4 is synthesized from guanosine triphosphate (GTP) through the activity of GTP-cyclohydrolase-1 (GCH-1), a rate-limiting step affecting the availability of BH4 in the cell.[60] Mice that are genetically deficient in GCH-1 activity demonstrate pulmonary hypertension spontaneously.[71] In contrast, GCH-1 overexpression protects mice from hypoxia-induced pulmonary hypertension.[72] BH4 is also regenerated from BH2 by dihydrofolate reductase in the cells.[73] Supplementation with BH4 increases NO availability and facilitates endothelium-dependent relaxation in hypoxia-induced pulmonary hypertension in piglets.[74] The developmental regulation of GCH-1 and its relationship to lung growth in fetal life require further investigation.

5

Regulation of NOS Activity through L-Arginine Availability

The endogenous arginine analogs, asymmetric dimethyl arginine (ADMA) and *N*-G-monomethyl-L-arginine (L-NMMA) also affect the availability and interaction of arginine with NOS. Plasma levels of these analogs are elevated in the presence of lung injury and pulmonary hypertension.[75] These analogs inhibit NO release and also cause uncoupling of NOS, leading to increased superoxide formation.[76] Levels of ADMA are regulated by protein arginine methyl transferases (PRMTs), which generate ADMA from protein methylation, and by the enzyme dimethyl arginine dimethyl amino hydrolase (DDAH), which metabolizes ADMA.[76] Activity of DDAH in particular regulates the ADMA levels tightly, indirectly affecting the activity of NOS.[77] DDAH activity is inhibited by oxidative stress and homocysteine, which modify the sulfhydryl group in its active site. Interestingly, NO also inhibits DDAH activity, creating feedback inhibition of NO synthesis.[77] Regulation of NOS activity by changes in the availability of ADMA during lung development remains unexplored. ADMA inhibits VEGF-induced angiogenesis in human umbilical vein endothelial cells in a NO-dependent manner.[78] Plasma levels of ADMA in umbilical cord venous blood are significantly higher than ADMA levels in venous blood during adult life, indicating higher levels during fetal life.[79,80] However, the significance of these observations to physiologically high fetal PVR or to lung development is unclear. The high ADMA levels may simply represent the high protein turnover in the fetus. Developmental changes in the activity of protein arginine methyl transferases and DDAH-1 during fetal lung growth also require further study.

L-Citrulline, the catalytic end product of NO synthesis, can be efficiently recycled in the cell by the enzymes argininosuccinate synthase and argininosuccinate lyase.[67] Although orally administered arginine is degraded by hepatic arginases, oral citrulline enters the circulation and helps raise plasma arginine levels by the recycling pathway. L-Citrulline also enters the cell more readily than L-arginine and may provide a therapeutic option to increase the L-arginine availability for NOS. L-Citrulline supplementation was previously shown to ameliorate hypoxia-induced pulmonary hypertension in piglets and to increase NO availability in these animals.[81] Preliminary studies in neonatal rats with O_2-induced lung injury suggest that L-citrulline supplementation reverses the impairment of alveolar growth in this model.[67]

A

Interaction of Antioxidant Enzyme Systems with Endogenous Nitric Oxide

The functional effects of NO depend on its biologic availability. NO in the cell is rapidly quenched by superoxide, which reacts with NO at a rate determined by the availability of SOD.[34] The bioavailability of NO is therefore very much dependent on the antioxidant defenses, primarily the SOD system. There are three isoforms of SOD within the cell—cytosolic copper-zinc SOD (SOD-1), mitochondrial manganese SOD (SOD-2), and extracellular copper-zinc SOD (SOD-3). The ability of SOD to scavenge O_2^- depends on the amount of available enzyme protein and post-translational modifications that can alter the reaction of O_2^- with SOD. The SOD isoforms show maturational increase toward term gestation, in parallel with the surfactant system.[82] The vulnerability of premature lung to injury is in part attributed to deficient SOD levels in the lung. O_2^- levels increase in the lung in response to both O_2 and barotrauma.[66,67] The facilitation of lung growth by NO is therefore indirectly dependent on the availability of SOD system relative to the levels of oxidative stress. Studies in ventilated neonatal lambs have demonstrated that exogenous recombinant human SOD can preserve NO availability and increase the expression of eNOS.[70] These studies point to a dynamic interaction between the NO-cGMP system and SOD in the lung. Reaction of NO with O_2^- results in the formation of peroxynitrite ($ONOO^-$), which can nitrate proteins and lead to cell apoptosis in high concentrations. Excess levels of peroxynitrite can impair angiogenesis through multiple mechanisms, including alteration of microtubules in the cytoskeleton and uncoupling of eNOS to amplify oxidative stress in the cell.[83]

Relationship of Oxygen Tension with NOS Function and Lung Growth during Fetal Life

Fetal oxygen tension facilitates lung mesenchymal and vascular growth. In contrast, premature exposure to postnatal oxygen tension, even normoxia, can inhibit epithelial-mesenchymal interactions and lung growth.[84] The signaling mechanisms involved in oxygen sensing by the lung are not clear. The oxygen-sensitive transcription factor hypoxia-inducible factor-1(HIF-1α) plays an important role in directing branching morphogenesis and lung vascular growth.[85] HIF-1α knockout mice show disrupted morphogenesis and enlarged vascular structures before death at E10.5.[85] The importance of fetal oxygen tension for lung growth has been demonstrated by studies of mouse lung explants in culture. Exposure to 3% oxygen promotes, and to 21% oxygen inhibits, branching morphogenesis and growth of vascular structures in these explants.[84] The specific oxygen-regulated genes that modulate lung growth have not been fully characterized yet. Genes that appear to function differently at fetal and postnatal O_2 tensions include HIF-1α, FGF9, hepatic nuclear factors (HNFs) 3 and 4, and TGF-β. HNF-3 and HIF-1α may co-modulate the differential expression of genes with changing O_2 concentrations.[86] Hypoxia also modulates the expression and activity of NOS isoforms, with targeted release of NO occurring in the epithelial and mesenchymal compartments in the periphery of growing lung at fetal PO_2.[47] TGF-β appears to downregulate NOS expression and may play an important role in targeting NOS expression to the peripheral areas of lung, where active airway branching and vasculogenesis occur, while turning off these signals in other areas.[5] Exposure to increased oxygen levels during fetal lung development may disrupt this selective and local modulation of NOS activity and expression in specific areas of the lung.[87] Exposure of premature lung to increased O_2 concentration during postnatal life can similarly disrupt the physiologic gradients established for angiogenic signals and growth of the gas exchange units in the lung through multiple mechanisms. Avoiding hyperoxia while preserving endogenous NOS activity may help reestablish growth signals in the premature lung.

Physiologic Role of Nitric Oxide in the Gas Exchange Function of the Lung

The role of NO in modulating basal vascular tone and changes in vessel diameter in response to diverse physiologic stimuli has been well recognized for more than 20 years.[34] In addition to its role in coordinating lung growth, NO plays a major role in the transition of lung function at birth. Release of NO occurs in the pulmonary circulation in response to well-recognized birth-related stimuli—oxygen, ventilation, and shear stress.[88-90] Inhibition of NO synthesis impairs pulmonary vasodilation in response to oxygen, shear stress, and endothelium-dependent vasodilators in fetal lambs.[88-90] NOS inhibition also impairs pulmonary vasodilation in response to ventilation in fetal lambs and leads to persistent elevation of PA pressure during postnatal life.[89] Although the pool of NO that regulates pulmonary vascular tone is assumed to be from eNOS in endothelial cells, the lung expresses all three NOS isoforms in the pulmonary epithelial cells. A dynamic role for airway-derived NO in the ventilation-perfusion matching during tidal respiration is suggested by a number of studies.[91,92] In vitro studies in rat lung pulmonary arteries demonstrated that bronchus-derived NO decreases the tone of PA.[91] Inhalation of airway-derived NO also contributes to basal pulmonary vascular tone. Measurement of pulmonary vascular resistance in adults using an indwelling PA catheter demonstrated that oral breathing is associated with higher pulmonary vascular resistance (PVR) than nasal breathing.[93] Breath NO levels were also higher during nasal breathing than oral breathing.[93] These studies demonstrate a functional role for airway-derived NO in modulating PVR during tidal respiration. Evidence from these and other studies indicates that locally, the blood flow through the capillaries is closely titrated to the expansion of alveolar space under the influence of both airway- and endothelium-derived NO.

In addition to regulating the local vascular tone, NO has multiple biologic effects that are required for the homeostasis of the air-blood barrier. These include maintaining endothelial barrier function, decreasing the adhesion of cells to the endothelium, maintaining surfactant function, and preventing apoptosis of endothelial and epithelial cells.[5] Although similar data are not available in neonates, nasal NO levels (median of 20 PPB) were found to be strikingly higher than lower airway NO levels (median of 4 PPB) measured in ventilated premature neonates.[94] The high nasal NO levels were observed even on the first day of life, before bacterial colonization occurs and when paranasal sinuses are only partially developed.[94] The nasal levels of NO measured in some babies in these studies were more than 100 parts per billion (0.1 parts per million), close to the therapeutically effective doses of inhaled NO.[94,95] The effect of NO inhaled from the upper airway in the growth of lungs in premature babies remains unknown, although the lower incidence of BPD among babies who did not receive mechanical ventilation may be partly related to the availability of endogenous, INO. Intubated babies are deprived of their own endogenous source of INO because an endotracheal tube bypasses the upper airway. In support of this possibility, knockout of iNOS, which is a major source of nasal/upper airway NO, is associated with an increase in basal PA pressure in mice.[40]

Altered Lung Architecture in BPD and Its Relation to NOS Signaling

Now, BPD is seen predominantly in premature babies born at less than 28 weeks of gestation,[5] in contrast to the pre-surfactant era, during which older premature babies also had significant incidence of this complication. The lung architecture in extremely premature babies that die of severe BPD shows growth arrest with alveolar simplification from a loss of septation and paucity of capillaries in the alveolar septa.[48,49] This pattern is different from the original BPD described in the era before the widespread use of prenatal steroids and postnatal surfactant. Babies in the previous era demonstrated marked lung injury, inflammation, and fibrosis.[5] The new presentation of BPD clearly represents arrested lung development affecting both epithelial and vascular compartments.[49] These observations point to the importance of understanding the nature of normal growth signals present in the developing lung and their alteration in premature babies.

The idea that restoring growth signals will lead to recovery of lung growth was suggested from studies in animal models. As previously summarized, both VEGF and its signaling agent, NO, have been studied in animal models of BPD. The expression of VEGF and eNOS is decreased in lung epithelial and vascular compartments in preterm infants with BPD[49] and in the ovine and primate models of BPD induced by ventilation of premature animals.[35,55,56] The expression of these two key factors is also decreased in neonatal rats exposed to hyperoxia injury.[13] Inhibition of VEGF receptors leads to decreased eNOS expression and to alveolar and vascular growth arrest reminiscent of BPD.[11] INO reverses the injury and restores lung growth in a number of these animal models, an observation that has led to clinical testing of this approach in premature babies as explained later.[13,46,55] Although recombinant human VEGF has shown the potential to increase lung growth in neonatal rats with hyperoxic injury, the lung growth is associated with greater vascular permeability and lung edema.[96] Similar effects were also seen in this model as a result of intratracheal gene therapy with an adenoviral vector containing VEGF gene.[97] Because these effects can be potentially detrimental to the gas exchange function of the premature lung, INO was investigated as a therapy to promote lung growth in premature infants.

Application of Inhaled Nitric Oxide to Restore Lung Growth in Premature Neonates

Studies done in animal models, as previously summarized, provided the biologic basis for application of INO therapy in premature neonates. BPD primarily represents a failure of normal alveolar and vascular growth during postnatal life in premature babies.[5,49] Because NO plays a major role in fetal lung development and restores lung growth in several animal models of lung injury, investigation of INO therapy to decrease BPD incidence in premature babies appears logical. As summarized previously, INO therapy decreased lung inflammation, stimulated alveolar growth, and reversed pulmonary hypertension in animal models.

On the basis of these findings, INO therapy was tested either early in the course of RDS to decrease lung injury or later in babies needing prolonged ventilation to prevent BPD. Both of these strategies have been tested in a number of large randomized trials (Table 5-2). A single-center study reported by Schreiber and associates[98] observed that INO therapy initiated in the first 3 days of life in premature babies of gestational age less than 34 weeks decreases the combined outcome of death/BPD.[98] However, two large multicenter trials reported subsequently by Kinsella and colleagues[99] and Mercier and associates[100] failed to show a decrease in the incidence of death/BPD in preterm babies treated in the first few days of life. Although these studies enrolled babies at different gestational ages and had different eligibility criteria, the concept for both of them was that early administration of INO prevents lung injury and enhances lung repair and growth. Both the trial reported by Kinsella and colleagues[99] and the European Multicenter NO trial described by Mercier and associates[100] enrolled nearly 800 babies each and found no difference in the outcome between placebo and treatment groups (see Table 5-2). The National Institute of Child Health and Human Development Neonatal Research Network trial reported by Van Meurs and coworkers[101] found that INO therapy given to preterm babies with severe RDS early in the course of their illness did not lower the incidence of death/BPD.[101] On the basis of large sample sizes (combined sample size of 2000 infants) and similar results from these three trials, INO therapy is unlikely to have an impact on the incidence of BPD when given to all premature babies early in the course of RDS. A subgroup of larger premature babies (>1000 g) in the Van Meurs and Kinsella trials showed decreases in the incidence of death/BPD when they received INO therapy. The European Nitric Oxide (EUNO) trial has specifically excluded these larger infants. Whether these larger infants, who are typically at the saccular stage of lung development, are more likely to have the beneficial effect from

Table 5-2 RANDOMIZED, CONTROLLED TRIALS OF INHALED NITRIC OXIDE (INO) IN PREMATURE INFANTS AND THEIR PRIMARY OUTCOME RESULTS*

Trial	Gestational Age of Subjects (wk)	Sample Size	Postnatal Age at Enrolment	Duration of NO Therapy	Effect of INO on Primary Outcome	Effect of INO in Subgroup Analyses
Schreiber et al[98]	<34	207	<72 hr	7 days	Increased rate of survival free of CLD from 36% to 51%	Improvement in survival free of BPD occurred in babies with OI < 6.94
Van Meurs et al[101]	<34	420	≤120 hr	Maximum 14 days, mean 76 hr	No effect on rate of death or BPD	Improvement in survival free of BPD in preterms > 1000 g
Kinsella et al[99]	≤34	793	<48 hr	Maximum 21 days; median 14 days	No effect on rate of death or BPD	Improvement in survival free of BPD in preterms > 1000 g
Mercier et al (European Nitric Oxide [EUNO])[100]	<29	800	<24 hr	Maximum 21 days; mean 16 days	No effect on rate of survival free of BPD	
Ballard et al[102]	≤32	582	7-21 days	Up to 24 days	Improved rate of survival without BPD from 37% to 44%	Improvement in rate of survival free of BPD from 28% to 49% for babies enrolled at age 7-14 days

BPD, bronchopulmonary dysplasia; CLD, chronic lung disease; INO, inhaled nitric oxide; OI, oxygenation index.
*Trials were selected if they had sample size > 200. Group.

INO requires further study. In contrast to these studies of early application of INO, Ballard and associates[102] reported that INO therapy given to premature babies needing ventilator support at 1 to 3 weeks of age improved the probability of survival free of BPD by 7%. Most of the improvement occurred in babies enrolled at 1 to 2 weeks of postnatal age if they required mechanical ventilation. This study raises the possibility that a more targeted approach to treating babies at a higher risk of BPD is more effective than a prophylactic approach, that is, treating all premature babies with RDS. A large trial of INO therapy targeting preterm infants born at less than 30 weeks gestational age who require ventilation at 1 to 2 weeks postnatal age is currently under way at a number of sites. This study will investigate whether INO is beneficial to this group as suggested by subgroup analysis of the Ballard trial.

Although INO induced lung growth in animal models, clinical trials so far show a lack of efficacy when INO is given to babies undergoing immediate postnatal transition. The reasons for the difference in results between animal models and clinical studies in premature babies are not clear. Some possible differences are that premature babies enrolled in clinical trials are typically born at earlier gestation than the animal models studied for INO therapy. Although premature infants most vulnerable to BPD are born at less than 28 weeks of (<0.7 term) gestation, one study examined ventilated premature baboons later than 0.7 term gestation.[55] The period of lung growth in humans spans a much longer time horizon than in rodents, sheep, and primates, lasting up to 8 years or longer (Fig. 5-7).[103,104] The duration of INO

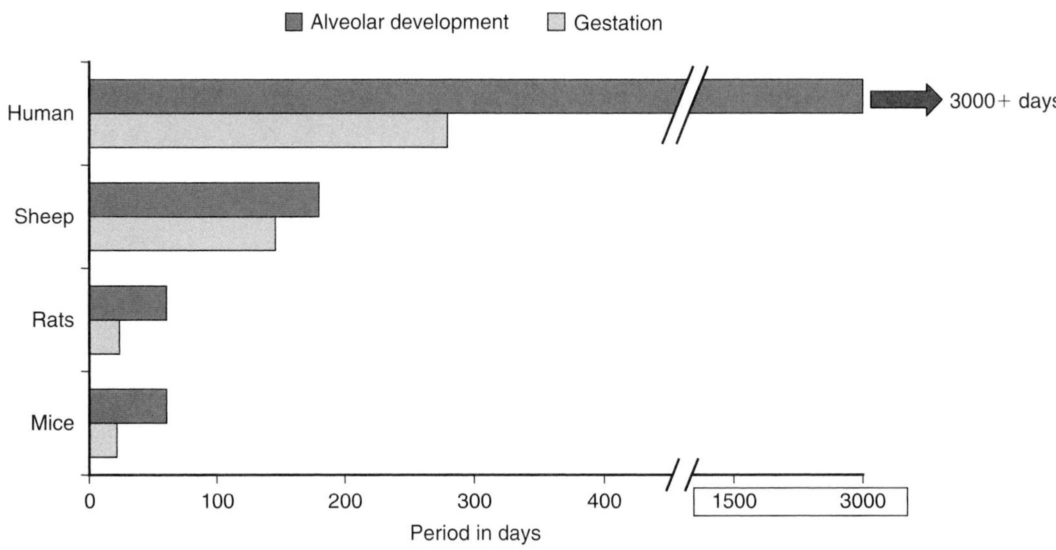

Figure 5-7 Comparative periods of gestation and lung growth for rodents, sheep, and humans. The graph shows length of gestation and the approximate postnatal period in days for completion of alveolar growth for comparison. The alveolar growth is completed in a few weeks after birth in rodents, but human lung growth continues into adult life (>8 years). The duration of nitric oxide therapy used in rodent, sheep, and primate studies (1-2 weeks) covers a larger proportion of lung growth for those species than the comparable duration used for human trials of inhaled NO (maximum 24 days).

therapy used in most clinical trials (<24 days) may be insufficient time for induction of lung growth (see Fig. 5-7; Table 5-2). The potential for restoring lung growth with longer administration of INO in premature babies requires further investigation. The apparent benefit of INO in larger preterm infants suggested by results of the subgroup analysis of the Van Meurs and Kinsella trials suggests that INO may be more beneficial when targeted to a specific stage of lung development. The baboon model of BPD targeted animals at the saccular stage, comparable to 27 to 30 weeks of human gestation.[55] Further studies are needed to verify these observations from the subgroup analyses. In addition, mortality and BPD were used as the outcome variables to define the efficacy of INO therapy in these trials. However, clinical definition of BPD as currently used may not be a sensitive indicator of changes in lung growth. Further clinical tools to assess the effect of INO on lung growth in premature babies are urgently needed. Finally, exogenous NO may not be as effective as restoring endogenous NOS activity in enhancing lung growth. Because NO has local effects on specific cell types, NO release is targeted to areas of active morphogenesis by NOS isoforms resident in the epithelial-endothelial interface to promote lung growth. Enhancing this process may require strategies to improve endogenous NOS function in the injured lung. Studies in mice demonstrated that BH4 and ascorbic acid attenuate the lung injury caused by high–tidal volume ventilation by recoupling NOS.[66] L-Citrulline appears to improve lung growth in oxygen-exposed neonatal rats by recoupling NOS enzyme.[67] Similar approaches to restore coupled activity of eNOS require further investigation in premature babies. Similarly, strategies to augment cGMP levels in the lung by use of PDE-V inhibitors or strategies to preserve endogenous NO by scavenging reactive oxygen species require further investigation.

Summary

Nitric oxide is a critical signaling molecule that plays an integral role along with a number of other angiogenic factors to promote the synchronized development of epithelial and vascular compartments in the lung. NO is both an upstream and downstream mediator for angiogenic signals, such as VEGF, angiopoietins, and Basic fibroblast growth factor (BFGF) and facilitates crosstalk between epithelial and endothelial cells to establish the air-blood interface. NO is also involved in maintaining integrity of the air-blood interface throughout postnatal life. The ability of NO to promote lung growth and repair after lung injury has been demonstrated in a number of animal models, including those involving rodents, sheep, and nonhuman primates. Application of INO therapy to accomplish the same goal in premature neonates with lung injury, however, had inconclusive results. Whether current strategies for the use of INO therapy in this population of babies can be improved by selecting specific sub-groups or different time point in the course of respiratory failure remains to be determined. Strategies to restore the normal catalytic function of endogenous NOS, preserve endogenous NO or increase cGMP levels to promote lung growth also require further investigation.

Acknowledgments

The author acknowledges the drawing for Figure 5-1 by Dr. Satyan Lakshminrusimha, Associate Professor of Pediatrics, University at Buffalo, New York, who retains the copyright for the drawing.

References

1. Shannon JM, Hyatt BA. Epithelial-mesenchymal interactions in the developing lung. *Annu Rev Physiol*. 2004;66:625-645.
2. De Mello DE, Sawyer D, Galvin N, Reid LM. Early fetal development of lung vasculature. *Am J Respir Cell Mol Biol*. 11997;6:5568-5581.
3. Hall SM, Hislop AA, Pierce CM, Haworth SG. Prenatal origins for human intrapulmonary arteries: formation and smooth muscle maturation. *Am J Respir Cell Mol Biol*. 2000;23:194-203.

3a. De Mello DE, Reid LM. Embryonic and early fetal development of human lung vasculature and its functional implications. *Pediatr Dev Pathol*. 2002;3:439-449.

4. Parera MC, Van Dooren M, Van Kempen M, et al. Distal angiogenesis: a new concept for vasculogenesis. *Am J Physiol Lung Cell Mol Biol*. 2005;288:L141-L146.
5. Stenmark RK, Abman SH. Lung vascular development: Implications for the pathogenesis of bronchopulmonary dysplasia. *Ann Rev Physiol*. 2005;67:623-661.
6. Han RN, Stewart DJ. Defective lung vascular development in endothelial nitric oxide synthase-deficient mice. *Trends Cardiovasc Med*. 2006;16:29-34.
7. Abman SH, Shanley PF, Accurso FJ. Failure of postnatal adaptation of the pulmonary circulation after chronic intrauterine pulmonary hypertension in fetal lambs. *J Clin Invest*. 1989; 83:184918-184958.
8. Morin FC 3rd. Ligating the ductus arteriosus before birth causes persistent pulmonary hypertension in the newborn lamb. *Pediatr Res*. 1989;25:245-250.
9. Wild LM, Nickerson PA, Morin FC 3rd. Ligating the ductus arteriosus before birth remodels the pulmonary vasculature of the lamb. *Pediatr Res*. 1989;25:251-257.
10. Grover TR, Parker TA, Balasubramaniam V, et al. Pulmonary hypertension impairs alveolarization and reduces lung growth in the ovine fetus. *Am J Physiol Lung Cell Mol Physiol*. 2005 Apr; 288:L648-L654.
11. Jakkula M, Le Cras TD, Gebb S, et al. Inhibition of angiogenesis decreases alveolarization in the developing rat lung. *Am J Physiol Lung Cell Mol Physiol*. 2000;279:L600-L607.
12. Delisser HM, Helmke BP, Cao G, et al. Loss of PECAM-1 function impairs alveolarization. *J Biol Chem*. 2006;281:8724-8731.
13. Lin YJ, Markham NE, Balasubramaniam V, et al. Inhaled nitric oxide enhances distal lung growth after exposure to hyperoxia in neonatal rats. *Pediatr Res*. 2005;58:22-29.
14. Truog WE, Xu D, Ekekezie II, Mabry S, et al. Chronic hypoxia and rat lung development: analysis by morphometry and directed microarray. *Pediatr Res*. 2008;64:56-62.
15. Zhang F, Tang Z, Hou X, et al. VEGF-B is dispensable for blood vessel growth but critical for their survival, and VEGF-B targeting inhibits pathological angiogenesis. *Proc Natl Acad Sci USA*. 2009;106:6152-6157.
16. Sun Y, Jin K, Childs JT, et al. Increased severity of cerebral ischemic injury in vascular endothelial growth factor-B-deficient mice. *J Cereb Blood Flow Metab*. 2004;24:1146-1152.
17. Ferrara N. Vascular endothelial growth factor. *Arterioscler Thromb Vasc Biol*. 20091 Jun; 29:789-791.
18. Ferrara N, Carver-Moore K, Chen H, et al. Heterozygous embryonic lethality induced by targeted inactivation of the VEGF gene. *Nature*. 1992;380:439-442.
19. Fong G, Rossant H, Gertenstein M, et al. Role of the Flt1 receptor tyrosine kinase in regulating the assembly of vascular endothelium. *Nature*. 1995;376:66-70.
20. Shalaby F, Rossant J, Yamaguchi TP, et al. Failure of blood-island formation and vasculogenesis in Flk-1-deficient mice. *Nature*. 1995;376:62-66.
21. Park JE, Keller GA, Ferrara N. The vascular endothelial growth factor (VEGF) isoforms: differential deposition into the subepithelial extracellular matrix and bioactivity of extracellular matrix bound VEGF. *Mol Biol Cell*. 1993;4:1317-1326.

22. Galambos C, Ng YS, Ali A, et al. Defective pulmonary development in the absence of heparin-binding vascular endothelial growth factor isoforms. *Am J Respir Cell Mol Biol*. 2002;27:194-203.
23. Akeson AL, Greenberg JM, Cameron JE, et al. Temporal and spatial regulation of VEGF-A controls vascular patterning in the embryonic lung. *Dev Biol*. 2003;264:443-455.
24. Jones N, Iljin K, Dumont DJ, Alitalo K. Tie receptors: new modulators of angiogenic and lymphangiogenic responses. *Nat Rev Mol Cell Biol*. 2001;2:257-267.
25. Dumont DJ, Gradwohl G, Fong GH, et al. Dominant-negative and targeted null mutations in the endothelial receptor tyrosine kinase, tek, reveal a critical role in vasculogenesis of the embryo. *Genes Dev*. 1994;8:1897-1909.
26. Sato TN, Tozawa Y, Deutsch U, et al. Distinct roles of the receptor tyrosine kinases Tie-1 and Tie-2 in blood vessel formation. *Nature*. 1995;376:70-74.
27. Suri C, Jones PF, Patan S, et al. Requisite role of angiopoietin-1, a ligand for the TIE2 receptor, during embryonic angiogenesis. *Cell*. 1996;87:1171-1180.
28. Gale NW, Thurston G, Hackett SF, et al. Angiopoietin-2 is required for postnatal angiogenesis and lymphatic patterning, and only the latter role is rescued by Angiopoietin-1. *Dev Cell*. 2002;411-423.
29. White AC, Lavine KJ, Ornitz DM. FGF9 and SHH regulate mesenchymal VEGFA expression and development of the pulmonary capillary network. *Development*. 2007;134:3743-3752.
30. Kostyk SK, Kourembanas S, Wheeler EL, et al. Basic fibroblast growth factor increases nitric oxide synthase production in bovine endothelial cells. *Am J Physiol*. 1995;269:H1583-H1589.
31. Yang HT, Yan Z, Abraham JA, Terjung RL. VEGF121 and bFGF-induced increase in collateral blood flow requires normal nitric oxide production. *Am J Physiol Heart Circ Physiol*. 2001 Mar;280:H1097-H1104.
32. Ng YS, Rohan R, Sunday ME, et al. Differential expression of VEGF isoforms in mouse during development and in the adult. *Dev Dyn*. 2001;220:112-121.
33. Greenberg JM, Thompson FY, Brooks SK, et al. Mesenchymal expression of vascular endothelial growth factors D and A defines vascular patterning in developing lung. *Dev Dyn*. 2002;224:144-153.
34. Sessa WC. Molecular control of blood flow and angiogenesis: role of nitric oxide. *J Thromb Haemost*. 2009;7(Suppl 1):35-37.
35. Afshar S, Gibson LL, Yuhanna IS, et al. Pulmonary NO synthase expression is attenuated in a fetal baboon model of chronic lung disease. *Am J Physiol Lung Cell Mol Physiol*. 2003;284:L749-L758.
36. Sherman TS, Chen Z, Yuhanna IS, et al. Nitric oxide synthase isoform expression in the developing lung epithelium. *Am J Physiol*. 1999;276:L383-L390.
37. Shaul PW. Regulation of vasodilator synthesis during lung development. *Early Hum Dev*. 1999;54:271-294.
38. Han RN, Babei S, Robb M, et al. Defective lung vascular development and fatal respiratory distress in eNOS deficient mice: a model of alveolar capillary dysplasia? *Circ Res*. 2004;94:1115-1123.
39. Fagan KA, McMurtry I, Rodman D. Nitric oxide synthase in pulmonary hypertension: lessons from knockout mice. *Physio Res*. 2000;49:539-548.
40. Fagan KA, Tyler RC, Sato K, et al. Relative contributions of endothelial, inducible and neuronal NOS to the tone in murine pulmonary circulation. *Am J Physiol Lung Cell Mol Physiol*. 1999;21:L472-L478.
41. Bloch KD, Filippov G, Sanchez LS, et al. Pulmonary soluble guanylate cyclase, a nitric oxide receptor, is increased during the perinatal period. *Am J Physiol*. 1997;272:L400-L406.
42. Sanchez LS, de la Monte SM, Filippov G, et al. Cyclic-GMP-binding, cyclic-GMP-specific phosphodiesterase (PDE5) gene expression is regulated during rat pulmonary development. *Pediatr Res*. 1998 Feb;43:163-168.
43. Dulak J, Jozkowicz A. Regulation of vascular endothelial growth factor synthesis by nitric oxide: facts and controversies. *Antioxid Redox Signal*. 2003;5:123-132.
44. Asikainen TM, Waleh NS, Schneider BK, et al. Enhancement of angiogenic effectors through hypoxia-inducible factor in preterm primate lung in vivo. *Am J Physiol Lung Cell Mol Physiol*. 2006;291:L588-L595.
45. Grover TR, Asikainen TM, Kinsella JP, et al. Hypoxia-inducible factors HIF-1alpha and HIF-2alpha are decreased in an experimental model of severe respiratory distress syndrome in preterm lambs. *Am J Physiol Lung Cell Mol Physiol*. 2007;292:L1345-L1351.
46. Tang JR, Markham NE, Lin YJ, et al. Inhaled nitric oxide attenuates pulmonary hypertension and improves lung growth in infant rats after neonatal treatment with a VEGF receptor inhibitor. *Am J Physiol Lung Cell Mol Physiol*. 2004;287:L344-L351.
47. Young SL, Evans K, Eu JP. Nitric oxide modulates branching morphogenesis in fetal rat lung explants. *Am J Physiol Lung Cell Mol Physiol*. 2002;282:L379-L385.
48. Jobe AH, Ikegami M. Mechanisms initiating lung injury in the preterm. *Early Hum Dev*. 1998;53:81-94.
49. Bhatt AJ, Pryhuber GS, Huyck H, et al. Disrupted pulmonary vasculature and decreased vascular endothelial growth factor, Flt-1, and TIE-2 in human infants dying with bronchopulmonary dysplasia. *Am J Respir Crit Care Med*. 2001;164:1971-1980.
50. Torday JS, Rehan VK. Developmental cell/molecular biologic approach to the etiology and treatment of bronchopulmonary dysplasia. *Pediatr Res*. 2007;62:2-7.
51. Willis BC, Liebler JM, Luby-Phelps K, et al. Induction of epithelial-mesenchymal transition in alveolar epithelial cells by transforming growth factor-beta1: potential role in idiopathic pulmonary fibrosis. *Am J Pathol*. 2005 May;166: 1321-1232.

52. Vyas-Read S, Shaul PW, Yuhanna IS, Willis BC. Nitric oxide attenuates epithelial-mesenchymal transition in alveolar epithelial cells. *Am J Physiol Lung Cell Mol Physiol*. 2007;293:L212-L221.
53. Balasubramaniam V, Maxey AM, Morgan DB, et al. Inhaled NO restores lung structure in eNOS-deficient mice recovering from neonatal hypoxia. *Am J Physiol Lung Cell Mol Physiol*. 2006;291:L119-L127.
54. Leuwerke SM, Kaza AK, Tribble CG, et al. Inhibition of compensatory lung growth in endothelial nitric oxide synthase-deficient mice. *Am J Physiol Lung Cell Mol Physiol*. 2002;282:L1272-L1278.
55. McCurnin DC, Pierce RA, Chang LY, et al. Inhaled NO improves early pulmonary function and modifies lung growth and elastin deposition in a baboon model of neonatal chronic lung disease. *Am J Physiol Lung Cell Mol Physiol*. 2005;288:L450-L459.
56. MacRitchie AN, Albertine KH, Sun J, et al. Reduced endothelial nitric oxide synthase in lungs of chronically ventilated preterm lambs. *Am J Physiol Lung Cell Mol Physiol*. 2001;281:L1011-L1020.
57. Kinsella JP, Parker TA, Galan H, et al. Effects of inhaled nitric oxide on pulmonary edema and lung neutrophil accumulation in severe experimental hyaline membrane disease. *Pediatr Res*. 1997;41:457-463.
58. Kanazawa H. Role of vascular endothelial growth factor in the pathogenesis of chronic obstructive pulmonary disease. *Med Sci Monit*. 2007 Nov;13:RA189-RA195.
59. Gutierrez HH, Nieves B, Chumley P, et al. Nitric oxide regulation of superoxide-dependent lung injury: oxidant-protective actions of endogenously produced and exogenously administered nitric oxide. *Free Radic Biol Med*. 1996;21:43-52.
60. Harrison DG, Chen W, Dikalov S, Li L. Regulation of endothelial cell tetrahydrobiopterin pathophysiological and therapeutic implications. *Adv Pharmacol*. 2010;60:107-132.
61. Garcia-Cardena G, Fan R, Shah V, et al. Dynamic activation of endothelial nitric oxide synthase by HSP90. *Nature*. 1998;392:821-824.
62. Pritchard KA, Ackerman AW, Gross ER, et al. Heat shock protein 90 mediates the balance of nitric oxide and superoxide anion from endothelial nitric oxide synthase. *J Biol Chem*. 2001;276:17621-17624.
63. Landmesser U, Dikalov S, Price SR, et al. Oxidation of tetrahydrobiopterin leads to uncoupling of endothelial cell nitric oxide synthase in hypertension. *J Clin Invest*. 2003 Apr;111:1201-1209.
64. Konduri GG, Bakhutashvili I, Eis A, Pritchard KA. Oxidant stress from uncoupled endothelial nitric oxide synthase impairs vasodilation in fetal lambs with persistent pulmonary hypertension. *Am J Physiol Heart Circ Physiol*. 2007;292:H1812-H1820.
65. Grobe AC, Wells SM, Benavidez E, et al. Increased oxidative stress in lambs with increased pulmonary blood flow and pulmonary hypertension: role of NADPH oxidase and endothelial NO synthase. *Am J Physiol Lung Cell Mol Physiol*. 2006;290:L1069-L1077.
66. Vaporidi K, Francis RC, Bloch KD, Zapol WM. Nitric oxide synthase 3 contributes to ventilator-induced lung injury. *Am J Physiol Lung Cell Mol Physiol*. 2010;299:L150-L159.
67. Vadivel A, Aschner JL, Rey-Parra GJ, et al. L-Citrulline attenuates arrested alveolar growth and pulmonary hypertension in oxygen-induced lung injury in newborn rats. *Pediatr Res*. 2010;68:519-525.
68. Teng RJ, Eis A, Bakhutashvili I, et al. Increased superoxide production contributes to the impaired angiogenesis of fetal pulmonary arteries with in utero pulmonary hypertension. *Am J Physiol Heart Circ Physiol*. 2009;297:L184-L195.
69. Davis JM, Parad RB, Michele T, et al. Pulmonary outcome at 1 year corrected age in premature infants treated at birth with recombinant human CuZn superoxide dismutase. *Pediatrics*. 2003;111:469-476.
70. Farrow KN, Lakshminrusimha S, Reda WJ, et al. Superoxide dismutase restores eNOS expression and function in resistance pulmonary arteries from neonatal lambs with persistent pulmonary hypertension. *Am J Physiol Lung Cell Mol Physiol*. 2008;295:L979-L987.
71. Nandi M, Miller A, Stidwill R, et al. Pulmonary hypertension in a GTP-cyclohydrolase 1-deficient mouse. *Circulation*. 2005;111:2086-2090.
72. Khoo JP, Zhao L, Alp NJ, et al. Pivotal role for endothelial tetrahydrobiopterin in pulmonary hypertension. *Circulation*. 2005;111:2126-2133.
73. Sugiyama T, Levy BD, Michel T. Tetrahydrobiopterin recycling, a key determinant of endothelial nitric-oxide synthase-dependent signaling pathways in cultured vascular endothelial cells. *J Biol Chem*. 2009;284:12691-12700.
74. Nandi M, Leiper J, Arrigoni F, et al. Developmental regulation of GTP-CH1 in the porcine lung and its relationship to pulmonary vascular relaxation. *Pediatr Res*. 2006;59:767-772.
75. Cooke JP. ADMA: its role in vascular disease. *Vasc Med*. 2005;10(Suppl 1):S11-S17.
76. Leiper J, Nandi M, Torondel B, et al. Disruption of methylarginine metabolism impairs vascular homeostasis. *Nat Med*. 2007;13:198-203.
77. Beltowski J, Kêdra A. Asymmetric dimethylarginine (ADMA) as a target for pharmacotherapy. *Pharmacol Reports*. 2006;58:159-178.
78. Fiedler LR, Bachetti T, Leiper J, et al. The ADMA/DDAH pathway regulates VEGF-mediated angiogenesis. *Arterioscler Thromb Vasc Biol*. 2009;29:2117-2124.
79. Maeda T, Yoshimura T, Okamura H. Asymmetric dimethylarginine, an endogenous inhibitor of nitric oxide synthase, in maternal and fetal circulation. *J Soc Gynecol Investig*. 2003;10:2-4.
80. Tsukahara H, Ohta N, Tokuriki S, Nishijima K et al. Determination of asymmetric dimethylarginine, an endogenous nitric oxide synthase inhibitor, in umbilical blood. *Metabolism*. 2008;57:215-220.

81. Ananthakrishnan M, Barr FE, Summar ML, et al. L-Citrulline ameliorates chronic hypoxia-induced pulmonary hypertension in newborn piglets. *Am J Physiol Lung Cell Mol Physiol.* 2009;297:L506-L511.
82. Frank L, Sosenko IR. Prenatal development of lung antioxidant enzymes in four species. *J Pediatrics.* 1987;110:106-110.
83. Teng RJ, Wu TJ, Bisig CG, et al. Nitrotyrosine impairs angiogenesis and uncouples eNOS activity of pulmonary artery endothelial cells isolated from developing sheep lungs. *Pediatr Res.* 2011 Feb;69:112-117.
84. Gebb SA, Fox K, Vaughn J, et al. Fetal oxygen tension promotes tenascin-C-dependent lung branching morphogenesis. *Dev Dyn.* 2005 Sep;234:1-10.
85. Kotch LE, Iyer NV, Laughner E, Semenza G. Defective vascularization of HIF-1alpha-null embryos is not associated with VEGF deficiency but with mesenchymal cell death. *Dev Biol.* 1999 May;15;209:254-367.
86. Land SC. Oxygen-sensing pathways and the development of mammalian gas exchange. *Redox Rep.* 2003;8:325-340.
87. Gebb SA, Jones PL. Hypoxia and lung branching morphogenesis. *Adv Exp Med Biol.* 2003;543:117-125.
88. Tiktinsky MH, Morin FC 3rd. Increasing oxygen tension dilates fetal pulmonary circulation via endothelium-derived relaxing factor. *Am J Physiol.* 1993;265:H376-H380.
89. Cornfield DN, Chatfield BA, McQueston JA, et al. Effects of birth-related stimuli on L-arginine-dependent pulmonary vasodilation in ovine fetus. *Am J Physiol.* 1992 May;262:H1474-H1481.
90. Abman SH, Chatfield BA, Hall SL, McMurtry IF. Role of endothelium-derived relaxing factor during transition of pulmonary circulation at birth. *Am J Physiol.* 1990;259:H1921-H1927.
91. Belik J, Pan J, Jankov RP, Tanswell AK. A bronchial epithelium-derived factor reduces pulmonary vascular tone in the newborn rat. *J Appl Physiol.* 2004;96:1399-1405.
92. Lakshminrusimha S, Russell JA, Gugino SF. Adjacent bronchus attenuates pulmonary arterial contractility. *Am J Physiol Lung Cell Mol Physiol.* 2006;291:L473-L478.
93. Settergren G, Angdin M, Astudill R, et al. Decreased pulmonary vascular resistance during nasal breathing: modulation by endogenous nitric oxide from the paranasal sinuses. *Acta Physiol Scand.* 1998;163:235-239.
94. Williams O, Rafferty GF, Hannam S, et al. Nasal and lower airway levels of nitric oxide in prematurely born infants. *Early Human Development.* 2003;72:67-73.
95. Leipala JA, Williams O, Sreekumar S, et al. Exhaled nitric oxide levels in infants with chronic lung disease. *Eur J Pediatr.* 2004;163:555-558.
96. Kunig AM, Balasubramaniam V, Markham NE, et al. Recombinant human VEGF treatment transiently increases lung edema but enhances lung structure after neonatal hyperoxia. *Am J Physiol Lung Cell Mol Physiol.* 2006;291:L1068-L1078.
97. Thébaud B, Ladha F, Michelakis ED, et al. Vascular endothelial growth factor gene therapy increases survival, promotes lung angiogenesis, and prevents alveolar damage in hyperoxia-induced lung injury: evidence that angiogenesis participates in alveolarization. *Circulation.* 2005 Oct; 18;112:2477-2486.
98. Schreiber MD, Gin-Mestan K, Marks JD, et al. Inhaled nitric oxide in premature infants with the respiratory distress syndrome. *N Engl J Med.* 2003;349:2099-2107.
99. Kinsella JP, Cutter GR, Walsh W, et al. Early inhaled nitric oxide therapy in premature newborns with respiratory failure. *N Engl J Med.* 2006;355:354-364.
100. Mercier JC, Hummler H, Durrmeyer X, et al. Inhaled nitric oxide for prevention of bronchopulmonary dysplasia in premature babies (EUNO): a randomized controlled trial. *Lancet.* 2010; 376:346-354.
101. Van Meurs KP, Wright LL, Ehrenkranz RA, et al. Inhaled nitric oxide for premature infants with severe respiratory failure. *N Engl J Med.* 2005;353:13-22.
102. Ballard RA, Truog WE, Cnaan A, et al. Inhaled nitric oxide in preterm infants undergoing mechanical ventilation. *N Engl J Med.* 2006 Jul;27;355:343-353.
103. Warburton D, Schwarz M, Tefft D, et al. The molecular basis of lung morphogenesis. *Mech Dev.* 2000;92:55-81.
104. Hyde DM, Blozis SA, Avdalovic MV et al. Alveoli increase in number but not size from birth to adulthood in rhesus monkeys. *Am J Physiol Lung Cell Mol Physiol.* 2007;293:L570-L579.

SECTION B

Lung Injury—Bronchopulmonary Dysplasia

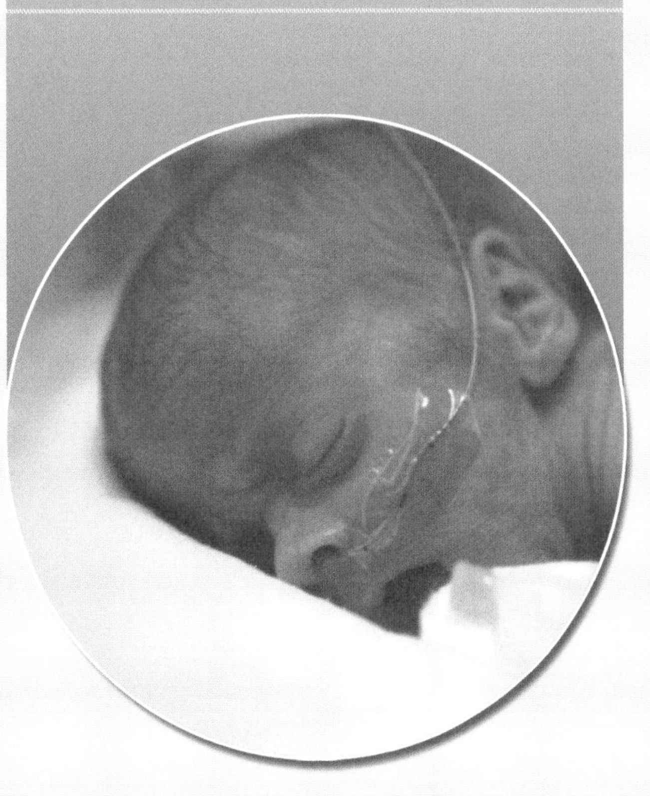

CHAPTER 6

Prenatal and Postnatal Microbial Colonization and Respiratory Outcome in Preterm Infants

Rose Marie Viscardi, MD

6

- Introduction
- Antenatal Infection and Pulmonary Outcomes
- Postnatal Microbial Colonization and Adverse Pulmonary Outcomes

Introduction

Bronchopulmonary dysplasia (BPD) was first described more than 40 years ago as a progression of characteristic chest radiographic findings that correlated with pathologic changes consisting of acute and chronic lung inflammation, fibrosis, and bronchial smooth muscle hypertrophy in premature, ventilator-dependent infants.[1,2] Although BPD remains one of the major morbidities of preterm birth, improvements in perinatal care such as antenatal steroids, exogenous surfactant, lung-protective ventilator strategies, and alternatives to mechanical ventilation have limited the disease to the most immature infants.[3] Compared with the lung histology observed in the ventilated preterm lung during the pre–exogenous surfactant era, the "new" BPD is characterized by more uniform inflation, fewer but larger alveoli, and less fulminant, but persistent inflammation.[4] Currently the incidence of "new" BPD is 30% in infants born at or before 28 weeks of gestation, but only 3% in infants born after 28 weeks.[5] Long-term sequelae include prolonged dependence on supplemental oxygen, reactive airway disease, risk for pulmonary infections, and neurodevelopmental delays.

There is accumulating evidence that the central event in BPD pathogenesis is the interruption of normal developmental signaling during early stages of lung development by lung injury and subsequent dysregulated inflammatory response, a complex process that is often initiated in utero by intrauterine infection and augmented postnatally by exposure to hyperoxia, volutrauma, and post-natal infection.[3] The objectives of this chapter are to describe (1) the consequences of fetal lung exposure to infection/inflammation in utero—and experimental evidence that provides insight into potential mechanisms for how this exposure alters lung developmental signaling—and of interactions with postnatal injurious stimuli; (2) the effects of postnatal infections in the preterm lung such as ventilator-associated pneumonia that may exacerbate lung injury, prolong hospitalization, and increase mortality; and (3) potential effects of these perinatally acquired infections on long-term pulmonary outcomes. The discussion focuses on the epidemiologic and experimental evidence that the genital mycoplasma species *Ureaplasma parvum* and *Ureaplasma urealyticum* contribute to neonatal lung injury and may affect long-term pulmonary outcomes in infants whose mothers were infected.

Antenatal Infection and Pulmonary Outcomes

Epidemiologic studies indicate that intrauterine infection is the leading cause of very early preterm birth.[6] The frequency of positive culture results in amniotic fluid and placental tissues along with histologic and biochemical evidence of intrauterine

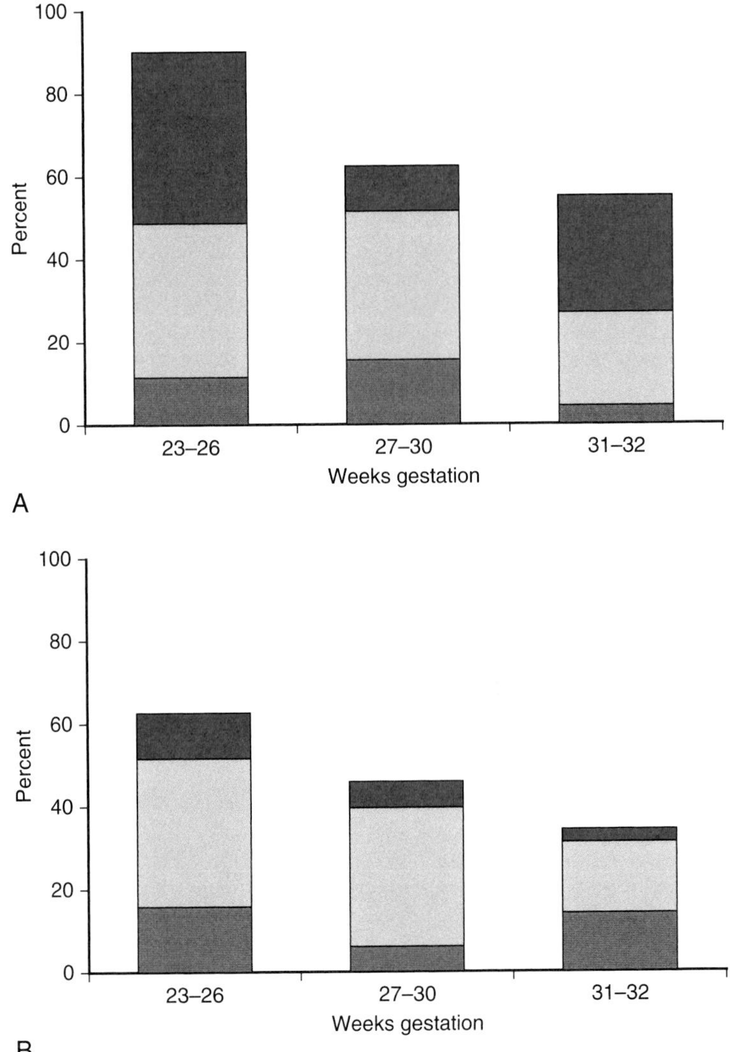

Figure 6-1 Distribution of maternal and fetal stages of histologic chorioamnionitis by gestational age. **A,** Maternal stages of histological chorioamnionitis are as follows: stage 1: polymorphonuclear neutrophils/leukocytes (PMNs) in subchorionic plate fibrin and/or membranous chorionic trophoblast layer (*gray*); stage 2: PMNs in chorionic plate or chorionic connective tissue and/or amnion (*pink*); and stage 3: necrotizing chorioamnionitis with degenerated neutrophils, thickened eosinophilic membrane, and amnionic epithelial degeneration (*red*). **B,** Fetal vasculitis stages are as follows: stage 1: PMNs in the wall of chorionic plate vessels or umbilical vein (*gray*); stage 2: PMNS in one or both umbilical arteries (*pink*); and stage 3: PMNs in concentric band(s) around one or more umbilical vessels accompanied by cellular debris, or eosinophilic precipitate, and necrotizing funisitis (*red*).[16] (From Viscardi RM, Muhumuza CK, Rodriguez A, et al. Inflammatory markers in intrauterine and fetal blood and CSF compartments are associated with adverse pulmonary and neurologic outcomes in preterm infants. *Pediatr Res.* 2004;55:1009-1017.)

inflammation among women with spontaneous preterm labor and premature preterm rupture of the membranes at less than 30 weeks of gestation is 70% to 80% and is inversely related to gestational age (Fig. 6-1).[5,7] The organisms most commonly isolated from amniotic fluid[8] and placentas[9,10] are the genital mycoplasmas *U. parvum*, *U. urealyticum*, and *Mycoplasma hominis*, and those less frequently isolated are gram-positive organisms (*Streptococcus* spp., *Staphylococcus* spp.), gram-negative organisms (*Escherichia. coli*, *Pseudomonas* spp.), anaerobes (e.g. *Bacteroides* spp.), and organisms associated with bacterial vaginosis. Analysis of amniotic fluid from women with preterm labor and intact membranes using advanced molecular techniques combined with culture demonstrated a greater prevalence (15%) and diversity (18 taxa) of microbes than culture or species-specific polymerase chain reaction (PCR) studies.[8] The microbes included a related group of fastidious bacteria, such as *Sneathia sanguinegens, Leptotrichia amnionii,* and an unassigned, uncultivated, and previously uncharacterized bacterium. Using culture-independent approaches such as analysis of the bacterial 16S ribosomal RNA gene[11,12] and denaturing gel electrophoresis (DGGE)[13] to analyze gastric and tracheal aspirates (TAs) to identify perinatally acquired microbes in preterm infants, other studies have identified at least 22 microbial species other than the *Mycoplasma* species, confirming the diversity of organisms potentially involved in intrauterine infection and it sequelae.

Histologic Chorioamnionitis and Pulmonary Outcomes

Chorioamnionitis has been defined by histologic criteria (presence of polymorphonuclear cells in choriodecidual space, fetal membranes, and/or cord), microbiologic criteria (positive results of culture or molecular detection methods), and/or biochemical criteria (elevated amniotic fluid cytokine and chemokine levels) as evidence of infection/inflammation in the intrauterine compartment.[14] Clinical chorioamnionitis defined by maternal fever, maternal and fetal tachycardia, uterine tenderness, foul-smelling vaginal discharge, and leukocytosis is present in less than 40% of cases of histologic chorioamnionitis,[5] indicating that the majority of intrauterine infections are subclinical.[15]

Standardization of placental pathology review has provided a framework for characterizing the stage or extent of polymorphonuclear cell infiltration and grading for severity.[16] In response to microbial invasion, maternal polymorphonuclear cells progress from infiltration of the subchorionic plate fibrin and/or membranous chorionic trophoblast layer (stage 1) to infiltration of the chorionic plate or chorionic connective tissue and/or amnion (stage 2) to necrotizing chorioamnionitis with degenerated neutrophils, thickened eosinophilic membrane, and amnionic epithelial degeneration (stage 3). A grade of inflammation is assigned to describe the number of neutrophils or presence of microabcesses.[16] It has been proposed that the presence of advanced maternal stage of necrotizing amnionitis is indicative of prolonged infection/inflammation.[16-18]

The fetal inflammatory response syndrome (FIRS) has been defined biochemically by elevated umbilical cord concentrations of cytokines (interleukin-1β [IL-1β], IL-6, and tumor necrosis factor-α [TNFα]).[5,19] However, this response also involves a broader inflammatory response, including upregulation of chemokines (IL-8, macrophage inflammatory protein-1β [MIP-1β], and RANTES [regulated upon activation, normal T cell expressed and secreted]), adhesion molecules (intracellular adhesion molecule-1 [ICAM-1], ICAM-3, and E-selectin), matrix metalloproteinases (MMP-1 and MMP-9), an angiogenic factor (vascular endothelial growth factor [VEGF]), and an acute-phase protein (C-reactive protein [CRP]), in venous blood in the first few days of life.[18] Histologically, the response is defined by fetal vasculitis/funisitis characterized by polymorphonuclear infiltration of the chorionic vessels or umbilical cord.[14] Stages of fetal vasculitis describe the progression from neutrophils in the wall of chorionic plate vessels or umbilical vein (stage 1) to one or both umbilical arteries (stage 2) to concentric bands around one or more umbilical vessel accompanied by cellular debris, or eosinophilic precipitate (stage 3, necrotizing funisitis).[16] Intensity of the inflammation is graded according to the number of neutrophils present.

Multiple epidemiologic studies have addressed the association of histologic chorioamnionitis with and without cord involvement with gestation-independent effects on neonatal pulmonary outcomes (summarized in a 2010 review[14]). In 1996,Watterberg and colleagues[20] observed that histologic chorioamnionitis was associated with a reduced risk for respiratory distress syndrome (RDS), but an increased risk for bronchopulmonary dysplasia (BPD) in a small cohort of mechanically ventilated preterm infants with birth weight less than 2000 g who were not exposed to antenatal steroids or exogenous surfactant. Subsequent studies over the past 15 years have found an association of chorioamnionitis with a reduced effect[21-24] or no effect[25-27] on RDS risk and an increased effect,[5,25,27] a decreased effect,[28] or no effect[22,26,29,30] on BPD risk.

Limitations of many of the studies include single-center cohorts with varying gestational age ranges, racial/ethnic distributions, and inclusion criteria, and sample sizes inadequately powered to analyze possible confounding or risk modification of gestational age and other important variables. For instance, Redline and associates[29] observed in a retrospective study that histologic chorioamnionitis tended to be higher in white infants and lower in African-American infants with BPD at 36 weeks postmenstrual age, suggesting that racial differences in response to chorioamnionitis may explain, in part, differences in study outcomes. Interpretation of these studies is also complicated by the potential selection bias of center-specific placental review criteria and nonstandardized criteria for chorioamnionitis diagnosis. A major challenge is the lack of a true "normal" comparison group, because many preterm placentas without chorioamnionitis have other lesions that may affect outcomes.[14]

It has been proposed that the timing, duration of exposure, and severity of chorioamnionitis affects neonatal pulmonary outcomes. In a cohort of 276 preterm infants born before 33 weeks of gestation at our institution, histologic chorioamnionitis was associated with 3.6-fold higher risk for BPD in infants born at 28 weeks gestation or earlier, but not in infants of 29 to 32 weeks gestation. Maternal stage of chorioamnionitis was significantly correlated with BPD severity[5] as defined by National Institutes of Health (NIH) consensus criteria.[3] Forty percent of the infants in whom moderate or severe BPD developed were exposed to longstanding or necrotizing amnionitis (stage 3) compared with 34% of infants in whom mild BPD developed and 19% infants without BPD (Fig. 6-2). Fetal vasculitis was not associated with BPD in this study. Subacute chorioamnionitis, a pathologic diagnosis distinct from acute chorioamnionitis, is characterized by mixed degenerative polymorphonuclear neutrophils/leukocytes (PMNs) and mononuclear cells in the chorionic plate with greatest severity involving the amnion.[31] In a study comparing 90 singleton placentas with stage 3 acute and subacute chorioamnionitis at 23 to32 weeks of gestation with gestational age– and birth weight–matched controls without chorioamnionitis, the presence of amniotic necrosis was independently associated

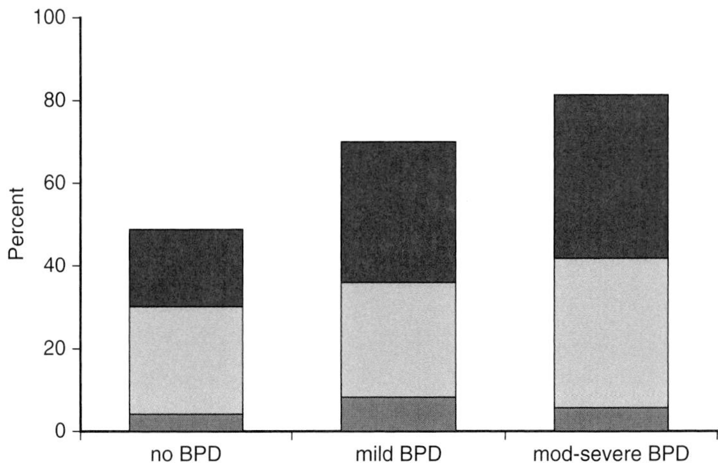

Figure 6-2 Relationship of severity of bronchopulmonary dysplasia (BPD) and maternal stage of chorioamnionitis. Percentages of study infants with mild, moderate-to-severe, and no BPD according to maternal involvement with chorioamnionitis by stages. Maternal stages are as described in Figure 6-1. BPD severity is defined according to National Institutes of Health (NIH) criteria.[3] (From Viscardi RM, Muhumuza CK, Rodriguez A, et al. Inflammatory markers in intrauterine and fetal blood and CSF compartments are associated with adverse pulmonary and neurologic outcomes in preterm infants. *Pediatr Res.* 2004;55:1009-1017.)

with BPD,[31] suggesting that longstanding or chronic inflammation contributes to lung injury in utero.

Although histologic chorioamnionitis may decrease the risk for RDS because of maturational effects in the fetal lung, it may also contribute to an increase in susceptibility to augmented postnatal lung injury. In a case-control study, Van Marter and coworkers[32] observed that histologic chorioamnionitis was associated with a decreased rate of BPD in infants undergoing ventilation for less than 1 week but an increased rate of BPD in infants undergoing prolonged ventilation or with postnatal sepsis. Furthermore, infants exposed to histologic chorioamnionitis with fetal vasculitis in another study had impaired responses to exogenous administration of surfactant, which contributed to both prolonged mechanical ventilation after surfactant administration and the development of BPD.[33] Peripheral blood leukocytosis (leukocyte count > 30,000/mm^3) in the first 2 days of life in chorioamnionitis-exposed infants has been found to increase the risk for BPD 4.6-fold but to decrease the risk for death.[34] Antenatal exposure to histologic chorioamnionitis may be an important response modifier of other postnatal interventions. Although there was no overall benefit of low-dose prophylactic hydrocortisone therapy in preterm infants in a randomized trial, the subgroup of chorioamnionitis-exposed infants in the treatment arm experienced significantly decreased mortality and improved survival without BPD in comparison with placebo-treated infants.[35]

6

Role of Infection-Mediated Cytokine Signaling in Bronchopulmonary Dysplasia

Clinical studies of biomarkers in intrauterine and pulmonary compartments and experimental animal and in vitro studies have demonstrated that the host inflammatory response to intrauterine microbial invasion is the link between antenatal infection and altered lung development. Amniotic fluid concentrations of proinflammatory cytokines IL-1β, IL-6, TNFα, and IL-8 were higher in pregnancies producing infants in whom BPD developed than in pregnancies producing infants without BPD.[36] The fetal inflammatory response characterized by placental vasculitis and/or elevated cord serum IL-6 concentrations was an independent risk factor for BPD.[19,37] Increased concentrations of IL-6 and IL-1β have been detected in TAs of preterm infants on the first day of life in association with prolonged rupture of the membranes[38] and histologic chorioamnionitis,[20,39] respectively. A series of longitudinal studies comparing the temporal changes in inflammatory mediators and their inhibitors in TAs from preterm infants with and without lung disease have shown that there is an imbalance in the levels of pro- and anti-inflammatory cytokines during the first week of life in infants in whom BPD develops.[40-43] The increase in expression of pulmonary proinflammatory cytokines, chemokines, adhesion molecules, proteases, and angiogenic factors in concert with a decreased capacity to downregulate this response in infants who experience BPD suggests that persistent endogenous generation of these factors might contribute to chronic lung injury and inflammation. Bose and coworkers[44] summarized the contribution of different aspects of the inflammatory response to BPD in an extensive review of TA biomarker studies.

Chronic Inflammation in the Immature Lung Alters Developmental Signaling and Fibrosis

Transforming growth factor-β1 (TGF-β1) is involved in lung morphogenesis, repair of lung injury, airway remodeling, lung fibrosis, and BPD.[45] TGF-β was detected at sites of lung injury in association with myofibroblast proliferation in lungs of infants dying with RDS, implicating TGF-β in the preterm lung response to injury.[46] TGF-β1 is elevated in TAs of infants who progress to BPD.[47] Overexpression of TGF-β1 in the lungs of newborn transgenic mice produces a phenotype similar to human BPD, with arrest of lung sacculation, epithelial differentiation, and vascular development.[48-50] TGF-β1–expressing adenoviral vectors were found to have similar effects in the newborn rodent lung.[45,51] Intra-amniotic endotoxin inoculation in pregnant sheep induced fetal lung TGF-β1 messenger RNA (mRNA) and protein expression and phosphorylation of protein Smad2, indicating TGF-β1 signaling.[52] These studies show that excessive TGF-β1 signaling during lung development contributes to the arrest of both alveolarization and fibrosis, both hallmarks of BPD.

In transgenic mice, overexpression of IL-1β, TNFα, IL,-6 or IL-11 was found to inhibit alveolarization, indicating that prolonged exposure of the preterm lung to a proinflammatory environment may contribute to abnormal alveolar septation.[3,53,54] Bry and coworkers[53] developed a bitransgenic mouse model in which the expression of mature human IL-1β is conditionally expressed in airway epithelial cells in the fetal and neonatal lung. In this model, IL-1β expression increased on E14.5, was maximal by E16.5 (pseudoglandular period), and decreased postnatally. Postnatal growth was impaired and mortality was higher in the IL-1β–expressing newborn mice. The lungs of these newborn mice demonstrated many features of the BPD phenotype, including disrupted alveolar septation and capillary development, and disordered deposition of α-smooth muscle actin and elastin in alveolar septa of distal air spaces.[53]

The effects of prolonged exposure to proinflammatory cytokines on alveolarization may be mediated by up-regulation of TGF-β1. Transient overexpression of TNFα[55] or IL-1β[56] in rat lung by adenoviral gene transfer produces lung fibrosis due to stimulation of TGF-β1, and induction of myofibroblasts. Absence of the β6 integrin subunit, an activator of TGF-β1, improves alveolar development in transgenic IL-1β–expressing newborn mice, implicating TGF-β signaling in the pathogenesis of BPD.[57] TNFα, IL-1β, and TGF-β1 are elevated in TAs of infants who progress to BPD.[40,41,47,58,59]

Taken collectively, these data indicate that prolonged exposure of the developing lung to proinflammatory, profibrotic factors may contribute to BPD by disrupting normal developmental signaling. The next section reviews the human and experimental evidence that the low-virulence pathogens *U. parvum* and *U. urealyticum* contribute to preterm birth and lung injury, and augment a dysregulated inflammatory response by stimulating the proinflammatory, profibrotic signaling pathways.

Role of Genital Mycoplasmas in Intrauterine Infection and Neonatal Lung Injury

The *Mollicute* class comprises at least 200 species; humans are the primary hosts for at least 17 of them. The organisms reside primarily in association with the mucosal surfaces of the urogenital and respiratory tracts. The four urogenital species belong to two different phylogenetic groups within the *Mollicute* class. *M. hominis* belongs to the Hominis group, whereas the *Ureaplasma* spp. and *Mycoplasma genitalium* belong to the Pneumoniae group.[60] *Ureaplasma* consists of 2 species and 14 serovars. *U. parvum* contains serovars 1, 3, 6, and 14, and *U. urealyticum* contains the remaining serovars.[61] The *Mycoplasma* species are the smallest self-replicating, free-living organisms. The *M. genitalium* genome is the smallest, with 580 kilo–base pairs (kbp), the *U. parvum* serovar 3 genome is the second smallest, with 751 kbp, and the newly sequenced *M. hominis* genome is 665 kbp.[60,62] Owing to their small genome size, the genital *Mycoplasma* species have limited biosynthetic capacities, requiring a parasitic relationship with a host. These species all lack cell walls and share 247 core coding sequences[60] but have distinct energy-generating pathways and pathogenic roles in human disease. *M. genitalium* utilizes glycolysis, but the *Ureaplasma* spp. and *M. hominis* hydrolyze urea and arginine, respectively, to generate adenosine triphosphate (ATP).[60,61] *M. genitalium* is associated with male urethritis and cervicitis but is not known to be a pathogen in infants. *M. hominis* is associated with pyelonephritis, bacterial vaginosis, pelvic inflammatory disease, and postpartum endometritis but has not been consistently associated with histologic chorioamnionitis or BPD.[13,61] It is much less commonly isolated as a single organism from amniotic fluid, chorioamnion, and neonatal tracheal and gastric aspirates than the *Ureaplasma* species.[13,61] The following section focuses on the evidence implicating the *Ureaplasma* species in neonatal lung disease.

Are There *Ureaplasma* Species- or Serovar-Specific Virulence Factors?

U. parvum is more commonly isolated from clinical vaginal,[63] amniotic fluid,[64] and infant respiratory specimens[12,65,66] and is the predominant species detected by PCR in newborn serum and/or cerebrospinal fluid (CSF) samples.[67] It has been proposed that some serovars have greater association with adverse pregnancy outcomes than others.[63,65,68] Abele-Horn and colleagues reported a higher rate of BPD in *U. urealyticum* respiratory tract colonized infants. In contrast, Katz and associates[63,69] observed no difference in prevalence of either species detected by PCR between infants with and without BPD. In a prospective study of respiratory secretions in infants born at less than 33 weeks of gestation, the distribution of *Ureaplasma* species and serovars was determined by real-time PCR using species- and serovar-specific primers/probes.[66,70] *U. parvum* was much more common (63%) than *U. urealyticum* (33%). Serovars 3 and 6 alone and in combination accounted for 96% of *U. parvum* isolates. *U. urealyticum* isolates were commonly a mixture of multiple serovars, serovar 11 either alone or combined with other serovars (59%) being the most common serovar. No individual species/serovars or serovar mixtures were associated with moderate to severe BPD. This finding supports the contention that *Ureaplasma* virulence is independent of species and serovar with regard to neonatal lung disease which nevertheless must be confirmed.

Previously proposed ureaplasmal virulence factors include immunoglobulin A (IgA) protease, urease, phospholipases A and C, and production of hydrogen peroxide.[62] These factors may allow the organism to evade mucosal immune defenses by degrading IgA and injuring mucosal cells through the local generation of ammonia, membrane phospholipid degradation and prostaglandin synthesis, and membrane peroxidation, respectively. Although functionally active IgA protease and phospholipase A and C have been found in *Ureaplasma* spp., the genes that code for these proteins have not been identified in the *U. parvum* serovar 3 genome.[62] The ureaplasmal enzymes may have unique gene sequences compared with analogous genes in other species.

The ureaplasmal MB antigen, which contains both serovar-specific and cross-reactive epitopes, is the predominant antigen recognized during ureaplasmal infections in humans. It exhibits highly variable size in vitro,[71] in clinical isolates in vivo,[72] and in an experimental ovine intra-amniotic infection model,[73] suggesting that antigen size variation may be another mechanism through which the organism evades host defenses.[61] Garcia-Castillo and coworkers[74] demonstrated that *Ureaplasma* isolates from patients with urethritis or chronic prostatitis formed biofilms in vitro, suggesting another means to evade the host immune response and alter antibiotic susceptibility.

Genetic diversity among ten clinical *U. parvum* isolates obtained from vaginal swabs was analyzed in one study by comparative genomic DNA hybridization to a DNA macroarray.[75] Although at least 538 genes (92%) were common to all the isolates, strain-specific genes mostly with unknown function represented 8% of the genome. One hypervariable plasticity region identified in this analysis had genetic features consistent with a putative pathogenicity island. Further genetic studies of the ureaplasmal genome are likely to identify virulence factors that may be novel therapeutic targets.

Potential Role of *Ureaplasma* Species in Preterm Birth and Intrauterine Inflammation

Because *Ureaplasma* is a commensal in the adult female genital tract, it has been regarded as being of low virulence. However, it has been associated with multiple obstetrical complications, including infertility, stillbirth, and preterm delivery.[61] *Ureaplasma* spp. are the organisms most commonly isolated from amniotic fluid obtained from women who present with preterm-onset labor (POL) with intact membranes,[76,77] preterm premature rupture of membranes (pPROM),[78] and short cervix associated with microbial invasion of the amniotic cavity,[79] as well as from infected placentas.[78] The prevalence of infected amniotic fluid with cultivated

Ureaplasma as the only microbe ranges from 6% to 9% for pregnancies complicated by POL with intact membranes[77,80] to 22% for a cohort of women with POL or pPROM.[81] Detection of cultivated *Ureaplasma* in placental chorion in pregnancies producing very low-birth-weight (VLBW) infants ranges from 6% to 10% in homogenized frozen tissue[9,10] to 28% in fresh tissue and is inversely related to gestational age.[82] Recovery of *Ureaplasma* from the chorion was reported to increase with duration of ruptured membranes, suggesting an ascending route of infection.[82] However, *Ureaplasma* has also been detected in 31% of infected placentas with duration of rupture of membranes less than 1 hour,[83] suggesting the possibility of a preexisting infection. Indeed, *Ureaplasma* species have been detected in amniotic fluid as early as the time of genetic amniocentesis (16-20 weeks) in up to 13% of asymptomatic women.[84-87] In one study, placentas with the lowest rate of *Ureaplasma* recovery were from women delivered for preeclampsia or intrauterine growth restriction.[82]

The presence of *Ureaplasma* as the only identified microbial isolate in the upper genital tract is significantly associated with chorioamnionitis and adverse pregnancy outcomes, including premature delivery, neonatal morbidity, and perinatal death.[77,78,81,82,88] Placentas colonized with *Ureaplasma* exhibit a characteristic bistriate inflammatory pattern with maternally derived neutrophils accumulating in the subchorion and amnion.[89] Experimental models of intrauterine *Ureaplasma* infection in mice,[90] sheep,[91,92] and nonhuman primates[93] have been described. Intra-amniotic inoculation of *U. parvum* was not found to stimulate preterm labor in mice or sheep but did stimulate progressive uterine contractions and preterm delivery in rhesus macaques inoculated at 136 days of gestation (80% term),[93] suggesting species differences in the host response or serovar differences in virulence. The rhesus macaque model is the first experimental model to definitely show a causal link between *Ureaplasma* intrauterine infection and preterm labor.

In the presence of pPROM, cultivated *Ureaplasma* as the sole microbe was associated with increases in levels of leukocytes and proinflammatory cytokines (IL-6, IL-1β, and TNFα) in amniotic fluid and increased concentrations of IL-6 in cord blood, indicating a robust inflammatory response to this infection.[94] Ureaplasmal bacterial load determined by quantitative PCR in amniotic fluid from women who delivered preterm was reported to be associated with histologic chorioamnionitis, preterm labor, PROM, and BPD.[64] The bacterial load correlated with amniotic fluid IL-8 concentrations. Although the majority of women in whom subclinical *Ureaplasma* amniotic cavity infection is detected midtrimester deliver at term,[87] those with elevated amniotic fluid IL-6 levels have increased risk for adverse pregnancy outcome, including fetal loss and preterm delivery.[95] In the rhesus *U. parvum* intrauterine infection model, uterine activity was preceded by a rise in amniotic fluid concentrations of leukocytes, inflammatory cytokines, prostaglandin (PG) E_2 and $PGF_{2\alpha}$, and matrix metalloproteinase 9 (MMP9), demonstrating that *Ureaplasma* alone stimulates the mediators of preterm labor.[93]

In vitro studies have provided additional evidence supporting the contention that *Ureaplasma* spp. stimulate inflammation in the intrauterine compartment. Estrada-Gutierrez G and colleagues[96] reported that plasma from placental whole blood (source of maternal circulating leukocytes) that had been pre-incubated with *U. parvum* serovar 3 clinical isolate stimulated IL-1β and PGE_2 secretion by chorioamnion explants.[96] High-inoculum (10^6 color changing units [CCU]/mL) but not low-inoculum (10^2 to 10^4 CCU/mL) heat-killed *U. urealyticum* serotype 8 stimulated production of TNFα, IL-10, and PGE_2 by choriodecidual explants in vitro. In contrast, heat-killed *U. parvum* serovar 1 laboratory reference strain failed to stimulate a significant increase in cytokine and PGE_2 response in fetal membrane explants derived from term placentas. The apparent low virulence of *Ureaplasma* in these in vitro studies may be due, in part, to the use of a laboratory reference strain rather than more virulent clinical isolates, or killed rather than live organisms. Alternatively, a decreased capacity to stimulate an inflammatory response in the intrauterine compartment may allow *Ureaplasma* infections to persist for long periods.

Table 6-1 CHARACTERISTIC CLINICAL AND LABORATORY FINDINGS IN *UREAPLASMA*-POSITIVE PRETERM INFANTS*

Clinical Presentation	Laboratory/ Radiographic Findings
Preterm onset of labor or preterm premature rupture of membranes[102]	Bistriate inflammatory pattern chorioamnionitis[89]
Gestational age <28 weeks[66]	Leukocytosis at birth[98,104,202]
Mild respiratory distress syndrome, but worsening gas exchange requiring increased respiratory support in 2nd week of life[65,102]	Early radiographic emphysematous changes[97,102,103]

*Superscript numbers indicate chapter references.

Ureaplasma Species and Neonatal Lung Injury

Ureaplasma respiratory tract colonization has been associated with higher incidence of pneumonia,[97,98] and BPD.[61,65,99,100] The rate of *Ureaplasma* respiratory tract colonization in infants of less than 1500 g birth weight ranges from 20% to 45%, depending on study entry criteria and frequency of sampling and detection methods.[99,101] In a cohort of infants of less than 33 weeks of gestation, *Ureaplasma* spp. were detected by combined culture/PCR one or more times in the first month of life in TAs or nasopharyngeal specimens in 35% of subjects.[67] Theilen and coworkers[102] concluded from their study that *Ureaplasma*-colonized infants are more likely to be born extremely preterm (<28 weeks of gestation) and to be delivered by spontaneous vaginal delivery following preterm labor or preterm premature rupture of membranes. Typically, such infants experience less respiratory distress in the first week of life with clinical deterioration in the second week, requiring increased oxygen and ventilatory support.[65,102] *Ureaplasma* respiratory tract colonization is associated with a peripheral blood leukocytosis[98] and early radiographic emphysematous changes of bronchopulmonary dysplasia (BPD).[97,102,103] These findings may be explained, in part, by an in utero onset of the inflammatory response and lung injury. Indeed, neonatal *Ureaplasma* respiratory colonization was found to be associated with BPD in infants exposed to antenatal histologic chorioamnionitis.[104] Clinical, radiographic, and laboratory characteristics of neonatal *Ureaplasma* respiratory tract colonization are summarized in Table 6-1 and Figure 6-3.

The contribution of *Ureaplasma* respiratory tract colonization to the development of BPD has been debated; however, a meta-analysis of 17 clinical studies published before 1995 supported a significant association between *Ureaplasma* respiratory tract colonization and development of BPD defined as oxygen dependence at 28 to 30 days postnatal age.[99] In a 2005 meta-analysis of 36 published studies involving almost 3000 preterm infants, Schelonka and associates[101] observed a significant association between *Ureaplasma* respiratory colonization and development of BPD, whether it was defined as oxygen dependence at 28 days (odds ratio [OR] 2.8; 95% confidence interval [CI] 2.3-3.5) or at 36 weeks postmenstrual age (PMA) (OR 1.6; 95% CI 1.1-2.3). Studies published since the last meta-analysis support the association of *Ureaplasma* respiratory colonization with BPD,[104,105] particularly for the subset of *Ureaplasma*-colonized infants exposed to chorioamnionitis and leukocytosis at birth.[104] Sung and coworkers[66] observed that in infants who had been mechanically ventilated for any duration and had a TA positive for *Ureaplasma* with or without a paired nasopharyngeal sample positive for the organism had a 7.9-fold higher risk (OR 7.86; 95% CI 1.31-47) for development of moderate to severe BPD than mechanically ventilated infants with a positive nasopharyngeal sample alone. This finding suggests that lower tract infection but not nasopharyngeal colonization augments lung injury in mechanically ventilated infants.

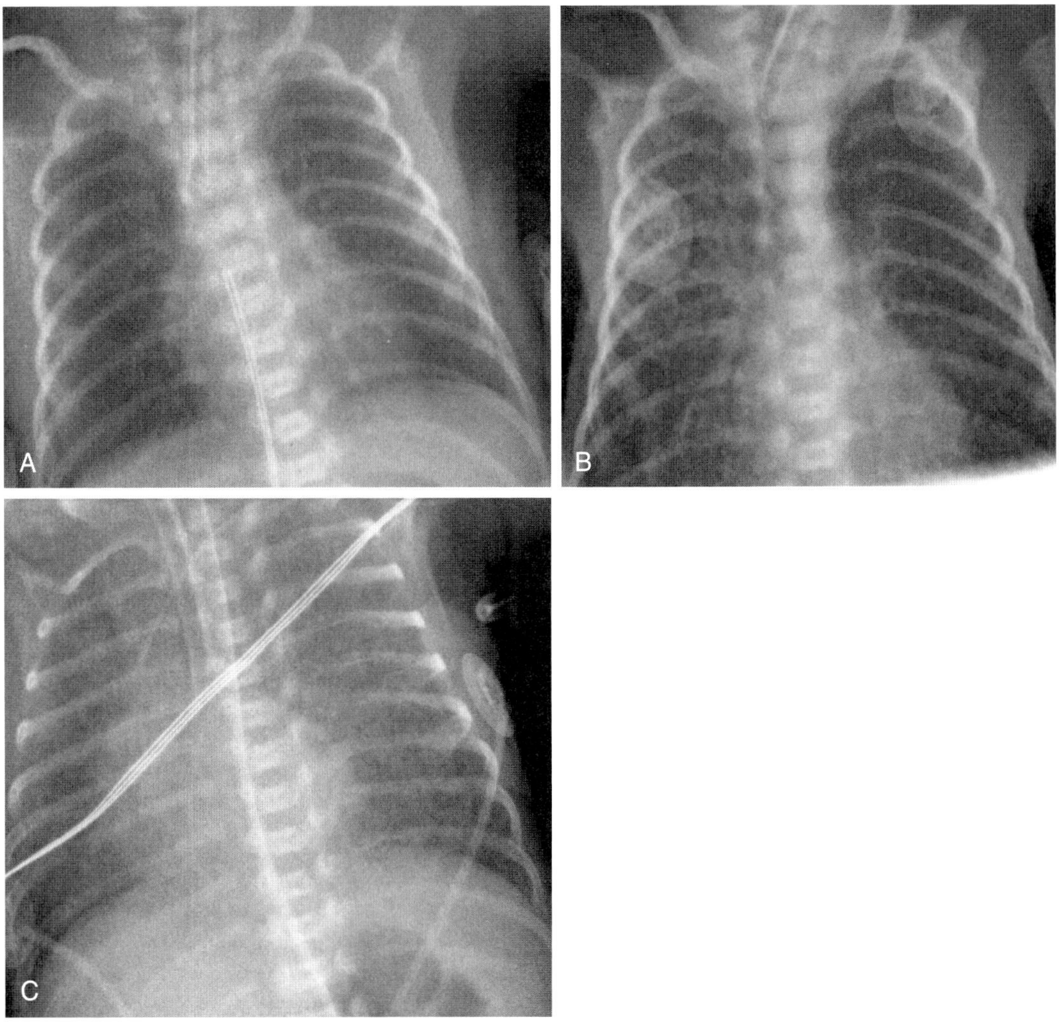

Figure 6-3 Characteristic chest radiographs of a preterm infant with *Ureaplasma* pneumonitis. **A,** Chest radiograph in the first day of life shows a mild ground-glass appearance consistent with respiratory distress syndrome (RDS). **B,** Chest radiograph at 2 weeks of age with early bronchopulmonary dysplasia (BPD) changes. **C,** Chest radiograph at 1 month of age showing progressive BPD with pulmonary edema or atelectasis.

Human and Experimental Evidence for the Role of Ureaplasma Species in Bronchopulmonary Dysplasia

Evidence from studies of human preterm infants[106-108] and from intrauterine infection models in mice,[90] sheep,[91,92] and nonhuman primates[93,109] show that *Ureaplasma* infection is proinflammatory and profibrotic and results in a BPD phenotype. In a review of lung pathology of archived autopsy specimens from *Ureaplasma*-infected preterm infants, gestational controls, and infants who died with pneumonia from other causes, the most striking findings in all members of the first group were (1) the presence of moderate to severe fibrosis, (2) increased myofibroblasts, (3) disordered elastin accumulation, and (4) increased numbers of TNFα– and (TGF-β1–immunoreactive cells.[107,108] The increase in fibrosis and elastic fiber accumulation in the distal lung correlated spatially and temporally with the presence of macrophages positive for TGF-β1, suggesting that these factors are closely linked. In two studies, my colleagues and I[107,108] found that severity of fibrosis score (Fig. 6-4A) and elastic fiber density (Fig. 6-4B) exhibited strong correlation with duration of ventilation in *Ureaplasma*-positive infants, suggesting that *Ureaplasma* infection augments the inflammatory response to volutrauma. Preterm infants with

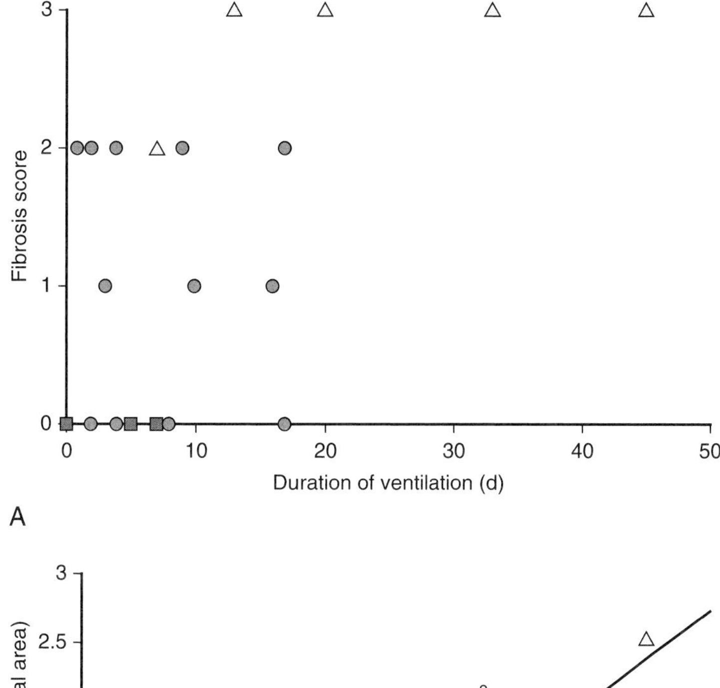

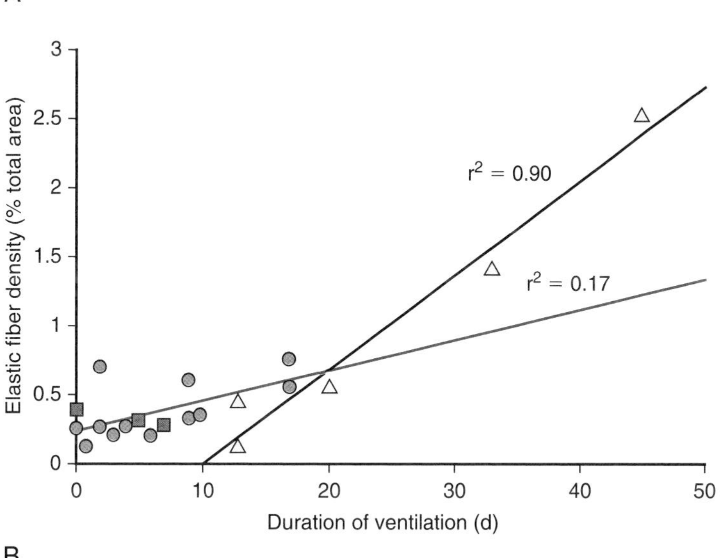

Figure 6-4 Relationship of fibrosis score (**A**) and elastic fiber density (**B**) with duration of ventilation (in days) in *Ureaplasma*-infected and noninfected preterm infants. The duration of ventilation (*x*-axis) and fibrosis score (**A**) or elastic fiber density (**B**) (*y*-axis) are shown for individual subjects in gestational controls (N = 3; *squares*), *Ureaplasma* pneumonia (N = 5; *triangles*), and other pneumonia cases (N = 11; *circles*). There was a significant correlation between duration of ventilation and fibrosis when both pneumonia groups were included ($P = 0.008$), but not within each group. Duration of ventilation was strongly correlated with elastic fiber density in the *Ureaplasma* pneumonia group ($r2 = 0.9$, $P = 0.015$), but not in other pneumonia group. (From Viscardi RM, Manimtim WM, Sun CCJ, et al. Lung pathology in premature infants with *Ureaplasma urealyticum* infection. *Pediatr Dev Pathol.* 2002;5:141-150; and Viscardi RM, Manimtim W, He JR, et al. Disordered pulmonary myofibroblast distribution and elastin expression in preterm infants with *Ureaplasma urealyticum* pneumonitis. *Pediatr Dev Pathol.* 2006;9: 143-151.)

Ureaplasma respiratory colonization have elevated TA concentrations of IL-1β, TNFα, and monocyte chemoattractant protein-1 (MCP-1) and increased neutrophil chemotactic activity during the first weeks of life in comparison with noncolonized infants.[106,110,111]

Experimental pneumonia models demonstrate the inflammatory response to *Ureaplasma* pulmonary infection. Intratracheal *Ureaplasma* inoculation caused an acute bronchiolitis in 140-day preterm baboons[112] and an acute interstitial pneumonia in newborn but not 14-day-old mice.[113] Hyperoxia exposure increased mortality and lung inflammation, and delayed pathogen clearance in *Ureaplasma*-inoculated newborn mice,[114] consistent with the hypothesis that *Ureaplasma* augments the inflammatory response to secondary stimuli. In a mouse *Ureaplasma* pneumonia model, intratracheal inoculation with *Ureaplasma* induced a prolonged inflammatory response, as indicated by a sustained recruitment of neutrophils and macrophages into the lung.[115]

Antenatal infection models provide insights into the effects of *Ureaplasma* on lung development. Experimental murine intrauterine *U. parvum* exposure stimulated fetal lung cytokine expression and augmented hyperoxia-induced lung injury.[90] Intra-amniotic *Ureaplasma* (serovar 1) inoculation 2 days prior to delivery at 125 days (67% of term gestation) in baboons caused an inflammatory response in the amniotic and fetal lung compartments and vertical transmission to the fetal lung that persisted up to 2 weeks postnatally in half of the antenatally exposed animals.[116] My colleagues and I[109] observed extensive fibrosis, an increase in the myofibroblast phenotype, increased expression of proinflammatory (TNFα, IL-1β) and profibrotic (TGF-β1; oncostatin M) cytokines, and the presence of macrophages as the predominant recruited leukocyte in lungs of *Ureaplasma*-exposed immature baboons in comparison with gestational controls and noninfected ventilated animals. After 14 days of ventilation, active TGF-β1 and TGF-β1 Smad signaling was higher in lung homogenates of *Ureaplasma*-infected animals than in gestational and ventilated controls (Fig. 6-5). Similarly, fetal sheep exposed to intra-amniotic *U. parvum* serovar 3 for 3 to 14 days prior to delivery at 124 days demonstrated increased fetal lung neutrophils after 3 days of exposure as well as reduced alveolar septa and elastin foci, and increased α-smooth muscle actin in arteries and bronchioli after 14 days.[117] This finding demonstrated that short-term intrauterine exposure to *Ureaplasma* induces an inflammatory response and altered structural lung development, a condition that may mimic the exposure with an ascending infection after rupture of membranes in the human condition.

Because subclinical *Ureaplasma* intrauterine infection has been detected early in human pregnancy, the effects of prolonged intrauterine exposure to this infection have been examined in animal models. In fetal sheep exposed to intra-amniotic *Ureaplasma* for periods up to 10 weeks, long-term exposure was associated with improvement in lung function but also with poor fetal growth, fetal acidemia, and evidence of fetal pulmonary inflammation.[91] Intra-amniotic inoculation of *U. parvum* serovar 3 or 6 at midgestation in fetal sheep did not result in preterm labor but did cause placental and fetal pulmonary inflammation and altered lung development whether delivery occurred preterm or at term.[92] However, after intra-amniotic inoculation of these serovars at 50 days of gestation, there was evidence of persistent infection, lung inflammation, increased surfactant, and improved lung volumes, but no significant effects on indices of air space and vascular morphology in fetuses delivered preterm at 125 days of gestation.[118] This finding suggests that effects on lung development are not sustained after prolonged exposure to *Ureaplasma* in utero in the sheep model. In contrast, in a study of rhesus macaques, a nonhuman primate, histologic changes in the fetal lungs depended on the duration of intrauterine exposure to *U. parvum*.[93] Infection exposure for less than 136 hours resulted in neutrophil infiltration without epithelial injury. With progressive duration of exposure, there was an influx of neutrophils and macrophages, epithelial necrosis, and alveolar type II cell proliferation. With exposure longer than 10 days, increased collagen and thickened alveolar walls were evident. These observations suggest that an early and prolonged exposure to *Ureaplasma*-mediated inflammation may be necessary to adversely affect lung development. Discrepancies among the experimental models may be due to species differences. Overall, the experimental models confirm that intra-amniotic *Ureaplasma* mimics many of the clinical features of the human infection.

The stimulatory effect of *Ureaplasma* on cytokine release has been confirmed in vitro. *Ureaplasma* has been reported to stimulate release of TNFα and IL-6 by alveolar macrophages from preterm infant TAs; production of cytokines and nitric oxide; upregulation of inducible nitric oxide synthase (iNOS); activation of nuclear

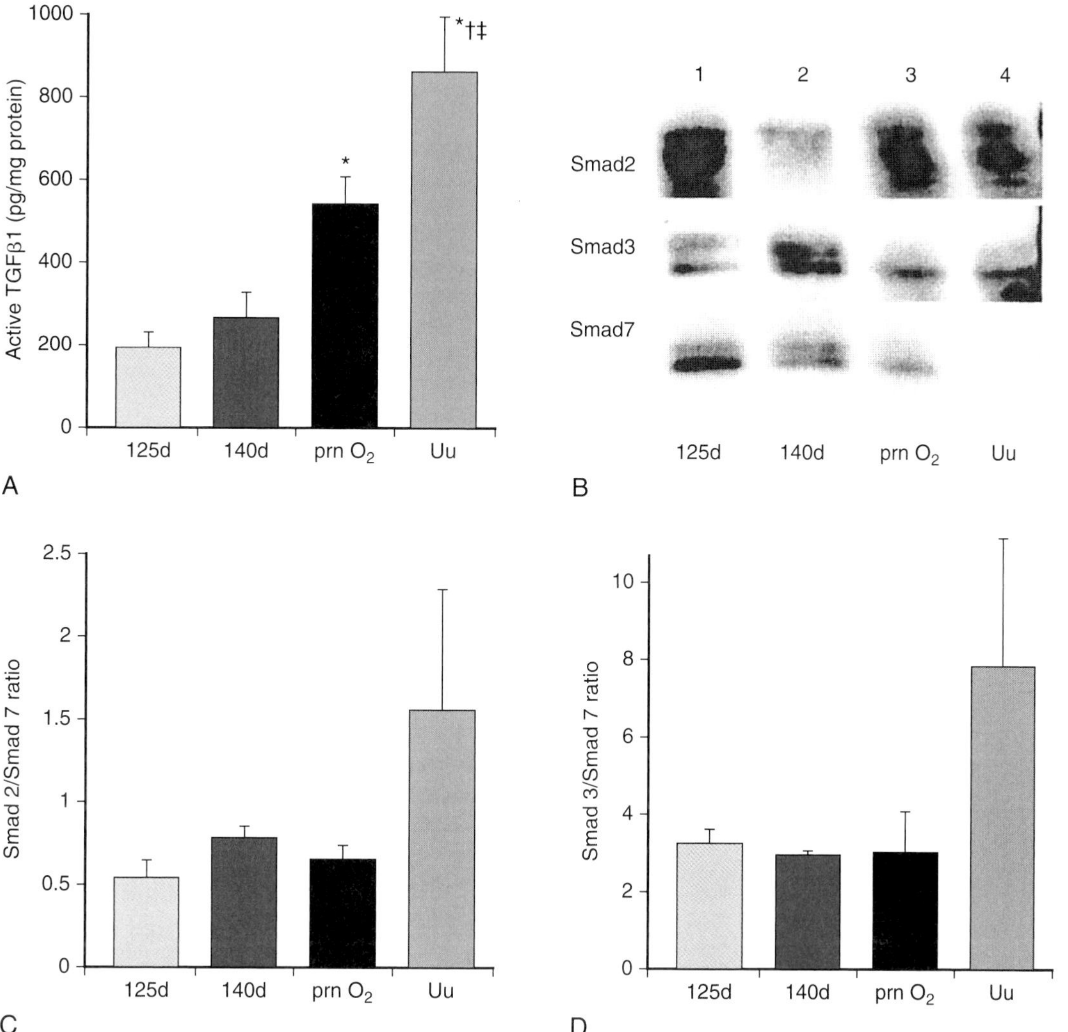

Figure 6-5 Levels of active transforming growth factor-β1 (TGF-β1) and ratios of proteins Smad2/Smad7 and Smad3/Smad7 in lung homogenates of gestational and ventilated controls and antenatally *U. parvum*–infected immature baboons. **A,** Lung homogenates from 125-day (d) and 140d gestational controls (GCs), consisting of a noninfected group and *Ureaplasma* (Uu) receiving oxygen as needed (prn) (N = 3 per group) were assayed for active TGF-β1 by enzyme-linked immunosorbent assay (ELISA). Results are expressed as mean ± SEM pg/mg lung homogenate protein. **B,** Aliquots of lung homogenates (N = 2 per group) were separated by sodium dodecyl sulfate polyacrylamide gel electrophoresis (SDS/PAGE) and immunoblotting performed with goat anti-Smad2, anti-Smad3, or anti-Smad7 antibodies. The amount of immunoreactive protein was quantitated by densitometry. Data are expressed as the mean ± SD ratio of the densitometry measurements of Smad2/Smad7 (**C**) or Smad3/Smad7 (**D**). $^{*}P < 0.05$ compared with 125d GCs; $^{\dagger}P < 0.05$ compared with 140d GCs; $^{\ddagger}P < 0.05$ compared with noninfected prn O_2 group. (From Viscardi RM, Atamas SP, Luzina IG, et al. Antenatal *Ureaplasma urealyticum* respiratory tract infection stimulates proinflammatory, profibrotic responses in the preterm baboon lung. *Pediatr Res.* 2006;60:141-146.)

factor-κB (NF-κB); and expression of VEGF and soluble and cell-associated ICAM-1 by human and mouse-derived monocytic cells.[119-121] *Ureaplasma* has also been found to induce apoptosis in A549 cells, a human alveolar type II cell line, and in THP-1 human acute monocytic leukemia cells.[122] These effects could be partially blocked by anti-TNFα monoclonal antibody,[121,122] implicating TNFα as a mediator of the host immune response to this infection that contributes to altered lung development. In cultured human monocytes, *Ureaplasma* stimulated release of TNFα and IL-8.[123] Moreover, in the presence of bacteria-endotoxic lipopolysaccharide (LPS), *Ureaplasma* greatly augmented monocyte production of

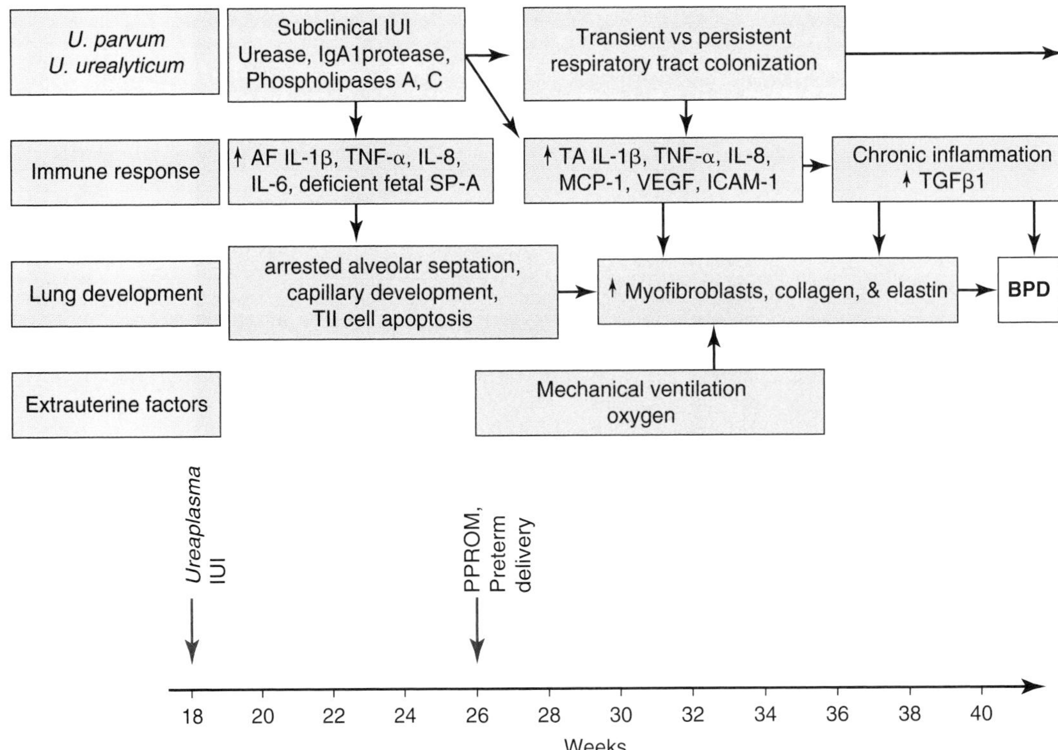

Figure 6-6 Proposed model for role of *Ureaplasma* infection in the pathogenesis of bronchopulmonary dysplasia (BPD). In this schematic, prolonged intra-amniotic exposure of the fetal lung to *Ureaplasma* infection and to maternally and fetally derived cytokines recruits inflammatory cells, and alters transforming growth factor-β1 (TGFβ1) developmental signaling in the lung. Postnatal exposure to ventilation and oxygen augments this proinflammatory response, leading to arrested alveolarization, disordered myofibroblast proliferation, and excessive deposition of collagen and elastin. AF, amniotic fluid; ICAM-1, intracellular adhesion molecule-1; IL, interleukin; MCP-1, monocyte chemoattractant protein-1; PPROM, preterm premature rupture of membranes; SP-A, surfactant protein-A; TA, tracheal aspirate [fluid]; TII, alveolar type II cells; TNF-α, tumor necrosis factor-α; IUI, intrauterine infection; VEGF, vascular endothelial growth factor. (From Viscardi RM, Hasday JD. Role of *Ureaplasma* species in neonatal chronic lung disease: Epidemiologic and experimental evidence. *Pediatr Res.* 2009;65:84R-89R.)

proinflammatory cytokines while blocking expression of anti-inflammatory cytokines (IL-6 and IL-10).

These data confirm that *Ureaplasma* infection contributes to chronic inflammation in the preterm lung. As shown in Figure 6-6, Viscardi and Hasday[123a] have proposed that *Ureaplasma* infection initiated in utero and augmented postnatally by exposure to volutrauma and oxygen elicits a sustained, dysregulated inflammatory response in the immature lung that impairs alveolarization and stimulates myofibroblast proliferation as well as excessive deposition of collagen and elastin.

Developmental Deficiencies in Innate Immunity Contribute to Susceptibility to *Ureaplasma* Infection and Dysregulated Inflammation

Immaturity of fetal host defense mechanisms may increase the susceptibility of the preterm lung to *Ureaplasma* infection and dysregulated inflammation. Surfactant protein A (SP-A), a product of the alveolar type II cell that is an important component of the lung's innate immune response, is deficient in the preterm lung. SP-A is critical for clearance of infection and limitation of inflammation in the lung.[124,125] My colleagues and I have shown that SP-A binds to *Ureaplasma* isolates in a calcium-dependent manner and enhances phagocytosis and bacterial killing by RAW264.7 cells, a murine macrophage cell line.[126,127] Furthermore, bacterial clearance was found to be delayed and the inflammatory response exaggerated in SP-A–deficient mice in comparison with wild-type mice inoculated intratracheally with *U. parvum*. Co-administration of purified human SP-A with the *Ureaplasma* inoculum to SP-A$^{-/-}$mice was reported to reduce the inflammatory response to the infection but not to improve the rate of bacterial clearance. SP-A deficiency of the preterm lung may contribute to the prolonged inflammatory response, lung injury, and risk for fibrosis in *Ureaplasma*-infected infants, giving it a role in the pathogenesis of BPD.

Other important components of the innate immune response are Toll-like receptors (TLRs) that respond to a broad range of pathogen-associated molecular patterns (PAMPs), including LPS, viral coat proteins, bacterial lipoproteins and glycolipids, viral RNA, and CpG-containing bacterial DNA.[128] Engagement of TLR proteins activates the expression of proinflammatory mediators by macrophages, neutrophils, dendritic cells, B cells, endothelial cells, and epithelial cells. TLR signaling activates the transcription factor NF-κB and subsequent upregulation of gene expression.

6

Studies by Peltier and associates[129] and Shimizu and colleagues[130] demonstrated that Triton X-114 detergent–extracted lipoproteins from *U. urealyticum* serovar 4 and *U. parvum* serovar 3 are responsible for NF-κB activation. Active lipoproteins identified for serovar 3 included the MB antigen.[130] The serovar 3 detergent extracts activated NF-κB through TLR2 cooperatively with TLR1 and TLR6,[130] whereas serovar 4 extracts activated both TLR2 and TLR4.[129] Further studies are needed to determine whether the different *Ureaplasma* species or serovars interact with different TLRs. If they do, this feature could explain, in part, differences in host responses to the different serovars.

Little is known concerning TLR expression during human lung development. In mice, TLR2 and TLR4 mRNA levels were barely detectable early in gestation, rising thereafter during late gestation and postnatally.[131] In fetal sheep lung, TLR2 and TLR4 mRNA levels increased throughout late gestation to reach half of adult levels at term but were induced by intra-amniotic LPS exposure.[132] In the immature baboon model, TLR2 and TLR4 mRNA and protein expression were low in nonventilated gestational controls delivered at 125 and 140 days, reached adult levels near term, and were increased in 125-day preterm baboons ventilated with oxygen for 21 days.[133] These data may explain, in part, the developmental susceptibility to *Ureaplasma* infection and interaction with other stimuli. Low TLR2 and TLR4 expression early in gestation may increase the susceptibility of the fetal lung to *Ureaplasma* infection and delay clearance, but postnatal exposures to mechanical ventilation, oxygen, and other infections may stimulate pulmonary TLR expression and enhance *Ureaplasma*-mediated inflammatory signaling.

Ureaplasma Diagnostic Methods

Because *Ureaplasma* spp. are susceptible to desiccation and are sensitive to temperature changes, attention to sample collection and processing are of utmost importance. Samples should be directly inoculated into 10B broth for transport on ice to the laboratory. The specimen should be inoculated in 10B broth with serial 1:10 dilutions, and on A8 agar and incubated in 5% CO_2 at 37° C. Cultures should be observed for up to 7 days for broth color change from yellow to pink, indicating pH change due to urease activity in the absence of turbidity. Any broth with color change should be subcultured on A8 agar. Colonies of *Ureaplasma* spp. are identified presumptively from their characteristic brown appearance on A8 agar in the presence of the $CaCl_2$ indicator. *Ureaplasma* can be differentiated from *M. hominis* by the larger size, lack of precipitate, and "fried-egg" appearance of *M. hominis*. The bacteria in culture usually grow within 24 to 48 hours. Because most clinical laboratories lack the expertise for culture of these organisms, specimens for culture may need to be shipped for processing to a reference laboratory, such as the University of Alabama Mycoplasma Diagnostic Laboratory.

Gel-based traditional[134-136] and real-time PCR[137-140] methods targeting the urease gene, the *mba* gene, or 16s rRNA gene have now been developed to discriminate between the two *Ureaplasma* species. Real-time PCR assays yield quantitative results and are more rapid, specific, and sensitive, and less subject to contamination than culture and traditional PCR methods. Availability of the genomic sequences for all 14 *Ureaplasma* serovars has enabled primers/probes to be designed that are specific for each serovar without any cross-reactions.[70]

Can Bronchopulmonary Dysplasia Be Prevented by Eradication of *Ureaplasma*?

Despite in vitro susceptibility of *Ureaplasma* to erythromycin,[141] trials of erythromycin therapy in the first few weeks of life in *Ureaplasma*-colonized preterm infants have failed to demonstrate efficacy to prevent BPD[142,143] or eradicate respiratory tract colonization.[144] The failure of this agent to prevent BPD in these studies may have been due to the small sample size of each study or to the initiation of erythromycin therapy too late to prevent the lung inflammation and injury that contribute to the pathogenesis of BPD.

The new 14-membered macrolides that are derivatives of erythromycin and the related 15-membered azalides have immunomodulatory effects, including effects on neutrophil function (e.g., chemotaxis, cell adhesion, oxidative burst, and phagocytosis) and inhibition of cytokine release[145] and nitric oxide production in vitro.[146] Macrolide antibiotics may exert immunomodulatory anti-inflammatory effects in the setting of infection, which may occur independently of a direct bactericidal effect.[147] In addition, azithromycin exhibits higher potency than erythromycin against clinical *Ureaplasma* isolates in vitro.[148] Pharmacokinetic studies in mice and humans have shown that azithromycin is preferentially concentrated in pulmonary epithelial lining fluid and alveolar macrophages.[149-151] Neutrophil recruitment and activation have been implicated in BPD pathogenesis,[152,153] so the experimental effects observed with azithromycin in vitro and in vivo indicate that this drug may be beneficial in the treatment of *Ureaplasma* infection and the prevention of BPD in preterm infants.

Because *Ureaplasma*-mediated lung injury may be initiated in utero and augmented postnatally by exposure to mechanical ventilation and hyperoxia, therapy to prevent BPD should be initiated as soon as possible after birth in infants at risk. Walls and associates[154] demonstrated that prophylaxis with azithromycin but not erythromycin improved outcomes and reduced inflammation in a murine neonatal *Ureaplasma* infection model. This finding suggests that azithromycin may be effective if administered immediately after birth. An initial single-dose pharmacokinetic study of 10 mg/kg azithromycin in infants born at 24 to 28 weeks of gestation suggested that this dose was well-tolerated but likely insufficient to maintain azithromycin concentrations above the MIC50 (minimum concentration that inhibits 50% of organisms) for *Ureaplasma*.[155] However, until additional pharmacokinetics and efficacy trials are conducted, a dosing regimen for azithromycin in neonates cannot be recommended.

Other Perinatally Acquired Microbes and Pulmonary Outcomes

Molecular methods have expanded the ability to detect microbes that are difficult to cultivate in clinical aspirates from preterm infants. By screening gastric and tracheal aspirates from infants born at or before 34 weeks of gestation for the presence of bacterial 16S rRNA genes and *Ureaplasma* by PCR, Beeton and coworkers[12] demonstrated that 77% of infants with chronic lung disease (CLD) tested positive, compared with 48% of infants with RDS, and 29% of term infants. There was a significant association between CLD and the presence of 16S rRNA genes and/or *Ureaplasma* and whether it was first detected within the first 3 days or after 3 days of age. Because *Ureaplasma* acquisition is by the vertical route, and horizontal transmission is unlikely, detection for the first time beyond the first few days of life likely represents chronic rather than new colonization. In this study, CLD infants were colonized more frequently than RDS infants with gram-negative organisms such as *E. coli, Haemophilus influenzae, Enterobacter* spp., and *Pseudomonas aeruginosa*.[12] Bacterial respiratory colonization is associated with increased levels of proinflammatory mediators such as, IL-1β, IL-6, and IL-8,[12,41] suggesting that prolonged infection-mediated inflammation contributes to the pathogenesis of BPD.

Chlamydia trachomatis has been investigated as a potential perinatally acquired pathogen contributing to BPD in preterm infants. In a series of 12 very preterm infants with confirmed *C. trachomatis* pneumonia, a common clinical biphasic course was identified.[156] After an early phase of disease indistinguishable from RDS with improving respiratory status during the first week of life, the infected infants demonstrated apnea, worsening respiratory signs, and chest radiographic evidence of lung hypoexpansion and fine reticular pattern during the second and third weeks of life. Numazaki and associates[157] reported that sera of 31% of infants with BPD that they screened, but of no controls without respiratory symptoms, tested positive for anti–*Chlamydia* IgM and that *C. trachomatis* was identified in autopsy lung tissue by immunohistochemistry in two seropositive infants who died. In multiple subsequent studies, *Chlamydia* was rarely detected, and this organism does not appear to be an important pathogen in neonatal lung disease in the preterm population in the United States.[105,158-161] However, *C. trachomatis* may be a more important pathogen in late-onset pneumonia in developing countries where sexually transmitted infections are common.[162]

Viruses as etiologic agents in neonatal lung disease have received less attention. The literature is mostly limited to case reports.[163,164] In a prospective study of 89 infants born at less than 30 weeks of gestation, TAs collected within the first week of life were analyzed by PCR for adenovirus, enterovirus, cytomegalovirus (CMV), parvovirus, *Mycoplasma* spp., and *Chlamydia* spp. and infants classified as having BPD at 28 days of life or 36 weeks PMA.[161] Of the viral genomes screened, only adenovirus was detected with increased frequency in infants with BPD at 28 days of life (27%) and 36 weeks PMA (29%) compared with infants without BPD at 28 days of life (3%) and 36 weeks PMA (6%). Cytomegalovirus and enterovirus were detected in one patient each. Over a 5 year period in a single institution, postnatally acquired cytomegalovirus was diagnosed in 32 preterm infants of less than 2000 g birth weight.[165] BPD developed in three quarters of the infected infants compared with 38% of controls matched for gestational age and birthweight. The cytomegalovirus-positive infants required more respiratory support than controls, and 9 (28%) had clinically apparent pneumonia.

Postnatal Microbial Colonization and Adverse Pulmonary Outcomes

Neonatal pneumonia is estimated to account for up to 10% of child mortality in the world. Onset is classified as either early, within the first 48 hours to 7 days, or late. Although early-onset disease is usually caused by perinatally acquired pathogens, late-onset disease may be caused by organisms colonizing the upper airway or from exogenous sources such as contaminated endotracheal tubes, suction equipment, ventilator circuits, and health care workers' hands. The importance of the contribution of health care–acquired infections in neonatal intensive care units (NICUs) to neonatal morbidity, mortality, length of stay, and hospital costs is increasingly recognized.[166,167] Ventilator-associated pneumonia (VAP) accounts for 6.8% to 32.2% of health care–acquired infections in neonates.[168-170] This section focuses on current knowledge about the epidemiology, diagnostic criteria, and preventive and therapeutic strategies for VAP in the neonatal population.

Ventilator-Associated Pneumonia in the Neonatal Intensive Care Unit

Diagnostic Criteria

Ventilator-associated pneumonia is defined as pneumonia that develops 48 hours or longer after initiation of mechanical ventilation.[169,170] Although the U.S. Centers for Disease Control and Prevention (CDC) and National Hospital Safety Network have developed specific criteria for VAP diagnosis in children less than 1 year of age, the criteria have not been validated in newborns. Pneumonia may be difficult to distinguish clinically and radiographically from other causes of neonatal lung disease, and diagnostic techniques used in adults are not commonly used in newborns, so diagnosing neonatal VAP is problematic. Current criteria are as follows: (1) mechanical ventilation for 48 hours or more preceding the onset of suspected VAP; (2) increase in oxygen and ventilatory requirements; (3) new infiltrates, consolidation, cavitation, or pneumatocele on at least 2 radiographs; and (4) at least three of the following signs or symptoms: temperature instability, wheezing, tachypnea, cough, abnormal heart rate, change in respiratory secretions, and abnormal peripheral white blood cell count.[171,172]

B

Although the VAP criteria do not include microbiologic identification of a pathogen from the lower respiratory tract, invasive testing is commonly used in adults with suspected VAP. Obtaining specimens from the lower respiratory tract for microbiologic examination by bronchoalveolar lavage (BAL) or protected specimen brush (PBS) is common in adults, but these techniques are not practical in neonates because of their small airway size. TAs are more often used in neonates but may be contaminated with oropharyngeal flora. Koksal and associates[173] performed nonbronchoscopic bronchoalveolar lavage through a sterile 6F or 8F catheter that was passed through the endotracheal tube and wedged in a bronchus to obtain specimens for culture in ventilated neonates with suspected pneumonia. In their series of 145 infants, 90% of infants with clinically diagnosed VAP had positive bronchoalveolar lavage culture results. No complications of this procedure were reported, but the sensitivity and specificity of this method in comparison with a gold standard, such as lung biopsy or tissue sample, are lacking.

In the clinical evaluation for neonatal VAP, TA culture and Gram stain are often used diagnostically and to guide antibiotic therapy. Alone, a positive TA result has low sensitivity, specificity, and positive predictive value because true infection is difficult to distinguish from airway colonization.[170] Cordero and colleagues[174] evaluated the relationship of TA purulence—defined as the number of PMNs per low-power field (LPF)—TA culture results, and clinical outcomes in a retrospective study of mechanically ventilated VLBW infants. TAs were culture-positive in 58% of nonpurulent samples, 94% of lightly purulent (<25 PMNs/LPF), and 100% of moderately to heavily purulent (≥25 PMNs/LPF) samples. Moderate/heavy purulence predicted culture-positive TAs infected with gram-negative bacilli with 70% sensitivity, 100% specificity, 100% predictive value, and 67% negative predictive value. However, VAP occurred in only 7% of VLBW infants without and in 5% with purulent TAs.[174] In a prospective cohort, purulent TAs were obtained in 46% of VAP cases as defined by National Nosocomial Infection Surveillance (NNIS) criteria.[166] In contrast, in a retrospective study in China, 92% of infants with VAP had purulent TAs, but only 53% had culture-positive TAs. Gram stain of TAs may be useful in predicting classes of pathogens in VAP cases. In a prospective study, the sensitivity and specificity of TA Gram stain were 82% and 100% for gram-positive organisms and 100% and 82% for gram-negative organisms.[175] However, whether the organism(s) present on TA Gram stain is the cause of the pneumonia is unknown. Despite these limitations, TAs are the only practical means of sampling the lower respiratory tract in neonates, and data from such sampling should be combined with clinical and radiographic findings for surveillance of VAP in the NICU population.

Risk Factors

Studies of neonatal VAP have identified specific risk factors in this age group. The risk of VAP is inversely related to birth weight and gestational age.[166,172,176-178] In a 2008 CDC-report, the rates of VAP in level III NICUs ranged from 2.6 cases/1000 ventilator-days among infants of less than 750 g birth weight, to 1.5 cases/1000 ventilator-days among infants of 1001 to 1500 g birth weight, and 0.9 cases/1000 ventilator-days among infants of more than 2500 g birth weight.[178] In a survey of NICUs from 19 children's hospitals, the reported VAP rate among infants of 1000 g or less birth weight was 3.5 cases/1000 ventilator-days, compared with 0.9 cases/1000 ventilator-days for infants of more than 2500 g birth weight.[179] In a report from a single institution, VAP rates were 6.5/1000 ventilator-days in infants born before 28 weeks of gestation compared to 4/1000 ventilator-days in infants born at or after 28 weeks of gestation.[166] Other risk factors for neonatal VAP are re-intubation, longer duration of mechanical ventilation, endotracheal suctioning, and opiate treatment.[177,180] Apisarnthanarak and colleagues[166] reported that the risk for VAP increased 11% for each additional week of mechanical ventilation in their study.[166] Previous bloodstream infection was identified as an independent risk factor for neonatal VAP.[166] Because the organisms isolated at time of VAP differed from the organisms isolated in the prior bloodstream infections in this study, the investigators suggested that previous bacteremia might be a surrogate for severity of illness in patients with VAP.

6

Microbiology

Because evaluation of the microbiology of neonatal VAP is based on TA cultures rather than invasive sampling of the lower airway, results may be difficult to interpret owing to possible contamination with oropharyngeal flora. Possibly because of the presence of oropharyngeal flora, TA culture results suggest that neonatal VAP is often polymicrobial.[166,181] Gram-negative (*Pseudomonas aeruginosa, E. coli, Klebsiella pneumoniae, Enterobacter* spp., and *Acinetobacter* spp.) and the gram-positive (*Staphylococcus aureus* and *Enterococcus* spp.) organisms are the predominant isolates in VAP cases.[166,177,181] Community-acquired methicillin-resistant *S. aureus* strains (CA-MRSA), differentiated from hospital-acquired strains by the presence of the genes for Panton-Valentine leukocidin (PVL) toxin and type IV staphylococcal chromosome cassette element, have been identified by molecular testing in neonates with necrotizing pneumonia.[182] Because CA-MRSA strains are susceptible to more classes of antibiotics than the hospital-acquired strains, review of antibiotic susceptibility testing of MRSA isolates may be helpful in differentiating the strains.

Pathogenesis

Lung defenses against invading pathogens include anatomic barriers such as the mucociliary lining of the respiratory tract, cough reflex, and innate and adaptive immune responses. The newborn is particularly susceptible to pneumonia because of greater permeability of the skin and mucous membranes and immaturity of the local and systemic immune systems. Intubation and mechanical ventilation prevent the cough reflex and injure the mucociliary lining of the respiratory tract, reducing the ability of the preterm lung to clear invading pathogens. It has been suggested that contaminated oral and gastric secretions that pool around the endotracheal tube cuff in adults gain access to lower respiratory tract by leaking around the cuff.[183] Because neonatal endotracheal tubes are uncuffed, the endotracheal tube may be a common entry for contaminated secretions, but the notion has yet to be proved in the NICU population. Elevation of the head of the bed is a measure used in adult ICUs to prevent aspiration of contaminated oropharyngeal/gastric secretions. In a small study in ventilated infants, Aly and coworkers[184] demonstrated that lateral positioning resulted in less tracheal colonization after 5 days of ventilation than supine positioning (30% vs. 87%, $P < 0.01$), providing support for aspiration of oropharyngeal secretions in the pathogenesis of neonatal VAP.

Gastric contents may also be an important source of pathogens implicated in VAP. Farhath and colleagues[185] reported that pepsin, a gastric marker, was detected in TAs of 92% of a cohort of ventilated neonates and was higher in TAs from infants in whom severe BPD developed, but their study did not evaluate an association with VAP.[185] Medications that reduce gastric acidity, such as histamine H_2 antagonists and antacids, may increase the risk for VAP by favoring stomach colonization with pathogens. In a single-institution study, 46% infants of less than 28 weeks of gestation were treated with H_2 antagonists, but such exposure was not significantly associated with VAP.[166] However, H_2 antagonist use has been associated with increased risk for late-onset gram-negative sepsis and necrotizing enterocolitis in VLBW infants.[186,187] Sucralfate, a medication for stress ulcer prophylaxis that does not affect gastric pH, has been shown to reduce VAP rates in adults.[169] This drug has not been evaluated in neonates for this indication. Currently, stress ulcer prophylaxis cannot be recommended to prevent VAP in preterm neonates.

External sources may be significant contributors to airway colonization and neonatal VAP. They include biofilm formation on endotracheal tubes and contamination of ventilator circuit condensate, suctioning equipment, nebulizers, and most importantly, health care workers' hands.[169,183] Implementation of a hand hygiene intervention in a Taiwanese NICU was reported to improve hand hygiene compliance and reduce the respiratory infection rate from 3.35/patient days pre-intervention to 1.06/patient days post-intervention ($P = 0.002$).[188] In a similar study in five NICUs in Northern Ireland, a quality improvement initiative focused on hand hygiene, was reported to have reduced the VAP rate by 38%.[189] These studies underscore the importance of hand hygiene compliance in the prevention of nosocomial infection in the NICU.

B

Outcomes

Infants with VAP experience longer durations of mechanical ventilation, longer hospital stays, and higher mortality.[166,177] The pathogen causing infection may determine the severity of infection and outcomes. More invasive organisms, such as *P. aeruginosa,*[190] enteric gram-negative bacteria,[172,191] and CA-MRSA,[182] may be associated with greater lung parenchymal injury, necrotizing pneumonia, and abscess formation. The impact of VAP on long-term pulmonary outcomes in survivors has not been investigated but likely augments pulmonary morbidity in infants with underlying lung disease such as BPD.

Prevention

Hand hygiene is the most effective intervention to prevent nosocomial infection in all age groups. Although there are specific recommendations for other interventions in adults, few are proven effective or are applicable to the neonatal population. Reducing exposure to mechanical ventilation is likely to be a significant change in practice that will affect neonatal VAP rates. Use of noninvasive means of respiratory support, such as nasal continuous positive airway pressure (NCPAP) and high-flow nasal cannula, reduced the risk for VAP.[192,193] A comparison of closed or in-line suctioning with open suction methods did not demonstrate superiority of either method. In-line suction may reduce environmental contamination, but the in-line catheter may become contaminated with oropharyngeal organisms.[183] Other potential interventions are wearing gloves when handling secretions, clearing oropharyngeal secretions before repositioning or removing the endotracheal tube, and draining accumulated ventilator circuit condensate to prevent aspiration. Whether side positioning or elevating the head is the best position to prevent VAP in mechanically ventilated newborns remains to be determined.

Effects of Antenatal Infection/Inflammation on Long-Term Pulmonary Outcomes

With increasing survival of extremely preterm births, there is accumulating evidence that prematurity, and particularly the development of BPD, are risk factors for chronic respiratory problems throughout childhood and into adulthood.[194,195] More severe respiratory symptoms result in higher rates of hospital admission in the first few years of life.[195] A meta-analysis of 19 studies of the association between prematurity and childhood asthma concluded that children born preterm have a 7% higher risk for development of asthma than children born at term.[196] Specifically, in a population-based study of Alaskan children younger than 10 years, the risk of asthma was inversely proportional to gestational age at birth but was not affected by small-for-gestational-age status.[197] This finding suggests that pathways contributing to prematurity may differ in their effects on lung development that extend beyond the perinatal period.

The association of chorioamnionitis exposure in utero and childhood asthma has been assessed in large population-based studies. In a retrospective cohort of

500,000 singletons born over a 16-year period in a health maintenance organization, Kaiser Permanente Southern California, Getahun and coworkers[198] analyzed the impact of prematurity and clinical chorioamnionitis on the risk of physician-diagnosed asthma in children younger than 8 years. Clinical chorioamnionitis exposure in children born preterm was independently associated with an increased risk for asthma among white, African-American, and Hispanic, but not Asian/Pacific Islander, subjects. In a prospective study of 1000 children in the Boston Birth Cohort, the highest rate of recurrent wheezing and physician-diagnosed asthma occurred in children born at less than 33 weeks of gestation with exposure to either clinical or histologic chorioamnionitis.[199] The effect of chorioamnionitis on wheezing and asthma was highest in very preterm African-American children. These studies suggest that exposure to microbes or resulting inflammation in the fetal lung contributes to airway remodeling and potentially to later airway hyperresponsiveness.

Ureaplasma respiratory tract colonization has also been proposed as an etiologic factor in reactive airway disease in young infants. Wheezing in infants and children younger than 3 years has been associated with isolation of *Ureaplasma* from the upper respiratory tract.[200] In a large study of almost 3000 women and their offspring in Sweden, maternal vaginal colonization with *Ureaplasma* during pregnancy was associated with a 2-fold higher risk for infant wheezing, defined as one or more hospitalizations for asthma during the first 3 years of life.[201] The investigators proposed that acquisition of microorganisms such as *Ureaplasma* spp. at birth affects the establishment of infant microflora and subsequent development of allergy and wheezing. Prospective studies of long-term pulmonary outcomes of preterm infants with *Ureaplasma* respiratory colonization with and without BPD are lacking. Long-term outcomes should be included in any therapeutic trial of neonatal interventions to eradicate *Ureaplasma* colonization.

Acknowledgments

This work was supported by NIH grants HL071113 and HL087166 and the American Heart Association.

References

1. Northway WH, Rosan RC, Porter DY. Pulmonary disease following respirator therapy of hyaline-membrane disease. *N Engl J Med*. 1967;276:357-368.
2. Bonikos DS, Bensch KG, Northway WH, et al. Bronchopulmonary dysplasia: the pulmonary pathologic sequel of necrotizing bronchiolitis and pulmonary fibrosis. *Hum Pathol*. 1976;7:643-666.
3. Jobe AH, Bancalari E. Bronchopulmonary dysplasia. *Am J Respir Crit Care Med*. 2001;163:1723-1729.
4. Husain AN, Siddiqui NH, Stocker JT. Pathology of arrested acinar development in postsurfactant bronchopulmonary dysplasia. *Hum Pathol*. 1998;29:710-717.
5. Viscardi RM, Muhumuza CK, Rodriguez A, et al. Inflammatory markers in intrauterine and fetal blood and cerebrospinal fluid compartments are associated with adverse pulmonary and neurologic outcomes in preterm infants. *Pediatr Res*. 2004;55:1009-1017.
6. Goldenberg RL, Hauth JC, Andrews WW. Intrauterine infection and preterm delivery. *N Engl J Med*. 2000;342:1500-1507.
7. Onderdonk AB, Hecht JL, McElrath TF, et al. Colonization of second-trimester placenta parenchyma. *Am J Obstet Gynecol*. 2008;199:52.e51-52.e10.
8. DiGiulio DB, Romero R, Amogan HP, et al. Microbial prevalence, diversity and abundance in amniotic fluid during preterm labor: a molecular and culture-based investigation. *PLoS One*. 2008;3:e3056.
9. Onderdonk AB, Delaney ML, DuBois AM, et al. Detection of bacteria in placental tissues obtained from extremely low gestational age neonates. *Am J Obstet Gynecol*. 2008;198:110.e111-110.e117.
10. Olomu IN, Hecht JL, Onderdonk AO, et al. Perinatal correlates of *Ureaplasma urealyticum* in placenta parenchyma of singleton pregnancies that end before 28 weeks of gestation. *Pediatrics*. 2009;123:1329-1336.
11. Oue S, Hiroi M, Ogawa S, et al. Association of gastric fluid microbes at birth with severe bronchopulmonary dysplasia. *Arch Dis Child Fetal Neonatal Ed*. 2009;94:F17-F22.
12. Beeton ML, Maxwell NC, Davies PL, et al. Role of pulmonary infection in the development of chronic lung disease of prematurity. *Eur Respir J*. 2011;37:1424-1430.
13. Payne MS, Goss KC, Connett GJ, et al. Molecular microbiological characterization of preterm neonates at risk of bronchopulmonary dysplasia. *Pediatr Res*. 2010;67:412-418.
14. Thomas W, Speer CP. Chorioamnionitis: important risk factor or innocent bystander for neonatal outcome? *Neonatology*. 2010;99:177-187.

B

15. Hecht JL, Onderdonk A, Delaney M, et al. Characterization of chorioamnionitis in 2nd-trimester C-section placentas and correlation with microorganism recovery from subamniotic tissues. *Pediatr Dev Pathol.* 2008;11:15-22.
16. Redline RW. Inflammatory responses in the placenta and umbilical cord. *Semin Fetal Neonatal Med.* 2006;11:296-301.
17. Redline RW, Wilson-Costello D, Borawski E, et al. Placental lesions associated with neurologic impairment and cerebral palsy in very low-birth-weight infants. *Arch Pathol Lab Med.* 1998; 122:1091-1098.
18. Hecht JL, Fichorova RN, Tang VF, et al. Relationship between neonatal blood protein concentrations and placenta histologic characteristics in extremely low GA newborns. *Pediatr Res.* 2011;69: 68-73.
19. Yoon BH, Romero R, Kim KS, et al. A systematic fetal inflammatory response and the development of bronchopulmonary dysplasia. *Am J Obstet Gynecol.* 1999;181:773-779.
20. Watterberg KL, Demers LM, Scott SM, et al. Chorioamnionitis and early lung inflammation in infants in whom bronchopulmonary dysplasia develops. *Pediatrics.* 1996;97:210-215.
21. Andrews WW, Goldenberg RL, Faye-Petersen O, et al. The Alabama Preterm Birth Study: polymorphonuclear and mononuclear cell placental infiltrations, other markers of inflammation, and outcomes in 23- to 32-week preterm newborn infants. *Am J Obstet Gynecol.* 2006;195: 803-808.
22. Kaukola T, Tuimala J, Herva R, et al. Cord immunoproteins as predictors of respiratory outcome in preterm infants. *Am J Obstet Gynecol.* 2009;200:100.e101-100.e108.
23. Lahra MM, Beeby PJ, Jeffery HE. Maternal versus fetal inflammation and respiratory distress syndrome: a 10-year hospital cohort study. *Arch Dis Child Fetal Neonatal Ed.* 2009;94:F13-F16.
24. Lee J, Oh KJ, Park CW, et al. The presence of funisitis is associated with a decreased risk for the development of neonatal respiratory distress syndrome. *Placenta.* 2011;32:235-240.
25. Ogunyemi D, Murillo M, Jackson U et al. The relationship between placental histopathology findings and perinatal outcome in preterm infants. *J Matern Fetal Neonatal Med.* 2003;13:102-109.
26. Richardson BS, Wakim E, daSilva O, et al. Preterm histologic chorioamnionitis: impact on cord gas and pH values and neonatal outcome. *Am J Obstet Gynecol.* 2006;195:1357-1365.
27. Zanardo V, Vedovato S, Suppiej A, et al. Histological inflammatory responses in the placenta and early neonatal brain injury. *Pediatr Dev Pathol.* 2008;11:350-354.
28. Lahra MM, Beeby PJ, Jeffery HE. Intrauterine inflammation, neonatal sepsis, and chronic lung disease: a 13-year hospital cohort study. *Pediatrics.* 2009;123:1314-1319.
29. Redline RW, Wilson-Costello D, Hack M. Placental and other perinatal risk factors for chronic lung disease in very low birth weight infants. *Pediatr Res.* 2002;52:713-719.
30. Kent A, Dahlstrom JE. Chorioamnionitis/funisitis and the development of bronchopulmonary dysplasia. *J Paediatr Child Health.* 2004;40:356-359.
31. Ohyama M, Itani Y, Yamanaka M, et al. Re-evaluation of chorioamnionitis and funisitis with a special reference to subacute chorioamnionitis. *Hum Pathol.* 2002;33:183-190.
32. van Marter LJ, Dammann O, Allred EN, et al. Chorioamnionitis, mechanical ventilation, and postnatal sepsis as modulators of chronic lung disease in preterm infants. *J Pediatr.* 2002;140: 171-176.
33. Been JV, Rours IG, Kornelisse RF, et al. Chorioamnionitis alters the response to surfactant in preterm infants. *J Pediatr.* 2010;156:10-15.e1.
34. Paul DA, Zook K, Mackley A, et al. Reduced mortality and increased BPD with histological chorioamnionitis and leukocytosis in very-low-birth-weight infants. *J Perinatol.* 2010;30:58-62.
35. Watterberg KL, Gerdes JS, Cole CH, et al. Prophylaxis of early adrenal insufficiency to prevent bronchopulmonary dysplasia: a multicenter trial. *Pediatrics.* 2004;114:1649-1657.
36. Yoon BH, Romero R, Jun JK, et al. Amniotic fluid cytokines (interleukin-6, tumor necrosis factor-α, interleukin-1β, and interleukin-8) and the risk for the development of bronchopulmonary dysplasia. *Am J Obstet Gynecol.* 1997;177:825-830.
37. Gomez R, Romero R, Ghezzi F, et al. The fetal inflammatory response syndrome. *Am J Obstet Gynecol.* 1998;179:194-202.
38. Grigg JM, Barber A, Silverman M. Increased levels of bronchoalveolar lavage fluid interleukin-6 in preterm ventilated infants after prolonged rupture of membranes. *Am Rev Respir Dis.* 1992; 145:782-786.
39. Kwong KY, Jones CA, Cayabyab R, et al. Differential regulation of IL-8 by IL-1β and TNFα in hyaline membrane disease. *J Clin Immunol.* 1998;18:71-80.
40. Bagchi A, Viscardi RM, Taciak V, et al. Increased activity of interleukin-6 but not tumor necrosis factor-α in lung lavage of premature infants is associated with the development of bronchopulmonary dysplasia. *Pediatr Res.* 1994;36:244-252.
41. Rindfleisch MS, Hasday JD, Taciak V, et al. Potential role of interleukin-1 in the development of bronchopulmonary dysplasia. *J Interferon Cytokine Res.* 1996;16:365-373.
42. Viscardi RM, Hasday JD, Gumpper KF, et al. Cromolyn sodium prophylaxis inhibits pulmonary proinflammatory cytokines in infants at high risk for bronchopulmonary dysplasia. *Am J Respir Crit Care Med.* 1997;156:1523-1529.
43. Jones CA, Cayabyab RG, Kwong KY, et al. Undetectable interleukin (IL)-10 and persistent IL-8 expression early in hyaline membrane disease: a possible developmental basis for the predisposition to chronic lung inflammation in preterm newborns. *Pediatr Res.* 1996;39:966-975.
44. Bose CL, Dammann CE, Laughon MM. Bronchopulmonary dysplasia and inflammatory biomarkers in the premature neonate. *Arch Dis Child Fetal Neonatal Ed.* 2008;93:F455-F461.

45. Warburton D, Tefft D, Mailleux A, et al. Do lung remodeling, repair, and regeneration recapitulate respiratory ontogeny? *Am J Respir Crit Care Med.* 2001;164:S59-S62.
46. Toti P, Buonocore G, Tanganelli P, et al. Bronchopulmonary dysplasia of the premature baby: an immunohistochemical study. *Pediatr Pulmonol.* 1997;24:22-28.
47. Lecart C, Cayabyab R, Buckley S, et al. Bioactive transforming growth factor-beta in the lungs of extremely low birthweight neonates predicts the need for home oxygen supplementation. *Biol Neonate.* 2000;77:217-223.
48. Zhou L, Dey CR, Wert SE, et al. Arrested lung morphogenesis in transgenic mice bearing an SP-C-TGF-beta 1 chimeric gene. *Dev Biol.* 1996;175:227-238.
49. Zeng X, Gray M, Stahlman MT, et al. TGF-beta1 perturbs vascular development and inhibits epithelial differentiation in fetal lung in vivo. *Dev Dyn.* 2001;221:289-301.
50. Vicencio AG, Lee CG, Cho SJ, et al. Conditional overexpression of bioactive transforming growth factor-beta1 in neonatal mouse lung: a new model for bronchopulmonary dysplasia? *Am J Respir Cell Mol Biol.* 2004;31:650-656.
51. Gauldie J, Galt T, Bonniaud P, et al. Transfer of the active form of transforming growth factor-beta 1 gene to newborn rat lung induces changes consistent with bronchopulmonary dysplasia. *Am J Pathol.* 2003;163:2575-2584.
52. Kunzmann S, Speer CP, Jobe AH, et al. Antenatal inflammation induced TGF-beta1 but suppressed CTGF in preterm lungs. *Am J Physiol Lung Cell Mol Physiol.* 2007;292:L223-L231.
53. Bry K, Whitsett JA, Lappalainen U. IL-1beta disrupts postnatal lung morphogenesis in the mouse. *Am J Respir Cell Mol Biol.* 2007;36:32-42.
54. Bry K, Hogmalm A, Backstrom E. Mechanisms of inflammatory lung injury in the neonate: lessons from a transgenic mouse model of bronchopulmonary dysplasia. *Semin Perinatol.* 2010;34:211-221.
55. Sime PJ, Marr RA, Gauldie D, et al. Transfer of tumor necrosis factor-alpha to rat lung induces severe pulmonary inflammation and patchy interstitial fibrogenesis with induction of transforming growth factor-beta1 and myofibroblasts. *Am J Pathol.* 1998;153:825-832.
56. Kolb M, Margetts P, Anthony D, et al. Transient expression of IL-1β induces acute lung injury and chronic repair leading to pulmonary fibrosis. *J Clin Invest.* 2001;107:1529-1536.
57. Hogmalm A, Sheppard D, Lappalainen U, et al. beta6 Integrin subunit deficiency alleviates lung injury in a mouse model of bronchopulmonary dysplasia. *Am J Respir Cell Mol Biol.* 2010;43:88-98.
58. Kotecha S, Wangoo A, Silverman M, et al. Increase in the concentration of transforming growth factor beta-1 in bronchoalveolar lavage fluid before development of chronic lung disease of prematurity. *J Pediatr.* 1996;128:464-469.
59. Jonsson B, Li YH, Noack G, et al. Downregulatory cytokines in tracheobronchial aspirate fluid from infants with chronic lung disease of prematurity. *Acta Paediatr.* 2000;89:1375-1380.
60. Pereyre S, Sirand-Pugnet P, Beven L, et al. Life on arginine for *Mycoplasma hominis*: clues from its minimal genome and comparison with other human urogenital mycoplasmas. *PLoS Genet.* 2009;5:e1000677.
61. Waites KB, Katz B, Schelonka RL. Mycoplasmas and ureaplasmas as neonatal pathogens. *Clin Microbiol Rev.* 2005;18:757-789.
62. Glass JI, Lefkowitz EJ, Glass JS, et al. The complete sequence of the mucosal pathogen *Ureaplasma urealyticum*. *Nature.* 2000;407:757-762.
63. Abele-Horn M, Wolff C, Dressel P, et al. Association of *Ureaplasma urealyticum* biovars with clinical outcome for neonates, obstetric patients, and gynecological patients with pelvic inflammatory disease. *J Clin Microbiol.* 1997;35:1199-1202.
64. Kasper DC, Mechtler TP, Reischer GH, et al. The bacterial load of *Ureaplasma parvum* in amniotic fluid is correlated with an increased intrauterine inflammatory response. *Diagn Microbiol Infect Dis.* 2010;67:117-121.
65. Hannaford K, Todd DA, Jeffrey H, et al. Role of *Ureaplasma urealyticum* in lung disease of prematurity. *Arch Dis Child Fetal Neonatal Ed.* 1999;81:F162-F167.
66. Sung TJ, Xiao L, Duffy L, et al. Frequency of *Ureaplasma* serovars in respiratory secretions of preterm infants at risk for bronchopulmonary dysplasia. *Pediatr Infect Dis J.* 2011;30:379-383.
67. Viscardi RM, Hashmi N, Gross GW, et al. Incidence of invasive *Ureaplasma* in VLBW infants: relationship to severe intraventricular hemorrhage. *J Perinatol.* 2008;28:759-765.
68. Grattard F, Soleihac B, De Barbeyrac B, et al. Epidemiologic and molecular investigations of genital mycoplasmas from women and neonates at delivery. *Pediatr Infect Dis J.* 1995;14:853-858.
69. Katz B, Patel P, Duffy L, et al. Characterization of ureaplasmas isolated from preterm infants with and without bronchopulmonary dysplasia. *J Clin Microbiol.* 2005;43:4852-4854.
70. Xiao L, Glass JI, Paralanov V, et al. Detection and characterization of human ureaplasma species and serovars by real-time PCR. *J Clin Microbiol.* 2010;48:2715-2723.
71. Zimmerman CU, Stiedl T, Rosengarten R, et al. Alternate phase variation in expression of two major surface membrane proteins (MBA and UU376) of *Ureaplasma parvum* serovar 3. *FEMS Microbiol Lett.* 2009;292:187-193.
72. Zheng X, Watson HL, Waites KB, et al. Serotype diversity and antigen variation among invasive isolates of *Ureaplasma urealyticum* from neonates. *Infect Immun.* 1992;60:3472-3474.
73. Knox CL, Dando SJ, Nitsos I, et al. The severity of chorioamnionitis in pregnant sheep is associated with *in vivo* variation of the surface-exposed multiple-banded antigen/gene of *Ureaplasma parvum*. *Biol Reprod.* 2010;83:415-426.

6

74. Garcia-Castillo M, Morosini MI, Galvez M, et al. Differences in biofilm development and antibiotic susceptibility among clinical *Ureaplasma urealyticum* and *Ureaplasma parvum* isolates. *J Antimicrob Chemother*. 2008;62:1027-1030.
75. Momynaliev K, Klubin A, Chelysheva V, et al. Comparative genome analysis of *Ureaplasma parvum* clinical isolates. *Res Microbiol*. 2007;158:371-378.
76. Gomez R, Ghezzi F, Romero R, et al. Premature labor and intra-amniotic infection. *Clin Perinatol*. 1995;22:281-342.
77. Yoon BH, Chang JW, Romero R. Isolation of *Ureaplasma urealyticum* from the amniotic cavity and adverse outcome in preterm labor. *Obstet Gynecol*. 1998;92:77-82.
78. Romero R, Yoon BH, Mazor M, et al. A comparative study of the diagnostic performance of amniotic fluid glucose, white blood cell count, interleukin-6, and Gram stain in the detection of microbial invasion in patients with preterm premature rupture of membranes. *Am J Obstet Gynecol*. 1993;169:839-851.
79. Hassan S, Romero R, Hendler I, et al. A sonographic short cervix as the only clinical manifestation of intra-amniotic infection. *J Perinat Med*. 2006;34:13-19.
80. Yoon BH, Romero R, Lim JH, et al. The clinical significance of detecting *Ureaplasma urealyticum* by the polymerase chain reaction in the amniotic fluid of patients with preterm labor. *Am J Obstet Gynecol*. 2003;189:919-924.
81. Kirchner L, Helmer H, Heinze G, et al. Amnionitis with *Ureaplasma urealyticum* or other microbes leads to increased morbidity and prolonged hospitalization in very low birth weight infants. *Eur J Obstet Gynecol Reprod Biol*. 2007;134:44-50.
82. Kundsin RB, Leviton A, Allred EN, et al. *Ureaplasma urealyticum* infection of the placenta in pregnancies that ended prematurely. *Obstet Gynecol*. 1996;87:122-127.
83. Dammann O, Allred EN, Genest DR, et al. Antenatal mycoplasma infection, the fetal inflammatory response and cerebral white matter damage in very-low-birthweight infants. *Paediatr Perinat Epidemiol*. 2003;17:49-57.
84. Gray DJ, Robinson HB, Malone J, et al. Adverse outcome in pregnancy following amniotic fluid isolation of *Ureaplasma urealyticum*. *Prenat Diagn*. 1992;12:111-117.
85. Horowitz S, Mazor M, Romero R, et al. Infection of the amniotic cavity with *Ureaplasma urealyticum* in the midtrimester of pregnancy. *J Reprod Med*. 1995;40:375-379.
86. Berg TG, Philpot KL, Welsh MS, et al. Ureaplasma/Mycoplasma-infected amniotic fluid: pregnancy outcome in treated and nontreated patients. *J Perinatol*. 1999;19:275-277.
87. Perni SC, Vardhana S, Korneeva I, et al. *Mycoplasma hominis* and *Ureaplasma urealyticum* in midtrimester amniotic fluid: association with amniotic fluid cytokine levels and pregnancy outcome. *Am J Obstet Gynecol*. 2004;191:1382-1386.
88. Witt A, Berger A, Gruber CJ, et al. Increased intrauterine frequency of *Ureaplasma urealyticum* in women with preterm labor and preterm premature rupture of the membranes and subsequent cesarean delivery. *Am J Obstet Gynecol*. 2005;193:1663-1669.
89. Namba F, Hasegawa T, Nakayama M, et al. Placental features of chorioamnionitis colonized with *Ureaplasma* species in preterm delivery. *Pediatr Res*. 2010;67:166-172.
90. Normann E, Lacaze-Masmonteil T, Eaton F, et al. A novel mouse model of *Ureaplasma*-induced perinatal inflammation: effects on lung and brain injury. *Pediatr Res*. 2009;65:430-436.
91. Moss TJ, Nitsos I, Ikegami M, et al. Experimental intrauterine *Ureaplasma* infection in sheep. *Am J Obstet Gynecol*. 2005;192:1179-1186.
92. Moss TJ, Knox CL, Kallapur SG, et al. Experimental amniotic fluid infection in sheep: effects of *Ureaplasma parvum* serovars 3 and 6 on preterm or term fetal sheep. *Am J Obstet Gynecol*. 2008;198:122 e121-e128.
93. Novy MJ, Duffy L, Axthelm MK, et al. *Ureaplasma parvum* or *Mycoplasma hominis* as sole pathogens cause chorioamnionitis, preterm delivery, and fetal pneumonia in rhesus macaques. *Reprod Sci*. 2009;16:56-70.
94. Yoon BH, Romero R, Chang JW, et al. Microbial invasion of the amniotic cavity with *Ureaplasma urealyticum* is associated with a robust host response in fetal, amniotic, and maternal compartments. *Am J Obstet Gynecol*. 1998;179:1254-1260.
95. Bashiri A, Horowitz S, Huleihel M, et al. Elevated concentrations of interleukin-6 in intra-amniotic infection with *Ureaplasma urealyticum* in asymptomatic women during genetic amniocentesis. *Acta Obstet Gynecol Scand*. 1999;78:379-382.
96. Estrada-Gutierrez G, Gomez-Lopez N, Zaga-Clavellina V, et al. Interaction between pathogenic bacteria and intrauterine leukocytes triggers alternative molecular signaling cascades leading to labor in women. *Infect Immun*. 2010;78:4792-4799.
97. Crouse DT, Odrezin GT, Cutter GR, et al. Radiographic changes associated with tracheal isolation of *Ureaplasma urealyticum* from neonates. *Clin Infect Dis*. 1993;17(suppl 1):S122-S130.
98. Panero A, Pacifico L, Roggini M, et al. *Ureaplasma urealyticum* as a cause of pneumonia in preterm infants: analysis of the white cell response. *Arch Dis Child*. 1995;73:F37-F40.
99. Wang EL, Ohlsson A, Kellner JD. Association of *Ureaplasma urealyticum* colonization with chronic lung disease of prematurity: Results of a metaanalysis. *J Pediatr*. 1995;127:640-644.
100. Castro-Alcaraz S, Greenberg EM, Bateman DA, et al. Patterns of colonization with *Ureaplasma urealyticum* during neonatal intensive care unit hospitalizations of very low birth weight infants and the development of chronic lung disease. *Pediatrics*. 2002;110:e45.
101. Schelonka RL, Katz B, Waites KB, et al. Critical appraisal of the role of *Ureaplasma* in the development of bronchopulmonary dysplasia with metaanalytic techniques. *Pediatr Infect Dis J*. 2005;24:1033-1039.

B

102. Theilen U, Lyon AJ, Fitzgerald T, et al. Infection with *Ureaplasma urealyticum*: is there a specific clinical and radiological course in the preterm infant? *Arch Dis Child Fetal Neonatal Ed.* 2004;89:F163-F167.
103. Pacifico L, Panero A, Roggini M, et al. *Ureaplasma urealyticum* and pulmonary outcome in a neonatal intensive care population. *Pediatr Infect Dis J.* 1997;16:579-586.
104. Honma Y, Yada Y, Takahashi N, et al. Certain type of chronic lung disease of newborns is associated with *Ureaplasma urealyticum* infection *in utero*. *Pediatr Int.* 2007;49:479-484.
105. Colaizy TT, Morris CD, Lapidus J, et al. Detection of ureaplasma DNA in endotracheal samples is associated with bronchopulmonary dysplasia after adjustment for multiple risk factors. *Pediatr Res.* 2007;61:578-583.
106. Patterson AM, Taciak V, Lovchik J, et al. *Ureaplasma urealyticum* respiratory tract colonization is associated with an increase in IL-1β and TNF-α relative to IL-6 in tracheal aspirates of preterm infants. *Pediatr Infect Dis J.* 1998;17:321-328.
107. Viscardi RM, Manimtim WM, Sun CCJ, et al. Lung pathology in premature infants with *Ureaplasma urealyticum* infection. *Pediatr Dev Pathol.* 2002;5:141-150.
108. Viscardi R, Manimtim W, He JR, et al. Disordered pulmonary myofibroblast distribution and elastin expression in preterm infants with *Ureaplasma urealyticum* pneumonitis. *Pediatr Dev Pathol.* 2006;9:143-151.
109. Viscardi RM, Atamas SP, Luzina IG, et al. Antenatal *Ureaplasma urealyticum* respiratory tract infection stimulates proinflammatory, profibrotic responses in the preterm baboon lung. *Pediatr Res.* 2006;60:141-146.
110. Groneck P, Goetze-Speer B, Speer CP. Inflammatory bronchopulmonary response of preterm infants with microbial colonisation of the airways at birth. *Arch Dis Child Fetal Neonatal Ed.* 1996;74: F51-F55.
111. Baier RJ, Loggins J, Kruger TE. Monocyte chemoattractant protein-1 and interleukin-8 are increased in bronchopulmonary dysplasia: relation to isolation of *Ureaplasma urealyticum*. *J Invest Med.* 2001;49:362-369.
112. Walsh WF, Butler J, Coalson J, et al. A primate model of *Ureaplasma urealyticum* infection in the premature infant with hyaline membrane disease. *Clin Infect Dis.* 1993;17(suppl 1):S158-S162.
113. Rudd PT, Cassell GH, Waites KB, et al. *Ureaplasma urealyticum* pneumonia: experimental production and demonstration of age-related susceptibility. *Infect Immun.* 1989;57:918-925.
114. Crouse DT, Cassell GH, Waites KB, et al. Hyperoxia potentiates *Ureaplasma urealyticum* pneumonia in newborn mice. *Infect Immun.* 1990;58:3487-3493.
115. Viscardi RM, Kaplan J, Lovchik JC, et al. Characterization of a murine model of *Ureaplasma urealyticum* pneumonia. *Infect Immun.* 2002;70:5721-5729.
116. Yoder BA, Coalson JJ, Winter VT, et al. Effects of antenatal colonization with *Ureaplasma urealyticum* on pulmonary disease in the immature baboon. *Pediatr Res.* 2003;54:797-807.
117. Collins JJ, Kallapur SG, Knox CL, et al. Inflammation in fetal sheep from intra-amniotic injection of *Ureaplasma parvum*. *Am J Physiol Lung Cell Mol Physiol.* 2010;299:L852-L860.
118. Polglase GR, Dalton RG, Nitsos I, et al. Pulmonary vascular and alveolar development in preterm lambs chronically colonized with *Ureaplasma parvum*. *Am J Physiol Lung Cell Mol Physiol.* 2010;299:L232-L241.
119. Li YH, Brauner A, Jonsson B et al. *Ureaplasma urealyticum*-induced production of proinflammatory cytokines by macrophages. *Pediatr Res.* 2000;48:114-119.
120. Li YH, Yan ZQ, Jensen JS, et al. Activation of nuclear factor kappaB and induction of inducible nitric oxide synthase by *Ureaplasma urealyticum* in macrophages. *Infect Immun.* 2000;68: 7087-7093.
121. Li YH, Brauner A, Jensen JS, et al. Induction of human macrophage vascular endothelial growth factor and intercellular adhesion molecule-1 by *Ureaplasma urealyticum* and downregulation by steroids. *Biol Neonate.* 2002;82:22-28.
122. Li YH, Chen M, Brauner A, et al. *Ureaplasma urealyticum* induces apoptosis in human lung epithelial cells and macrophages. *Biol Neonate.* 2002;82:166-173.
123. Manimtim WM, Hasday JD, Hester L, et al. *Ureaplasma urealyticum* modulates endotoxin-induced cytokine release by human monocytes derived from preterm and term newborns and adults. *Infect Immun.* 2001;69:3906-3915.
123a. Viscardi RM, Hasday JD. Role of *Ureaplasma* species in neonatal chronic lung disease: Epidemiologic and experimental evidence. *Pediatr Res.* 2009;65:84R-89R.
124. LeVine AM, Kurak KE, Bruno MD, et al. Surfactant protein-A-deficient mice are susceptible to *Pseudomonas aeruginosa* infection. *Am J Respir Cell Mol Biol.* 1998;19:700-708.
125. LeVine AM, Kurak KE, Wright JR, et al. Surfactant protein-A binds group B streptococcus enhancing phagocytosis and clearance from lungs of surfactant protein-A-deficient mice. *Am J Respir Cell Mol Biol.* 1999;20:279-286.
126. Famuyide ME, Hasday JD, Carter HC, et al. Surfactant protein-A limits *Ureaplasma*-mediated lung inflammation in a murine pneumonia model. *Pediatr Res.* 2009;66:162-167.
127. Okogbule-Wonodi AC, Chesko KL, Famuyide ME, et al. Surfactant protein-A enhances ureaplasmacidal activity in vitro. *Innate Immun.* 2010;17:145-151.
128. Kaisho T, Akira S. Pleiotropic function of Toll-like receptors. *Microbes Infect.* 2004;6:1388-1394.
129. Peltier MR, Freeman AJ, Mu HH, et al. Characterization of the macrophage-stimulating activity from *Ureaplasma urealyticum*. *Am J Reprod Immunol.* 2007;57:186-192.
130. Shimizu T, Kida Y, Kuwano K. *Ureaplasma parvum* lipoproteins, including MB antigen, activate NF-{kappa}B through TLR1, TLR2 and TLR6. *Microbiology.* 2008;154:1318-1325.

6

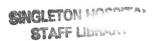

131. Harju K, Glumoff V, Hallman M. Ontogeny of Toll-like receptors Tlr2 and Tlr4 in mice. *Pediatr Res.* 2001;49:81-83.
132. Hillman NH, Moss TJ, Nitsos I, et al. Toll-like receptors and agonist responses in the developing fetal sheep lung. *Pediatr Res.* 2008;63:388-393.
133. Awasthi S, Cropper J, Brown KM. Developmental expression of Toll-like receptors-2 and -4 in preterm baboon lung. *Dev Comp Immunol.* 2008;32:1088-1098.
134. Robertson JA, Vekris A, Bebear C, et al. Polymerase chain reaction using 16S rRNA gene sequences distinguishes the two biovars of *Ureaplasma urealyticum*. *J Clin Microbiol.* 1993;31: 824-830.
135. Blanchard A, Hentschel J, Duffy L, et al. Detection of *Ureaplasma urealyticum* by polymerase chain reaction in the urogenital tract of adults, in amniotic fluid, and in the respiratory tract of newborns. *Clin Infect Dis.* 1993;17(suppl 1):S148-S153.
136. Kong F, Ma Z, James G, et al. Species identification and subtyping of *Ureaplasma parvum* and *Ureaplasma urealyticum* using PCR-based assays. *J Clin Microbiol.* 2000;38:1175-1179.
137. Yi J, Yoon BH, Kim EC. Detection and biovar discrimination of *Ureaplasma urealyticum* by real-time PCR. *Mol Cell Probes.* 2005;19:255-260.
138. Yoshida T, Ishiko H, Yasuda M, et al. Polymerase chain reaction-based subtyping of *Ureaplasma parvum* and *Ureaplasma urealyticum* in first-pass urine samples from men with or without urethritis. *Sex Transm Dis.* 2005;32:454-457.
139. Cao X, Jiang Z, Wang Y, et al. Two multiplex real-time TaqMan polymerase chain reaction systems for simultaneous detecting and serotyping of *Ureaplasma parvum*. *Diagn Microbiol Infect Dis.* 2007;59:109-111.
140. Cao X, Wang Y, Hu X, et al. Real-time TaqMan polymerase chain reaction assays for quantitative detection and differentiation of *Ureaplasma urealyticum* and *Ureaplasma parvum*. *Diagn Microbiol Infect Dis.* 2007;57:373-378.
141. Renaudin H, Bebear C. Comparative in vitro activity of azithromycin, clarithromycin, erythromycin and lomefloxacin against *Mycoplasma pneumoniae, Mycoplasma hominis* and *Ureaplasma urealyticum*. *Eur J Clin Microbiol Infect Dis.* 1990;9:838-841.
142. Bowman ED, Dharmalingam A, Fan WQ, et al. Impact of erythromycin on respiratory colonization of *Ureaplasma urealyticum* and the development of chronic lung disease in extremely low birth weight infants. *Pediatr Infect Dis J.* 1998;17:615-620.
143. Jonsson B, Rylander M, Faxelius G. *Ureaplasma urealyticum*, erythromycin and respiratory morbidity in high-risk preterm neonates. *Acta Paediatr.* 1998;87:1079-1084.
144. Baier RJ, Loggins J, Kruger TE. Failure of erythromycin to eliminate airway colonization with ureaplasma urealyticum in very low birth weight infants. *BMC Pediatr.* 2003;3:10.
145. Rubin BK. Macrolides as biologic response modifiers. *J Respir Dis.* 2002;23:S31-S38.
146. Ianaro A, Ialenti A, Maffia P, et al. Anti-inflammatory activity of macrolide antibiotics. *J Pharmacol Exp Ther.* 2000;292:156-163.
147. Tsai WC, Standiford TJ. Immunomodulatory effects of macrolides in the lung: lessons from in-vitro and in-vivo models. *Curr Pharm Des.* 2004;10:3081-3093.
148. Duffy LB, Crabb D, Searcey K, et al. Comparative potency of gemifloxacin, new quinolones, macrolides, tetracycline and clindamycin against Mycoplasma spp. *J Antimicrob Chemother.* 2000;45(suppl 1):29-33.
149. Girard AE, Cimochowski CR, Faiella JA. Correlation of increased azithromycin concentrations with phagocyte infiltration into sites of localized infection. *J Antimicrob Chemother.* 1996;37(suppl C): 9-19.
150. Patel KB, Xuan D, Tessier PR, et al. Comparison of bronchopulmonary pharmacokinetics of clarithromycin and azithromycin. *Antimicrob Agents Chemother.* 1996;40:2375-2379.
151. Capitano B, Mattoes HM, Shore E, et al. Steady-state intrapulmonary concentrations of moxifloxacin, levofloxacin, and azithromycin in older adults. *Chest.* 2004;125:965-973.
152. Auten RL, Ekekezie II. Blocking leukocyte influx and function to prevent chronic lung disease of prematurity. *Pediatr Pulmonol.* 2003;35:335-341.
153. Liao L, Ning Q, Li Y, et al. CXCR2 blockade reduces radical formation in hyperoxia-exposed newborn rat lung. *Pediatr Res.* 2006;60:299-303.
154. Walls SA, Kong L, Leeming HA, et al. Antibiotic prophylaxis improves *Ureaplasma*-associated lung disease in suckling mice. *Pediatr Res.* 2009;66:197-202.
155. Hassan HE, Othman AA, Eddington ND, et al. Pharmacokinetics, safety, and biologic effects of azithromycin in extremely preterm infants at risk for *Ureaplasma* colonization and bronchopulmonary dysplasia. *J Clin Pharmacol.* 2010;51:1264-1275.
156. Sollecito D, Midulla M, Bavastrelli M, et al. *Chlamydia trachomatis* in neonatal respiratory distress of very preterm babies: biphasic clinical picture. *Acta Paediatr.* 1992;81:788-791.
157. Numazaki K, Chiba S, Kogawa K, et al. Chronic respiratory disease in premature infants caused by *Chlamydia trachomatis*. *J Clin Pathol.* 1986;39:84-88.
158. Wang EE, Frayha H, Watts J, et al. Role of *Ureaplasma urealyticum* and other pathogens in the development of chronic lung disease of prematurity. *Pediatr Infect Dis J.* 1988;7:547-551.
159. Garland SM, Bowman ED. Role of *Ureaplasma urealyticum* and *Chlamydia trachomatis* in lung disease in low birth weight infants. *Pathology.* 1996;28:266-269.
160. Da Silva O, Gregson D, Hammerberg O. Role of *Ureaplasma urealyticum* and *Chlamydia trachomatis* in development of bronchopulmonary dysplasia in very low birth weight infants. *Pediatr Infect Dis J.* 1997;16:364-369.

B

161. Couroucli XI, Welty SE, Ramsay PL, et al. Detection of microorganisms in the tracheal aspirates of preterm infants by polymerase chain reaction: association of adenovirus infection with bronchopulmonary dysplasia. *Pediatr Res*. 2000;47:225-232.
162. Duke T. Neonatal pneumonia in developing countries. *Arch Dis Child Fetal Neonatal Ed*. 2005;90:F211-F219.
163. Sun CC, Duara S. Fatal adenovirus pneumonia in two newborn infants, one case caused by adenovirus type 30. *Pediatr Pathol*. 1985;4:247-255.
164. Montone KT, Furth EE, Pietra GG, et al. Neonatal adenovirus infection: a case report with in situ hybridization confirmation of ascending intrauterine infection. *Diagn Cytopathol*. 1995;12: 341-344.
165. Sawyer MH, Edwards DK, Spector SA. Cytomegalovirus infection and bronchopulmonary dysplasia in premature infants. *Am J Dis Child*. 1987;141:303-305.
166. Apisarnthanarak A, Holzmann-Pazgal G, Hamvas A, et al. Ventilator-associated pneumonia in extremely preterm neonates in a neonatal intensive care unit: characteristics, risk factors, and outcomes. *Pediatrics*. 2003;112:1283-1289.
167. Safdar N, Dezfulian C, Collard HR, et al. Clinical and economic consequences of ventilator-associated pneumonia: a systematic review. *Crit Care Med*. 2005;33:2184-2193.
168. Sohn AH, Garrett DO, Sinkowitz-Cochran RL, et al. Prevalence of nosocomial infections in neonatal intensive care unit patients: Results from the first national point-prevalence survey. *J Pediatr*. 2001;139:821-827.
169. Foglia E, Meier MD, Elward A. Ventilator-associated pneumonia in neonatal and pediatric intensive care unit patients. *Clin Microbiol Rev*. 2007;20:409-425.
170. Garland JS, Uhing MR. Strategies to prevent bacterial and fungal infection in the neonatal intensive care unit. *Clin Perinatol*. 2009;36:1-13.
171. Langley JM, Bradley JS. Defining pneumonia in critically ill infants and children. *Pediatr Crit Care Med*. 2005;6:S9-S13.
172. Bradley JS. Considerations unique to pediatrics for clinical trial design in hospital-acquired pneumonia and ventilator-associated pneumonia. *Clin Infect Dis*. 2010;51(suppl 1):S136-S143.
173. Koksal N, Hacimustafaoglul M, Celebi S, et al. Nonbronchoscopic bronchoalveolar lavage for diagnosing ventilator-associated pneumonia in newborns. *Turk J Pediatr*. 2006;48:213-220.
174. Cordero L, Sananes M, Dedhiya P, et al. Purulence and gram-negative bacilli in tracheal aspirates of mechanically ventilated very low birth weight infants. *J Perinatol*. 2001;21:376-381.
175. Katayama Y, Minami H, Enomoto M, et al. Usefulness of Gram staining of tracheal aspirates in initial therapy for ventilator-associated pneumonia in extremely preterm neonates. *J Perinatol*. 2010;30:270-274.
176. Cordero L, Ayers LW, Miller RR, et al. Surveillance of ventilator-associated pneumonia in very-low-birth-weight infants. *Am J Infect Control*. 2002;30:32-39.
177. Yuan TM, Chen LH, Yu HM. Risk factors and outcomes for ventilator-associated pneumonia in neonatal intensive care unit patients. *J Perinat Med*. 2007;35:334-338.
178. Edwards JR, Peterson KD, Andrus ML, et al. National Healthcare Safety Network (NHSN) Report, data summary for 2006 through 2007, issued November 2008. *Am J Infect Control*. 2008;36:609-626.
179. Stover BH, Shulman ST, Bratcher DF, et al. Nosocomial infection rates in US children's hospitals' neonatal and pediatric intensive care units. *Am J Infect Control*. 2001;29:152-157.
180. Da Silva PS, Neto HM, de Aguiar VE, et al. Impact of sustained neuromuscular blockade on outcome of mechanically ventilated children. *Pediatr Int*. 2010;52:438-443.
181. Webber S, Wilkinson AR, Lindsell D, et al. Neonatal pneumonia. *Arch Dis Child*. 1990;65:207-211.
182. Yee-Guardino S, Kumar D, Abughali N, et al. Recognition and treatment of neonatal community-associated MRSA pneumonia and bacteremia. *Pediatr Pulmonol*. 2008;43:203-205.
183. Garland JS. Strategies to prevent ventilator-associated pneumonia in neonates. *Clin Perinatol*. 2010;37:629-643.
184. Aly H, Badawy M, El-Kholy A, et al. Randomized, controlled trial on tracheal colonization of ventilated infants: can gravity prevent ventilator-associated pneumonia? *Pediatrics*. 2008;122: 770-774.
185. Farhath S, He Z, Nakhla T, et al. Pepsin, a marker of gastric contents, is increased in tracheal aspirates from preterm infants who develop bronchopulmonary dysplasia. *Pediatrics*. 2008;121: e253-259.
186. Graham PL 3rd, Begg MD, Larson E, et al. Risk factors for late onset gram-negative sepsis in low birth weight infants hospitalized in the neonatal intensive care unit. *Pediatr Infect Dis J*. 2006;25: 113-117.
187. Guillet R, Stoll BJ, Cotten CM, et al. Association of H2-blocker therapy and higher incidence of necrotizing enterocolitis in very low birth weight infants. *Pediatrics*. 2006;117:e137-e142.
188. Won SP, Chou HC, Hsieh WS, et al. Handwashing program for the prevention of nosocomial infections in a neonatal intensive care unit. *Infect Control Hosp Epidemiol*. 2004;25:742-746.
189. Rogers E, Alderdice F, McCall E, et al. Reducing nosocomial infections in neonatal intensive care. *J Matern Fetal Neonatal Med*. 2010;23:1039-1046.
190. Cordero L, Sananes M, Coley B, et al. Ventilator-associated pneumonia in very low-birth-weight infants at the time of nosocomial bloodstream infection and during airway colonization with *Pseudomonas aeruginosa*. *Am J Infect Control*. 2000;28:333-339.

191. Cordero L, Ayers L, Davis K. Neonatal airway colonization with Gram-negative bacilli: association with severity of bronchopulmonary dysplasia. *Pediatr Infect Dis J*. 1997;16:18-23.
192. Hentschel J, Brungger B, Studi K, et al. Prospective surveillance of nosocomial infections in a Swiss NICU: low risk of pneumonia on nasal continuous positive airway pressure? *Infection*. 2005;33:350-355.
193. Holleman-Duray D, Kaupie D, Weiss MG. Heated humidified high-flow nasal cannula: use and a neonatal early extubation protocol. *J Perinatol*. 2007;27:776-781.
194. Greenough A. Long-term pulmonary outcome in the preterm infant. *Neonatology*. 2008;93: 324-327.
195. Doyle LW, Anderson PJ. Adult outcome of extremely preterm infants. *Pediatrics*. 2010;126: 342-351.
196. Jaakkola JJ, Ahmed P, Ieromnimon A, et al. Preterm delivery and asthma: a systematic review and meta-analysis. *J Allergy Clin Immunol*. 2006;118:823-830.
197. Gessner BD, Chimonas MA. Asthma is associated with preterm birth but not with small for gestational age status among a population-based cohort of Medicaid-enrolled children <10 years of age. *Thorax*. 2007;62:231-236.
198. Getahun D, Strickland D, Zeiger RS, et al. Effect of chorioamnionitis on early childhood asthma. *Arch Pediatr Adolesc Med*. 2010;164:187-192.
199. Kumar R, Yu Y, Story RE, et al. Prematurity, chorioamnionitis, and the development of recurrent wheezing: a prospective birth cohort study. *J Allergy Clin Immunol*. 2008;121:878-884.e6.
200. Pinna GS, Skevaki CL, Kafetzis DA. The significance of *Ureaplasma urealyticum* as a pathogenic agent in the paediatric population. *Curr Opin Infect Dis*. 2006;19:283-289.
201. Benn CS, Thorsen P, Jensen JS, et al. Maternal vaginal microflora during pregnancy and the risk of asthma hospitalization and use of antiasthma medication in early childhood. *J Allergy Clin Immunol*. 2002;110:72-77.
202. Ohlsson A, Wang E, Vearncombe M. Leukocyte counts and colonization with *Ureaplasma urealyticum* in preterm neonates. *Clin Infect Dis*. 1993;17(suppl 1):S144-S147.

B

CHAPTER 7

Influence of Nutrition on Neonatal Respiratory Outcomes

Cristina T. Navarrete, MD, and Ilene R.S. Sosenko, MD

7

- **Preterm Infant Nutrition**
- **Growth Failure, Undernutrition, and Pulmonary Consequences**
- **Adequate Nutrition to Support Lung Growth and Function: How Specific Nutrients May Influence Pulmonary Outcome**
- **Conclusion**

The process of providing nutrients to maintain homeostasis in a premature infant, allowing similar in utero growth rates and body composition to continue, is complicated and not easily achieved in the clinical setting. The hurdles that are inherent to prematurity and that are ingrained in current clinical practices need to be surmounted.[1] Foremost is the inability of the premature infant to benefit from the late-gestation accumulation of fuel stores in the form of glycogen and adipose tissue. This absence of any rapidly mobilizable energy stores makes the establishment of proper nutrient intake after preterm birth an urgent matter. Second, the immaturity of the infant's metabolic capabilities produces many instances of intolerance to different nutritional regimens. The neonate's inability to immediately use the gastrointestinal tract mandates the use of parenteral nutrition with its numerous limitations and complications. Third, the presence of acute clinical instability often downgrades the importance of nutritional needs. The volumes of parenteral nutrition solutions are often displaced by increasing amounts of medication drips in critically ill infants. Last, the clinician's misconceptions about and inattention to nutrition may hinder the consistent delivery of adequate nutrients. The widespread misperception that the infant can sustain metabolic function despite suboptimal nutrient delivery and concerns about parenteral nutrition toxicities mistakenly "justify" delayed initiation and the slow progression of nutrition practices.

Suboptimal nutrient delivery compromises the function of all organ systems and affects growth negatively. The respiratory system is no exception. Undernutrition has detrimental effects on lung growth and function, and its presence may be a further disadvantage to the already metabolically compromised premature infant. Preterm infant respiratory conditions may be ameliorated by the provision of enough nutrients to support the processes of ventilation, lung growth, and repair, antioxidant defenses, and the ability to ward off infections. The improved survival and extension of neonatal care to lower gestational ages,[2] during the period when the most rapid phase of growth occurs, highlight the emergence of the relatively new morbidity called *postnatal growth retardation*[3] (also called extrauterine growth restriction[4]). Progressively more preterm infants are being discharged from the neonatal intensive care unit with anthropometric measures below the 10th percentile, and increasingly, relationships among nutrition, early growth patterns, various morbidities, and longevity are being defined.

Pulmonary morbidity in the form of bronchopulmonary dysplasia (BPD), also called chronic lung disease (CLD), is another major complication in the preterm infant population. Although the epidemiology and degree of severity of this condition have changed over the years,[5] the incidence remains the same owing to the rising numbers of very preterm births.[2,6,7] Among very low-birth-weight (VLBW; <1500 g) infants, who are at greatest risk for this disease, published reports state an incidence anywhere from 3% to as much as 60%[2,5,8] in various centers, with a wide variability because of differing definitions of diagnostic criteria and diverse postnatal management styles. In addition, patient susceptibility contributes to this wide variability. It is known that the risk rises with decreasing gestational age at birth,[2,5] although why some preterm infants are capable of easy adaptation to early birth and survive without complications, and others do not, is still unknown. In particular, we do not understand why some preterm infants of similar low gestational age require prolonged periods of ventilator support and oxygen supplementation but others require very little support, if any.

It is assumed that the growth and development of the respiratory system are largely programmed in utero and are interrupted by preterm birth. Increasingly, BPD is being demonstrated histopathologically as a failure or disorder in the alveolarization process,[9,10] the stage in lung development that occurs in the last part of gestation and extends to the first years of life. Although multiple prenatal and postnatal factors influence lung growth and alveolar development,[11] some of them (e.g., adequate nutritional intake) are conveniently under the control of the medical professional. This chapter discusses different nutritional approaches that may positively or negatively influence respiratory outcomes.

Preterm Infant Nutrition

The objective of human gestation is to produce viability at birth. This objective is supported by the highly regulated active and facilitated transfer of nutrients from the mother through the placenta to the fetus for promotion of programmed growth and development. Because the rates of fetal nutrient transfer and consequent fetal growth for normal pregnancies are regarded as ideal, the current goal for optimal postnatal nutrition is the provision of nutrients to approximate the rate of growth and composition of weight gain for a normal fetus of the same postmenstrual age.[12]

It is widely known that fetal nutrient transfer is not easily duplicated ex utero[13] and that metabolic demands are very different in the postnatal state. Thus, some experts believe that the standard of aiming for intrauterine growth rates may not be appropriate.[14] Fetal nutrient accretion is divided mostly between the energy costs of basal metabolism and growth of the fetus, but after birth, the infant has to allocate both exogenous nutrient supply and endogenous nutrient reserves for energy that is essential to cover not just the higher basal metabolic needs but also activity, thermogenesis, excretory losses, and, if present, the stress of illness (e.g., respiratory failure, sepsis). With the interruption of placental nutrient supply at birth, the premature infant is further disadvantaged by having limited endogenous energy reserves that are normally accumulated during the final trimester of gestation. From the seminal chemical analysis of fetuses by Widdowson, it is extrapolated that although approximately 15% of the body weight of a full-term infant is represented by fat and about 2% is glycogen reserves, a 24-week preterm infant has only 1.7% fat by weight and an unmeasurable glycogen reserve.[15] Hence, this lack of energy reserve makes it vital to establish immediate postnatal nutritional intake or risk the onset of "metabolic" shock and recalcitrant nutrient deficits.[13] Thureen and Hay[16] aptly declared that "the nutritional requirements of the preterm infant do not end with birth." However, because of the perceived illness severity of these infants, nutritional needs are not always a high priority for clinicians.[14,17]

Recommendations for preterm infant nutrition continue to evolve as perinatal care extends to lower gestational ages. In 1985 the American Academy of Pediatrics Committee on Nutrition produced recommendations for low-birth-weight (LBW; <2500 g) infant nutrition,[18] which was modified in 1999 by a National Institute of Child Health and Human Development workshop to extend the recommendations to the nutritional needs of the extremely low-birth-weight (ELBW; <1000 g) infant (Table 7-1).[19] Because most of these recommendations are based on "healthy"

Table 7-1 SELECTED SUGGESTED RECOMMENDATIONS FOR DAILY NUTRIENT INTAKES FOR EXTREMELY LOW-BIRTH-WEIGHT INFANTS (<1000 g) PRETERM INFANTS*

	Transitional Phase		Stable and Growing Phase		
Source	Parenteral	Enteral	Parenteral	Enteral	Comments
Energy (kcal/kg/day)	35-90	110-120	105-115	130-150	
Water (mL/kg/day)	80-140	80-140	120-150	150-200	
Carbohydrate: Glucose (mg/kg/min)	5-7 mg/kg/min initially, to progress to 10-11 mg/kg/min[16]		5-7 mg/kg/min initially, to progress to 10-11 mg/kg/min[16]		Plasma glucose target >60 and <120 mg/dL[16]
Carbohydrate (g/kg/day)	6-12	3.8-11.2	13-17	9-20	
Protein: amino acids (g/kg/day)	3-4	3.6-3.8	3.5-4	3.8-4.4	
Fat: Lipids (g/kg/day)	0.5-1, up to 3[16]	unspecified	3-4	6.2-8.4	Maintain serum triglyceride levels <150 to 250 mg/dL
Vitamin A (IU)	700-1500	700-1500	700-1500	700-1500	BPD prophylaxis: 5,000 IU IM 3×/wk for 4 wks for ventilated extremely low-birth-weight infants[114]
Vitamin D (IU)	40-160	150-400	40-160	150-400	
Vitamin E (IU)	3.5	6-12	2.8-3.5	6-12[121]	Maximum enteral 25 IU
Vitamin C (mg/kg/day)	15-25	18-24	15-25	18-24	
Calcium (mg/kg/day)	60-90	120-230	60-80[116]	100-220	
Phosphorus (mg/kg/day)	47-70	60-140	45-60	60-140	
Zinc (µg/kg/day)	150	500-800	400	1000-3000	
Selenium (µg/kg/day)	0, 1.3	1.3	1.5-4.5	1.3-4.5	Up to 7 µg/kg/day to approximate levels in breastfed infants[126]
Copper (µg/kg/day)	0, 20	120	20	120-150	
Manganese (µg/kg/day)	0, 0.75	0.75	1	0.7-7.75	

*Superscript numbers indicate chapter references.
Adapted from Kleinman RE, editor; AAP Committee on Nutrition. *Pediatric Nutrition Handbook*. 6th ed. Elk Grove Village, IL: American Academy of Pediatrics; 2009; and Appendix. In: Tsang RC, Uauy R, Koletzko B, Zlotkin SH, eds. *Nutrition of the Preterm Infant: Scientific Basis and Practical Guidelines*. 2nd ed. Cincinnati, OH: Digital Education Publishing; 2005:417-418.

preterm infants and designed to provide nutrients during the stable growing period, there is no clear recommendation for the nutritional support of the more immature, clinically unstable preterm infant. Until recently, these infants at birth were kept predominantly without enteral intake and started on an intravenous supply of low-volume plain dextrose in water or fluids containing very small amounts of dextrose, protein, and lipids that were gradually increased over the first weeks of life. The proportions of the macronutrients delivered contrast with those in normal fetal nutrient delivery (high glucose and lipid, and low amino acid).[16] Different investigators have suggested that the current nutritional recommendations and practices inevitably produce negative energy and protein balance and poor postnatal growth[13,14]; as mentioned previously, this new condition in preterm infants is called postnatal growth retardation[3] and extrauterine growth restriction (EUGR).[4] However, other researchers have reported that merely ensuring the provision of early nutrition, protein, and calories at current recommendations to VLBW infants would prevent the acquisition of early nutrient deficits and would consequently improve postnatal growth.[20,21] Early and "aggressive" (above current recommendations) nutritional strategies are increasingly being given top priority.[22,23]

B

Undernutrition, Growth Failure, and Pulmonary Consequences

Extrauterine growth restriction is defined as growth values less than or equal to the 10th percentile of intrauterine growth expectation based on estimated postmenstrual age in premature neonates at the time of hospital discharge.[4] The incidence of postnatal growth failure in VLBW infants ranges between 43% and 97%[2,4,8] in various centers, with a wide variability due to the use of different reference growth charts and nonstandard nutritional strategies. Growth failure in VLBW infants results from the complex interaction of many factors, including morbidities affecting nutrient requirements, endocrine abnormalities, central nervous system damage, difficulties in suck and swallow coordination, and administration of drugs that affect nutrient metabolism,[24] but inadequate nutrition (≈45%), especially during the first weeks of life, is largely responsible.[13] The consequences of EUGR are not fully known, in large part because it is difficult to separate the effects of the many other concurrent problems of prematurity (e.g., necrotizing enterocolitis, BPD, intracranial hemorrhage).[25]

Malnutrition (or undernutrition), as defined by the World Health Organization, is the cellular imbalance between supply of nutrients and energy and the body's demand to ensure growth, maintenance, and specific functions.[26] Malnutrition can be a consequence of either inadequate or excessive nutrient quantity and/or quality. Globally, malnutrition is recognized to have profound effects primarily on somatic growth and on functional development of the brain. In the premature infant population, analysis of growth velocities during the initial neonatal intensive care unit (NICU) hospitalization of VLBW infants shows that after data are controlled for possible confounders (such as small for gestational age, BPD, intraventricular hemorrhage, sepsis, and postnatal steroid exposure), poor rates of weight gain (presumably from suboptimal nutrition) exert a significant and independent effect on neurodevelopmental outcomes (cerebral palsy and developmental indices) at 18 to 22 months corrected age.[14,27]

The effects of malnutrition, however, are not limited to the brain. It can affect the entire body, and its consequences for the respiratory system are substantial. In the developing VLBW infant, the potential pulmonary effects of undernutrition are numerous (Table 7-2).[28]

Effect of Undernutrition on Lung Growth and Development

Growth, particularly weight gain, is traditionally the preferred means of assessing adequacy of nutritional support. To match intrauterine growth, a postnatal weight gain of 15 to 20 g/kg/day is conventionally accepted for the premature infant. The ultimate goal of adequate preterm infant weight gain is the body composition of a

Table 7-2 POTENTIAL PULMONARY EFFECTS OF UNDERNUTRITION IN VLBW INFANTS

Lung growth and development	Decreased lung biosynthesis, decreased surface area Alveolar loss or "nutritional" emphysema
Respiratory muscle function	Diaphragm and other respiratory muscle fatigue
Lung function	Fewer structural proteins in extracellular matrix Altered surfactant production Decreased stability of chest wall
Protection from hyperoxia	Decreased antioxidant defense systems (glutathione, vitamin E, vitamin C, polyunsaturated fatty acids)
Infection susceptibility	Decreased cellular and humoral defenses
Alveolar fluid balance	Decreased plasma oncotic pressure Diminished alveolar fluid clearance
Control of breathing	Diminished response to hypoxia

Modified from Thureen P, Hay W: Conditions requiring special nutritional management. In Tsang RC, Uauy R, Koletzko B, Zlotkin S, editors. Nutrition of the Preterm Infant: Scientific Basis and Practical Guidelines, 2nd ed. Cincinnati, OH, Digital Educational Publishing, 2005, pp 383-411.

7

healthy term infant with proper distribution of lean body mass and fat mass. Growth of this metabolically active body mass (lean body mass component) needs an appropriate lung surface area to meet its needs for gas exchange. In humans, this is accomplished for lung growth by an increase in lung surface area, initially in terms of a rise in the number of alveoli until early childhood[29,30] and later by an increase in alveolar size/dimension.

Different fetal and postnatal animal models of undernutrition consistently affect both somatic and lung growth.[31] Undernutrition in fetal sheep[32] and in mature and immature mice,[33,34] rats,[33,35,36] and rabbits[37] as well as starvation in adult humans[38] cause alveolar loss or enlargement, also called "nutritional" emphysema. This presentation of "nutritional" emphysema has similarities to the alveolar simplification seen in BPD. Slow postnatal growth rates in preterm sheep also result in lower alveolar numbers and reduced surface area for gas exchange in relation to lung or body weight, and this pattern persists into maturity.[39] In preterm humans, the presence of fetal growth restriction independently raises the risk for CLD,[40] with VLBW infants growing at the lowest quartiles having BPD more often than infants growing at the highest growth quartile.[27] Because EUGR may be analogous to intrauterine or fetal growth restriction, it is conceivable that EUGR per se may also raise the risk for BPD. The pathogenesis of BPD is multifactorial, but it is plausible that inadequate energy secondary to undernutrition can limit the occurrence of biochemical and molecular events necessary for vital lung cell signaling, cell multiplication, differentiation, and growth, and extracellular matrix structural protein deposition. This possibility may explain the occurrence of BPD in some preterm infants who were minimally exposed to BPD-promoting factors such as oxygen, mechanical ventilation, and infection/inflammation.[41,42]

As an alternative to the hypothesis that undernourishment leads to the development of an emphysema-like condition, the lung's response to caloric restriction could reflect an evolutionarily conserved adaptation to diminished oxygen consumption during food scarcity.[38,43] Whereas established BPD is associated with poor somatic growth,[44,45] this poor growth may be merely a marker of disease severity, because infants who ultimately demonstrate BPD are sicker and likely more undernourished initially.[14] Conversely, poor growth could be secondary to BPD per se, producing higher metabolic needs from increased work of breathing[46] and from episodes of hypoxemia that may be growth limiting.[47] If lung growth and surface area are limited, the systemic provision of adequate levels of oxygen may be diminished, perpetuating the limitation of growth even further.

Effect of Undernutrition on Respiratory Muscle Function

The energy source of muscle is either glycogen or fatty acids (FAs), from intrinsic stores or from circulating fuels like glucose and free FAs, which are broken down to produce adenosine triphosphate (ATP). The diaphragm is the major muscle of respiration, utilizing 10% of basal metabolic rate in "healthy" preterm infants.[48] When energy supply is limited, muscle contractility may be compromised, leading to ineffective activity or, in the case of the diaphragm muscle, respiratory failure. In undernourished adult patients without lung disease, respiratory muscle strength, maximum voluntary ventilation, and vital capacity are reduced.[49] Undernutrition causes a decrease in diaphragm strength and endurance partially related to a loss of muscle mass.[49-51] In addition, two studies in rats found that undernutrition induces a significant decrease in mitochondrial oxygen consumption[52] and that a reduction in muscle insulin-like growth factor-1 (IGF-I) expression is associated with muscle fiber atrophy.[53] Branched-chain amino acids have been shown to improve diaphragm function in vitro, and when parenteral protein solutions were enriched with branched-chain amino acids, apnea events in preterm infants were decreased.[54]

Mechanical ventilation has been the basis of the respiratory care of the premature infant, and prolonged dependence is associated with disuse atrophy of the diaphragm. Allowing infants to breathe spontaneously with minimal, noninvasive support in the form of continuous positive airway pressure (CPAP), however, is evolving as the preferred mode in select preterm infants (e.g., with good ventilatory drive).[2,55] CPAP alters the shape of the diaphragm and increases its activity.[56] Hence, the provision of adequate energy substrate to sustain diaphragm and other respiratory muscle function may be more important than ever.

Effect of Undernutrition on Lung Function

The extracellular matrix of the lung, composed mainly of collagen and elastin fibers, provides the template for normal parenchymal cell architecture on which efficient gas exchange depends. In addition, the organization and amount of this extracellular matrix account for much of the mechanical behavior of the lung parenchyma (tensile strength and lung elasticity) during the respiratory cycle. During lung growth, deposition of newly created connective tissue in this scaffold is essential. The preservation of this intricate connective tissue scaffold depends on the lung's capacity to prevent enzymatic disruption of the component matrix proteins. Specifically, the integrity of the normal connective tissue skeleton of the lung is determined by the maintenance of a balance between proteases (released by inflammatory cells) capable of cleaving these structural elements (e.g., matrix metalloproteinases) and specific protease inhibitors (e.g., tissue inhibitors of metalloproteinases).[57] The breakdown of connective tissue fibers leads to emphysema, and the same connective tissue fibers are affected by undernutrition. In a young rat starvation model, hydroxyproline (a collagen biomarker) and elastin levels in the lung were found to be reduced, with associated loss of tissue elastic forces evident in pressure-volume curves.[51,58]

In addition to the connective tissue skeleton that contributes to lung function, surfactant is a very important contributor. Surfactant decreases surface tension at the air-liquid interface in the alveoli, provides lung stability (promotes expansion at inspiration and prevents collapse at expiration), and reduces the risk of infection. It contains about 80% phospholipids, 8% neutral lipids, and 12% protein.[59] The principal classes of phospholipids are saturated and unsaturated phosphatidylcholine compounds, phosphatidylglycerol, and phosphatidylinositol. FA moieties of the phospholipids may be derived from circulating long-chain free FAs or through de novo synthesis from glucose.[60] Different experimental animal models of undernutrition showed reduced numbers of lamellar bodies, multilamellated structures, and lipid vacuoles in type II pneumocytes[51] and decreased dipalmitoyl phosphatidylcholine content of lung lavage fluid[61] and the lung phospholipid pool.[62] Despite the reduction in surfactant components, changes in lung mechanics were insignificant.

The rigid thoracic cage contains the lungs and together with the muscles of respiration creates the negative pressure and elastic recoil necessary for ventilation.

Inadequate ossification of the bony skeleton, including the thoracic cage, is common after preterm birth. An easily distorted and compliant chest wall in combination with a poorly compliant lung parenchyma in association with significant lung disease sets the infant up for inefficient ventilation.[63] Normal bone calcium deposition and consequent improved rigidity is frequently impaired with the onset of metabolic bone disease (osteopenia or, in its advanced stage, rickets) of prematurity. Metabolic bone disease is a frequent complication of preterm birth secondary to inadequate prenatal accretion and then inadequate provision of calcium and phosphorus in postnatal nutrition along with exposure to calcium-wasting medications like furosemide and glucocorticoids.[64] Complicating rib fractures in advanced rickets make breathing efforts even more inefficient,[65] increasing the risk for respiratory failure and prolonged ventilator dependence.

Effect of Undernutrition on the Antioxidant System

The balance between the production of reactive oxygen species (ROS) and the antioxidant defense system is important for homeostasis. Developmentally, the increases in various antioxidant enzymes and antioxidants (e.g., Cu-Zn–superoxide dismutase [SOD], Mn-SOD, and vitamins E and C) occur late in gestation to prepare the infant for birth and exposure to the oxygen-rich environment ex utero.[66] The underdevelopment of both enzymatic and nonenzymatic (from interrupted maternal transfer) antioxidant defense systems in preterm infants tips the balance towards increased ROS, producing oxidant stress that is aggravated further by frequent exposure to ROS-generating conditions such as hyperoxia and inflammation.

The provision of supplemental oxygen continues to be an integral part of neonatal care, although its use has become more judicious because of its association with oxygen toxicity and morbidities such as retinopathy of prematurity (ROP) and BPD.[5,10] BPD is considered among the oxygen radical diseases of the newborn. Lungs of infants with respiratory disorders have reduced staining for Cu-Zn–SOD.[66] High concentrations of oxygen induce lung inflammation, which may lead to chronic fibrotic and destructive changes, as the production of ROS and release of chemotactic factors lead to release of inflammatory mediators and proteolytic enzymes. In adult animal models of hyperoxia, fasting increased susceptibility to hyperoxic injury. Fasted mice had decreased lung concentrations of the tripeptide antioxidant glutathione,[67] of which cysteine, glutamate, and glycine are precursors. In newborn rat pups, the presence of undernutrition during hyperoxic exposure had an additive detrimental effect on somatic and lung growth and lethality (56% of the undernourished pups died in O_2, compared with 27% of the normally nourished pups).[31] Although elevations in antioxidant enzyme values were demonstrated in this study, it is speculated that protection from O_2–free radical toxicity is a complex phenomenon and that other vital factors (in addition to the endogenous antioxidant enzyme systems) are required to provide optimal protection against the detrimental effects of prolonged O_2 treatment.

Effect of Undernutrition on Infection Susceptibility

Undernutrition is known to alter pulmonary defense mechanisms, compromising epithelial cell integrity and clearance mechanisms, allowing easier access by pathogens, and jeopardizing cellular and humoral immune function, and thereby decreasing the ability of the host to eliminate pathogens. Thus, undernutrition predisposes to infections. Globally, undernourished children frequently succumb to repeated upper[68] and lower[69] respiratory tract infections. Animal models of malnutrition have also demonstrated decreased alveolar macrophage count,[70] phagocytosis, and microbial killing.[71] Newborn rats deprived of adequate protein antenatally were found to develop reduced alveolar macrophage function, which could be reversed by postnatal protein supplementation.[72]

Individual components of surfactant, specifically surfactant proteins A and D, have important roles in the innate immune response and in defense against microbes.[73] As already mentioned, undernutrition has an effect on surfactant, although whether it has any specific impact on surfactant proteins is unknown.

Effect of Undernutrition on Alveolar Fluid Balance

Pulmonary edema is due to the movement of excess fluid into the interstitial or alveolar space as a result of the alteration in one or more of Starling's forces, a change either in hydrostatic or oncotic pressure gradients or in membrane permeability. In experimental animal models of hyperoxic or hypoxic exposure, anorexia, weight loss, and lung injury, characterized by pulmonary edema and decreased lung water clearance, developed.[74,75] The edema was partially or fully reversed by the provision of continuous enteral feeding,[74] refeeding, or treatment with the amino acid glutamate.[76]

Effect of Undernutrition on Control of Breathing

B

The incidence of sudden infant death syndrome is increased in individuals with evidence of intrauterine growth restriction[77]; however there is little information on the postnatal effects of growth restriction or undernutrition on the control of breathing. In growth-restricted lambs, the ventilatory response to progressive hypoxia was found to be related to birth weight, whereas the response to hypercapnia was not.[78]

Adequate Nutrition to Support Lung Growth and Function

The following paragraphs offer a brief description of the importance of each nutritional component on lung growth, pulmonary physiology, and pathophysiology.

Energy

Energy is required for body function and growth and is obtained from food sources. In a preterm infant with negligible energy stores (as described previously), energy is gained from nutritional intake, expended as needed, and then stored if in excess. Energy expenditure is negatively related to gestational age and is positively related to energy intake, weight gain, and postnatal age.[79-81] Expert committees estimate that a daily energy intake of approximately 120 to 130 kcal/kg is sufficient to meet the metabolic demands of a healthy premature infant and to allow for growth rates comparable to intrauterine growth rates.[82] A review of nutritional intakes in a preterm infant cohort showed that for every 1-kcal/day increase in total energy intake, there was a 0.34-g/day increase in weight, a 0.003-cm/day increase in length, and a 0.002-cm/day increase in head circumference.[83]

It is unknown whether these estimates of energy intake are also applicable to sick and unstable low-gestation infants. Whether energy expenditure changes during respiratory illness is unclear. Severity of illness was not found to correlate to energy expenditure in studies of some ventilated preterm infants,[80,81] but increased metabolic rates were observed in others.[84] No measures are available in non–ventilator-dependent infants with respiratory distress, so the advantage of adjusting energy intake for increased respiratory distress is undefined. Because infants with established BPD have higher energy expenditure and poorer rates of weight gain,[45] energy intake targets are commonly raised. What is clear is that the process of respiration requires energy and deficient energy intakes impinge on respiration and may cause respiratory failure. Conversely, excessive intake may be counterproductive by increasing fat stores and energy expenditure for lipogenesis.

Water and Fluid Volume

Water is essential for life because it carries nutrients to cells, removes waste products, and makes up the physiochemical milieu that allows cellular work to occur.[85] Growth requires water intake into new tissues or cells. The ideal weight gain of 15 to 20 g/kg/day (new tissue generation) is 65% to 80% water mass (10-12 mL/kg/day).[85] Water is the major compound of enteral and parenteral nutrition. Daily recommended intakes vary according to gestational age, postnatal age, and fluid balance. Intakes are conventionally limited during the first few days of life, when normal fluid shifts and weight loss occur. A large retrospective analysis showed that higher fluid intake and less weight loss during the first 10 days of life were associated with an increased risk of BPD.[86]

There is an association between the presence of a patent ductus arteriosus (PDA) and an increased risk for BPD. The acute pulmonary effects of a PDA include pulmonary edema (and occasionally hemorrhage), worsened lung mechanics, and deterioration in gas exchange with hypoxemia and hypercapnia.[87] Also the greater pulmonary blood flow can trigger an inflammatory cascade that promotes BPD. One meta-analysis found that fluid restriction significantly reduced the risk of PDA and showed a trend toward reducing BPD risk.[88] Therefore, common clinical practice is to limit fluid intake when a PDA is suspected or when BPD is established. An unwanted consequence of limiting fluid intake is inadvertent delivery of insufficient calories because of inadequate caloric intake from unadjusted dilutions (continued provision of dilute or minimally concentrated fluids).

Macronutrients

Macronutrients are the classes of chemical compounds that represent the largest quantities in the diet and that provide bulk energy. Carbohydrate and fat provide the energy needed to meet the demands of all organ systems, including the cardiorespiratory system. When provided in adequate amounts, they spare proteins to support cell maturation, remodeling, growth, activity of enzymes, and transport proteins for all body organs.

Carbohydrates

Glucose, the primary circulating form of carbohydrate, is the major source of energy. It is the final pathway for the metabolism and oxidation of all carbohydrates as well as an important carbon source for de novo synthesis of amino acids and FAs. The rates of endogenous hepatic glucose production are 8 to 9 mg/kg/min in preterm infants and 5 mg/kg/min in term infants.[89] These levels are considered to be enough to meet most of the energy requirements of the brain only. Consequently, they are the lower limits of glucose intakes aimed for initially. Levels required for energy needs plus growth may be as high as 12 to 13 mg/kg/min.

Oxidation of carbohydrates results in a higher rate of carbon dioxide production for the same amount of oxygen consumed (respiratory quotient [RQ] 1.0) in comparison with fat (RQ 0.7) and protein (RQ 0.8).[90] Hence, administration of high-glucose loads should be made cautiously in conditions in which there is difficulty in carbon dioxide elimination (e.g., respiratory failure, BPD). Also, high or excessive carbohydrate intakes above the amount that can be oxidized for energy and stored as glycogen leads only to increased lipogenesis,[91] a process with inherent increased carbon dioxide production (RQ 5 to 8), altered fat deposition,[92] and obesity. Efforts should be made to maintain proper ratios of nonprotein energy to protein energy to avoid weight gain secondary to fat mass rather than lean body mass, and yet to avoid utilization of protein as an energy source and not for net protein growth, which can occur at low nonprotein caloric intakes (<60 kcal/kg/day).[93]

Fats

Lipids provide a concentrated form of energy and supply essential FAs, which are important for normal growth and development of the nervous system, retina, and immune system. Intravenous lipids commonly used in the clinical setting are composed of vegetable oil (soybean or a combination of soybean and safflower oil) emulsified with egg phospholipids and glycerol. A 20% intravenous (IV) fat emulsion is typically started at 0.5 to 1 g fat/kg on the first day of life, usually at the same time amino acids are started to prevent essential fatty acid deficiency and provide a more generous source of calories. The lipid emulsion is advanced as tolerated in incremental rates of 0.5 to 1 g/kg/day to a typical maximum of 3 g/kg/day, infused over 24 hours. Excessive or rapid infusion of large doses of fat emulsion has been correlated with an increase in alveolar-arteriolar diffusion gradient in adults but not in preterm infants.[94]

Long-chain polyunsaturated FAs (LCPUFAs) contained in lipid emulsions are readily incorporated in a dose-dependent manner into cell phospholipid membranes and other tissues, where they are involved in cell signaling, the production of eicosanoids involved in inflammation, blood vessel tone, platelet aggregation, and modulation of the immune system. The main LCPUFAs are the ω-6FAs (e.g., linoleic acid) and ω-3FAs. Mediators arising from ω-6FAs (thromboxane A_2, leukotrienes B_4, C_4, and D_4, prostaglandins D_2, E_2, and F_2, and prostacyclin I_2) have a primarily pro-inflammatory effect, whereas those arising from ω-3FAs (thromboxane A_3, leukotrienes B_5, C_5, and D_5, prostaglandins D_3, E_3, and F_3, and prostacyclin I_3) are less potent and have reduced inflammatory activity.[95] ω-6FAs and ω-3FAs share metabolic pathways and thus interact with each other through a complex system involving substrate availability, competition for the same metabolic enzymes for synthesis and membrane incorporation, as well as powerful negative feedback of the end products.[96] Thus, docosahexaenoic acid and eicosapentaenoic acid in the family of ω-3FAs interfere with arachidonic acid (ω-6FA) and downregulate associated inflammatory eicosanoids, making the ratio of ω-6FAs to ω-3FAs, the n6:n3 ratio, an important marker in the regulation of inflammatory mediators.[97]

Vegetable-derived oils (e.g., soybean oil in Intralipid) are rich in ω-6FAs but not ω-3FAs. Because of the anti-inflammatory property of ω-3FAs, their potential role in different pathologies secondary to inflammation (including pulmonary disorders) is being defined.[98] In a hyperoxic lung injury model in neonatal rats, dams fed a diet rich in fat emulsion (Intralipid; high in ω-6FAs) produced newborn rats with high lung PUFA levels and marked protection against oxygen toxicity[99]; provision of fish oil (high in ω-3FAs) was shown to give the same protection.[100] Although not directly compared, the clinicopathologic scores (combination of clinical status, histopathologic presence of lung edema, hemorrhage, and atelectasis) in the lungs was better in offspring of ω-3FA–fed mothers than in offspring of ω-6FA–fed mothers. In a different animal model, feeding of ω-3FAs resulted in decreased oxidative stress in the liver associated with lower activity of superoxide dismutase and glutathione peroxidase.[101] Newer fish oil–based intravenous fat emulsions (e.g., Omegaven) and dietary preparations are being utilized to avoid the proinflammatory properties of ω-6FA–rich soy-based oils; however their effect on inflammation-based neonatal pulmonary pathologies is still unknown, and their effect on prolongation of bleeding times may be a disadvantage.[102]

Despite the advantage against hyperoxic damage, LCPUFAs are susceptible to lipid peroxidation, and excessive intakes may reduce antioxidant capacity and enhance susceptibility to oxidative damage. Hence, newer approaches to lipid administration are leaning towards limiting lipid amounts to the minimum necessary to prevent essential fatty acid deficiency and to provide just enough to meet caloric needs.

Proteins

Protein requirements for the neonate are inversely related to gestational age and size as a result of the more rapid growth rates and greater protein losses in the smaller, more premature infants.[103] The early provision of protein within the first minutes to hours after birth is critical to attainment of positive nitrogen balance and accretion, because premature babies lose about 1% of their protein stores daily.[104] Studies suggest that at least 1 g/kg/day of amino acids can decrease catabolism.[105] Current aggressive protein intake strategies include starting protein at rates appropriate for gestational age: 3.5-4 g/kg/day for infants less than 30 weeks gestational age, 2.5 to 3.5 g/kg/day for infants 30 to 36 weeks gestational age, and 2.5 g/kg/day for infants more than 36 weeks gestational age.[103] Studies show that early and aggressive provision of protein and adequate nonprotein energy within the first few days of life is safe and effective at providing protein to meet accretion needs and facilitate intrauterine growth rates.[106] In addition, albumin synthesis is upregulated rapidly if amino acids are administered immediately after birth.[107] Albumin is a key element in the regulation of plasma oncotic pressure and has antioxidant activity secondary to its ligand- and free radical–binding capacities.[108] Caution is necessary to avoid excessive protein intake, which has been shown to induce metabolic stress from protein overload, reduced neurodevelopmental outcomes, and, ironically, growth failure.[109]

Micronutrients

Micronutrients are so called because they are needed in only minuscule amounts. These nutrients are the "magic wands" that enable the body to produce enzymes, hormones, and other substances essential for proper metabolism of macronutrients. As tiny as the amounts are, however, the consequences of their absence are severe. Most of the micronutrients are transferred to the fetus late in gestation; thus the preterm infant fails to receive them, and as a result, most preterm infants are born with micronutrient deficiencies. Although an adequate well-balanced nutritional intake is essential, specific manipulations of micronutrients that may be scarce in the preterm infant population may play a role in protecting them from development of BPD.

Vitamins

Vitamin A

Vitamin A is a fat-soluble micronutrient involved in the growth and differentiation of epithelial tissues. It influences the orderly growth and differentiation of epithelial cells by regulating membrane structure and function. Retinol is the major circulating form, and retinol-binding protein is the transport protein. Retinol is among the substances transplacentally transferred late in gestation; hence preterm infants are born with low plasma retinol levels[110,111] and decreased retinol stores in the liver and lungs.[112] In one study, infants who eventually progressed to BPD were noted to have lower values of plasma retinol at birth and weeks later despite receiving the recommended intakes.[111] Initial clinical trials involving supplementation showed inconsistencies in pulmonary outcomes due to underdosage and loss en route by photodegradation and adherence to plastic tubing.[113] In a multicenter study reported by Tyson and colleagues,[114] retinol supplementation in ELBW ventilated infants, consisting of 5000 IU of vitamin A given intramuscularly three times per week for 4 weeks, resulted in a modest but significant decrease in oxygen requirement at 36 weeks postmenstrual age or death. For every 14 to 15 ELBW infants supplemented in this study, 1 infant survived without chronic lung disease.[114] Current practice surveys reveal inconsistent application of vitamin A in clinical practice because of its perceived small benefit and the need for an intramuscular administration route.[115]

Vitamin D

Vitamin D is a fat-soluble vitamin with the primary function of maintaining serum calcium and phosphorus concentrations. Also among the substances transplacentally transferred late in gestation, it must be provided by dietary or parenteral supplementation because its production from sun exposure is not an option in the hospitalized preterm infant. Once enteral or parenteral supplemental vitamin D enters the circulation, it associates with vitamin D–binding protein. Depending on the preparation, hydroxylation has to occur first in the liver and then in the kidneys into the most active or hormonal form, $1,25(OH)_2D$. From 24 weeks of gestation on, the infant is capable of enzymatic conversion to the active form of vitamin D. The role of vitamin D in the multifactorial metabolic bone disease of prematurity is still undefined. At preterm birth, the newborn's serum 25(OH) D level is 50% to 70% of the maternal serum level. Supplementation of the parent compound of vitamin D at 30 to 400 IU/kg/day results in substantial plasma 25(OH)D levels.[116] All infant formulas and human milk fortifiers in the United States are fortified with about 400 IU/L of vitamin D.

Vitamin E

Vitamin E (α-tocopherol) is a fat-soluble vitamin that has eight naturally occurring isomers. It has antioxidant properties that may help prevent injury related to lipid peroxidation by scavenging free radicals. Vitamin E can be incorporated into cell membranes in proportion to the content of PUFAs, making cells more resistant to oxygen-induced injury.[117] Stored in the liver, adipose tissue and skeletal muscles, vitamin E is integrated into lipid droplets and cell membranes at the cellular level. The limited proportion of adipose tissue in preterm infants limits total body vitamin E levels. The possibility that vitamin E may have a role in prevention of oxidation-related injury of pulmonary cell membranes has prompted clinical trials involving its supplementation.[118,119] However, supplementation of vitamin E in preterm neonates does not prevent BPD.

Vitamin E plays a prominent role in respiratory and peripheral muscle function. Deficiency of vitamin E increases lipid peroxidation and glutathione oxidation in the rat diaphragm.[120] In addition, vitamin E deficiency is associated with impaired in vitro force generation of the diaphragm. Inspiratory resistive breathing (a technique for loading the respiratory muscles) induced impairment in in vitro force generation and increased oxidized glutathione levels in the diaphragm in vitamin E deficient rats.[120] The provision of 2.8-3.5 IU/kg/day of vitamin E parenterally and 6-12 IU/kg/day enterally is recommended to maintain normal plasma levels and tissue stores.[121]

Vitamin C

Vitamin C (ascorbic acid), a water-soluble vitamin with both antioxidant and pro-oxidant properties (when available in high amounts in the presence of free iron in vitro), is essential to connective tissue formation. A randomized controlled trial of VLBW infants to one of three levels of ascorbic acid supplementation (low, low then high, or high) during the first 28 days of life showed no difference in pulmonary outcomes.[122] Although the difference is statistically insignificant, the proportion of surviving infants with oxygen requirement at 36 weeks postmenstrual age in the high supplementation group (19%) was half that in the low supplementation group (41%).[122] Current recommended intake based on available parenteral multivitamin preparations is 32 mg/kg/day.

Trace Elements

Important microelements or trace elements in human nutrition are zinc, copper, selenium, chromium, molybdenum, manganese, iodine, and iron. Although they quantitatively represent a small fraction of the total mineral content of the human body, they play key roles in several metabolic pathways. Preterm infants may have trace element deficiencies due to low stores at birth, even if clinical manifestations are absent, because major transfer of these substances occurs late in gestation. Very little is known about the metabolism of trace elements in the nutrition of preterm infants, and even less about their effect on the respiratory system.

Selenium functions partly as a component of proteins, including enzymes such as glutathione peroxidases, that play an important role in preventing free radical formation and oxygen toxicity. There are no data on fetal selenium accretion rates through direct chemical analysis of fetuses. Poor selenium and glutathione peroxidase levels in VLBW infants were found to be associated with increased incidence of BPD.[123,124] Although a clinical trial of selenium supplementation (7 μg/kg/day parenterally or 5 μg /kg/day orally from week 1 to 36 weeks postmenstrual age or discharge home) did not improve outcomes, the investigators noted that lower maternal and neonatal prerandomization selenium levels were associated with higher respiratory morbidity.[125] Current recommendation is to provide 2 μg/kg/day. However, to maintain concentrations closer to umbilical cord blood levels, 3 μg/kg/day is suggested. To increase concentrations above umbilical cord blood levels and bring them closer to those of breastfed full-term infants, 5 to 7 μg/kg/day of selenium is recommended.[126]

Manganese is a cofactor for the antioxidant enzyme mitochondrial SOD and is involved in activation of enzymes involved in synthesis of mucopolysaccharides necessary for growth and maintenance of connective tissue, cartilage, and bone.[127] Zinc is important for growth, cell differentiation, and the metabolism of proteins, carbohydrates, and lipids. It is also a cofactor, along with copper, in cytoplasmic

SOD. Despite the demonstration of low levels of all trace elements, except for copper, in preterm infants receiving currently suggested trace element doses in parenteral nutrition, there are no studies of the effect of giving higher doses to preterm infants at risk for deficiencies.

Other Nutrients

Calcium/Phosphorus

Bone and rib cage formation requires protein and energy for collagen matrix synthesis, and an adequate intake of calcium and phosphorus is necessary for proper mineralization. Calcium is actively transported across the placenta to the fetus with a 1:4 maternal-to-fetal gradient so that calcium levels are higher in the fetus to meet the high demand of the developing skeleton. It has been estimated that fetal accretion in the last trimester is approximately 100 to 120 mg/kg/day for calcium and 50 to 65 mg/kg/day for phosphorus.[64] Interruption of the placental supply of calcium at birth stimulates the release of parathyroid hormone (PTH) to maintain calcium homeostasis. PTH stimulates the reabsorption of calcium and excretion of phosphorus in the kidneys and bone reabsorption of calcium. Without any dietary intake, preterm infants are started on parenteral nutrition containing calcium in the form of inorganic salts and phosphorus as inorganic sodium or potassium phosphate. Owing to limits in solubility, the goal of parenteral calcium and phosphorus provision is to maintain normal serum levels and not to match in utero accretion rates. At best, about 60% of intrauterine mineralization is provided by 60 to 80 mg/kg/day of parenteral calcium and 58 to 60 mg/kg/day of parenteral phosphorus,[116] provided that amino acid intake is more than 2 to 2.25 g/kg/day and the volume of infusate is higher than 100 mL/kg/day. Rates closer to in utero accretion are attainable via assimilation from fortified human milk or preterm milk formula, explaining the urgency for the establishment of enteral nutrition. Current recommendations for the stable growing preterm are 100 to 160 mg/kg/day of calcium and 60 to 90 mg/kg/day of phosphorus,[128] to account for the relative absorptive inefficiency of the developing gut. Preterm human milk contains 31 mg of calcium and 20 mg of phosphorus per 100 kcal; with 70% calcium and 80% phosphorus absorption, it provides about a third of in utero accretion rates.[129] Fortified preterm human milk provides 91 mg of calcium and 53 mg of phosphorus per 100 kcal, attaining about two thirds of in utero accretion rates.

Surfactant Precursors

Inositol is a six-carbon sugar present in several biologic compounds, such as phosphatidylinositol found in surfactant and breast milk. Prior to the availability of exogenous surfactant, a trial of parenteral supplementation for preterm infants with respiratory distress showed that inositol supplementation (80 mg/kg/day of IV inositol for 5 days) was associated with longer survival and lower incidence of BPD.[130] A systematic review confirmed the same findings.[131] With the availability of exogenous surfactant replacement therapy, however, no subsequent randomized control trials have been conducted.

Individual Amino Acids

The supplementation of individual amino acids has not demonstrated positive results. Cysteine (glutathione precursor) supplementation in VLBW infants was found to improve plasma levels but not to stimulate glutathione synthesis.[132] Supplementation using the cysteine precursor *N*-acetylcysteine was reported to have no effect on the rates of death and BPD in preterm infants.[133,134] In fetal rat lung type II pneumocytes, glutamine is oxidized preferentially over glucose for energy metabolism.[135] Glutamine supplementation has been shown to reduce the risk of sepsis and mortality in critically ill adult surgical patients,[136] but its supplementation in VLBW infants had no effect.[137] Whether glutamine has any effect on pulmonary morbidity is unknown.

Conclusion

Nutrition is a therapeutic tool and a crucial aspect of neonatal care. All organs, including those in the respiratory system, have nutritional needs. Biochemical and physiologic functions require energy for basic cellular function, multiplication, repair, gene expression, and enzyme production. Dietary protein is needed to provide amino acids for synthesis of body proteins and enzymes with various functional roles. Micronutrients are essential in many metabolic functions in the body as components and cofactors in enzymatic processes. Nutritional quantity and quality ultimately affect all cells in the body.

The lung is vulnerable to adverse exposures during fetal development. There are differing windows of susceptibility, depending on the lung's developmental stage. Preterm birth interrupts in utero lung development, so as the lung continues to develop after birth, postnatal exposures, including nutrition, may significantly influence lung growth, especially because these exposures occur during the period of rapid alveolarization. Once the basic structure of the respiratory system has been realized during this critical phase, the development of lung function and anatomy follows a more or less fixed course and exhibits tracking well into adolescence and adulthood. As such, the lung function an individual is born with or, in the case of the preterm infant, the lung function developed through the neonatal intensive care unit experience, is a major determinant of lung function throughout life.

References

1. Bloom BT, Mulligan J, Arnold C, et al. Improving growth of very low birth weight infants in the first 28 days. *Pediatrics*. 2003;112(1 Pt 1):8-14.
2. Stoll BJ, Hansen NI, Bell EF, et al. Neonatal outcomes of extremely preterm infants from the NICHD Neonatal Research Network. *Pediatrics*. 2010;126:443-456.
3. Cooke RJ, Ainsworth SB, Fenton AC. Postnatal growth retardation: a universal problem in preterm infants. *Arch Dis Child Fetal Neonatal Ed*. 2004;89:F428-F430.
4. Clark RH, Thomas P, Peabody J. Extrauterine growth restriction remains a serious problem in prematurely born neonates. *Pediatrics*. 2003;111:986-990.
5. Bancalari E, Claure N, Sosenko IR. Bronchopulmonary dysplasia: changes in pathogenesis, epidemiology and definition. *Semin Neonatol*. 2003;8:63-71.
6. Goldenberg RL, Culhane JF, Iams JD, Romero R. Epidemiology and causes of preterm birth. *Lancet*. 2008;371:75-84.
7. Lawn JE, Gravett MG, Nunes TM, et al. Global report on preterm birth and stillbirth (1 of 7): definitions, description of the burden and opportunities to improve data. *BMC Pregnancy Childbirth*. 2010;10(suppl 1):S1.
8. Lemons JA, Bauer CR, Oh W, et al. Very low birth weight outcomes of the National Institute of Child Health and Human Development Neonatal Research Network, January 1995 through December 1996. NICHD Neonatal Research Network. *Pediatrics*. 2001;107:E1.
9. Jobe AJ. The new BPD: an arrest of lung development. *Pediatr Res*. 1999;46:641-643.
10. Jobe AH. The new BPD. *NeoReviews* 2006;7:e531-e544.
11. Kotecha S. Lung growth: implications for the newborn infant. *Arch Dis Child Fetal Neonatal Ed*. 2000;82:F69-F74.
12 Kleinman RE, ed. *AAP Committee on Nutrition: Pediatric Nutrition Handbook*. 6th ed. Elk Grove Village, IL: American Academy of Pediatrics; 2009.
13. Embleton NE, Pang N, Cooke RJ. Postnatal malnutrition and growth retardation: an inevitable consequence of current recommendations in preterm infants? *Pediatrics*. 2001;107:270-273.
14. Ehrenkranz RA, Younes N, Lemons JA, et al. Longitudinal growth of hospitalized very low birth weight infants. *Pediatrics*. 1999;104:280-289.
15. Sosenko IR, Frank L. Nutritional influences on lung development and protection against chronic lung disease. *Semin Perinatol*. 1991;15:462-468.
16. Thureen PJ, Hay WW. Nutritional requirements of the very low birth weight infant. In: Neu J, ed. *Gastroenterology and Nutrition: Neonatology Questions and Controversies*. St Louis: Saunders Elsevier; 2008:208-222.
17. Ehrenkranz RA. Early nutritional support for ELBW Infants: Influence of severity of illness. Pediatric Academic Societies'. *Annual Meeting*. 2007;61:6282.83, E-PAS2007:616282.23.
18. American Academy of Pediatrics Committee on Nutrition. Nutritional needs of low-birth-weight infants. *Pediatrics*. 1985;75:976-986.
19. Hay WW Jr, Lucas A, Heird WC, et al. Workshop summary: nutrition of the extremely low birth weight infant. *Pediatrics*. 1999;104:1360-1368.
20. Herrmann KR. Early parenteral nutrition and successful postnatal growth of premature infants. *Nutr Clin Pract*. 2010;25:69-75.

21. Madden J, Kobaly K, Minich NM, et al. Improved weight attainment of extremely low-gestational-age infants with bronchopulmonary dysplasia. *J Perinatol*. 2010;30:103-111.
22. Wilson DC, Cairns P, Halliday HL, et al. Randomised controlled trial of an aggressive nutritional regimen in sick very low birthweight infants. *Arch Dis Child Fetal Neonatal Ed*. 1997;77: F4-F11.
23. Ehrenkranz RA. Early nutritional support and outcomes in ELBW infants. *Early Hum Dev*. 2010;86(suppl 1):21-25.
24. De Curtis M, Rigo J. Extrauterine growth restriction in very-low-birthweight infants. *Acta Paediatr*. 2004;93:1563-1568.
25. Heird WC. Determination of nutritional requirements in preterm infants, with special reference to 'catch-up' growth. *Semin Neonatol*. 2001;6:365-375.
26. World Health Organization. Malnutrition—The Global Picture. Available at http://www.who.int/home-page/
27. Ehrenkranz RA, Dusick AM, Vohr BR, et al. Growth in the neonatal intensive care unit influences neurodevelopmental and growth outcomes of extremely low birth weight infants. *Pediatrics*. 2006;117:1253-1261.
28. Thureen P, Hay, W. Conditions requiring special nutritional management. In: Tsang RC, Uauy R, Koletzko B, Zlotkin S, eds. *Nutrition of the Preterm Infant: Scientific Basis and Practical Guidelines*. 2nd ed. Cincinnati, OH: Digital Educational Publishing; 2005:383-411.
29. Rao L, Tiller C, Coates C, et al. Lung growth in infants and toddlers assessed by multi-slice computed tomography. *Acad Radiol*. 2010;17:1128-1135.
30. Balinotti JE, Tiller CJ, Llapur CJ, et al. Growth of the lung parenchyma early in life. *Am J Respir Crit Care Med*. 2009;179:134-137.
31. Frank L, Groseclose E. Oxygen toxicity in newborn rats: the adverse effects of undernutrition. *J Appl Physiol*. 1982;53:1248-1255.
32. Maritz GS, Cock ML, Louey S, et al. Fetal growth restriction has long-term effects on postnatal lung structure in sheep. *Pediatr Res*. 2004;55:287-295.
33. Massaro D, Massaro GD, Baras A, et al. Calorie-related rapid onset of alveolar loss, regeneration, and changes in mouse lung gene expression. *Am J Physiol Lung Cell Mol Physiol*. 2004;286: L896-L906.
34. Das RM. The effects of intermittent starvation on lung development in suckling rats. *Am J Pathol*. 1984;117:326-332.
35. Sahebjami H, Wirman JA. Emphysema-like changes in the lungs of starved rats. *Am Rev Respir Dis*. 1981;124:619-624.
36. Kerr JS, Riley DJ, Lanza-Jacoby S, et al. Nutritional emphysema in the rat. Influence of protein depletion and impaired lung growth. *Am Rev Respir Dis*. 1985;131:644-650.
37. Mataloun MM, Rebello CM, Mascaretti RS, et al. Pulmonary responses to nutritional restriction and hyperoxia in premature rabbits. *J Pediatr (Rio J)*. 2006;82:179-185.
38. Coxson HO, Chan IH, Mayo JR, et al. Early emphysema in patients with anorexia nervosa. *Am J Respir Crit Care Med*. 2004;170:748-752.
39. Maritz G, Probyn M, De Matteo R, et al. Lung parenchyma at maturity is influenced by postnatal growth but not by moderate preterm birth in sheep. *Neonatology*. 2008;93:28-35.
40. Bose C, Van Marter LJ, Laughon M, et al. Fetal growth restriction and chronic lung disease among infants born before the 28th week of gestation. *Pediatrics*. 2009;124:e450-e458.
41. Kinsella JP, Greenough A, Abman SH. Bronchopulmonary dysplasia. *Lancet*. 2006;367: 1421-1431.
42. Laughon M, Bose C, Allred EN, et al. Antecedents of chronic lung disease following three patterns of early respiratory disease in preterm infants. *Arch Dis Child Fetal Neonatal Ed*. 2010;96: F114-F120.
43. Massaro D, Massaro GD. Hunger disease and pulmonary alveoli. *Am J Respir Crit Care Med*. 2004;170:723-724.
44. Markestad T, Fitzhardinge PM. Growth and development in children recovering from bronchopulmonary dysplasia. *J Pediatr*. 1981;98:597-602.
45. Kurzner SI, Garg M, Bautista DB, et al. Growth failure in infants with bronchopulmonary dysplasia: nutrition and elevated resting metabolic expenditure. *Pediatrics*. 1988;81:379-384.
46. Kurzner SI, Garg M, Bautista DB, et al. Growth failure in bronchopulmonary dysplasia: elevated metabolic rates and pulmonary mechanics. *J Pediatr*. 1988;112:73-80.
47. Groothuis JR, Rosenberg AA. Home oxygen promotes weight gain in infants with bronchopulmonary dysplasia. *Am J Dis Child*. 1987;141:992-995.
48. Guslits BG, Gaston SE, Bryan MH, et al. Diaphragmatic work of breathing in premature human infants. *J Appl Physiol*. 1987;62:1410-1415.
49. Arora NS, Rochester DF. Respiratory muscle strength and maximal voluntary ventilation in undernourished patients. *Am Rev Respir Dis*. 1982;126:5-8.
50. Dias CM, Passaro CP, Cagido VR, et al. Effects of undernutrition on respiratory mechanics and lung parenchyma remodeling. *J Appl Physiol*. 2004;97:1888-1896.
51. Dias CM, Passaro CP, Antunes MA, et al. Effects of different nutritional support on lung mechanics and remodelling in undernourished rats. *Respir Physiol Neurobiol*. 2008;160:54-64.
52. Matecki S, Py G, Lambert K, et al. Effect of prolonged undernutrition on rat diaphragm mitochondrial respiration. *Am J Respir Cell Mol Biol*. 2002;26:239-245.
53. Lewis MI, Li H, Huang ZS, et al. Influence of varying degrees of malnutrition on IGF-I expression in the rat diaphragm. *J Appl Physiol*. 2003;95:555-562.

7

54. Blazer S, Reinersman GT, Askanazi J, et al. Branched-chain amino acids and respiratory pattern and function in the neonate. *J Perinatol*. 1994;14:290-295.
55. Mahmoud R, Roehr CC, Schmalisch G. Current methods in non-invasive ventilatory support for neonates. *Pediatr Respir Rev*. 2011;12:196-205.
56. Rehan VK, Laiprasert J, Nakashima JM, et al. Effects of continuous positive airway pressure on diaphragm dimensions in preterm infants. *J Perinatol*. 2001;21:521-524.
57. Parks WC, Shapiro SD. Matrix metalloproteinases in lung biology. *Respir Res*. 2001;2:10-19.
58. Sahebjami H, MacGee J. Effects of starvation on lung mechanics and biochemistry in young and old rats. *J Appl Physiol*. 1985;58:778-784.
59. Jobe AH. Pulmonary surfactant therapy. *N Engl J Med*. 1993;328:861-868.
60. Batenburg JJ. Surfactant phospholipids: synthesis and storage. *Am J Physiol*. 1992;262: L367-L385.
61. Guarner V, Tordet C, Bourbon JR. Effects of maternal protein-calorie malnutrition on the phospholipid composition of surfactant isolated from fetal and neonatal rat lungs. Compensation by inositol and lipid supplementation. *Pediatr Res*. 1992;31:629-635.
62. Lechner AJ, Winston DC, Bauman JE. Lung mechanics, cellularity, and surfactant after prenatal starvation in guinea pigs. *J Appl Physiol*. 1986;60:1610-1614.
63. Gerhardt T, Bancalari E. Chestwall compliance in full-term and premature infants. *Acta Paediatr Scand*. 1980;69:359-364.
64. Rigo J, De Curtis M, Pieltain C, et al. Bone mineral metabolism in the micropremie. *Clin Perinatol*. 2000;27:147-170.
65. Glasgow JF, Thomas PS. Rachitic respiratory distress in small preterm infants. *Arch Dis Child*. 1977;52:268-273.
66. Dobashi K, Asayama K, Hayashibe H, et al. Immunohistochemical study of copper-zinc and manganese superoxide dismutases in the lungs of human fetuses and newborn infants: developmental profile and alterations in hyaline membrane disease and bronchopulmonary dysplasia. *Virchows Arch A Pathol Anat Histopathol*. 1993;423:177-184.
67. Deneke SM, Lynch BA, Fanburg BL. Effects of low protein diets or feed restriction on rat lung glutathione and oxygen toxicity. *J Nutr*. 1985;115:726-732.
68. Zaman K, Baqui AH, Yunus M, et al. Malnutrition, cell-mediated immune deficiency and acute upper respiratory infections in rural Bangladeshi children. *Acta Paediatr*. 1997;86:923-927.
69. Cunha AL. Relationship between acute respiratory infection and malnutrition in children under 5 years of age. *Acta Paediatr*. 2000;89:608-609.
70. Skerrett SJ, Henderson WR, Martin TR. Alveolar macrophage function in rats with severe protein calorie malnutrition. Arachidonic acid metabolism, cytokine release, and antimicrobial activity. *J Immunol*. 1990;144:1052-1061.
71. Martin TR, Altman LC, Alvares OF. The effects of severe protein-calorie malnutrition on antibacterial defense mechanisms in the rat lung. *Am Rev Respir Dis*. 1983;128:1013-1019.
72. Schuit KE, Krebs RE, Rohn D, Steele V. Effect of fetal protein malnutrition on the postnatal structure and function of alveolar macrophages. *J Infect Dis*. 1982;146:498-505.
73. Sano H, Kuroki Y. The lung collectins, SP-A and SP-D, modulate pulmonary innate immunity. *Mol Immunol*. 2005;42:279-287.
74. Factor P, Ridge K, Alverdy J, Sznajder JI. Continuous enteral nutrition attenuates pulmonary edema in rats exposed to 100% oxygen. *J Appl Physiol*. 2000;89:1759-1765.
75. Sakuma T, Hida M, Nambu Y, et al. Effects of hypoxia on alveolar fluid transport capacity in rat lungs. *J Appl Physiol*. 2001;91:1766-1774.
76. Sakuma T, Zhao Y, Sugita M, et al. Malnutrition impairs alveolar fluid clearance in rat lungs. *Am J Physiol Lung Cell Mol Physiol*. 2004;286:L1268-L1274.
77. Oyen N, Skjaerven R, Little RE, Wilcox AJ. Fetal growth retardation in sudden infant death syndrome (SIDS) babies and their siblings. *Am J Epidemiol*. 1995;142:84-90.
78. Moss TJ, Davey MG, McCrabb GJ, Harding R. Development of ventilatory responsiveness to progressive hypoxia and hypercapnia in low-birth-weight lambs. *J Appl Physiol*. 1996;81:1555-1561.
79. Hulzebos CV, Sauer PJ. Energy requirements. *Semin Fetal Neonatal Med*. 2007;12:2-10.
80. Bauer K, Laurenz M, Ketteler J, Versmold H. Longitudinal study of energy expenditure in preterm neonates <30 weeks' gestation during the first three postnatal weeks. *J Pediatr*. 2003;142: 390-396.
81. DeMarie MP, Hoffenberg A, Biggerstaff SL, et al. Determinants of energy expenditure in ventilated preterm infants. *J Perinat Med*. 1999;27:465-472.
82. Kashyap S, Schulze KF. Energy requirements and protein-energy metabolism and balance in preterm and term infants. In: Thureen P, Hay W, eds. *Neonatal Nutrition and Metabolism*. Cambridge, UK: Cambridge University Press; 2006:134-146.
83. Collins CT, Gibson RA, Miller J, et al. Carbohydrate intake is the main determinant of growth in infants born <33 weeks' gestation when protein intake is adequate. *Nutrition*. 2008;24:451-457.
84. Wahlig TM, Gatto CW, Boros SJ, et al. Metabolic response of preterm infants to variable degrees of respiratory illness. *J Pediatr*. 1994;124:283-288.
85. Costarino ATJ, Baumgart, S. Water as nutrition. In: Tsang RC, Lucas A, Uauy R, Zlotkin S, eds. *Nutritional Needs of the Preterm Infant: Scientific Basis and Practical Guidelines*. New York: Williams & Wilkins; 1993:1-14.
86. Oh W, Poindexter BB, Perritt R, et al. Association between fluid intake and weight loss during the first ten days of life and risk of bronchopulmonary dysplasia in extremely low birth weight infants. *J Pediatr*. 2005;147:786-790.

87. Bancalari E, Claure N, Gonzalez A. Patent ductus arteriosus and respiratory outcome in premature infants. *Biol Neonate*. 2005;88:192-201.
88. Bell EF, Acarregui MJ. Restricted versus liberal water intake for preventing morbidity and mortality in preterm infants. *Cochrane Database Syst Rev*. 2008:CD000503.
89. Parimi P, Kalhan, SC. Carbohydrates including oligosaccharides and inositol. In: Tsang RC, Uauy R, Koletzko B, Zlotkin S, eds. *Nutrition of the Preterm Infant: Scientific Basis and Practical Guidelines*. 2nd ed. Cincinnati, OH: Digital Educational Publishing; 2005:81-95.
90. Sauer PJ, Van Aerde JE, Pencharz PB, et al. Glucose oxidation rates in newborn infants measured with indirect calorimetry and [U-13C]glucose. *Clin Sci (Lond)*. 1986;70:587-593.
91. Van Aerde JE, Sauer PJ, Pencharz PB, et al. Effect of replacing glucose with lipid on the energy metabolism of newborn infants. *Clin Sci (Lond)*. 1989;76:581-588.
92. Uthaya S, Thomas EL, Hamilton G, et al. Altered adiposity after extremely preterm birth. *Pediatr Res*. 2005;57:211-215.
93. Duffy B, Gunn T, Collinge J, Pencharz P. The effect of varying protein quality and energy intake on the nitrogen metabolism of parenterally fed very low birthweight (less than 1600 g) infants. *Pediatr Res*. 1981;15:1040-1044.
94. Brans YW, Dutton EB, Andrew DS, et al. Fat emulsion tolerance in very low birth weight neonates: effect on diffusion of oxygen in the lungs and on blood pH. *Pediatrics*. 1986;78:79-84.
95. Waitzberg DL, Torrinhas RS. Fish oil lipid emulsions and immune response: what clinicians need to know. *Nutr Clin Pract*. 2009;24:487-499.
96. Arterburn LM, Hall EB, Oken H. Distribution, interconversion, and dose response of n-3 fatty acids in humans. *Am J Clin Nutr*. 2006;83(suppl):1467S-1476S.
97. Calder PC. n-3 polyunsaturated fatty acids, inflammation, and inflammatory diseases. *Am J Clin Nutr*. 2006;83(suppl 6):1505S-1519S.
98. Schwartz J. Role of polyunsaturated fatty acids in lung disease. *Am J Clin Nutr*. 2000;71(suppl): 393S-396S.
99. Sosenko IR, Innis SM, Frank L. Intralipid increases lung polyunsaturated fatty acids and protects newborn rats from oxygen toxicity. *Pediatr Res*. 1991;30:413-417.
100. Sosenko IR, Innis SM, Frank L. Menhaden fish oil, n-3 polyunsaturated fatty acids, and protection of newborn rats from oxygen toxicity. *Pediatr Res*. 1989;25:399-404.
101. Yeh SL, Chang KY, Huang PC, Chen WJ. Effects of n-3 and n-6 fatty acids on plasma eicosanoids and liver antioxidant enzymes in rats receiving total parenteral nutrition. *Nutrition*. 1997;13: 32-36.
102. Simopoulos AP. Summary of the NATO advanced research workshop on dietary omega 3 and omega 6 fatty acids: biological effects and nutritional essentiality. *J Nutr*. 1989;119:521-528.
103. Hay WW, Thureen P. Protein for preterm infants: how much is needed? How much is enough? How much is too much? *Pediatr Neonatol* 2010;51:198-207.
104. Denne SC, Poindexter BB. Evidence supporting early nutritional support with parenteral amino acid infusion. *Semin Perinatol*. 2007;31:56-60.
105. Thureen PJ, Hay WW, Jr. Intravenous nutrition and postnatal growth of the micropremie. *Clin Perinatol*. 2000;27:197-219.
106. Poindexter BB, Langer JC, Dusick AM, Ehrenkranz RA. Early provision of parenteral amino acids in extremely low birth weight infants: relation to growth and neurodevelopmental outcome. *J Pediatr*. 2006;148:300-305.
107. van den Akker CH, te Braake FW, Schierbeek H, et al. Albumin synthesis in premature neonates is stimulated by parenterally administered amino acids during the first days of life. *Am J Clin Nutr*. 2007;86:1003-1008.
108. Roche M, Rondeau P, Singh NR, et al. The antioxidant properties of serum albumin. *FEBS Lett*. 2008;582:1783-1787.
109. Kalhoff H, Manz F, Kiwull P, Kiwull-Schone H. Food mineral composition and acid-base balance in preterm infants. *Eur J Nutr*. 2007;46:188-195.
110. Shenai JP, Chytil F, Jhaveri A, Stahlman MT. Plasma vitamin A and retinol-binding protein in premature and term neonates. *J Pediatr*. 1981;99:302-305.
111. Hustead VA, Gutcher GR, Anderson SA, Zachman RD. Relationship of vitamin A (retinol) status to lung disease in the preterm infant. *J Pediatr*. 1984;105:610-615.
112. Shenai JP, Chytil F. Vitamin A storage in lungs during perinatal development in the rat. *Biol Neonate*. 1990;57:126-132.
113. Silvers KM, Sluis KB, Darlow BA, et al. Limiting light-induced lipid peroxidation and vitamin loss in infant parenteral nutrition by adding multivitamin preparations to Intralipid. *Acta Paediatr*. 2001;90:242-249.
114. Tyson JE, Wright LL, Oh W, et al. Vitamin A supplementation for extremely-low-birth-weight infants. National Institute of Child Health and Human Development Neonatal Research Network. *N Engl J Med*. 1999;340:1962-1968.
115. Ambalavanan N, Kennedy K, Tyson J, Carlo WA. Survey of vitamin A supplementation for extremely-low-birth-weight infants: is clinical practice consistent with the evidence? *J Pediatr*. 2004; 145:304-307.
116. Atkinson SA, Tsang R. Calcium, magnesium, phosphorus and vitamin D. In: Tsang RC, Uauy R, Koltzko B, Zlotkin S, eds. *Nutrition of the Preterm Infant: Scientific Basis and Practical Guidelines*. 2nd ed. Cincinnati, OH: Digital Educational Publishing; 2005:245-275.
117. Burton GW, Traber MG. Vitamin E: antioxidant activity, biokinetics, and bioavailability. *Annu Rev Nutr*. 1990;10:357-382.

B

118. Watts JL, Milner R, Zipursky A, et al. Failure of supplementation with vitamin E to prevent bronchopulmonary dysplasia in infants less than 1,500 g birth weight. *Eur Respir J*. 1991;4:188-190.
119. Ehrenkranz RA, Ablow RC, Warshaw JB. Effect of vitamin E on the development of oxygen-induced lung injury in neonates. *Ann N Y Acad Sci*. 1982;393:452-466.
120. Anzueto A, Andrade FH, Maxwell LC, et al. Diaphragmatic function after resistive breathing in vitamin E-deficient rats. *J Appl Physiol*. 1993;74:267-271.
121. Greene HL, Hambidge KM, Schanler R, Tsang RC. Guidelines for the use of vitamins, trace elements, calcium, magnesium, and phosphorus in infants and children receiving total parenteral nutrition: report of the Subcommittee on Pediatric Parenteral Nutrient Requirements from the Committee on Clinical Practice Issues of the American Society for Clinical Nutrition. *Am J Clin Nutr*. 1988; 48:1324-1342.
122. Darlow BA, Buss H, McGill F, et al. Vitamin C supplementation in very preterm infants: a randomised controlled trial. *Arch Dis Child Fetal Neonatal Ed*. 2005;90:F117-F122.
123. Sluis KB, Darlow BA, George PM, et al. Selenium and glutathione peroxidase levels in premature infants in a low selenium community (Christchurch, New Zealand). *Pediatr Res*. 1992;32: 189-194.
124. Darlow BA, Inder TE, Graham PJ, et al. The relationship of selenium status to respiratory outcome in the very low birth weight infant. *Pediatrics*. 1995;96:314-319.
125. Darlow BA, Winterbourn CC, Inder TE, et al. The effect of selenium supplementation on outcome in very low birth weight infants: a randomized controlled trial. The New Zealand Neonatal Study Group. *J Pediatr*. 2000;136:473-480.
126. Darlow BA, Austin NC. Selenium supplementation to prevent short-term morbidity in preterm neonates. *Cochrane Database Syst Rev*. 2003;(4):CD003312.
127. Zlotkin SH, Atkinson S, Lockitch G. Trace elements in nutrition for premature infants. *Clin Perinatol*. 1995;22:223-240.
128. Rigo J, Pieltain C, Salle B, Senterre J. Enteral calcium, phosphate and vitamin D requirements and bone mineralization in preterm infants. *Acta Paediatr*. 2007;96:969-974.
129. Abrams SA. In utero physiology: role in nutrient delivery and fetal development for calcium, phosphorus, and vitamin D. *Am J Clin Nutr*. 2007;85:604S-607S.
130. Hallman M, Bry K, Hoppu K, et al. Inositol supplementation in premature infants with respiratory distress syndrome. *N Engl J Med*. 1992;326:1233-1239.
131. Howlett A, Ohlsson A. Inositol for respiratory distress syndrome in preterm infants. *Cochrane Database Syst Rev*. 2003;(4):CD000366.
132. te Braake FW, Schierbeek H, Vermes A, et al. High-dose cysteine administration does not increase synthesis of the antioxidant glutathione preterm infants. *Pediatrics*. 2009;124:e978-e984.
133. Sandberg K, Fellman V, Stigson L, et al. *N*-Acetylcysteine administration during the first week of life does not improve lung function in extremely low birth weight infants. *Biol Neonate*. 2004;86:275-279.
134. Ahola T, Lapatto R, Raivio KO, et al. *N*-Acetylcysteine does not prevent bronchopulmonary dysplasia in immature infants: a randomized controlled trial. *J Pediatr*. 2003;143:713-719.
135. Fox RE, Hopkins IB, Cabacungan ET, Tildon JT. The role of glutamine and other alternate substrates as energy sources in the fetal rat lung type II cell. *Pediatr Res*. 1996;40:135-141.
136. Novak F, Heyland DK, Avenell A, et al. Glutamine supplementation in serious illness: a systematic review of the evidence. *Crit Care Med*. 2002;30:2022-2029.
137. Poindexter BB, Ehrenkranz RA, Stoll BJ, et al. Parenteral glutamine supplementation does not reduce the risk of mortality or late-onset sepsis in extremely low birth weight infants. *Pediatrics*. 2004;113:1209-1215.

CHAPTER 8

Patent Ductus Arteriosus and the Lung: Acute Effects and Long-Term Consequences

Eduardo Bancalari, MD, Ilene R.S. Sosenko, MD, and
Nelson Claure, MSc, PhD

8

- Why Does the Ductus Arteriosus Remain Open in Preterm Infants?
- Surfactant Treatment and PDA
- Systemic Consequences of PDA
- Pulmonary Consequences of PDA
- PDA and Bronchopulmonary Dysplasia
- Management of PDA and Respiratory Outcome
- Respiratory Management of Infants with PDA
- Summary

During fetal development the ductus arteriosus plays a critical role by allowing most of the blood returning to the right heart to bypass the pulmonary circulation while maintaining fetal systemic blood flow. In the normal infant born at term the ductus closes during the first hours after birth. However, in the very premature infant the ductus frequently remains open for longer periods, and as the pulmonary vascular resistance falls, there is an increasing systemic-to-pulmonary shunt that can result in a significant rise in pulmonary blood flow and a fall in systemic blood flow. The increase in pulmonary blood flow through an immature pulmonary vascular bed can have a number of immediate and long-term consequences on the structure and function of the still developing cardiovascular and respiratory systems. This chapter addresses some of the short- and long-term respiratory consequences of patent ductus arteriosus (PDA) in preterm infants.

Why Does the Ductus Arteriosus Remain Open in Preterm Infants?

Although in most term infants the ductus arteriosus closes within hours after birth, in the very premature infant the ductus frequently closes considerably later or fails to undergo spontaneous closure. Part of the reason is the elevated sensitivity of the immature ductal tissue to the dilating effects of prostaglandins (PGs) and its low sensitivity to the constrictive effects of oxygen.[1] The more immature the infant the more striking the differences in sensitivity. As a result, the ductus of the smaller preterm infant can remain open for many days or weeks, and in many cases, even when it may constrict initially, it can reopen later. This reopening is frequently associated with clinical deterioration induced by an episode of systemic infection or other event associated with a systemic inflammatory response, such as pneumonia or necrotizing enterocolitis. The incidence of a PDA is also increased in infants who are exposed antenatally to magnesium sulfate administered to the mother to delay delivery or to treat hypertension[2]; persistency of ductal patency after indomethacin therapy has been observed in infants who were exposed to infection and inflammatory mediators before birth.[3]

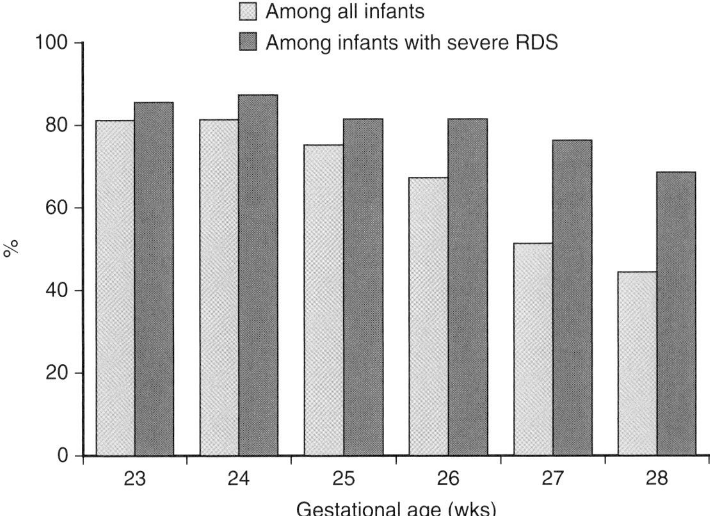

Figure 8-1 Incidence of patent ductus arteriosus (PDA) at University of Miami-Jackson Memorial Medical Center (UM-JMMC) from 2003-2009 in infants born at 28 or less weeks of gestation. Data show that the incidence of PDA is inversely related to gestational age as well as a higher incidence among infants with severe respiratory distress syndrome (RDS) (defined as the need for >30% inspired oxygen and for mechanical ventilation during days 1 to 3).

The incidence of a PDA is inversely related to gestational age and this relationship is even more striking in preterm infants with respiratory failure (Fig. 8-1). Some statistics indicate that more than 70% of preterm infants born before 28 weeks of gestation are exposed to therapeutic interventions to close the PDA and that decreased efficacy of such medical treatment at earlier gestational ages leads to a greater need for surgical ligation (Fig. 8-2).[4]

Despite multiple studies evaluating the effects of antenatal corticosteroids on neonatal outcomes, only a few have evaluated the effect of these agents on the PDA.

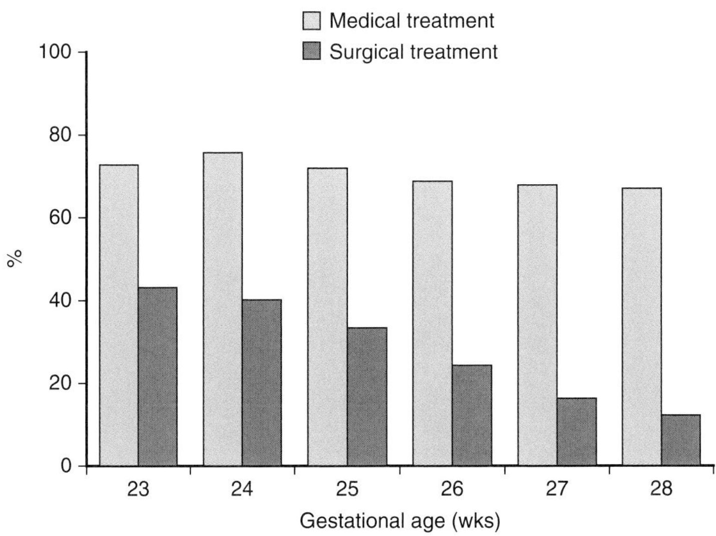

Figure 8-2 Treatment of patent ductus arteriosus (PDA) in the National Institute of Child Health and Human Development (NICHD) neonatal research network from 2003 to 2007. Data show that more than 70% of all infants with PDA received medical treatment at relatively constant rates for all gestational ages. The need for surgical ligation of the PDA was higher among infants of lower gestational age. (From Stoll BJ, Hansen NI, Bell EF, et al. Neonatal outcomes of extremely preterm infants from the NICHD Neonatal Research Network. *Pediatrics.* 2010;126:443-456.)

Evidence in experimental animals demonstrates a constrictive effect of glucocorticoids on the ductus and an increased responsiveness of the ductal muscle to oxygen.[5,6] When premature infants were exposed to corticosteroids at least 24 hours prior to preterm delivery, the incidence of symptomatic PDA and PDA requiring treatment was significantly reduced.[7-9] This effect was not observed when the steroids were administered to the mother less than 24 hours before delivery. There is also an association between lower cortisol levels in preterm infants during the first week after birth and a higher incidence of PDA.[10] This finding may be explained by the fact that cortisol decreases the sensitivity of the ductal tissue to the dilatory effects of PGs.

Surfactant Treatment and PDA

With the introduction of exogenous surfactant therapy, the clinical presentation and incidence of PDA in premature infants with respiratory distress syndrome (RDS) have been modified. Whereas surfactant itself has no effect on ductal contractility, the rapid improvement in Pa_{O_2} observed after surfactant administration can result in a rapid fall in pulmonary vascular resistance, producing an earlier clinical presentation of PDA in preterm infants and in experimental animals.[11-15] This finding may explain the observation in a meta-analysis of several randomized trials that prophylactic administration of synthetic surfactant seems to increase the incidence of symptomatic PDA[16] as well as the possible association between surfactant administration and the development of pulmonary hemorrhage in infants with left-to-right ductal shunting.[13,17,18] There is also a relationship between a large ductal diameter with significant shunting and pulmonary hemorrhage.[19,20] Data from trials of exogenous administration of surfactant, when pooled, demonstrate an increased rate of symptomatic PDA and a higher risk of pulmonary hemorrhage, a serious complication that is associated with both significant mortality and an increased risk of chronic respiratory morbidity.[21-23]

Systemic Consequences of PDA

The consequences of PDA in preterm infants depend on the size of the ductus and the magnitude of left-to-right shunting. The latter is determined by the difference in pressures between the systemic and pulmonary circulations. The left-to-right shunting results in increased pulmonary blood flow, volume overload of the left heart chambers, and decreases in systemic flow and perfusion. Although the left ventricle has the ability to increase its output, systemic blood flow distribution may be compromised by the decline in diastolic blood pressure as well as local vasoconstriction in different organs,[24] resulting in decreased organ perfusion. This may explain many of the systemic manifestations of a significant PDA, such as renal dysfunction, poor gastrointestinal function, and necrotizing enterocolitis.[25,26] A significant PDA can also compromise cerebral blood flow, producing ischemia and contributing to the development of brain injury.[27,28]

Pulmonary Consequences of PDA

Acute Effects

Premature birth is frequently complicated by respiratory failure due to inadequate surfactant with or without pneumonia. The increased pulmonary blood flow from ductal shunting can have a significant negative effect on the underlying disease process; in fact, delayed recovery from the initial respiratory failure has been reported in infants with PDA.[29-34] Because low plasma oncotic pressure and increased capillary permeability are common in premature infants with respiratory distress, the increase in pulmonary blood flow and microvascular pressure can lead to increased interstitial and alveolar edema.[35] Initially there is a compensatory increase in pulmonary lymph flow,[36] so that a patent ductus may not have a major hemodynamic effect during the first 24 to 72 hours. However, if the ductus remains patent beyond this time, with ductal flow increasing because of the falling pulmonary vascular resistance, the likelihood of edema increases significantly along with alterations in lung mechanics and gas exchange.[37,38] In a group of premature infants who underwent surgical ligation of PDA, a rapid improvement in lung compliance was reported and was found to be most striking among those infants with worse baseline lung mechanics.[39] Similar improvement in lung mechanics was also reported in infants with respiratory distress when the ductus was closed with indomethacin.[40,41] In comparison with infants with asymptomatic PDA and infants with spontaneous ductal closure, infants requiring treatment for symptomatic PDA had lower dynamic lung compliance and required respiratory support with higher mean airway pressures.[42] The lower compliance and increased pulmonary resistance in infants with significant PDA explains why many of these infants have hypoventilation and hypercarbia and require higher ventilator settings to maintain arterial blood gas levels.

Infants with a significant increase in pulmonary blood flow often demonstrate pulmonary edema that in more severe cases can lead to hemorrhagic pulmonary edema, which can manifest as frank pulmonary hemorrhage, frequently resulting in a dramatic deterioration in respiratory function and gas exchange.

PDA and Lung Inflammation

A new understanding of the development of bronchopulmonary dysplasia (BPD) has been its association with evidence of a significant inflammatory response in the airways and in the lung tissue.[43,44] Infants in whom BPD develops have been found to have elevated values of various cytokines, lipid mediators, and inflammatory cells, which may be implicated in the pathogenesis.[45,46] Infants and experimental animals with infection have increased levels of cytokines and inflammatory cells in blood and in bronchoalveolar lavage fluid.[47,48] Of interest, elevated tumor necrosis factor-α (TNF-α) values were observed in infants with sepsis and with PDA, particularly when both sepsis and PDA were temporally related.[49] Because TNF-α induces sequestration of neutrophils in the lungs, elevated TNF-α values can result in pulmonary vascular injury and edema, whereas the subsequent inflammatory response and vascular damage associated with elevated TNF-α levels may exacerbate the pulmonary edema that results from the increased pulmonary capillary pressure produced by the PDA.

Infants with pulmonary hemorrhage were found to have increased levels of lung inflammatory cytokines and monocyte chemoattractant chemokines.[50] However, it is not known whether the increase in inflammatory cytokines and chemokines results from the hemorrhage itself or is a consequence of the greater pulmonary blood flow. Among those infants in whom pulmonary hemorrhage developed, there was a higher incidence of PDA and they were more likely to require supplemental oxygen at 28 days of life and at 36 weeks postmenstrual age (PMA).

Activated neutrophils are also associated with inflammation. They induce free radical formation, catalyzed by the enzyme myeloperoxidase (MPO), generating hypochlorides, that can produce surfactant dysfunction and lung tissue injury. In a study of infants with RDS, PDA closure with indomethacin was found to be associated with a decline in myeloperoxidase in the tracheoalveolar fluid (TAF),[51] and a reduction in serum and tracheoalveolar fluid polymorphonuclear leukocytes.[52] Platelet-activating factor (PAF) can increase pulmonary vascular resistance[53-55] and induce airway constriction.[56,57] Increased levels of platelet-activating factor have been found in tracheal aspirates of infants with BPD.[58] Of interest, a study in a small group of infants reported increased levels of platelet-activating factor during symptomatic PDA.[59]

Evidence that early adrenal insufficiency is associated with lung inflammation and increased incidence of PDA and BPD was reported by Watterberg and colleagues.[10] In this study, cortisol levels in the first week of life were lower in infants with PDA. In addition, cortisol levels correlated inversely with levels of tracheal interleukins and proteins, signs of increased lung inflammation and microvascular protein leak. In fact, infants who had lower cortisol levels required prolonged supplemental oxygen and had an increased incidence of BPD. Whereas glucocorticoids can affect PDA closure, cortisol plays a central role in the ability of the body to attenuate its response to inflammation; cortisol is also a potent inhibitor of inflammatory edema.[60-63] These findings suggest that early adrenal insufficiency may be an explanation for the association of PDA, increased lung inflammation, and adverse respiratory outcome. Inadequate adrenal function associated with a higher incidence of PDA and increased susceptibility to lung inflammation, protein leak, edema, and possibly infection may play an important role in the development of BPD.

Long-Term Consequences

Effects of Increased Pulmonary Blood Flow on Vascular and Alveolar Development

Although the patency of the ductus in the fetus protects the developing pulmonary circulation from overflow, the persistence of ductal patency after birth exposes the pulmonary vessels to higher driving pressures and excessive blood flow, which can negatively affect the development of the pulmonary vasculature. Lung injury in the premature infant is not limited only to air spaces and conducting airways but also includes the immature pulmonary vasculature, and in fact, inadequate structural development and function of the pulmonary vessels are major features of BPD.[64]

Constriction of the ductus arteriosus in utero results in an increase in blood flow through the pulmonary vessels and exposure to higher vascular pressure. This condition can be a consequence of antenatal exposure to PG inhibitors.[65,66] Vascular remodeling resulting in a postnatal increase in pulmonary vascular resistance[67,68] and alterations in alveolar development can be caused by elevated blood flow through an immature pulmonary bed.[69-71] In experimental animal models of surgical aortopulmonary shunts, significant postnatal pulmonary hypertension and increased reactivity of the pulmonary vessels were found.[72]

When fetuses were exposed to indomethacin in utero, the result was a decreased effectiveness of prostaglandin inhibitor therapy for ductal closure after birth.[73-75] In fact, an increase in respiratory morbidity and BPD has been reported after maternal indomethacin administration for tocolysis.[76-78] It is important to note that the studies reporting these findings included not only extremely low-birth-weight infants, but also infants born at more advanced gestations. Characteristic of more mature infants is a lower risk of respiratory morbidity; however, the fetal ductus in infants of more advanced gestations is actually more sensitive to the effects of in utero PG inhibition.[79,80] Therefore the increased pulmonary blood flow in the more mature fetus produced by antenatal indomethacin may raise the risk of respiratory morbidity among these more mature infants, who would otherwise not have significant respiratory disease.

The presence of a systemic-to-pulmonary communication after birth results in an increase in blood flow through an immature pulmonary vascular bed that can produce marked vascular lesions with intimal fibrosis and medial hypertrophy.[81,82] Significant anatomic changes in the small pulmonary arteries are observed in experimental animals after exposure to high concentrations of inspired oxygen and increased pulmonary blood flow that result in an increase in pulmonary vascular resistance and abnormal vasoreactivity.[83,84] Similar features are commonly observed in infants with severe BPD who have experienced prolonged supplemental oxygen exposure and hemodynamically significant PDA.[85-88]

In addition, examination of the lung vasculature that has been exposed to greater shear and stretch has shown profound alterations in pulmonary vascular bed structure and cellular function. Endothelial injury occurs secondary to the increase in blood flow or pressure and results in disruption of the regulation of pulmonary vascular tone and growth. When experimental animals were exposed to increased pulmonary blood flow and hypertension, they showed alteration of the genetic regulatory cascade of endothelin-1 (ET-1).[89] In fact, preterm infants in whom BPD developed had elevated values of endothelin-1 in tracheoalveolar fluid early after birth,[90] a finding that correlated with an increase in the pro-inflammatory cytokine interleukin-8. Of note, infants with severe pulmonary hypertension have also been found to have elevated endothelin-1 values.[91]

Both vascular endothelial growth factor (VEGF) and transforming growth factor-β (TGF-β) are key to lung development and function. Whereas VEGF is a cell specific mediator of angiogenesis and vasculogenesis, TGF-β regulates cell growth and differentiation in the airways and pulmonary vasculature. Fetal lambs with increased pulmonary blood flow and hypertension show reduced VEGF expression shortly after birth.[92] Reduced expression of VEGF is also seen in preterm infants with severe RDS and in infants with BPD.[93,94] Unlike VEGF expression, TGF-β expression is increased in animals exposed to increased pulmonary blood flow[95] and in infants with BPD.[96,97] Thus, expressions of both VEGF and TGF-β are affected by increased pulmonary blood flow and intravascular pressure, which may play a significant role in lung morphologic and functional alterations.

Studies in preterm baboons support the deleterious effect of increased pulmonary blood flow on lung development. Preterm baboons that underwent early pharmacologic closure of the PDA with ibuprofen at day 3 were found to have better alveolar development and improved alveolar surface area than animals in whom the PDA remained open.[98] Interestingly, and perhaps paradoxically, this advantage in lung development was not observed in animals undergoing surgical PDA closure on day 6.[99]

PDA and Bronchopulmonary Dysplasia

Despite the strong experimental evidence that increased flow and pressure in the developing pulmonary vasculature can produce severe morphologic and functional alterations in the immature lung, there is still no conclusive evidence regarding the role of PDA in the pathogenesis of BPD. The respiratory morbidity associated with a PDA is caused not only by the increase in pulmonary blood flow and edema as well as indicators of lung inflammation; in addition, most premature infants presenting with symptomatic PDA require mechanical ventilation and/or supplemental oxygen. For this reason infants with PDA are exposed to multiple factors that increase the risk of lung injury, and these factors become important confounders in the reported association between PDA and increased risk for BPD.[49,100,101] The negative effects of PDA on lung function were documented by Cotton and associates[102] with the demonstration of a longer duration of mechanical ventilation in infants with symptomatic PDA than in those without PDA.[102] In addition, these researchers reported a decreased duration of mechanical ventilation with early surgical PDA closure.[103] A subsequent trial of early pharmacologic PDA closure with indomethacin also revealed a reduction in incidence of BPD.[104]

From an epidemiologic standpoint, several studies have found a rising incidence of BPD with increased survival of extremely preterm infants, many of whom actually had mild or no initial RDS.[105-109] Of extremely low-birth-weight infants in whom BPD develop, a significant proportion actually come from this subgroup of “low-risk” infants who were not exposed initially to high inspired oxygen concentrations and positive-pressure ventilation, both of which are well-established risk factors for BPD. Multivariate logistic analysis showed an increased risk of BPD in infants with symptomatic PDA and episodes of sepsis.[101] Interestingly, the BPD risk was even greater when the PDA and sepsis occurred simultaneously, suggesting an interaction between these two events. Also associated with marked increase in BPD risk were the occurrence of symptomatic PDA after the first week and a longer duration of symptomatic PDA (Fig. 8-3).

This interaction of a symptomatic PDA and infection was evaluated in preterm infants born at less than 1000 g in another prospective study.[49] Results indicated that episodes of late PDA reopening were more frequent in infected infants; in addition, there was an elevated risk for failed PDA closure when sepsis and PDA were temporally related. As in the previous study, the BPD risk was increased by PDA and by sepsis and more strikingly when the two occurred simultaneously. It has been reported that infants with infection and those with PDA had higher levels of

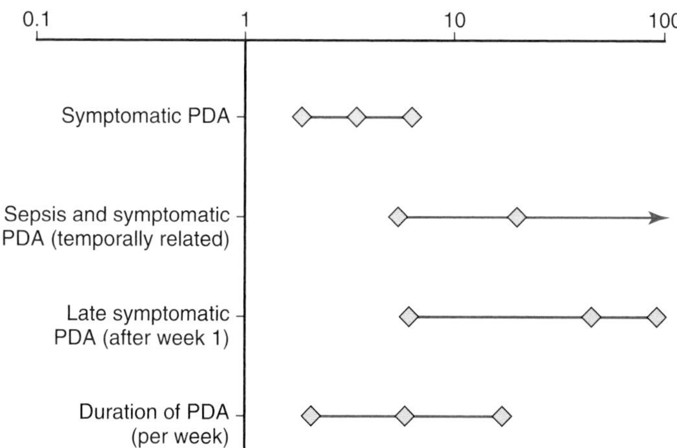

Figure 8-3 Odds ratios for development of bronchopulmonary dysplasia (BPD). Multivariate logistic regression analysis shows increased risk for development of BPD with the occurrence of patent ductus arteriosus (PDA), with PDA that is temporally related to sepsis, with symptomatic PDA lasting more than 1 week, and with the duration of PDA. (From Rojas MA, Gonzalez A, Bancalari E, et al. Changing trends in the epidemiology and pathogenesis of neonatal chronic lung disease. *J Pediatr.* 1995;126: 605-610.)

6-ketoprostaglandin F1α as well as elevated values of TNF-α. Elevated values of 6-ketoprostaglandin F1α in infected infants were found to be associated with increased rate of late PDA and unresponsiveness to indomethacin.[3] These data indicate that infection adversely influences PDA outcome by increasing the risk of ductal reopening and failure of closure.[110-115] These findings have been confirmed in larger population-based studies of very low-birth-weight infants born in the post-surfactant era.[116,117] These two studies also suggested a role for PDA in the pathogenesis of BPD, particularly in infected infants.

Despite the experimental and epidemiologic evidence supporting the role of the PDA in the pathogenesis of lung injury, there are scarce data from prospective clinical trials to confirm this association.

Management of PDA and Respiratory Outcome

Different strategies to close the PDA have been investigated in an attempt to reduce its adverse consequences. Clearly, closure of the PDA by surgical or pharmacologic means is associated with rapid improvement in lung mechanics.[39-41] Several randomized trials have compared early PDA closure with delayed treatment—that is, treatment given when signs of left heart failure are present. Even when the time difference between early and late closure was relatively small, six of eight studies demonstrated that early PDA closure was associated with decreased pulmonary morbidity.[104,118-124] When Clyman[125] conducted a meta-analysis of these studies, results indicated that infants who received early PDA treatment were at lower risk of BPD and had shorter duration of mechanical ventilation than those receiving delayed treatment. In contrast, Van Overmeire and colleagues[126] did not find significant differences in respiratory outcome between infants with RDS and PDA who received indomethacin "early" (on day 3 ± 0.5) and "late" (on day 7 ± 1.7). However, in this study infants were relatively mature and half of the patients in the "late" treatment group had spontaneous PDA closure by day 9, suggesting that even the late-treated infants were not exposed to the effects of the PDA for very long.

Prophylactic indomethacin for the prevention of PDA has been extensively investigated.[127-133] In most of these studies prophylactic indomethacin was started on the first day after birth, even before the onset of PDA symptoms. As expected, most of these reports found a significant reduction in the incidence of PDA and need for surgical ligation with indomethacin prophylaxis. Surprisingly, the most dramatic effect of prophylactic indomethacin was a reduction in incidence of severe intracranial hemorrhage. However, in terms of pulmonary outcome, pooled data from two meta-analyses failed to demonstrate a decrease in long-term pulmonary morbidity when prophylactic indomethacin treatment (given prior to PDA symptoms) was compared with later treatment (given after the PDA became symptomatic).[125,134] It is important to note that most infants randomly assigned to the control arms of these trials were exposed to a relatively short period of increased pulmonary blood flow because indomethacin was administered soon after the symptoms of PDA appeared. Because the effects of PDA on pulmonary outcome appear to be related to the duration of ductal patency, the relatively early PDA closure in the control groups may have protected against further lung damage. Another explanation for the findings is that the potential benefits of early PDA closure may have been negated by the detrimental effects of indomethacin on renal function and fluid retention,[135] which contributed to deterioration in lung function, particularly in those infants who did not have PDA but still received prophylactic indomethacin. A meta-analysis of six randomized controlled trials comparing ibuprofen with indomethacin for PDA closure showed that PDA treatment with intravenous ibuprofen after 24 hours of life was associated with a higher risk of BPD than treatment using indomethacin (relative risk [RR] 1.28; 95% confidence interval [CI] 1.03-1.60.[136] However, no significant difference in BPD incidence was found between infants who received indomethacin and those who received placebo.

B

In an extensive analysis of the literature, Benitz[137] concluded that there was no clear evidence that routine medical or surgical closure of the ductus was beneficial in preterm infants. However this conclusion is not entirely supported by the results of the review that showed a significant decrease in death or chronic lung disease in infants who received early treatment in comparison with those treated late for symptomatic PDA.

The main argument of those proposing a conservative approach to interventions to close the PDA is the fact that in many cases, the ductus will close spontaneously, and waiting for spontaneous closure prevents the unnecessary use of drugs or surgery, both of which are associated with significant complications. However, the spontaneous PDA closure rate depends on gestational age, being much lower in the infant with birth weight less than 1000 g, who is at higher risk of severe BPD. There is no experimental or clinical evidence that the persistence of an open ductus confers any benefit in the clinical course of premature infants. Therefore, the risk:benefit ratio must be measured in each individual case; in other words, the possible negative consequences of a persistent open ductus must be measured against the complications associated with the interventions to close it. Without definitive data, the approach to PDA treatment must be addressed for the individual infant, with the gestational age, clinical course, size, and hemodynamic consequences of the ductal shunt as well as the potential side effects of the interventions to close the PDA taken into account.

Most infants who have PDA and experience BPD are extremely premature, but surprisingly few studies have focused their analysis on this population. When Mahony and associates[120] compared the effects of early and late medical treatment of PDA, early treatment did not result in a lower oxygen dependency in the overall population. However, stratified birth weight analysis showed early treatment was associated with a significantly shorter duration of oxygen need in infants with birth weight less than 1000 grams.

Studies that evaluated the effect of short versus prolonged indomethacin therapy did not show consistent effects on PDA closure or on respiratory outcome, but the strategies that have led to more effective PDA closure also resulted in lower respiratory morbidity.[138-140]

As mentioned previously, sepsis negatively influences PDA as a result of many factors. Sepsis can induce ductal reopening, is associated with treatment failure, and can also interfere with PDA management because septic infants often have associated complications such as thrombocytopenia and renal failure, which may be considered contraindications to surgical or pharmacologic intervention.

When pharmacologic treatment is contraindicated or fails, surgical ligation of the PDA is generally used as a second alternative. As with medical treatment, the potential benefits of surgical closure must be weighed against potential side effects of the surgical procedure. The effect of surgical PDA closure on lung mechanics is an immediate improvement, with a rapid increase in compliance[39] most likely due to the sudden reduction in pulmonary blood flow, blood volume, and interstitial lung fluid. Despite these positive hemodynamic and pulmonary changes from surgical PDA ligation, a significant number of infants suffer a deterioration in clinical condition following surgery.[141,142] This deterioration, manifested by higher inspired oxygen requirement and arterial hypotension, occurs mostly in smaller infants who had prolonged PDA.[143,144] The mechanisms for this deterioration may be related to surgical trauma, to left ventricular dysfunction due to immediate increase in afterload, or to sudden reduction in pulmonary blood flow after ductal closure.[145]

Because no trials have compared continued medical management of hemodynamically significant PDA with surgical closure when medical management has been ineffective, the benefits and side effects of surgical ligation on respiratory function remain unclear. However, reports have suggested significantly worse neurologic and pulmonary outcomes in infants who underwent PDA ligation than in those who had successful pharmacologic closure or needed no treatment.[146-148] A number of other complications have been associated with PDA ligation, all of which can be associated with an increase in respiratory morbidity, including compromised cerebral oxygen supply, diaphragmatic paralysis due to phrenic nerve injury, chylothorax, scoliosis, and vocal cord paralysis.[149-151]

In a 2007 reanalysis of the results of a randomized controlled clinical trial done many years ago to compare early PDA ligation with expectant management, Clyman and associates[146] found that infants who underwent PDA ligation during the first days of life had almost a threefold higher risk for development of BPD than the controls.

An interesting observation published recently by Schmidt and coworkers[152] showed that caffeine, administered to decrease apnea and favor successful weaning from mechanical ventilation in premature infants, was found to lower the incidence of PDA, decrease the need for PDA ligation, and also decrease the incidence of BPD in comparison with placebo. The mechanisms for these beneficial effects are not clear, but in addition to stimulating central respiratory activity, caffeine may be functioning through its weak diuretic effect or through its anti-inflammatory properties.

Thus, the persistence of a PDA in a preterm infant can be associated with acute and long-term deleterious effects on lung development and function. Strong epidemiologic data suggest that a long-lasting PDA is correlated with increased risk of BPD; however, the few prospective clinical trials of ductal closure have failed to confirm this association. Although the effects of the ductus on lung development and function are likely related to the size of the ductus and duration and magnitude of left-to-right shunting, few of the studies have evaluated these parameters, underscoring the need for additional large randomized trials to evaluate the effect of different PDA management strategies on respiratory, cardiovascular, and neurologic outcomes.

Respiratory Management of Infants with PDA

Ductal patency does not have a significant effect on the respiratory system shortly after birth,[125] but as the pulmonary vascular resistance declines during the first hours, left-to-right shunting increases; it is at this time that infants often show deterioration in lung function requiring increased respiratory support. A very common finding in these infants is an increase in arterial carbon dioxide tension requiring higher ventilator rates and peak airway pressures. A possible mechanism for this observation is that elevations of circulating PGE_2 that induce ductal patency may also lead to inhibition of the respiratory center, contributing to the hypoventilation.[153,154]

A common strategy used to attempt to reduce the left-to-right ductal shunting consists of an increase in positive end-expiratory pressure (PEEP). In animal models of hyaline membrane disease, institution of PEEP reduced the left-to-right ductal flow.[155] In addition, higher PEEP is thought to prevent alveolar and small airway closure and severe pulmonary edema, although actual data on the effects of this intervention are lacking and the possible benefits of a higher PEEP in preterm infants could be offset by the negative effects on cardiac function, venous return, and respiratory mechanics. In a study to evaluate the hemodynamic effects of different levels of PEEP in infants with a symptomatic PDA, Fajaro and coworkers[156] showed that the application of a higher level of PEEP did not consistently reduce ductal left-to-right shunting.

Regarding oxygenation, there are opposite effects of an increase or decrease in oxygen tension on the ductus and the pulmonary vasculature. Ductal patency is to some extent the result of a reduced sensitivity of the ductal tissue to oxygen. Although a rise in alveolar oxygen tension can increase left-to-right ductal shunting through a reduction in pulmonary vascular resistance, it simultaneously can produce constriction of the ductus arteriosus and reduce the shunt.[157] Therefore changes in oxygenation can have opposite effects, with higher Pao_2 favoring PDA closure but at the same time reducing pulmonary vascular resistance and increasing left-to-right shunting if the ductus remains open.

Summary

Persistent ductus arteriosus is a very common event in preterm infants. The greater pulmonary blood flow due to systemic-to-pulmonary shunting that occurs as the pulmonary vascular resistance decreases after birth can have significant negative cardiovascular and respiratory consequences. Acute pulmonary effects include pulmonary edema and occasionally pulmonary hemorrhage, worsening lung mechanics, and deterioration in gas exchange with hypoxemia and hypercapnia. The increased pulmonary blood flow can also damage the immature capillary endothelium and trigger an inflammatory cascade within the lung that can lead to reduced alveolar and capillary formation. These pathologic effects, plus the need for longer and more aggressive mechanical ventilation, can explain the reported association between a hemodynamically significant PDA and an increased risk for BPD in extremely premature infants.

References

1. Clyman RI. Mechanisms regulating the ductus arteriosus. *Biol Neonate*. 2006;89:330-335.
2. del Moral T, Gonzalez-Quintero VH, Claure N, et al. Antenatal exposure to magnesium sulfate and the incidence of patent ductus arteriosus in extremely low birth weight infants. *J Perinatol*. 2007;27:154-157.
3. Kim ES, Kim EK, Choi CW, et al. Intrauterine inflammation as a risk factor for persistent ductus arteriosus patency after cyclooxygenase inhibition in extremely low birth weight infants. *J Pediatr*. 2010;157:745-750.
4. Stoll BJ, Hansen NI, Bell EF, et al. Neonatal outcomes of extremely preterm infants from the NICHD Neonatal Research Network. *Pediatrics*. 2010;126:443-456.
5. Momma K, Nishihara S, Ota Y. Constriction of the fetal ductus by glucocorticoid hormones. *Pediatr Res*. 1981;15:19-21.
6. Clyman RI, Mauray F, Roman C, et al. Glucocorticoids alter the sensitivity of the lamb ductus arteriosus to prostaglandin E2. *J Pediatr*. 1981;98:126-128.
7. Clyman RI, Ballard PL, Sniderman S, et al. Prenatal administration of betamethasone for prevention of patent ductus arteriosus. *J Pediatr*. 1981;98:123-126.
8. Waffarn F, Siassi B, Cabal LA, Schmidt PL. Effect of antenatal glucocorticoids on the clinical closure of the ductus arteriosus. *Am J Dis Child*. 1983;137:336-338.
9. Morales WJ, Angel JL, O'Brien WF, Knuppel RA. Use of ampicillin and corticosteroids in premature rupture of membranes: a randomized study. *Obstet Gynecol*. 1989;73:721-726.
10. Watterberg KL, Scott S, Backstrom C, et al. Links between early adrenal function and respiratory outcome in preterm infants: airway inflammation and patent ductus arteriosus. *Pediatrics*. 2000;105:320-324.
11. Shimada S, Raju TNK, Bhat R, et al. Treatment of patent ductus arteriosus after exogenous surfactant in baboons with hyaline membrane disease. *Pediatr Res*. 1989;26:565-569.
12. Clyman RI, Jobe A, Heymann MA, et al. Increased shunt through the patent ductus arteriosus after surfactant replacement therapy. *J Pediatr*. 1982;100:101-107.
13. Kaapa P, Seppanen M, Kero P, Saraste M. Pulmonary hemodynamics after synthetic surfactant replacement in neonatal respiratory distress syndrome. *J Pediatr*. 1993;123:115-119.
14. Reller MD, Buffkin DC, Colasurdo MA, et al. Ductal patency in neonates with respiratory distress syndrome: a randomized surfactant trial. *Am J Dis Child*. 1991;145:1017-1020.

15. Reller MD, Rice MJ, McDonald RW. Review of studies evaluating ductal patency in the premature infant. *J Pediatr*. 1993;122:S59-S62.
16. Soll RF. Prophylactic synthetic surfactant for preventing morbidity and mortality in preterm infants. *Cochrane Database Syst Rev*. 2010;(1):CD001079.
17. Clyman RI, Jobe A, Heymann MA, et al. Increased shunt through the patent ductus arteriosus after surfactant replacement therapy. *J Pediatr*. 1982;100:101-107.
18. Garland J, Buck R, Weinberg M. Pulmonary hemorrhage risk in infants with a clinically diagnosed patent ductus arteriosus: a retrospective cohort study. *Pediatrics*. 1994;94:719-723.
19. Kluckow M, Evans N. Ductal shunting, high pulmonary blood flow, and pulmonary hemorrhage. *J Pediatr*. 2000;137:68-72.
20. Gonzalez A, Hummler H, Sosenko I, et al. Surfactant administration, patent ductus arteriosus and pulmonary hemorrhage in premature infants <1000 g. *Pediatr Res*. 1994;35:227A.
21. Raju TNK, Langenberg P. Pulmonary hemorrhage and exogenous surfactant therapy: a metaanalysis. *J Pediatr*. 1993;123:606-610.
22. Pappin A, Shenker N, Hack M, Redline RW. Extensive intraalveolar pulmonary hemorrhage in infants dying after surfactant therapy. *J Pediatr*. 1994;124:621-626.
23. Pandit PB, O'Brien K, Asztalos E, et al. Outcome following pulmonary hemorrhage in very low birthweight neonates treated with surfactant. *Arch Dis Child Fetal Neonatal Ed*. 1999;81: F40-F44.
24. Shimada S, Kasai T, Hoshi A, et al. Cardiocirculatory effects of patent ductus arteriosus in extremely low-birth-weight infants with respiratory distress syndrome. *Pediatr Int*. 2003;45:255-262.
25. Shimada S, Kasai T, Konishi M, Fujiwara T. Effects of patent ductus arteriosus on left ventricular output and organ blood flows in preterm infants with respiratory distress syndrome treated with surfactant. *J Pediatr*. 1994;125:270-277.
26. Meyers RL, Alpan G, Lin E, Clyman RI. Patent ductus arteriosus, indomethacin, and intestinal distension: effects on intestinal blood flow and oxygen consumption. *Pediatr Res*. 1991;29: 569-574.
27. Martin CG, Snider AR, Katz SM, et al. Abnormal cerebral blood flow patterns in preterm infants with large patent ductus arteriosus. *J Pediatr*. 1982;101:587-593,
28. Perlman JM, Hill A, Volpe J. The effect of patent ductus arteriosus on flow velocity in the anterior cerebral arteries: ductal steal in the premature infant. *J Pediatr*. 1981;99:767-771.
29. Thibeault DW, Emmanouilides GC, Nelson R et al. Patent ductus arteriosus complicating the respiratory distress syndrome in preterm infants. *J Pediatr*. 1975;86:120-126.
30. Dudell GG, Gersony WM. Patent ductus arteriosus in neonates with severe respiratory disease. *J Pediatr*. 1984;104:915-920.
31. Jacob J, Gluck L, DiSessa T, et al. The contribution of PDA in the neonate with severe RDS. *J Pediatr*. 1980;96:79-87.
32. Kitterman JA, Edmunds LH, Gregory GA, et al. Patent ductus arteriosus in premature infants. Incidence, relation to pulmonary disease and management. *N Engl J Med*. 1972;287:473-477.
33. Neal WA, Bessinger FB Jr, Hunt CE, Lucas RV Jr. Patent ductus arteriosus complicating respiratory distress syndrome. *J Pediatr*. 1975;86:127-132.
34. Siassi B, Emmanouilides GC, Cleveland RJ, Hirose F. Patent ductus arteriosus complicating prolonged assisted ventilation in respiratory distress syndrome. *J Pediatr*. 1969;74:11-19.
35. Alpan G, Scheerer R, Bland R, Clyman R. Patent ductus arteriosus increases lung fluid filtration in preterm lambs. *Pediatr Res*. 1991;30:616-621.
36. Alpan G, Mauray F, Clyman RI. Effect of patent ductus arteriosus on water accumulation and protein permeability in the premature lungs of mechanically ventilated premature lambs. *Pediatr Res*. 1989;26:570-575.
37. Perez Fontan JJ, Clyman RI, Mauray F, et al. Respiratory effects of a patent ductus arteriosus in premature newborn lambs. *J Appl Physiol*. 1987;63:2315-2324.
38. Krauss AN, Fatica N, Lewis BS, et al. Pulmonary function in preterm infants following treatment with intravenous indomethacin. *Am J Dis Child*. 1989;143:78-81.
39. Gerhardt T, Bancalari E. Lung compliance in newborns with patent ductus arteriosus before and after surgical ligation. *Biol Neonate*. 1980;38:96-105.
40. Yeh TF, Thalji A, Luken L, et al. Improved lung compliance following indomethacin therapy in premature infants with persistent ductus arteriosus. *Chest*. 1981;80:698-700.
41. Stefano JL, Abbasi S, Pearlman SA, et al. Closure of the ductus arteriosus with indomethacin in ventilated neonates with respiratory distress syndrome: effects of pulmonary compliance and ventilation. *Am Rev Respir Dis*. 1991;143:236-239.
42. Heldt GP, Personen E, Merritt TA, et al. Closure of the ductus arteriosus and mechanics of breathing in preterm infants after surfactant replacement. *Pediatr Res*. 1989;25:305-310.
43. Speer CP. Inflammation and bronchopulmonary dysplasia. *Semin Neonatol*. 2003;8:29-38.
44. Jobe AH, Bancalari E. Bronchopulmonary dysplasia. *Am J Respir Crit Care Med*. 2001;163: 1723-1729.
45. Bagghi A, Viscardi RM, Taciak V, et al. Increased activity of interleukin-6 but not tumor necrosis factor-alpha in lung lavage of premature infants associated with the development of bronchopulmonary dysplasia. *Pediatr Res*. 1994;36:244-252.
46. Groneck P, Gotze-Speer B, Oppermann M, et al. Association of pulmonary inflammation and increased microvascular permeability during the development of bronchopulmonary dysplasia: A sequential analysis of inflammatory mediators in respiratory fluids of high-risk preterm neonates. *Pediatrics*. 1994;93:712-718.

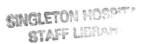

47. Girardin EP, Berner ME, Grau GE, et al. Serum tumor necrosis factor in newborns at risk for infections. *Eur J Pediatr*. 1990;149:645-647.
48. de Bont ES, Martens A, van Raan J, et al. Diagnostic value of tumor necrosis factor (TNF) and interleukin-6 (IL-6) in newborns with sepsis. *Acta Paediatr*. 1994;83:696-699.
49. Gonzalez A, Sosenko IR, Chandar J, et al. Influence of infection on patent ductus arteriosus and chronic lung disease in premature infants weighing 1000 grams or less. *J Pediatr*. 1996;128:470-478.
50. Baier RJ, Loggins J, Kruger TE. Increased interleukin-8 and monocyte chemoattractant protein-1 concentrations in mechanically ventilated preterm infants with pulmonary hemorrhage. *Pediatr Pulmonol*. 2002;34:131-137.
51. Varsilla E, Hallman M, Venge P, Andersson S. Closure of patent ductus arteriosus decreases pulmonary myeloperoxidase in premature infants with respiratory distress syndrome. *Biol Neonate*. 1995;67:167-171.
52. Nakamura T, Takasaki J, Ogawa Y. Inflammatory changes in the lungs of premature infants with symptomatic patent ductus arteriosus. *Pediatr Int*. 2002;44:363-367.
53. Hamasaki Y, Mojarad M, Saga H, et al. Platelet activating factor raises airway and systemic vascular pressure and induces edema in lungs perfused with platelet free solution. *Am Rev Respir Dis*. 1984;129:742-746.
54. Ibe BO, Hibler S, Raj JU. Platelet-activating factor modulates pulmonary vasomotor tone in the perinatal lamb. *J Appl Physiol*. 1998;85:1079-1085.
55. Clavijo LC, Carter MB, Matheson PJ, et al. PAF increases vascular permeability without increasing pulmonary arterial pressure in the rat. *J Appl Physiol*. 2001;90:261-268.
56. Cuss FM, Dixon CM, Barnes PJ. Effects of inhaled platelet activating factor on pulmonary function and bronchial responsiveness in man. *Lancet*. 1986;2:189-192.
57. Smith LJ, Rubin AH, Patterson R. Mechanism of platelet activating factor-induced bronchoconstriction in humans. *Am Rev Respir Dis*. 1988;137:1015-1019.
58. Stenmark KR, Eyzaguirre M, Wescott JY, et al. Potential role of eicosanoids and PAF in the pathophysiology of bronchopulmonary dysplasia. *Am Rev Respir Dis*. 1987;136:770-772.
59. Koyama N, Ogawa Y, Kamiya K, et al. Increased platelet activating factor in the tracheal aspirates from neonates with patent ductus arteriosus. *Clin Chim Acta*. 1993;215:73-79.
60. Munck A, Guyre PM, Holbrook NJ. Physiological functions of glucocorticoids in stress and their relation to pharmacological agents. *Endocr Rev*. 1984;5:25-44.
61. Chrousos GP The hypothalamic-pituitary-adrenal axis and immune-mediated inflammation. *N Engl J Med*. 1995;332:1351-1362.
62. Goujon E, Parnet P, Laye S, et al. Adrenalectomy enhances pro-inflammatory cytokines gene expression, in the spleen, pituitary and brain of mice in response to lipopolysaccharide. *Brain Res Mol Brain Res*. 1996;36:53-62.
63. Farsky SP, Sannomiya P, Garcia-Leme J. Secreted glucocorticoids regulate leukocyte-endothelial interactions in inflammation. A direct vital microscopic study. *J Leukoc Biol*. 1995;57:379-386.
64. Abman SH. Pulmonary hypertension in chronic lung disease of infancy. Pathogenesis, pathophysiology and treatment. In: Bland RD, Coalson JJ, eds. *Chronic lung disease of infancy*. New York: Dekker; 2000.
65. Heymann MA, Rudolph AM. Effects of acetylsalicylic acid on the ductus arteriosus and circulation in fetal lambs in utero. *Circ Res*. 1976;38:418-422.
66. Levin DL, Fixler DE, Morriss FC, Tyson J. Morphologic analysis of the pulmonary vascular bed in infants exposed in utero to prostaglandin synthetase inhibitors. *J Pediatr*. 1978;92:478-483.
67. Levin DL, Hyman AI, Heymann MA, Rudolph AM. Fetal hypertension and the development of increased pulmonary vascular smooth muscle: a possible mechanism for persistent pulmonary hypertension of the newborn infant. *J Pediatr*. 1978;92:265-269.
68. Morin FC. Ligation the ductus arteriosus before birth causes persistent pulmonary hypertension in the newborn lamb. *Ped Research*. 1989;25:245-250.
69. Demello D, Murphy JD, Aonowitz MJ, et al. Effects of indomethacin in utero on the pulmonary vasculature of the newborn guinea pig. *Pediatr Res*. 1987;22:693-697.
70. Herget J, Hampi V, Povysilova V, Slavik Z. Long-term effects of prenatal indomethacin administration on the pulmonary circulation in rats. *Eur Respir J*. 1995;8:209-215.
71. Bustos R, Ballejo G, Guissi G, et al. Inhibition of fetal lung maturation by indomethacin in pregnant rabbits. *J Perinat Med*. 1978;6:240-245.
72. Reddy VM, Meyrick B, Wong J, et al. Aortopulmonary shunts: in utero placement of aortopulmonary shunts: A model of postnatal pulmonary hypertension with increased pulmonary blood flow in lambs. *Circulation*. 1995;92:606-613.
73. Norton ME, Merril J, Cooper BA, et al. Neonatal complications after the administration of indomethacin for preterm labor. *N Engl J Med*. 1993;329:1602-1607.
74. Major CA, Lewis DF, Harding JA, et al. Tocolysis with indomethacin increases the incidence of necrotizing enterocolitis in the low birth weight neonate. *Am J Obstet Gynecol*. 1994;170:102-106.
75. Hammerman C, Glaser J, Kaplan M, et al. Indomethacin tocolysis increases postnatal patent ductus arteriosus. *Pediatrics*. 1998;102:1202-1205.
76. Eronen M, Psonen E, Kurki T, et al. Increased incidence of bronchopulmonary dysplasia after antenatal administration of indomethacin to prevent preterm labor. *J Pediatr*. 1994;124:782-788.
77. Van Overmeire B, Slootmaekers V, De Loor J, et al. The addition of indomethacin to betamimetics for tocolysis: any benefit for the neonate? Eur J Obstet Gynec *Reprod Biol*. 1998;77:41-45.

78. Panter KR, Hannah ME, Amankwah KS, et al. The effect of indomethacin tocolysis in preterm labor on perinatal outcome: a randomised placebo-controlled trial. *Br J Obstet Gynaec.* 1999;106: 467-473.
79. Moise KJ Jr. Effect of advancing gestational age on the frequency of fetal ductal constriction in association with maternal indomethacin use. *Am J Obstet Gynec.* 1993;168:1350-1353.
80. Van den Veyver IB, Moise KJ Jr, Ou CN, Carpenter RJ Jr. The effect of gestational age and fetal indomethacin levels on the incidence of constriction of the fetal ductus arteriosus. *Obstet Gynec.* 1993;82:500-503.
81. Broccard AF, Hotchkiss JR, Kuwayama N, et al. Consequences of vascular flow on lung injury induced by mechanical ventilation. *Am J Respir Crit Care Med.* 1998;157:1935-1942.
82. Corno AF, Tozzi P, Genton CY, von Segesser LK. Surgically induced unilateral pulmonary hypertension: time related analysis of a new experimental model. *Eur Resp J Cardiothorac Surg.* 2003;23:513-517.
83. Jones R, Zapol WM, Reid LM. Pulmonary artery remodeling and pulmonary hypertension after exposure to hyperoxia for 7 days. *Am J Pathol.* 1984;117:273-285.
84. Jones R, Jacobson M, Steudel W. Alpha smooth muscle actin and microvascular precursor smooth muscle cells in pulmonary hypertension. *Am J Respir Cell Mol Bio.* 1999;20:582-594.
85. Hislop AA, Haworth SG. Pulmonary vascular damage and the development of cor pulmonale following hyaline membrane disease. *Pediatr Pulmonol.* 1990;9:152-161.
86. Goodman G, Perkin RM, Anas NG, et al. Pulmonary hypertension in infants with bronchopulmonary dysplasia. *J Pediatr.* 1988;112:67-72.
87. Halliday HL, Dumpit FM, Brady JP. Effects of inspired oxygen on echocardiographic assessment of pulmonary vascular resistance and myocardial contractility in BPD. *Pediatrics.* 1980;65:536-540.
88. Abman SH, Wolfe RR, Accurso FJ, et al. Pulmonary vascular response to oxygen in infants with severe bronchopulmonary dysplasia. *Pediatrics.* 1985;75:80-84.
89. Black SM, Bekker JM, Johengen MJ, et al. Altered regulation of the ET-1 cascade in lambs with increased pulmonary blood flow and pulmonary hypertension. *Ped Research.* 2000;47:97-106.
90. Niu JO, Mushi UK, Siddiq MM, Parton LA. Early increase in endothelin-1 in tracheal aspirates of preterm infants: Correlation with bronchopulmonary dysplasia. *J Pediatr.* 1998;132:965-970.
91. Rosenberg AA, Kennaugh J, Koppenhafer SL, et al. Elevated immunoreactive endothelin-1 levels in newborns with persistent pulmonary hypertension. *J Pediatr.* 1993;123:109-114.
92. Grover TR, Parker TA, Zenge JP, et al. Intrauterine hypertension decreases lung VEGF expression and VEGF inhibition causes pulmonary hypertension in the ovine fetus. *Am J Physiol Lung Cell Mol Physiol.* 2003;284:L508-L517.
93. Bhatt AJ, Pryhuber GS, Huyck H, et al. Disrupted pulmonary vasculature and decreased vascular endothelial growth factor, Flt-1, and TIE-2 in human infants dying with bronchopulmonary dysplasia. *Am J Respir Crit Care Med.* 2001;164:1971-1980.
94. Lassus P, Turanlahti M, Heikkila P, et al. Pulmonary vascular endothelial growth factor and Flt-1 in fetuses, in acute and chronic lung disease, and in persistent pulmonary hypertension of the newborn. *Am J Respir Crit Care Med.* 2001;164:1981-1987.
95. Mata-Greenwood E, Meyrick B, Steinhorn RH, et al. Alteration in TGF-B1 expression in lambs with increased pulmonary blood flow and pulmonary hypertension. *Am J Physiol Lung Cell Mol Physiol.* 2003;285:L209-L221.
96. Kotecha S, Wangoo A, Silverman M, Shaw RJ. Increase in the concentration of transforming growth factor beta-1 in bronchoalveolar lavage fluid before development of chronic lung disease of prematurity. *J Pediatr.* 1996;128:464-469.
97. Lecart C, Cayabyab R, Buckley S, et al. Bioactive transforming growth factor-beta in the lungs of extremely low birthweight neonates predicts the need for home oxygen supplementation. *Biol Neonate.* 2000;77:217-223.
98. McCurnin D, Seidner S, Chang LY, et al. Ibuprofen-induced patent ductus arteriosus closure: physiologic, histologic, and biochemical effects on the premature lung. *Pediatrics.* 2008;121:945-956.
99. Chang LY, McCurnin D, Yoder B, et al. Ductus arteriosus ligation and alveolar growth in preterm baboons with a patent ductus arteriosus. *Pediatr Res.* 2008;63:299-302.
100. Brown ER. Increased risk of bronchopulmonary dysplasia in infants with patent ductus arteriosus. *J Pediatr.* 1979;95:865-866.
101. Rojas MA, Gonzalez A, Bancalari E, et al. Changing trends in the epidemiology and pathogenesis of neonatal chronic lung disease. *J Pediatr.* 1995;126:605-610.
102. Cotton RB, Stahlman MT, Kovar I, Catterton WZ. Medical management of small preterm infants with symptomatic patent ductus arteriosus. *J Pediatr.* 1978;92:467-473.
103. Cotton RB, Stahlman MT, Bender HW, et al. Randomized trial of early closure of symptomatic patent ductus arteriosus in small preterm infants. *J Pediatr.* 1978;93:647-651.
104. Merritt TA, Harris JP, Roghmann K, et al. Early closure of the patent ductus arteriosus in very low-birth-weight infants: a controlled trial. *J Pediatr.* 1981;99:281-286.
105. Wung JT, Koons AH, Driscoll JM, James LS. Changing incidence of bronchopulmonary dysplasia. *J Pediatr.* 1979;95:845-847.
106. O'Brodovich HM, Mellins RB: Bronchopulmonary dysplasia: unresolved neonatal acute lung injury. *Am Rev Respir Dis.* 1985;132:694-709.
107. Heneghan MA, Sosulski R, Baquero JM. Persistent pulmonary abnormalities in newborns: the changing picture of bronchopulmonary dysplasia. *Pediatr Radiol.* 1986;16:180-184.
108. Parker RA, Lindstrom DP, Cotton RB. Improved survival accounts for most, but not all, of the increase in bronchopulmonary dysplasia. *Pediatrics.* 1992;90:663-668.

B

109. Charafeddine L, D'Angio CT, Phelps DL. Atypical chronic lung disease patterns in neonates. *Pediatrics*. 1999;103:759-765.
110. Hutchison A, Ogletree M, Palme J, et al. Plasma 6-keto-prostaglandin F1 and thromboxane B2 in sick preterm neonates. *Prostaglandins Leukotrienes and Medicine*. 1985;18:163-181.
111. Lucas M, Mitchell A. Plasma prostaglandins in preterm neonates before and after treatment for patent ductus arteriosus. *Lancet*. 1978;2:130-132.
112. Hammerman C, Zaia W, Berger S, et al. Prostaglandin levels: predictors of indomethacin responsiveness. *Pediatr Cardiol*. 1986;7:61-65.
113. Lamont RF, Rose M, Elder MG. Effect of bacterial products on prostaglandin E production by amnion cells. *Lancet*. 1985;2:1331-1333.
114. Fletcher JR. The role of prostaglandins in sepsis. *Scand J Infect Dis*. 1982;31(Suppl):55-60.
115. Runkle B, Goldberg RN, Streitfeld MM, et al. Cardiovascular changes in group B streptococcal sepsis in the piglet: response to indomethacin and relationship to prostacyclin and thromboxane A2. *Pediatr Res*. 1984;18:874-878.
116. Marshall DD, Kotelchuck M, Young TE, et al. Risk factors for chronic lung disease in the surfactant era: a North Carolina population-based study of very low birth weight infants. *Pediatrics*. 1999;104:1345-1350.
117. Cavazza A, Tagliabue P, Fedeli T, et al; Investigators of the Italian Group of Neonatal Pneumology. Impact of chronic lung disease on very low birth weight infants: a collaborative study of the Italian Group of Neonatal Pneumology. *Ital J Pediatr*. 2004;30:393-400.
118. Gersony WM, Peckham GJ, Ellison RC, et al. Effects of indomethacin in premature infants with patent ductus arteriosus: results of a national collaborative study. *J Pediatr*. 1983;102:895-906.
119. Cotton RB, Hickey DE, Graham TP, Stahlman MT. Effect of early indomethacin on ventilatory status of preterm infants with symptomatic patent ductus arteriosus. *Pediatr Res*. 1980;14:442.
120. Mahony L, Carnero V, Brett C, et al. Prophylactic indomethacin therapy for patent ductus arteriosus in very-low-birth-weight infants. *N Engl J Med*. 1982;306:506-510.
121. Kaapa P, Lanning P, Koivisto M. Early closure of patent ductus arteriosus with indomethacin in preterm infants with idiopathic respiratory distress syndrome. *Acta Paediatr Scand*. 1983;72:179-184.
122. Weesner KM, Dillard RG, Boyle RJ, Block SM. Prophylactic treatment of asymptomatic patent ductus arteriosus in premature infants with respiratory distress syndrome. *South Med J*. 1987;80:706-708.
123. Pongiglione G, Marasini M, Silvestri G, et al. Early treatment of patent ductus arteriosus in premature infants with severe respiratory distress syndrome. *Pediatric Cardiol*. 1988;9:91-94.
124. Mahony L, Caldwell RL, Girod DA, et al. Indomethacin therapy on the first day of life in infants with very low birth weight. *J Pediatr*. 1985;106:801-805.
125. Clyman RI. Recommendations for the postnatal use of indomethacin: An analysis of four separate treatment strategies, *J Pediatr*. 1996;128:601-607.
126. Van Overmeire B, Van de Brock H, Van Laer P, et al. Early versus late indomethacin treatment for patent ductus arteriosus in premature infants with respiratory distress syndrome. *J Pediatr*. 2001;138(205):11.
127. Rennie JM, Doyle J, Cooke RWI. Early administration of indomethacin to preterm infants. *Arch Dis Child*. 1986;61:233-238.
128. Vincer M, Allen A, Evans JR, et al. Early intravenous indomethacin prolongs respiratory support in very low birthweight infants. *Acta Paediatr Scand*. 1987;76:894-897.
129. Krueger E, Mellander M, Bratton D, Cotton R. Prevention of symptomatic patent ductus arteriosus with a single dose of indomethacin. *J Pediatr*. 1987;111:749-754.
130. Setzer-Bandstra E, Montalvo BM, Goldberg R, et al. Prophylactic indomethacin for prevention of intraventricular hemorrhage in premature infants. *Pediatrics*. 1988;82:533-542.
131. Bada HS, Green RS, Pourcyrous M, et al. Indomethacin reduces the risks of severe intraventricular hemorrhage. *J Pediatr*. 1989;115:631-637.
132. Ment LR, Oh W, Ehrenkranz RA, et al. Low-dose indomethacin and prevention of intraventricular hemorrhage: a multicenter randomized trial. *Pediatrics*. 1994;93:543-550.
133. Schmidt B, Davis P, Moddemann D, et al. and the TIPP investigators. Long-term effects of indomethacin prophylaxis in extremely-low-birth-weight infants. *New Engl J Med*. 2001;344:1966-1972.
134. Fowlie PW, Davis PG, McGuire W. Prophylactic intravenous indomethacin for preventing mortality and morbidity in preterm infants. *Cochrane Database Syst Rev*. 2005.
135. Cifuentes RF, Olley PM, Balfe JW et al. Indomethacin and renal function in premature infants with persistent ductus arteriosus. *J Pediatr*. 1979;95:583-587.
136. Jones LJ, Craven PD, Attia J, et al. Network meta-analysis of indomethacin versus ibuprofen versus placebo for PDA in preterm infants. *Arch Dis Child Fetal Neonatal Ed*. 2011;96:F45-F52.
137. Benitz WE. Treatment of persistent patent ductus arteriosus in preterm infants: time to accept the null hypothesis? *J Perinatol*. 2010;30:241-252.
138. Hammerman C, Aramburo MJ. Prolonged indomethacin therapy for the prevention of recurrences of patent ductus arteriosus. *J Pediatr*. 1990;117:771-776.
139. Tammela O, Ojala R, Livainen T, et al. Short versus prolonged indomethacin therapy for patent ductus arteriosus in preterm infants. *J Pediatr*. 1999;134:552-557.
140. Lee J, Rajadurai VS, Tan KW, et al. Randomized trial of prolonged low-dose versus conventional-dose indomethacin for treating patent ductus arteriosus in very low birth weight infants. *Pediatrics*. 2003;112:345-350.

141. Merritt TA, DiSessa TG, Feldman BH, et al. Closure of the patent ductus arteriosus with ligation and indomethacin: a consecutive experience. *J Pediatr.* 1978;93:639-646.
142. Cassady G, Crouse DT, Kirklin JW, et al. A randomized, controlled trial of very early prophylactic ligation of the ductus arteriosus in babies who weighed 1000 g or less at birth. *N Engl J Med.* 1989;320:1511-1516.
143. Nagle MG, Peyton MD, Harrison LH Jr, Elkins RC. Ligation of patent ductus arteriosus in very low birth weight infants. *Am J Surg.* 1981;142:681-686.
144. Moin F, Kennedy KA, Moya FR. Risk factors predicting vasopressor use after patent ductus arteriosus ligation. *Am J Perinatol.* 2003;20:313-320.
145. Taylor AF, Morrow WR, Lally KP, et al. Left ventricular dysfunction following ligation of the ductus arteriosus in the preterm baboon. *J Surg Res.* 1990;48:590-596.
146. Kabra NS, Schmidt B, Roberts RS, et al. Trial of Indomethacin Prophylaxis in Preterms Investigators. Neurosensory impairment after surgical closure of patent ductus arteriosus in extremely low birth weight infants: results from the Trial of Indomethacin Prophylaxis in Preterms. *J Pediatr.* 2007;150:229-234.
147. Clyman R, Cassady G, Kirklin JK, et al. The role of patent ductus arteriosus ligation in bronchopulmonary dysplasia: reexamining a randomized controlled trial. *J Pediatr.* 2009;154:873-876.
148. Madan JC, Kendrick D, Hagadorn JI, Frantz ID 3rd; National Institute of Child Health and Human Development Neonatal Research Network. Patent ductus arteriosus therapy: impact on neonatal and 18-month outcome. *Pediatrics.* 2009;123:674-681.
149. Lemmers PM, Molenschot MC, Evens J, et al. Is cerebral oxygen supply compromised in preterm infants undergoing surgical closure for patent ductus arteriosus? *Arch Dis Child Fetal Neonatal Ed.* 2010;95:F429-F434.
150. Roclawski M, Sabiniewicz R, Potaz P, et al. Scoliosis in patients with aortic coarctation and patent ductus arteriosus: does standard posterolateral thoracotomy play a role in the development of the lateral curve of the spine? *Pediatr Cardiol.* 2009;30:941-945.
151. Benjamin JR, Smith PB, Cotten CM, et al. Long-term morbidities associated with vocal cord paralysis after surgical closure of a patent ductus arteriosus in extremely low birth weight infants. *J Perinatol.* 2010;30:408-413.
152. Schmidt B, Roberts RS, Davis P, et al, Caffeine for Apnea of Prematurity Trial Group. Caffeine therapy for apnea of prematurity. *N Engl J Med.* 2006;354:2112-2121.
153. Guerra FA, Savich RD, Wallen LD, et al. Prostaglandin E2 causes hypoventilation and apnea in newborn lambs. *J Appl Physiol.* 1988;64:2160-2166.
154. Hoch B, Berhard M. Central apnoea and endogenous prostaglandins in neonates. *Acta Paediatr.* 2000;89:1364-1368.
155. Cotton RB, Lindstrom DP, Kanarek KS, et al. Effect of positive-end-expiratory-pressure on right ventricular output in lambs with hyaline membrane disease. *Acta Paediatr Scand.* 1980;69:603-606.
156. Fajardo F, Buzzella B, Sattar S, et al. Effect of PEEP on left to right shunt and superior vena cava flow in preterm infants with a patent ductus arteriosus. *Society for Pediatric Research E-PAS.* 2009;4346:294.
157. Skinner JR, Hunter S, Poets CF, et al. Haemodynamic effects of altering arterial oxygen saturation in preterm infants with respiratory failure. *Arch Dis Child Fetal Neon Ed.* 1999;80:F81-F87.

CHAPTER 9

Role of Stem Cells in Neonatal Lung Injury

Karen C. Young, MD, and Cleide Suguihara, MD, PhD

9

- **Stem Cells**
- **Exogenous Stem Cells for Lung Repair**
- **Mechanisms of Stem Cell Repair**
- **Lung Bioengineering**
- **Endogenous Lung Stem Cells**
- **Endogenous Circulating Stem Cells**
- **Conclusion**

The lungs are remarkably complex organs with more than 40 different cell types uniquely organized to facilitate gas transport and exchange. This intrinsic complexity along with low cell turnover has led to challenges in the understanding of lung stem cell biology.[1,2] Nevertheless, real progress has been made in the past decade, and reports now indicate that after injury, the damaged lung epithelium has the capacity to repair itself with a population of resident epithelial progenitor cells, with a possible minor contribution from bone marrow–derived stem cells. More data, albeit sparse, is also available on the molecular mechanisms that regulate the balance between stem cell self-renewal and differentiation, and their impact on disease pathogenesis.[3-9] Stem cell–based therapies have now proved to be efficacious in several preclinical models of adult and neonatal lung disease, although reports suggest the effect to be mainly paracrine-mediated. Conversely, agents that negatively modulate stem cell migration to the lung may potentially alleviate lung fibrosis. The utilization of stem cells to deliver gene therapy and bioengineer functional lung tissue has also been the focus of extensive promising research, and an attractive alternative to embryonic stem cells, induced pluripotent stem (iPS) cells generated from mature somatic cells may be a therapeutic strategy for genetic lung diseases such as cystic fibrosis. Clinical trials utilizing stem cell–based therapies are also under way in chronic obstructive pulmonary disease as well as pulmonary hypertension (PH). This chapter reviews the advances in lung stem cell biology and discusses stem cell–based therapies for lung disease and their implications for the neonate.

Stem Cells

Stem cells have the ability both to replenish themselves through self-renewal and to differentiate into mature progeny.[10-12] They may divide symmetrically or asymmetrically, giving rise to a stem cell and a more committed progenitor cell (Fig. 9-1).[13,14] They may also be classified as totipotent, pluripotent, or multipotent (Fig. 9-2).[14] *Totipotent* stem cells are capable of differentiating into all adult and embryonic tissues, including extraembryonic tissues such as trophectoderm.[15,16] In mammals, only the zygote and the first-cleavage blastomeres are totipotent.[16] *Pluripotent* stem cells are capable of differentiating into derivatives of all three germ layers (ectoderm,

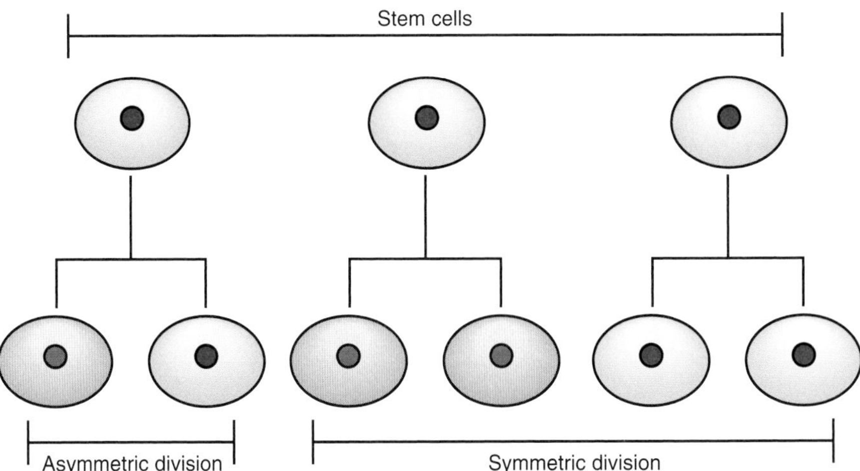

Figure 9-1 Stem cell division. Stem cells may divide asymmetrically or symmetrically. During symmetric division, each stem cell divides and produces two daughter stem cells or two differentiated daughter progeny. Alternatively, during asymmetric division, each stem cell produces one differentiated daughter progeny and one stem cell.

mesoderm, and endoderm) and are typically derived from embryos at different embryonic stages of development.[17] *Multipotent* stem cells are able to differentiate into multiple cell types of one lineage.[18,19] The most prominent example remains hematopoietic stem cells (HSCs), which are capable of differentiating into all the cell types of the hematopoietic system.[20]

Stem cells may also be categorized as embryonic or adult stem cells. Embryonic stem cells are derived from blastocysts in the developing embryo and are pluripotent.[21] Adult stem cells are found in adult tissues in specialized microenvironments known as *niches*.[22,23] These cells are typically multipotent and, after an asymmetric cell division, produce a population of transit-amplifying progenitor cells.[24] These cells act as intermediates between dedicated stem cells and a mature differentiated cell. They proliferate more rapidly than dedicated stem cells and can

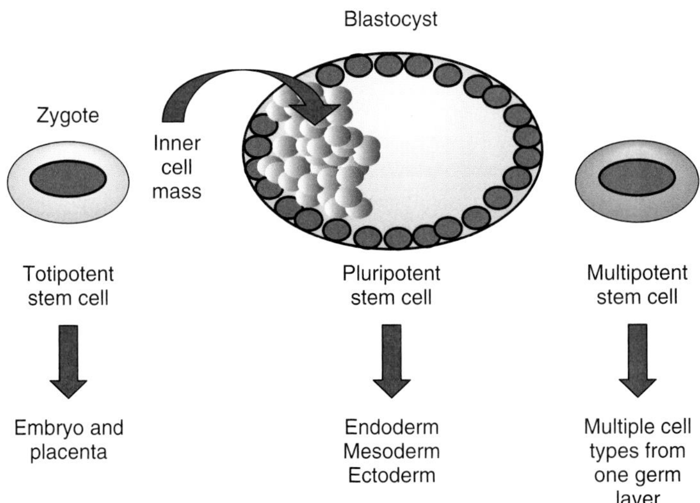

Figure 9-2 Stem cell potency. Totipotent stem cells (zygote or first-cleavage blastomeres) can give rise to all cells in the embryo and placenta. Pluripotent stem cells (e.g., embryonic stem cells) can give rise to the entire embryo and all cell lineages (endoderm, mesoderm and ectoderm). Multipotent stem cells typically give rise to cells in one cell lineage.

renew themselves over the short term. Within tissues, there may also be facultative stem cells; they are normally quiescent differentiated cells but after injury, they may self-renew and give rise to other differentiated progeny.[2,25]

Exogenous Stem Cells for Lung Repair

Embryonic Stem Cells

Embryonic stem cells (ESCs) are self-renewable, pluripotent cells derived from the inner cell mass of a blastocyst-stage embryo.[26] These cells are characterized by nearly unlimited self-renewal, and during differentiation in vitro, they develop into cellular derivatives of endodermal, mesodermal, and ectodermal origin.[26] This unequaled capacity of ESCs to develop into all somatic cell types was first suggested in 1961 by Kleinsmith and Pierce,[27] who developed the first pluripotent cells in culture from germ cell tumors. They showed that single embryonal carcinoma cells transferred to a new host could reform a complex teratocarcinoma that could be retransplanted to another host. Several decades later, the first embryonic stem cells were isolated from mice and humans.[28-30] These discoveries not only led to a tremendous increase in knowledge of the signals that direct cell fate but also opened the door for the possible use of ESCs in regenerative medicine.

The potential use of ESCs in the treatment of lung diseases has evoked extensive interest in developing techniques that support the differentiation of ESCs into lung cells. The derivation of lung cells from ESCs has, however, been difficult. Unlike cellular derivatives from the mesodermal or ectodermal germ layers, the differentiation of ESCs into endoderm has been complex. Indeed, it was only in 2002 that ESCs cultured in specialized media were shown to differentiate into type 2 alveolar epithelial cells.[31] The derived cells expressed surfactant protein C (SP-C) and had a few lamellar bodies, but the yield was low. Since then, multiple protocols attempting to improve the differentiation efficiency has been developed via either embryonic body (EB) formation[32] or co-culture of EBs with pulmonary mesenchyme.[33,34] Co-culture of EB with lung mesenchyme obtained at embryonic day 11.5 (E11.5) resulted in the generation of cells that formed pseudoglandular structures and early lung cells that expressed thyroid transcription factor-1 (TTF-1), a marker of lung epithelial cell fate commitment. Moreover, when ESCs were cultured under air-liquid interface conditions, the cells were shown to give rise to fully differentiated airway epithelium, composed of basal, ciliated, intermediate, and Clara cells, similar to those of native tracheobronchial airway epithelium.[35]

An even more efficient strategy has been to recapitulate in vitro some of the crucial differentiation cues that promote cell lineage commitment in vivo. Exposure of early differentiating embryonic bodies to activin A, a member of the Nodal signaling family, enhanced the specification of distal lung epithelium and yielded cells with a phenotype most closely resembling that of lung-committed progenitor cells present in the foregut endoderm and the early lung buds during embryonic development.[36] Even more efficient was a strategy involving transduction of a human embryonic stem cell line with an SP-C promoter–driven neomycin expression cassette.[37] This strategy was shown to develop an essentially pure (>99%) population of type 2 alveolar epithelial cells. These cells exhibited lamellar body formation, expressed surfactant proteins A, B, and C, α_1-antitrypsin, and the cystic fibrosis transmembrane conductance receptor, and synthesized and secreted complement proteins C3 and C5.[37]

The use of ESCs in preclinical models of neonatal or adult lung injury has been limited, however, by both ethical and tumor transformation concerns.[38,39] The transplantation of a pure population of pulmonary progenitor cells or mature type II alveolar epithelial (AEC2) cells derived from human ESCs in vitro could provide an alternative strategy to regenerate endogenous lung cells destroyed by injury and disease. Because alveolar type II epithelial cells are able to differentiate into alveolar type I epithelial (AEC1) cells, the therapeutic potential of a pure population of type II alveolar epithelial cells derived from ESCs could be very promising. Indeed,

B

ESC-derived type II alveolar cells transplanted into the lungs of mice subjected to bleomycin-induced acute lung injury were reported to behave like normal primary alveolar type II cells, differentiating into cells expressing phenotypic markers of alveolar type I epithelial cells.[40] There were no tumorigenic side effects, and lung injury was abrogated in the mice transplanted with the ESCs-derived type II alveolar cells, as demonstrated by recovery of body weight and arterial blood oxygen saturation, decreased collagen deposition, and increased survival.[40] Moreover, up to 20% of the total SP-C–expressing cells appeared to be of ESC origin.[40] It is not clear, however, whether the reparative effects were from structural engraftment or, alternatively, whether the ESC-derived cells triggered the release of growth factors that improved the lung microenvironment or expanded the endogenous lung progenitor and stem cell compartments. Nevertheless, these findings hold tremendous promise for the field of ESC-derived cells for lung repair. It should be cautioned that ESCs are not protected against T lymphocyte–mediated cytotoxicity, so cellular derivatives of ESCs may be rejected after implantation.[41]

Induced Pluripotent Stem Cells

Another consideration for neonatal lung repair could be the transplantation of autologous iPS cells.[42] These cells are derived by direct reprogramming of mature somatic cells to an embryonic pluripotent state unidentifiable from ESCs.[43,44] Currently, there are no published reports of preclinical or clinical use of iPS cells in lung diseases; however, neurons and pancreatic cells derived from reprogrammed fibroblasts have been shown to improve Parkinson's disease and diabetes, respectively.[45,46] Moreover, Somers and colleagues[47] reported the generation of iPS cells from dermal or liver fibroblasts from patients with cystic fibrosis and α_1-antitrypsin deficiency.[47] Potentially, the administration of gene-corrected iPS cell–derived lung epithelial progenitor cells could be a potent strategy for inherited diseases, such as surfactant protein deficiencies, cystic fibrosis, and α_1-antitrypsin deficiency.[47] Further research into the in vitro reprogramming of somatic cells to iPS cells must be performed in order to improve efficiency and avoid oncogenesis.

Umbilical Cord Stem Cells

Since the 1990s, umbilical cord–derived stem cells have been extensively explored as a source of stem cells for organ repair.[48-51] These cells are highly attractive because they are free from the ethical concerns about ESCs and with the hematopoietic stem cell compartment in cord blood is less mature and has a higher proliferative potential than that of adult stem cells[52]; both properties may translate into greater stem cell plasticity. There is also the added advantage of several non-hematopoietic stem cell populations being present within the umbilical cord. These include endothelial colony–forming cells (ECFCs)[53] and multipotent mesenchymal stromal cells (MSCs).[54-56] Interestingly, although the yield of MSCs from cord blood has been reported to be low,[57] cord-derived MSCs have a relatively high proliferation rate[57] and can be successfully differentiated into mature adipocytes, epithelial cells,[58] osteoblasts,[59] chondrocytes,[60] skeletal myocytes, cardiomyocytes,[61] neurons,[62] and endothelial cells.[63]

Although cord-derived stem cells have been shown to improve neurologic deficit following stroke,[64] improve ventricular function after myocardial infarction,[65] increase limb perfusion after ischemia,[66] and reduce glucose levels in preclinical diabetic models,[67] the use of cord-derived stem cells for neonatal lung repair is only now been investigated. In fact, to date only two published studies have evaluated cord-derived stem cells in lung injury models. In one study, human umbilical cord-derived MSCs obtained from Wharton's jelly were administered systemically to mice with bleomycin-induced lung injury.[68] The administration of cord stem cells significantly reduced inflammation and inhibited the expression of transforming growth factor-β (TGF-β), interferon-γ (IFN-γ), and the pro-inflammatory cytokines macrophage migratory inhibitory factor (MIF) and tumor necrosis factor-α (TMF-α). Collagen concentration in the lung was also significantly reduced by cord-derived stem cells, but engraftment was limited. Similarly, in a preclinical model of bronchopulmonary dysplasia (BPD), the intratracheal transplantation of human cord–derived MSCs to newborn rat pups significantly attenuated hyperoxia-induced lung injury, and the protective effect was associated with a downregulation in the expression of inflammatory and fibrotic genes.[69] There was also little convincing evidence of engraftment. Currently, two clinical phase 1 studies are listed on *clinical trials.gov* that are both evaluating the safety and efficacy of umbilical cord stem cells in treating preterm patients with BPD. More basic investigations, however, are needed to elucidate the therapeutic efficacy of administering term in comparison with preterm umbilical cord–derived stem cells in models of neonatal lung injury, as well as the dosage, the optimal timing, and the route of administration. Clearly, compared with term umbilical cord blood, preterm umbilical cord blood is richer in hematopoietic progenitors, and precursors from preterm umbilical cord blood can be extensively expanded ex vivo.[52,70,71] Autologous preterm umbilical cord–derived stem cells may not necessarily be the best umbilical cord blood source for treatment of BPD, however, because progenitor cells from preterm umbilical cord blood compared to term cord blood has been shown to be more susceptible to hyperoxic damage.[72]

Bone Marrow–Derived Stem cells

The bone marrow (BM) is a mesodermally derived tissue consisting of a complex hematopoietic cellular component supported by a microenvironment composed of stromal cells embedded in a complex extracellular matrix.[73] Albeit engraftment now known to be a rare occurrence, several studies have documented, in multiple lung injury models, the engraftment of unfractioned BM-derived cells as well as purified specific marrow-derived stem populations.[74-84]

Type of Bone Marrow–Derived Stem Cells

The BM-derived stem cell populations are HSCs, MSCs, and endothelial progenitor cells (EPCs).

Hematopoietic Stem Cells

Hematopoietic stem cells are defined as cells that are capable of self-renewal and that differentiate into all mature hematopoietic cells in the body. Although these undifferentiated cells are extremely rare, HSCs have been shown to home to the injured lung and to engraft.[78] In a landmark study, Krause and associates[85] utilized a single stem cell to demonstrate high-level engraftment of type II pneumocytes in the lungs of lethally irradiated mice. Additionally, after human HSC transplantation, significant rates of epithelial and endothelial chimerism have been detected in the recipient lung.[76] This engraftment rate of HSCs has now been challenged,[86] and most reports suggest that although this phenomenon does occur, engraftment is perhaps a rare event.

Mesenchymal Stem Cells

The possibility that mesenchymal stem cells, also called multipotent mesenchymal stromal cells, can regenerate the injured lung has gained increasing attention over the past decade.[87] Compared with other adult stem cells, MSCs are a very attractive population for organ repair and regeneration because they are easily expanded and genetically manipulated. In addition, MSCs appear to be immunoprivileged cells, in that they constitutively express low levels of human leukocyte antigen (HLA) class I molecules and do not express either HLA class II molecules or the co-stimulatory molecules CD40, CD80, and CD86, which are essential for activation of T lymphocyte–mediated immune responses.[88]

Originally characterized in 1968 by Friedenstein and colleagues,[89] MSCs were described as a population of BM stromal cells that were adherent, fibroblastic in appearance, and clonogenic. Later studies demonstrated that MSCs could be isolated from several human tissues,[90] including, lung,[91] liver,[92] adipose tissue,[93] dental pulp,[94] placenta,[95] and human cord blood.[56] These cells were shown to have the capacity not only to differentiate into mesoderm but also to differentiate into cells of endodermal and ectodermal origins.[87]

Unfortunately, there are no specific cell markers for MSCs. Hence studies have been plagued by nonuniformity relating to the techniques used for their isolation, culture, characterization as well as to their nomenclature. This situation has led to significant issues in interpreting and comparing studies. In order to control these disparities, the International Society of Cellular Therapy in 2006 established the following minimal criteria for defining MSCs: (1) adherence to plastic under standard tissue culture conditions; (2) expression of cell surface markers CD105, CD90, and CD73, and no expression for HLA-DR, CD79a, CD45, CD34, CD14, CD19 or CD11b; and (3) the capacity to differentiate into osteoblasts, chondroblasts, and adipocytes under appropriate in vitro conditions.[96]

B

In terms of BPD, rodent models of hyperoxia-induced lung injury suggest that MSCs are decreased in the lungs after exposure to hyperoxia.[97] However, increased numbers of MSCs in the tracheal aspirate of preterm infants were shown in one study to predict a greater than 25-fold higher risk for BPD,[98] and autocrine production of TGF-β1 was suggested by another study to drive the lung MSCs toward myofibroblastic differentiation.[99] A possible explanation for these contradictory findings could be that increased numbers of MSCs in the lung in the early stage of disease may be an endogenous reparative response that is depleted in later stages of the disease. Interestingly, bone marrow–derived MSCs were shown not to undergo myofibroblastic differentiation AFTER exposure to TGF-β1.[99]

Endothelial Progenitor Stem Cells

EPCs were first described by Asahara and coworkers[100] in 1997. This group described a population of peripheral blood mononuclear cells that could differentiate into endothelial cells. These cells expressed the hematopoietic stem marker CD34 as well as the endothelial cell marker VEGFR2 and were shown to contribute to revascularization and the salvage of ischemic hindlimbs.[100] Since then, various different markers have been used to identify this population, and the exact source for these cells remains controversial. Regardless of such questions, however, EPCs are known to mobilize from the BM into the peripheral blood in response to tissue ischemia and to differentiate into mature endothelial cells.[51,101] Moreover, data now suggest that EPCs may contribute to physiologic neovascularization in the normal lung.[102]

The quantity of circulating EPCs has been linked to adult lung disease outcome. In patients with acute lung injury, a reduced number of circulating EPCs has been associated with worse outcome. Similarly, patients with end-stage chronic lung disease had reduced circulating EPCs,[103] and patients with idiopathic pulmonary fibrosis showed a marked EPC depletion, that was most severe in the presence of PH.[104] In terms of the role of EPCs in neonatal hyperoxia-induced lung injury, data show that preterm cord blood–derived EPCs are more sensitive to hyperoxia than cord EPCs obtained from term infants.[72] Moreover, hyperoxia exposure was found to decrease murine BM-derived lung endothelial progenitor cells,[105] and cord EPCs have been shown to be decreased in preterm infants in whom BPD develops,[106] suggesting a potential role for EPCs as a therapeutic strategy.

Bone Marrow–Derived Stem Cells and Lung Disease

Efficacy in Lung Injury

BM-derived cells have been shown in preclinical studies to be efficacious in reducing lung injury. MSCs are now perhaps the cell type most frequently tested. Indeed, despite rare engraftment, recent in vivo and in vitro studies suggest that MSCs may have beneficial effects in acute lung injury induced by bacterial pneumonia,[107] endotoxin,[108] hyperoxia,[97] cecal ligation, and puncture-induced sepsis.[109,110] These therapeutic effects have been attributed mainly to the potent anti-inflammatory and immunomodulatory characteristics of MSCs as well as to their constitutive secretion of growth factors (angiopoietin-1, keratinocyte growth factor, hepatocyte growth factor), which not only improve alveolar fluid clearance but also restore endothelial cell integrity.[111-116] MSCs administered systemically or directly into the air spaces 1 hour or 4 hours after the intrapulmonary administration of *Escherichia coli* endotoxin was shown to improve survival, decrease pulmonary edema, and increase the secretion of anti-inflammatory cytokines, with minimal engraftment.[108] Furthermore, transfection of MSCs with human angiopoieitin-1 even further reduced the severity of the lung injury.[117] Similarly, in ex vivo perfused human lung, intrabronchial instillation of MSCs 1 hour after endotoxin-induced injury restored alveolar fluid clearance, and in primary cultures of human alveolar epithelial cells, human allogeneic mesenchymal stem cells were shown to restore the increase in epithelial permeability to protein caused by exposure to inflammatory cytokines. These beneficial effects of MSCs on lung epithelial permeability were in part secondary to increased angiopoeitin-1 secretion.[118] Also, intratracheal administration of MSCs into lung tissue affected by elastase-induced emphysema was shown to ameliorate the severity of the disease, and this effect was associated with increased expression of hepatocyte growth factor (HGF) and epidermal growth factor (EGF).[115]

9

Similar benefits were also demonstrated in models of neonatal hyperoxia-induced lung injury. In a seminal study by van Haaften and colleagues,[97] exposure of neonatal rats to hyperoxia was associated with a decrease in circulating and resident lung MSCs. Intratracheal delivery of MSCs not only restored alveolar and vascular structure but also improved survival and exercise tolerance with minimal engraftment. [97] In another study, MSC-derived conditioned media prevented hyperoxia-induced alveolar epithelial cell apoptosis and enhanced endothelial cord formation, suggesting a mainly paracrine effect.[97] In a similar study reported by Aslam and coworkers,[119] intravenous administration of MSCs improved alveolarization and decreased PH in neonatal mice, but the administration of MSC-conditioned medium had a more pronounced reparative effect. In our own laboratory, we have collected preliminary data suggesting that the reparative effects of MSC-conditioned medium and MSC are similar in hyperoxia-induced neonatal lung injury (Fig. 9-3). Also, a BM-derived population of angiogenic cells was shown in another study to improve vascular development and alveolarization in a neonatal murine model of hyperoxia-induced lung injury.[120] Interestingly, although a significant fraction of the transplanted cells engrafted into the damaged lungs and were evident up to 8 weeks later, they did not actually differentiate into endothelial or epithelial cells. Whether the engrafted transplanted cells were secreting factors to improve the tolerance of the neonatal lung to hyperoxia is still being investigated.

Lung Fibrosis

Pulmonary fibrosis is a feature of severe BPD. The possibility that BM-derived stem cells could prevent or reverse pulmonary fibrosis has now been extensively investigated in murine bleomycin-induced models of pulmonary fibrosis.[121,122] In fact, in one of the earliest in vivo studies utilizing plastic-adherent BM cells in a fibrotic lung model, there was significant engraftment of donor cells in the lungs of mice with bleomycin-induced fibrosis, and these cells expressed markers of type 1 epithelial cells.[74] Although most later studies have not demonstrated this significant

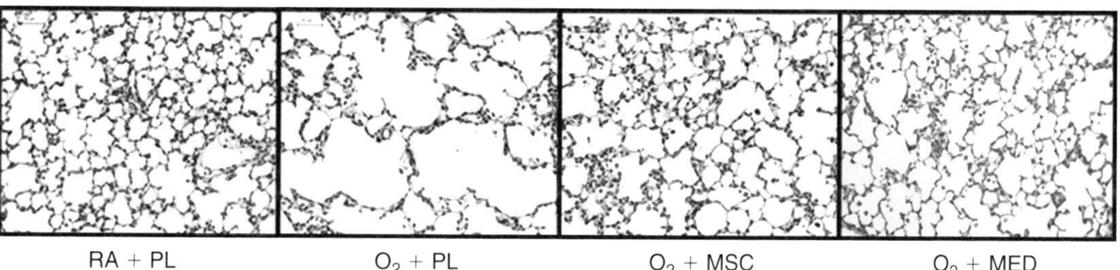

Figure 9-3 Mesenchymal stem cells (MSCs) and MSC-conditioned medium (MED) improve hyperoxia-induced alveolar simplification. Lung sections demonstrating similar improvement in alveolar structure after administration of intratracheal MSC and MED to neonatal rats with hyperoxia-induced lung injury. PL, Placebo; RA, Room Air.

engraftment of MSCs, several investigators have now shown that MSC administration immediately after bleomycin exposure results in significant reductions in inflammation, collagen deposition, and mortality.[123-125] This finding suggests that the effect of MSCs in improving bleomycin-induced fibrosis is due to the paracrine secretion of growth factors and cytokines that ultimately stimulate host repair and regeneration. In fact Ortiz and colleagues[124] showed that interleukin-1α receptor antagonist at least partly mediated the protective effects of MSCs in bleomycin-induced fibrosis. It is interesting, however, to note that the administration of MSCs at day 7 after bleomycin exposure in this study did not have any protective effects. Similarly, another study reported that donor cells injected immediately into the lung after irradiation injury could differentiate into functional lung cells but those injected at the later stage, after irradiation, participate in the fibrotic process.[126] These data suggest that the reparative effects of MSCs are directly modulated by the microenvironment of injured tissue. In the acute injury phase, the regulatory effect of microenvironment is to accelerate cell proliferation and differentiation to participate in the repair of injured tissue. In addition, abundant necrotic cells will vacate space for the engrafted cells. In the middle and later stages of fibrosis, the microenvironment, characterized by markedly increased TGF-β1 expression, might induce MSCs to differentiate into myofibroblasts, which then participate in lung fibrosis. MSCs may therefore be less efficacious in established fibrotic diseases but their use may be highly beneficial as a preventive strategy. A therapeutic modality for established fibrotic disease may actually involve antagonizing the mobilization of stem cells.

Pulmonary Hypertension

Pulmonary hypertension remains a significant cause of morbidity and mortality in humans and is especially severe in term neonates who have been exposed to hypoxia, sepsis, or meconium aspiration or preterm neonates with severe BPD. Evidence now suggests that both intratracheally and systemically administered MSCs can attenuate monocrotaline-induced PH and decrease right ventricular hypertrophy.[127,128] Moreover, the intravenous administration of BM-derived MSCs obtained from donor rats suffering from PH into recipient rats with PH was found to decrease right ventricular systolic pressure, pulmonary arteriolar narrowing, alveolar septum thickening, and improved right ventricular function, suggesting that autologous MSCs may be beneficial in patients with PH.[129] Similarly, the use of MSCs as a vector to deliver endothelial nitric oxide synthase[130] or prostacyclin synthase[131] resulted in even further improvements in PH. It is not clear whether the improvements in monocrotaline-induced PH are the result of its anti-inflammatory properties or of the release of growth factors that enhance neovascularization. This latter property may be actually quite beneficial in preterm neonates, whose PH may in part be secondary to vascular pruning.

EPCs have also been shown to be quite efficacious in preclinical models of idiopathic PH.[132] Although the mechanism of action of these cells in PH is still unclear, it is possible that EPCs have vasodilatory and antiproliferative properties. In a randomized study by Wang and colleagues,[133] the effects of intravenous autologous EPCs in patients with idiopathic pulmonary arterial hypertension (IPAH) was compared with conventional therapy. After 12 weeks of follow-up, the changes in 6-minute walk distance and hemodynamics were significantly better for the EPC-treated group.[133] There were no safety issues during the study. A second study of EPC therapy for pulmonary arterial hypertension, the Pulmonary Hypertension And Cell Therapy (PHACeT) Trial, is under way in Canada (ClinicalTrials.gov). This is a safety study, and its primary endpoint is the tolerability of cell transplantation in patients with pulmonary arterial hypertension that is refractory to all standard therapies.

Airway Disease

Neonates with BPD may have extensive airway remodeling, such as seen in patients with refractory asthma. MSCs are known to be immunomodulatory as well as anti-inflammatory and as such have been investigated in preclinical models of airway disease. Human MSCs given after induction of airway disease has been shown to dramatically decrease the pathology and airway inflammation associated with the murine ovalbumin model of chronic asthma.[134] Whether MSCs may also reverse epithelial-mesenchymal miscommunication, which occurs in asthma and other airway diseases, needs to be further explored.

Chronic Obstructive Pulmonary Disease

Several studies have documented the efficacy of BM-derived cells in ameliorating elastase-induced emphysema.[115,135] Shigemura and coworkers[135] demonstrated that autologous transplantation of adipose tissue–derived MSC ameliorates pulmonary emphysema in rats, and accelerates alveolar and vascular regeneration after lung volume reduction surgery in rats with emphysema.[135] MSCs have also been shown to decrease elastase-induced emphysematous damage through the release of soluble humoral factors rather than by engraftment in the lung tissue.[115] Thus far, these findings have translated into a clinical trial for chronic obstructive pulmonary disease (COPD). Findings from phase 1 of the trial did not raise any apparent safety concerns, and treated patients had a decrease in C-reactive protein levels.

Mechanisms of Stem Cell Repair

Engraftment or Paracrine

Although engraftment and differentiation of bone marrow–derived cells is more evident in rapidly growing neonates, embryos, fetuses, or adult animals with severely injured tissues, it is now clear that engraftment may not be the principal mechanism of stem cell repair.[136-141] In fact, several studies utilizing MSCs to regenerate the injured lung have shown that although these cells do indeed have the ability to conform to a specific identity in response to local host factors, the engraftment and differentiation of MSCs into lung epithelial cells in vivo is very uncommon.[97,119,122] Evidence now points to the possibility that MSCs function as pericytes[142,143] at sites of local damage, inhibiting immunosurveillance and establishing a regenerative microenvironment. This effect is achieved not only by cell-cell crosstalk but also by the secretion of several soluble growth factors and the immunomodulatory properties of MSCs.[144,145] These properties are as follows: (1) suppression of T-cell cytokine secretion and cytotoxicity[146-148]; (2) inhibition of B-cell proliferation and differentiation, thus reducing antibody formation[149]; (3) suppression of natural killer cell proliferation, cytokine production, and cytotoxicity[150]; and (4) inhibition of dendritic cell maturation and activation.[151] Finally, another distinct possibility is that MSCs may partially restore the endogenous stem cell pool, leading to increased genesis of alveolar cells for the resolution of disrupted alveolar surfaces, thereby augmenting the repair process. This generation of lung stem cells may explain how low levels of MSC engraftment in the lung can have a beneficial effect.

Lung Bioengineering

Tissue engineering is the creation of living, physiologic three-dimensional tissues or organs utilizing specific combinations of cells, scaffolds, and cell signals.[152] Although, the complex architecture of the lung has made lung bioengineering very challenging, the utilization of several innovative in vivo and ex vivo approaches has allowed for a resurgence of this approach in the lung regeneration field. Lung tissue has now been created by seeding of fetal lung cells on several three-dimensional matrices or scaffolds. These include sterile gelatin sponge (Gelfoam) scaffolds,[153] collagen,[154] polyglycolic acid, and basement membrane matrix (Matrigel). In 2010, Peterson and colleagues[155] published an innovative procedure that removes cellular components of the lung but leaves behind a scaffold of extracellular matrix that retains the hierarchical branching structures of airways and vasculature.[155] The decellularized lung is then placed into a specialized bioreactor and reperfused with several cell types.

The investigators reported that the seeded epithelium displayed remarkable hierarchical organization within the matrix and that the seeded endothelial cells efficiently repopulated the vascular compartment. In vitro, the mechanical characteristics of the engineered lungs were similar to those of native lung tissue, and when implanted into rats in vivo for short intervals (45 to 120 minutes), the engineered lungs participated in gas exchange, thus demonstrating the potential translation of this approach to the bedside.

Although data using stem cells are thus far quite sparse, one group demonstrated that a population of somatic lung progenitor cells cultured on synthetic polymer could form alveolar cell–like structures when implanted subcutaneously in nude mice.[156] Another report documents the successful transplantation of an engineered main bronchus into a patient with bronchial stenosis secondary to tuberculosis.[157] In this study, a segment of a cadaveric trachea was decellularized and seeded with the patient's epithelial cells and MSC-derived chondrocytes. Following transplantation of the trachea into the patient, the luminal surface was not distinguishable from adjacent tissue on bronchoscopy. These findings suggest that stem cells could potentially enhance lung bioengineering techniques and open new avenues for lung regenerative therapy.

B

Endogenous Lung Stem Cells

The postnatal lung contains stem cells capable of reconstituting the lung following injury[25,158] (Fig. 9-4). These resident lung-committed stem cells are, however, limited in their differentiation potential, have potency restricted to the cell lineages found only in the lung and topographically, and are localized to specific anatomic regions and tissue microenvironments known as *niches*.[159,160] Within the proximal gas-conducting system (the trachea as well as main bronchi), a distinct population of undifferentiated basal cells that express p63 and cytokeratins 5 and 14 have been shown to function as stem cells.[161-165] These basal cells self-renew and give rise to ciliated as well as secretory cells[165,166] under steady-state conditions and after injury.

Within the distal conducting airways (the bronchioles), Clara cells are known to self-renew and to differentiate into ciliated cells.[167,168] There are also different Clara cell subpopulations with different proliferative capacity and lineage potential.[169,170] One Clara cell subpopulation is resistant to the toxin naphthalene, which normally poisons the cytochrome P450 enzyme found in Clara cells.[170] These resistant cells, which have been termed variant Clara cells, and located around the neuroendocrine bodies and at the bronchoalveolar duct junction. Variant Clara cells are quiescent in the steady state, but following naphthalene-induced injury they proliferate quite rapidly.[171] Another subpopulation of Clara cells found at the bronchoalveolar junction are bronchoalveolar stem cells (BASCs).[172] These cells express both SP-C and

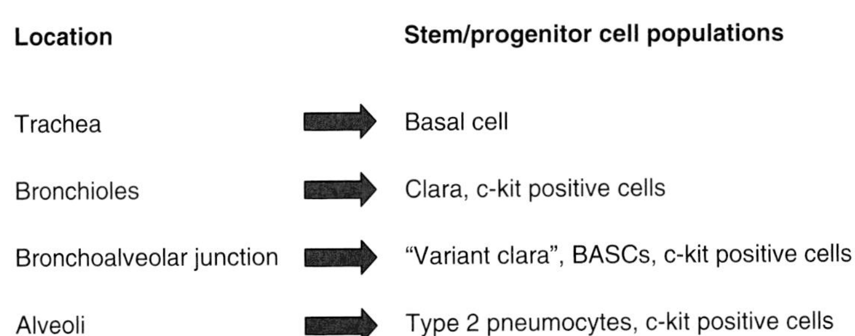

Location
Stem/progenitor cell populations
Trachea
Basal cell
Bronchioles
Clara, c-kit positive cells
Bronchoalveolar junction
"Variant clara", BASCs, c-kit positive cells
Alveoli
Type 2 pneumocytes, c-kit positive cells

Figure 9-4 Schematic showing the locations of lung progenitor cells. Within the trachea, basal cells are putative progenitor cells. Clara cells located within bronchioles and "variant" Clara cells found mainly at the bronchoalveolar junction also function as epithelial progenitors. Type 2 pneumocytes within the alveoli are progenitors for type 1 pneumocytes. c-kit–positive stem cell populations are localized mainly to the distal bronchiole and alveoli. BASCs, bronchoalveolar stem cells.

Clara cell secretory protein (CCSP). They are also resistant to naphthalene and proliferate rapidly after naphthalene injury. These cells not only self-renew but also, in specialized culture media, give rise to cells that express pro-SP-C, aquaporin 5, and CCSP, suggesting that BASCs could give rise to cells in the conducting portion as well as the gas exchange portion of the lung. Another progenitor population that express the embryonic stem cell marker Oct-4 have also been identified in the neonatal lung.[173] Like BASCs, these Oct-4–positive (Oct-4$^+$) cells were found to be present at the bronchoalveolar junction and to give rise to AEC2 and AEC1 cells. The role of these BASCS and Oct-4$^+$ progenitor cells in injury and homeostasis is not yet clear. Moreover, whether the BASCs and Oct-4$^+$ cells are just variant Clara cells is still being investigated.

In the neonate with alveolar injury, the AEC2 cells have been shown in vivo and in vitro to be the progenitor cell for regeneration of AEC1 cells.[174-177] There also appear to be different subpopulations of AEC2 cells with different regenerative potentials. Indeed, whole-lung and primary cultures of adult rat AEC2 cells indicate that there is a hyperoxia-resistant subpopulation of telomerase-positive AEC2 cells that expand in response to injury.[178] Later studies also suggest that there is a clear difference between hyperoxic AEC2 cells that are telomerase-positive and E-cadherin–positive and those that are E-cadherin–negative.[179] AEC2 cells vulnerable to the most long-term DNA-damaging effects of hyperoxia were reported to express high surface levels of telomerase as well as E-cadherin, and conversely, those cells that had telomerase but low levels of E-cadherin expression during hyperoxia were significantly less likely to undergo damage in culture and were relatively more proliferative.[179] Telomerase is a ribonucleoprotein that stabilizes the telomeres of chromosomes in actively growing cells, and the ability of a cell to divide over an indefinite lifespan may require the expression of telomerase. Interestingly, telomerase-null mice have been shown to have greater susceptibility to hyperoxia-induced alveolar injury as compared to wild type mice.[180]

Several questions, however, still remain. Whether the basal stem cells in the proximal conducting airway, the Clara cells in the distal conducting airway, and the BASCs at the bronchoalveolar junction cells are actually just transit-amplifying progenitor cells, acting as intermediates for a more dedicated stem cell, is not entirely clear. It is quite interesting, however, that Kajstura and associates[181] demonstrated the presence of a population of undifferentiated stem cells testing positive for the stem cell antigen c-kit nested in niches of the distal airways of human lungs (Fig. 9-5). These cells were self-renewing, clonogenic, and multipotent in vitro, and after being injected into damaged mouse lung in vivo, these human c-kit–positive lung stem cells formed human bronchioles, alveoli, and pulmonary vessels that integrated structurally and functionally with the damaged organ.[181] Results of this seminal study actually suggest that there is a resident c-kit–positive, dedicated lung stem cell population capable of regenerating the conducting and gas-exchange regions of the lung. Certainly, lineage-tracing experiments are necessary to track the fate of these cells and to establish their function in development and repair. Moreover, determining whether these endogenous stem cell populations are decreased qualitatively and quantitatively in preterm infants at increased risk for BPD will be quite interesting. The molecular mechanisms that drive these endogenous stem cells towards stem cell quiescence or activity also need to be clarified. Further studies are needed to identify the stem cells resident in the lung vasculature[182] and mesenchyme,[91] their roles in lung maintenance, and their interactions with epithelial cells.

Endogenous Circulating Stem Cells

Endogenous circulating BM-derived stem cells may contribute to both lung injury and lung repair. Early evidence of the potential involvement of BM-derived stem cells in lung homeostasis and repair was provided by reports of significant epithelial and endothelial chimerism in the recipient lung after hematopoietic stem cell transplantation.[183,184] Following lung transplantation in which donors and recipients are of opposite genders, examination of airway biopsy specimens of the transplanted

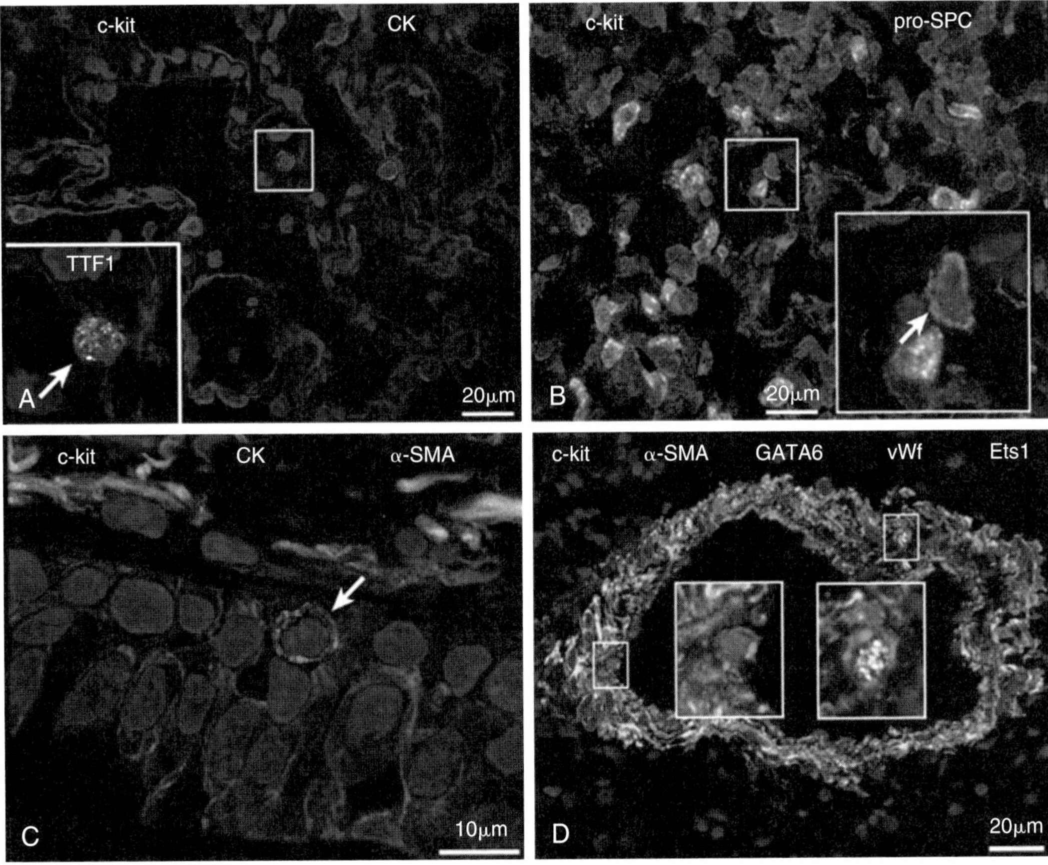

Figure 9-5 Human lung c-kit–positive stem cells and committed cells. **A,** An epithelial progenitor located in the alveolar wall (pan-cytokeratin [CK]) is shown at higher magnification in the *inset*; this progenitor cell retains the stem cell antigen c-kit and expresses the epithelial transcription factor thyroid transcription factor (TTF1: *white*). **B,** An epithelial precursor within the alveolar wall is shown at higher magnification in the inset. This cell is positive for c-kit and pro-surfactant protein C (pro-SPC) (*white*). **C,** Another epithelial precursor positive for c-kit and pan-CK (*arrow*) is apparent in the bronchiolar epithelium. **D,** Endothelial and smooth muscle progenitors located in the arteriolar wall are illustrated at higher magnification in the *insets*. These progenitor cells are c-kit–positive and express the gene *Ets1* or *GATA6*. von Willebrand factor (vWf), α-smooth muscle actin (α-SMA). (From Kajstura J, Rota M, Hall SR, et al. Evidence for human lung stem cells. *N Engl J Med.* 2011;364:1795-1806; see color image online.)

organs showed recipient-derived airway epithelial cells as well as AEC2 cells.[185] BM-derived, CD45$^+$ CXCR4$^+$ cytokeratin 5$^+$ cells have been identified in the peripheral blood of both mice and humans; in mice, these cells populated the proximal airway epithelium after sex-mismatched tracheal and BM transplantation.[186] Similarly, BM-derived cells expressing CCSP were shown to preferentially home to naphthalene-damaged airways.[187]

Circulating progenitor cells with fibroblast-like features[188,189] have been associated with pulmonary fibrosis,[188,190-193] PH,[194] and asthma.[195-197] Fibrocytes have been shown to traffic to the lungs after irradiation exposure[198] and after bleomycin challenge.[79] Moreover, in comparison with control subjects, patients with idiopathic pulmonary fibrosis (IPF) have higher levels of circulating fibrocytes, and the mean survival of patients with the disease and in whom fibrocytes accounted for more than 5% of total blood leukocytes was 7.5 months, compared with 27 months in those with fibrocyte levels less than 5% of total leukocytes.[199] In patients with asthma, fibrocytes were also identified in the airways, and the numbers of these cells increased following antigen challenge.[195] Moreover, the percentage of circulating fibrocytes was higher in patients with chronic obstructive asthma than in patients with asthma without chronic airway obstruction and in normal controls.[200] In neonatal calves with chronic hypoxia–induced PH, fibrocytes were also increased in the pulmonary vascular wall.[201] The recruitment of BM-derived cells to the lung is mediated by the chemokine stromal derived factor-1 (SDF-1/CXCL12) and interestingly, neutralization of SDF-1 has been shown to decrease established pulmonary fibrosis[187,191] as well as chronic hypoxia–induced PH.[202] These findings suggest that strategies that reduce the migration of fibrocytes may be beneficial in idiopathic pulmonary fibrosis and PH.

Conclusion

Although the use of stem cells to regenerate the injured neonatal lung is still in its embryonic phase, the potential of stem cell–based therapies to improve the outcome of preterm patients at risk for BPD has generated significant excitement. Stem cells not only improve alveolarization and vascular development in animal models of BPD but also increase functional capacity. There are, however, several challenges that must be overcome prior to the clinical use of such therapies. The possibility of ectopic tissue formation as well as the potential tumorigenicity of exogenous stem cells must be excluded. Certainly, the effects of neonatal lung disease on the endogenous populations of lung stem cells need to be clarified. The ideal timing of cell administration, the best population of cells to use, the most suitable candidates, the most efficacious dosing, the best route, and long-term safety must be carefully and systematically evaluated. Yet, despite these outstanding issues, the overwhelming data showing the reparative capacity of stem cells in lung disease suggest that this therapy holds substantial promise for preterm infants with BPD.

Acknowledgments

This review is supported in part by grants from the National Institute of Health (KY), the Florida Biomedical Research Grant Program (KY), the Batchelor Research Foundation (KY), and Project New Born (CS).

References

1. Bowden DH. Cell turnover in the lung. *Am Rev Respir Dis*. 1983;128:S46-S48.
2. Rawlins EL, Okubo T, Que J. Epithelial stem/progenitor cells in lung postnatal growth, maintenance, and repair. *Cold Spring Harb Symp Quant Biol*. 2008;73:291-295.
3. Tian Y, Zhang Y, Hurd L, et al. Regulation of lung endoderm progenitor cell behavior by miR302/367. *Development*. 2011;138:1235-1245.
4. Cohen ED, Ihida-Stansbury K, Lu MM, et al. Wnt signaling regulates smooth muscle precursor development in the mouse lung via a tenascin C/PDGFR pathway. *J Clin Invest*. 2009;119:2538-2549.
5. Zhang Y, Goss AM, Cohen ED, et al. A Gata6-Wnt pathway required for epithelial stem cell development and airway regeneration. *Nat Genet*. 2008;40:862-870.
6. Konigshoff M, Eickelberg O. WNT signaling in lung disease: A failure or a regeneration signal? *Am J Respir Cell Mol Biol*. 2010;42:21-31.
7. Harris-Johnson KS, Domyan ET, Vezina CM, Sun X. β-Catenin promotes respiratory progenitor identity in mouse foregut. *Proc Natl Acad Sci*. 2009;106:16287-16292.
8. Whitsett J. A lungful of transcription factors. *Nat Gen*. 1998;20:7-8.
9. Maeda Y, Dave V, Whitsett JA. Transcriptional control of lung morphogenesis. *Physiol Rev*. 2007;87:219-244.
10. Goss AM, Morrisey EE. Wnt signaling and specification of the respiratory endoderm. *Cell Cycle*. 2010;9:10-11.
11. Weissman IL. Stem cells: Units of development, units of regeneration, and units in evolution. *Cell*. 2000;100:157-168.
12. Morrison SJ, Shah NM, Anderson DJ. Regulatory mechanisms in stem cell biology. *Cell*. 1997;88:287-298.
13. Till JE, McCulloch EA, Siminovitch L. a stochastic model of stem cell proliferation, based on the growth of spleen colony-forming cells. *Proc Natl Acad Sci U S A*. 1964;51:29-36.
14. Smith A. A glossary for stem-cell biology. *Nature*. 2006;441:1060.
15. Kelly SJ. Studies of the developmental potential of 4- and 8-cell stage mouse blastomeres. *J Exp Zool*. 1977;200:365-376.
16. Modlinski JA. The fate of inner cell mass and trophectoderm nuclei transplanted to fertilized mouse eggs. *Nature*. 1981;292:342-343.
17. Donovan PJ, Gearhart J. The end of the beginning for pluripotent stem cells. *Nature*. 2001;414:92-97.

B

18. Rawlins EL, Okubo T, Xue Y. The role of Scgb1a1+ Clara cells in the long-term maintenance and repair of lung airway, but not alveolar, epithelium. *Cell Stem Cell*. 2009;4:525-534.
19. Lathja LG. *Stem Cells*. Edinburgh: Churchill Livingstone; 1983.
20. Wu AM, Siminovitch L, Till JE, McCulloch EA. Evidence for a relationship between mouse hemopoietic stem cells and cells forming colonies in culture. *Proc Natl Acad Sci U S A*. 1968;59: 1209-1215.
21. Thomson JA, Itskovitz-Eldor J, Shapiro SS, et al. Embryonic stem cell lines derived from human blastocysts. *Science*. 1998;282:1145-1147.
22. Moore KA, Lemischka IR. Stem cells and their niches. *Science*. 2006;311:1880-1885.
23. Li L, Xie T. Stem cell niche: structure and function. *Annu Rev Cell Dev Biol*. 2005;21:605-631.
24. Potten CS, Loeffler M. Stem cells: attributes, cycles, spirals, pitfalls and uncertainties. Lessons for and from the crypt. *Development*. 1990;110:1001-1020.
25. Rawlins EL, Hogan BL. Epithelial stem cells of the lung: privileged few or opportunities for many? *Development*. 2006;133:2455-2465.
26. Wobus AM, Boheler KR. Embryonic stem cells: Prospects for developmental biology and cell therapy. *Physiological Reviews*. 2005;85:635-678.
27. Kleinsmith LJ, Pierce Jr GB. Multipotentiality of single embryonal carcinoma cells. *Cancer Res*. 1964;24:1544-1551.
28. Brook FA, Gardner RL. The origin and efficient derivation of embryonic stem cells in the mouse. *Proc Natl Acady Sci*. 1997;94:5709-5712.
29. Martin GR. Isolation of a pluripotent cell line from early mouse embryos cultured in medium conditioned by teratocarcinoma stem cells. *Proc Natl Acad Sci U S A*. 1981;78:7634-7638.
30. Evans MJ, Kaufman MH. Establishment in culture of pluripotential stem cells from mouse embryos. *Nature*. 1982;291:154.
31. Ali NN, Edgar AJ, Samadikuchaksaraei A, et al. Derivation of type II alveolar epithelial cells from murine embryonic stem cells. *Tissue Eng*. 2002;8:541.
32. Samadikuchaksaraei A, Bishop AE. Derivation and characterization of alveolar epithelial cells from murine embryonic stem cells in vitro. *Methods Mol Biol*. 2006;330:233-248.
33. Denham M, Cole TJ, Mollard R. Embryonic stem cells form glandular structures and express surfactant protein C following culture with dissociated fetal respiratory tissue. *Am J Physiol Lung Cell Mol Physiol*. 2006;290:L1210-L1215.
34. Vranken BEV, Romanska HM, Polak JM, et al. Coculture of embryonic stem cells with pulmonary mesenchyme: A microenvironment that promotes differentiation of pulmonary epithelium. *Tissue Eng*. 2005;11:1177-1187.
35. Coraux C, Nawrocki-Raby B, Hinnrasky J, et al. Embryonic stem cells generate airway epithelial tissue. *Am J Respir Cell Mol Biol*. 2005;32:87-92.
36. Rippon HJ, Polak JM, Qin M. Derivation of distal lung epithelial progenitors from murine embryonic stem cells using a novel 3-step differentiation protocol. *Stem Cells*. 2006;24:1389.
37. Wang D, Haviland DL, Burns AR, et al. A pure population of lung alveolar epithelial type II cells derived from human embryonic stem cells. *Proc Natl Acad Sci U S A*. 2007;104:4449-4454.
38. Blum B, Bar-Nur O, Golan-Lev T, Benvenisty N. The anti-apoptotic gene survivin contributes to teratoma formation by human embryonic stem cells. *Nat Biotechnol*. 2009;27:281-287.
39. Blum B, Benvenisty N. The tumorigenicity of human embryonic stem cells. *Adv Cancer Res*. 2008;100:133-158.
40. Wang D, Morales JE, Calame DG, et al. Transplantation of human embryonic stem cell-derived alveolar epithelial type II cells abrogates acute lung injury in mice. *Mol Ther*. 2010;18: 625-634.
41. Wu DC, Boyd AS, Wood KJ. Embryonic stem cells and their differentiated derivatives have a fragile immune privilege but still represent novel targets of immune attack. *Stem Cells*. 2008;26: 1939-1950.
42. Wetsel RA, Wang D, Calame DG. Therapeutic potential of lung epithelial progenitor cells derived from embryonic and induced pluripotent stem cells. *Annu Rev Med*. 2011;62:95-105.
43. Takahashi K, Yamanaka S. Induction of pluripotent stem cells from mouse embryonic and adult fibroblast cultures by defined factors. *Cell*. 2006;126:663-676.
44. Lengner CJ. iPS cell technology in regenerative medicine. *Anna N Y Acad Scis*. 2010;1192:38-44.
45. Wernig M, Zhao J-P, Pruszak J, et al. Neurons derived from reprogrammed fibroblasts functionally integrate into the fetal brain and improve symptoms of rats with Parkinson's disease. *Proc Natl Acad Sci*. 2008;105:5856-5861.
46. Alipio Z, Liao W, Roemer EJ, et al. Reversal of hyperglycemia in diabetic mouse models using induced-pluripotent stem (iPS)-derived pancreatic Î2-l'ke cells. *Proc Natl Acad Sci U S A*. 2010;107:13426-13431.
47. Somers A, Jean J-C, Sommer CA, et al. Generation of transgene-free lung disease-specific human induced pluripotent stem cells using a single excisable lentiviral stem cell cassette. *Stem Cells*. 2010;28:1728-1740.
48. Broxmeyer HE, Douglas GW, Hangoc G, et al. Human umbilical cord blood as a potential source of transplantable hematopoietic stem/progenitor cells. *Proc Natl Acad Sci U S A*. 1989;86: 3828-3832.
49. Arien-Zakay H, Lazarovici P, Nagler A. Tissue regeneration potential in human umbilical cord blood. *Best Pract Res Clin Haematol*. 2010;23:291-303.
50. Murohara T, Ikeda H, Duan J, et al. Transplanted cord blood-derived endothelial precursor cells augment postnatal neovascularization. *J Clin Invest*. 2000;105:1527-1536.

51. Kalka C, Masuda H, Takahashi T, et al. Transplantation of ex vivo expanded endothelial progenitor cells for therapeutic neovascularization. *Proc Natl Acad Sci U S A*. 2000;97:3422-3427.
52. Wyrsch A, dalle Carbonare V, Jansen W, et al. Umbilical cord blood from preterm human fetuses is rich in committed and primitive hematopoietic progenitors with high proliferative and self-renewal capacity. *Exp Hematol*. 1999;27:1338-1345.
53. Ingram DA, Mead LE, Tanaka H, et al. Identification of a novel hierarchy of endothelial progenitor cells using human peripheral and umbilical cord blood. *Blood*. 2004;104:2752-2760.
54. Lee OK, Kuo TK, Chen W-M, et al. Isolation of multipotent mesenchymal stem cells from umbilical cord blood. *Blood*. 2004;103:1669-1675.
55. Erices A, Conget P, Minguell JJ. Mesenchymal progenitor cells in human umbilical cord blood. *Br J Haematol*. 2000;109:235-242.
56. Romanov YA, Svintsitskaya VA, Smirnov VN. Searching for alternative sources of postnatal human mesenchymal stem cells: Candidate MSC-like cells from umbilical cord. *Stem Cells*. 2003;21:105-110.
57. Kern S, Eichler H, Stoeve J, et al. Comparative analysis of mesenchymal stem cells from bone marrow, umbilical cord blood, or adipose tissue. *Stem Cells*. 2006;24:1294-1301.
58. Sueblinvong V, Loi R, Eisenhauer PL, et al. Derivation of lung epithelium from human cord blood-derived mesenchymal stem cells. *Am J Respir Crit Care Med*. 2008;177:701-711.
59. Toai T, Thao H, Thao N, et al. In vitro culture and differentiation of osteoblasts from human umbilical cord blood. *Cell Tissue Banking*. 2010;11:269-280.
60. Baksh D, Yao R, Tuan RS. Comparison of proliferative and multilineage differentiation potential of human mesenchymal stem cells derived from umbilical cord and bone marrow. *Stem Cells*. 2007;25:1384-1392.
61. Wang H-S, Hung S-C, Peng S-T, et al. Mesenchymal stem cells in the Wharton's jelly of the human umbilical cord. *Stem Cells*. 2004;22:1330-1337.
62. Weiss ML, Medicetty S, Bledsoe AR, et al. Human umbilical cord matrix stem cells: Preliminary characterization and effect of transplantation in a rodent model of Parkinson's disease. *Stem Cells*. 2006;24:781-792.
63. Wu KH, Zhou B, Lu SH, et al. In vitro and in vivo differentiation of human umbilical cord derived stem cells into endothelial cells. *J Cell Biochem*. 2007;100:608-616.
64. Chen J, Sanberg PR, Li Y, et al. Intravenous administration of human umbilical cord blood reduces behavioral deficits after stroke in rats. *Stroke*. 2001;32:2682-2688.
65. Leor J, Guetta E, Feinberg MS, et al. Human umbilical cord blood-derived CD133+ cells enhance function and repair of the infarcted myocardium. *Stem Cells*. 2006;24:772-780.
66. Pesce M, Orlandi A, Iachininoto MG, et al. Myoendothelial differentiation of human umbilical cord blood-derived stem cells in ischemic limb tissues. *Circ Res*. 2003;93:e51-e62.
67. Denner L, Bodenburg Y, Zhao JG, et al. Directed engineering of umbilical cord blood stem cells to produce C-peptide and insulin. *Cell Proliferation*. 2007;40:367-380.
68. Moodley Y, Atienza D, Manuelpillai U, et al. Human umbilical cord mesenchymal stem cells reduce fibrosis of bleomycin-induced lung injury. *Am J Pathol*. 2009;175:303-313.
69. Chang YS, Oh W, Choi SJ, et al. Human umbilical cord blood-derived mesenchymal stem cells attenuate hyperoxia-induced lung injury in neonatal rats. *Cell Transplant*. 2009;18:869-886.
70. Dimitriou H, Perdikogianni C, Stiakaki E, et al. The impact of mode of delivery and gestational age on cord blood hematopoietic stem/progenitor cells. *Ann Hematol*. 2006;85:381-385.
71. Javed MJ, Mead LE, Prater D, et al. Endothelial colony forming cells and mesenchymal stem cells are enriched at different gestational ages in human umbilical cord blood. *Pediatr Res*. 2008;64:68-73.
72. Baker CD, Ryan SL, Ingram DA, et al. Endothelial colony-forming cells from preterm infants are increased and more susceptible to hyperoxia. *Am J Respir Crit Care Med*. 2009;180:454-461.
73. Rafii S, Shapiro F, Rimarachin J, et al. Isolation and characterization of human bone marrow microvascular endothelial cells: hematopoietic progenitor cell adhesion. *Blood*. 1994;84:10-19.
74. Kotton DN, Ma BY, Cardoso WV, et al. Bone marrow-derived cells as progenitors of lung alveolar epithelium. *Development*. 2001;128:5181-5188.
75. Kleeberger W, Versmold A, Rothamel T, et al. Increased chimerism of bronchial and alveolar epithelium in human lung allografts undergoing chronic injury. *Am J Pathol*. 2003;162:1487-1494.
76. Suratt BT, Cool CD, Serls AE, et al. Human pulmonary chimerism after hematopoietic stem cell transplantation. *Am J Respir Crit Care Med*. 2003;168:318-322.
77. Rojas M, Xu J, Woods CR, et al. Bone marrow-derived mesenchymal stem cells in repair of the injured lung. *Am J Respir Cell Mol Biol*. 2005;33:145-152.
78. Aliotta JM, Keaney P, Passero M, et al. Bone marrow production of lung cells: the impact of G-CSF, cardiotoxin, graded doses of irradiation, and subpopulation phenotype. *Exp Hematol*. 2006;34:230-241.
79. Hashimoto N, Jin H, Liu T. Bone marrow-derived progenitor cells in pulmonary fibrosis. *J Clin Invest*. 2004;113:243.
80. Krause DS. Engraftment of bone marrow-derived epithelial cells. *Ann N Y Acad Sci*. 2005;1044:117-124.
81. Kotton DN, Fabian AJ, Mulligan RC. Failure of bone marrow to reconstitute lung epithelium. *Am J Respir Cell Mol Biol*. 2005;33:328-334.
82. Bruscia EM, Price JE, Cheng EC, et al. Assessment of cystic fibrosis transmembrane conductance regulator (CFTR) activity in CFTR-null mice after bone marrow transplantation. *Proc Natl Acad Sci U S A*. 2006;103:2965-2970.

83. Bruscia EM, Ziegler EC, Price JE, et al. Engraftment of donor-derived epithelial cells in multiple organs following bone marrow transplantation into newborn mice. *Stem Cells*. 2006;24: 2299-2308.
84. Harris RG, Herzog EL, Bruscia EM, et al. Lack of a fusion requirement for development of bone marrow-derived epithelia. *Science*. 2004;305:90-93.
85. Krause DS, Theise ND, Collector MI, et al. Multi-organ, multi-lineage engraftment by a single bone marrow-derived stem cell. *Cell*. 2001;105:369-377.
86. Wagers AJ, Sherwood RI, Christensen JL, Weissman IL. Little evidence for developmental plasticity of adult hematopoietic stem cells. *Science*. 2002;297:2256-2259.
87. Phinney DG, Prockop DJ. Concise review: Mesenchymal stem/multipotent stromal cells: the state of transdifferentiation and modes of tissue repair-current views. *Stem Cells*. 2007;25:2896-2902.
88. Patel SA, Sherman L, Munoz J, Rameshwar P. Immunological properties of mesenchymal stem cells and clinical implications. *Arch Immunol Ther Exp (Warsz)*. 2008;56:1-8.
89. Friedenstein AJ, Petrakova KV, Kurolesova AI, Frolova GP. Heterotopic of bone marrow. Analysis of precursor cells for osteogenic and hematopoietic tissues. *Transplantation*. 1968;6:230-247.
90. Young HE, Mancini ML, Wright RP, et al. Mesenchymal stem cells reside within the connective tissues of many organs. *Developmental Dynamics*. 1995;202:137-144.
91. Lama VN, Smith L, Badri L, et al. Evidence for tissue-resident mesenchymal stem cells in human adult lung from studies of transplanted allografts. *J Clin Invest*. 2007;117:989-996.
92. Campagnoli C, Roberts IA, Kumar S, et al. Identification of mesenchymal stem/progenitor cells in human first-trimester fetal blood, liver, and bone marrow. *Blood*. 2001;98:2396-2402.
93. Zuk PA, Zhu M, Mizuno H, et al. Multilineage cells from human adipose tissue: implications for cell-based therapies. *Tissue Eng*. 2001;7:211-228.
94. Pierdomenico L, Bonsi L, Calvitti M, et al. Multipotent mesenchymal stem cells with immunosuppressive activity can be easily isolated from dental pulp. *Transplantation*. 2005;80:836-842.
95. Zhang Y, Li C, Jiang X, et al. Human placenta-derived mesenchymal progenitor cells support culture expansion of long-term culture-initiating cells from cord blood CD34+ cells. *Expl Hematol*. 2004;32:657-664.
96. Dominici M, Le Blanc K, Mueller I, et al. Minimal criteria for defining multipotent mesenchymal stromal cells. The International Society for Cellular Therapy position statement. *Cytotherapy*. 2006;8:315-317.
97. van Haaften T, Byrne R, Bonnet S, et al. Airway delivery of mesenchymal stem cells prevents arrested alveolar growth in neonatal lung injury in rats. *Am J Respir Crit Care Med*. 2009;180: 1131-1142.
98. Popova AP, Bozyk PD, Bentley JK, et al. Isolation of tracheal aspirate mesenchymal stromal cells predicts bronchopulmonary dysplasia. *Pediatrics*. 2010;126:e1127-e1133.
99. Popova AP, Bozyk PD, Goldsmith AM, et al. Autocrine production of TGF-B1 promotes myofibroblastic differentiation of neonatal lung mesenchymal stem cells. *Am J Physiol Lung Cell Mol Physiol*. 2010;298:L735-L743.
100. Asahara T, Murohara T, Sullivan A, et al. Isolation of putative progenitor endothelial cells for angiogenesis. *Science*. 1997;275:964-966.
101. Tepper OM, Capla JM, Galiano RD, et al. Adult vasculogenesis occurs through in situ recruitment, proliferation, and tubulization of circulating bone marrow-derived cells. *Blood*. 2005;105: 1068-1077.
102. Asahara T, Masuda H, Takahashi T, et al. Bone marrow origin of endothelial progenitor cells responsible for postnatal vasculogenesis in physiological and pathological neovascularization. *Circ Res*. 1999;85:221-228.
103. Fadini GP, Schiavon M, Cantini M, et al. Circulating progenitor cells are reduced in patients with severe lung disease. *Stem Cells*. 2006;24:1806-1813.
104. Fadini GP, Schiavon M, Rea F, et al. Depletion of endothelial progenitor cells may link pulmonary fibrosis and pulmonary hypertension. *Am J Respir Crit Care Med*. 2007;176:724-725.
105. Balasubramaniam V, Mervis CF, Maxey AM, et al. Hyperoxia reduces bone marrow, circulating, and lung endothelial progenitor cells in the developing lung: implications for the pathogenesis of bronchopulmonary dysplasia. *Am J Physiol- Lung Cell Mol Physiol*. 2007;292:L1073-L1084.
106. Borghesi A, Massa M, Campanelli R, et al. Circulating endothelial progenitor cells in preterm infants with bronchopulmonary dysplasia. *Am J Respir Crit Care Med*. 2009;180:540-546.
107. Krasnodembskaya A, Song Y, Fang X, et al. Antibacterial effect of human mesenchymal stem cells is mediated in part from secretion of the antimicrobial peptide LL-37. *Stem Cells*. 2010;28: 2229-2238.
108. Gupta N, Su X, Popov B, et al. Intrapulmonary delivery of bone marrow-derived mesenchymal stem cells improves survival and attenuates endotoxin-induced acute lung injury in mice. *J Immunol*. 2007;179:1855-1863.
109. Nemeth K, Leelahavanichkul A, Yuen PST, et al. Bone marrow stromal cells attenuate sepsis via prostaglandin E2-dependent reprogramming of host macrophages to increase their interleukin-10 production. *Nat Med*. 2009;15:42-49.
110. Mei SH, Haitsma JJ, Dos Santos CC, et al. Mesenchymal stem cells reduce inflammation while enhancing bacterial clearance and improving survival in sepsis. *Am J Respir Crit Care Med*. 2010;182:1047-1057.
111. Fang X, Neyrinck AP, Matthay MA, Lee JW. Allogeneic human mesenchymal stem cells restore epithelial protein permeability in cultured human alveolar type II cells by secretion of angiopoietin-1. *J Biol Chem*. 2010;285:26211-26222.

B

112. Zhao YD, Ohkawara H, Vogel SM, et al. Bone marrow-derived progenitor cells prevent thrombin-induced increase in lung vascular permeability. *Am J Physiol Lung Cell Mol Physiol*. 2010;298: L36-L44.
113. Lee JW, Fang X, Gupta N, et al. Allogeneic human mesenchymal stem cells for treatment of E. coli endotoxin-induced acute lung injury in the ex vivo perfused human lung. *Proc Natl Acad Sci U S A*. 2009;106:16357-16362.
114. Mei SHJ, McCarter SD, Deng Y, et al. Prevention of LPS-induced acute lung injury in mice by mesenchymal stem cells overexpressing angiopoietin 1. *PLoS Med*. 2007;4:e269.
115. Katsha AM, Ohkouchi S, Xin H, et al. Paracrine factors of multipotent stromal cells ameliorate lung injury in an elastase-induced emphysema model. *Mol Ther*. 2011;19:196-203.
116. Lee JW, Fang X, Krasnodembskaya A, et al. Concise review: Mesenchymal stem cells for acute lung injury: role of paracrine soluble factors. *Stem Cells*. 2011;29:913-919
117. Xu J, Qu J, Cao L, et al. Mesenchymal stem cell-based angiopoietin-1 gene therapy for acute lung injury induced by lipopolysaccharide in mice. *J Pathol*. 2008;214:472-481.
118. Fang X, Neyrinck AP, Matthay MA, Lee JW. Allogeneic human mesenchymal stem cells restore epithelial protein permeability in cultured human alveolar type ii cells by secretion of angiopoietin-1. *J Biol Chem*. 2010;285:26211-26222.
119. Aslam M, Baveja R, Liang OD, et al. Bone marrow stromal cells attenuate lung injury in a murine model of neonatal chronic lung disease. *Am J Respir Crit Care Med*. 2009;180:1122-1130.
120. Balasubramaniam V, Ryan SL, Seedorf GJ, et al. Bone marrow-derived angiogenic cells restore lung alveolar and vascular structure after neonatal hyperoxia in infant mice. *Am J Physiol Lung Cell Mol Physiol*. 2010;298:L315-L323.
121. Rojas M, Xu J, Woods CR, et al. Bone marrow-derived mesenchymal stem cells in repair of the injured lung. *Am J Respir Cell Mol Biol*. 2005;33:145-152.
122. Ortiz LA, Gambelli F, McBride C, et al. Mesenchymal stem cell engraftment in lung is enhanced in response to bleomycin exposure and ameliorates its fibrotic effects. *Proc Natl Acad Sci U S A*. 2003;100:8407-8411.
123. Ortiz LA, Gambelli F, McBride C, et al. Mesenchymal stem cell engraftment in lung is enhanced in response to bleomycin exposure and ameliorates its fibrotic effects. *Proc Natl Acad Sci U S A*. 2003; 100:8407-8411.
124. Ortiz LA, Dutreil M, Fattman C, et al. Interleukin 1 receptor antagonist mediates the antiinflammatory and antifibrotic effect of mesenchymal stem cells during lung injury. *Proc Natl Acad Sci U S A*. 2007;104:11002-11007.
125. Lee SH, Jang AS, Kim YE, et al. Modulation of cytokine and nitric oxide by mesenchymal stem cell transfer in lung injury/fibrosis. *Respir Res*. 2010;11:16.
126. Yan X, Liu Y, Han Q, et al. Injured microenvironment directly guides the differentiation of engrafted Flk-1+ mesenchymal stem cell in lung. *Exp Hematol*. 2007;35:1466-1475.
127. Umar S, de Visser YP, Steendijk P, et al. Allogeneic stem cell therapy improves right ventricular function by improving lung pathology in rats with pulmonary hypertension. *Am J Physiol Heart Circ Physiol*. 2009;297:H1606-H1616.
128. Baber SR, Deng W, Master RG, et al. Intratracheal mesenchymal stem cell administration attenuates monocrotaline-induced pulmonary hypertension and endothelial dysfunction. *Am J Physiol Heart Circ Physiol*. 2007;292:H1120-H1128.
129. Umar S, de Visser YP, Steendijk P, et al. Allogeneic stem cell therapy improves right ventricular function by improving lung pathology in rats with pulmonary hypertension. *Am J Physiol Heart Circ Physiol*. 2009;297:H1606-H1616.
130. Kanki-Horimoto S, Horimoto H, Mieno S, et al. Implantation of mesenchymal stem cells overexpressing endothelial nitric oxide synthase improves right ventricular impairments caused by pulmonary hypertension. *Circulation*. 2006;114:I-181-I-185.
131. Takemiya K, Kai H, Yasukawa H, et al. Mesenchymal stem cell-based prostacyclin synthase gene therapy for pulmonary hypertension rats. *Basic Res Cardiol*. 2009;105:409-417.
132. Zhao YD, Courtman DW, Deng Y, et al. Rescue of monocrotaline-induced pulmonary arterial hypertension using bone marrow-derived endothelial-like progenitor cells: Efficacy of combined cell and eNOS gene therapy in established disease. *Circ Res*. 2005;96:442-450.
133. Wang XX, Zhang FR, Shang YP, et al. Transplantation of autologous endothelial progenitor cells may be beneficial in patients with idiopathic pulmonary arterial hypertension: a pilot randomized controlled trial. *J Am Coll Cardiol*. 2007;49:1566-1571.
134. Bonfield TL, Koloze M, Lennon DP, et al. Human mesenchymal stem cells suppress chronic airway inflammation in the murine ovalbumin asthma model. *Am J Physiol Lung Cell Mol Physiol*. 2010;299:L760-L770.
135. Shigemura N, Okumura M, Mizuno S, et al. Autologous transplantation of adipose tissue-derived stromal cells ameliorates pulmonary emphysema. *Am J Transpl*. 2006;6:2592-2600.
136. Kopen GC, Prockop DJ, Phinney DG. Marrow stromal cells migrate throughout forebrain and cerebellum, and they differentiate into astrocytes after injection into neonatal mouse brains. *Proc Natl Acad Sci U S A*. 1999;96:10711-10716.
137. Pereira RF, O'Hara MD, Laptev AV, et al. Marrow stromal cells as a source of progenitor cells for nonhematopoietic tissues in transgenic mice with a phenotype of osteogenesis imperfecta. *Proc Natl Acad Sci U S A*. 1998;95:1142-1147.
138. Munoz-Elias G, Marcus AJ, Coyne TM, et al. Adult bone marrow stromal cells in the embryonic brain: engraftment, migration, differentiation, and long-term survival. *J Neurosci*. 2004;24: 4585-4595.

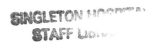

139. Pochampally RR, Neville BT, Schwarz EJ, et al. Rat adult stem cells (marrow stromal cells) engraft and differentiate in chick embryos without evidence of cell fusion. *Proc Natl Acad Sci U S A.* 2004;101:9282-9285.
140. Wu Y, Chen L, Scott PG, Tredget EE. Mesenchymal stem cells enhance wound healing through differentiation and angiogenesis. *Stem Cells.* 2007;25:2648-2659.
141. Sasaki M, Abe R, Fujita Y, et al. Mesenchymal stem cells are recruited into wounded skin and contribute to wound repair by transdifferentiation into multiple skin cell type. *J Immunol.* 2008;180:2581-2587.
142. Caplan AI. All MSCs are pericytes? *Cell Stem Cell.* 2008;3:229-230.
143. da Silva Meirelles L, Caplan AI, Nardi NB. In search of the in vivo identity of mesenchymal stem cells. *Stem Cells.* 2008;26:2287-2299.
144. Krampera M, Cosmi L, Angeli R, et al. Role for interferon-gamma in the immunomodulatory activity of human bone marrow mesenchymal stem cells. *Stem Cells.* 2006;24:386-398.
145. Nauta AJ, Fibbe WE. Immunomodulatory properties of mesenchymal stromal cells. *Blood.* 2007;110:3499-3506.
146. Meisel R, Zibert A, Laryea M, et al. Human bone marrow stromal cells inhibit allogeneic T-cell responses by indoleamine 2,3-dioxygenase-mediated tryptophan degradation. *Blood.* 2004;103: 4619-4621.
147. Zappia E, Casazza S, Pedemonte E, et al. Mesenchymal stem cells ameliorate experimental autoimmune encephalomyelitis inducing T-cell anergy. *Blood.* 2005;106:1755-1761.
148. Krampera M, Glennie S, Dyson J, et al. Bone marrow mesenchymal stem cells inhibit the response of naive and memory antigen-specific T cells to their cognate peptide. *Blood.* 2003;101: 3722-3729.
149. Corcione A, Benvenuto F, Ferretti E, et al. Human mesenchymal stem cells modulate B-cell functions. *Blood.* 2006;107:367-372.
150. Sotiropoulou PA, Perez SA, Gritzapis AD, et al. Interactions between human mesenchymal stem cells and natural killer cells. *Stem Cells.* 2006;24:74-85.
151. Nauta AJ, Kruisselbrink AB, Lurvink E, et al. Mesenchymal stem cells inhibit generation and function of both CD34+-derived and monocyte-derived dendritic cells. *J Immunol.* 2006;177: 2080-2087.
152. Griffith LG. Emerging design principles in biomaterials and scaffolds for tissue engineering. In: Sipe JD, Kelley CA, McNicol LA, eds. *Reparative Medicine: Growing Tissues and Organs.* New York: New York Academy of Sciences; 2002.
153. Andrade CF, Wong AP, Waddell TK, et al. Cell-based tissue engineering for lung regeneration. *Am J Physiol Lung Cell Mol Physiol.* 2007;292:L510-L518.
154. Sugihara H, Toda S, Miyabara S, et al. Reconstruction of alveolus-like structure from alveolar type II epithelial cells in three-dimensional collagen gel matrix culture. *Am J Pathol.* 1993;142: 783-792.
155. Petersen TH, Calle EA, Zhao L, et al. Tissue-engineered lungs for in vivo implantation. *Science.* 2010;329:538-541.
156. Cortiella J, Nichols JE, Kojima K, et al. Tissue-engineered lung: An in vivo and in vitro comparison of polyglycolic acid and pluronic F-127 hydrogel/somatic lung progenitor cell constructs to support tissue growth. *Tissue Eng.* 2006;12:1213-1225.
157. Macchiarini P, Jungebluth P, Go T, et al. Clinical transplantation of a tissue-engineered airway. *Lancet.* 2008;372:2023-2030.
158. Kim CF. Paving the road for lung stem cell biology: bronchioalveolar stem cells and other putative distal lung stem cells. *Am J Physiol Lung Cell Mol Physiol.* 2007;293:L1092-L1098.
159. Watt FM, Hogan BL, Brigid LM. Out of Eden: Stem cells and their niches. *Science.* 2000;287: 1427-1430.
160. Morrison SJ, Shah NM, Anderson DJ. Regulatory mechanisms in stem cell biology. *Cell.* 1997;88:287-298.
161. Rock JR, Onaitis MW, Rawlins EL. Basal cells as stem cells of the mouse trachea and human airway epithelium. *Proc Natl Acad Sci U S A.* 2009;106:12771-12775.
162. Hong KU, Reynolds SD, Watkins S, et al. Basal cells are a multipotent progenitor capable of renewing the bronchial epithelium. *Am J Pathol.* 2004;164:577-588.
163. Hong KU, Reynolds SD, Watkins S, et al. In vivo differentiation potential of tracheal basal cells: evidence for multipotent and unipotent subpopulations. *Am J Physiol Lung Cell Mol Physiol.* 2004;286:L643-L649.
164. Schoch KG, Lori A, Burns KA, et al. A subset of mouse tracheal epithelial basal cells generates large colonies in vitro. *Am J Physiol Lung Cell Mol Physiol.* 2004;286:L631-L642.
165. Rock JR, Randell SH, Hogan BL. Airway basal stem cells: a perspective on their roles in epithelial homeostasis and remodeling. *Dis Model Mech.* 2010;3:545-556.
166. Borthwick DW, Shahbazian M, Todd Krantz Q, et al. Evidence for stem-cell niches in the tracheal epithelium. *Am J Respir Cell Mol Biol.* 2001;24:662-670.
167. Rawlins EL, Okubo T, Xue Y, et al. The role of Scgb1a1+ Clara cells in the long-term maintenance and repair of lung airway, but not alveolar, epithelium. *Cell Stem Cell.* 2009;4:525-534.
168. Evans MJ, Cabral-Anderson LJ, Freeman G. Role of the Clara cell in renewal of the bronchiolar epithelium. *Lab Invest.* 1978;38:648-653.
169. Giangreco A, Reynolds SD, Stripp BR. Terminal bronchioles harbor a unique airway stem cell population that localizes to the bronchoalveolar duct junction. *Am J Pathol.* 2002;161:173-182.

B

170. Hong KU, Reynolds SD, Giangreco A, et al. Clara cell secretory protein-expressing cells of the airway neuroepithelial body microenvironment include a label-retaining subset and are critical for epithelial renewal after progenitor cell depletion. *Am J Respir Cell Mol Biol*. 2001;24:671-681.
171. Reynolds SD, Giangreco A, Power JH. Neuroepithelial bodies of pulmonary airways serve as a reservoir of progenitor cells capable of epithelial regeneration. *Am J Pathol*. 2000;156:269.
172. Kim CF, Jackson EL, Woolfenden AE. Identification of bronchioalveolar stem cells in normal lung and lung cancer. *Cell*. 2005;121:823-835.
173. Ling T-Y, Kuo M-D, Li C-L, et al. Identification of pulmonary Oct-4+ stem/progenitor cells and demonstration of their susceptibility to SARS coronavirus (SARS-CoV) infection in vitro. *Proc Natl Acad SciU S A*. 2006;103:9530-9535.
174. Adamson IY, Bowden DH. The type 2 cell as progenitor of alveolar epithelial regeneration. A cytodynamic study in mice after exposure to oxygen. *Lab Invest*. 1974;30:35-42.
175. Tryka AF, Witschi H, Gosslee DG, et al. Patterns of cell proliferation during recovery from oxygen injury: Species differences. *Am Rev Respir Dis*. 1986;133:1055-1059.
176. Adamson IY, Bowden DH. The type 2 cell as progenitor of alveolar epithelial regeneration. A cytodynamic study in mice after exposure to oxygen. *Lab Invest*. 1974;30:35.
177. Adamson IY, Bowden DH. Derivation of type 1 epithelium from type 2 cells in the developing rat lung. *Lab Invest*. 1975;32:736.
178. Driscoll B, Buckley S, Bui KC, et al. Telomerase in alveolar epithelial development and repair. *Am J Physiol Lung Cell Mol Physiol*. 2000;279:L1191-L1198.
179. Reddy R, Buckley S, Doerken M, et al. Isolation of a putative progenitor subpopulation of alveolar epithelial type 2 cells. *Am J Physiol Lung Cell Mol Physiol*. 2004;286:L658-L667.
180. Lee J, Reddy R, Barsky L, et al. Lung alveolar integrity is compromised by telomere shortening in telomerase-null mice. *Am J Physiol Lung Cell Mol Physiol*. 2009;296:L57-L70.
181. Kajstura J, Rota M, Hall SR, et al. Evidence for human lung stem cells. *N Engl J Med*. 2011; 364:1795-1806.
182. Alvarez DF, Huang L, King JA, et al. Lung microvascular endothelium is enriched with progenitor cells that exhibit vasculogenic capacity. *Am J Physiol Lung Cell Mol Physiol*. 2008;294:L419-L430.
183. Suratt BT, Cool CD, Serls AE, et al. Human pulmonary chimerism after hematopoietic stem cell transplantation. *Am J Respir Crit Care Med*. 2003;168:318.
184. Mattsson J, Jansson M, Wernerson A. Lung epithelial cells and type II pneumocytes of donor origin after allogeneic hematopoietic stem cell transplantation. *Transplantation*. 2004;78:154.
185. Kleeberger W, Versmold A, Rothamel T. Increased chimerism of bronchial and alveolar epithelium in human lung allografts undergoing chronic injury. *Am J Pathol*. 2003;162:1487.
186. Gomperts BN, Belperio JA, Rao PN, et al. Circulating progenitor epithelial cells traffic via CXCR4/CXCL12 in response to airway injury. *J Immunol*. 2006;176:1916-1927.
187. Wong AP, Keating A, Lu WY, et al. Identification of a bone marrow-derived epithelial-like population capable of repopulating injured mouse airway epithelium. *J Clin Invest*. 2009;119:336-348.
188. Bucala R, Spiegel LA, Chesney J. Circulating fibrocytes define a new leukocyte subpopulation that mediates tissue repair. *Mol Med*. 1994;1:71.
189. Quan TE, Cowper S, Wu SP. Circulating fibrocytes: collagen-secreting cells of the peripheral blood. *Int J Biochem Cell Biol*. 2004;36:598.
190. Strieter RM, Keeley EC, Hughes MA, et al. The role of circulating mesenchymal progenitor cells (fibrocytes) in the pathogenesis of pulmonary fibrosis. *J Leukoc Biol*. 2009;86:1111-1118.
191. Phillips RJ, Burdick MD, Hong K, et al. Circulating fibrocytes traffic to the lungs in response to CXCL12 and mediate fibrosis. *J Clin Invest*. 2004;114:438-446.
192. Moore BB, Murray L, Das A, et al. The role of CCL12 in the recruitment of fibrocytes and lung fibrosis. *Am J Respir Cell Mol Biol*. 2006;35:175-181.
193. Gomperts BN, Strieter RM. Stem cells and chronic lung disease. *Annu Rev Med*. 2007;58: 285-298.
194. Nikam VS, Schermuly RT, Dumitrascu R, et al. Treprostinil inhibits the recruitment of bone marrow-derived circulating fibrocytes in chronic hypoxic pulmonary hypertension. *EurRespir J*. 2010;36:1302-1314.
195. Schmidt M, Sun G, Stacey MA. Identification of circulating fibrocytes as precursors of bronchial myofibroblasts in asthma. *J Immunol*. 2003;171:380.
196. Nihlberg K, Larsen K, Hultgardh-Nilsson A, et al. Tissue fibrocytes in patients with mild asthma: a possible link to thickness of reticular basement membrane? *Respir Res*. 2006;7:50.
197. Saunders R, Siddiqui S, Kaur D, et al. Fibrocyte localization to the airway smooth muscle is a feature of asthma. *J Allergy Clin Immunol*. 2009;123:376-384.
198. Epperly MW, Guo H, Gretton JE. Bone marrow origin of myofibroblasts in irradiation pulmonary fibrosis. *Am J Respir Cell Mol Biol*. 2003;29:213.
199. Moeller A, Gilpin SE, Ask K, et al. Circulating fibrocytes are an indicator of poor prognosis in idiopathic pulmonary fibrosis. *Am J Respir Crit Care Med*. 2009;179:588-594.
200. Wang C-H, Huang C-D, Lin H-C, et al. Increased circulating fibrocytes in asthma with chronic airflow obstruction. *Am J Respir Crit Care Med*. 2008;178:583-591.
201. Frid MG, Brunetti JA, Burke DL, et al. Hypoxia-induced pulmonary vascular remodeling requires recruitment of circulating mesenchymal precursors of a monocyte/macrophage lineage. *Am J Pathol*. 2006;168:659-669.
202. Young KC, Torres E, Hatzistergos KE, et al. Inhibition of the SDF-1/CXCR4 axis attenuates neonatal hypoxia-induced pulmonary hypertension. *Circ Res*. 2009;104:1293-1301.

CHAPTER 10

New Developments in the Pathogenesis and Prevention of Bronchopulmonary Dysplasia

Ilene R.S. Sosenko, MD, and Eduardo Bancalari, MD

10

- New Developments in Clinical Presentation
- New Developments in Understanding of BPD Pathogenesis
- New Developments in Prevention and Management of BPD
- Future Directions in Prevention of BPD
- Conclusion

Whereas markedly improved survival of extremely low-birth-weight infants (LBW) is a major success of current day neonatology, the success has been tempered by the fact that these infants have an unacceptably high risk for complications such as the chronic lung damage of bronchopulmonary dysplasia (BPD). The incidence of BPD ranges between 15% and 50% in infants weighing less than 1500 g at birth and increases with decreasing gestational age (Fig. 10-1).[1,2] BPD was originally described by Northway and colleagues[3] in 1967. Over the past four decades its clinical picture has changed, and both clinical research and translational research have yielded greater understanding of the pathogenesis and potential approaches to therapy and prevention of BPD. Unfortunately, studies have also raised caution that some potential approaches to BPD, such as limitation of inspired oxygen, might actually be deleterious to the outcome of the vulnerable premature infant,[4] and that proposed therapies, such as inhaled nitric oxide, may lack the effectiveness they once promised.[5] Nonetheless, ongoing research continues to offer great promise about reaching the future goal of eradicating and/or ameliorating the chronic lung complication known as BPD.

New Developments in Clinical Presentation

When Northway and colleagues[3] originally described and named the process they called bronchopulmonary dysplasia (BPD), they reported chronic lung damage in premature infants who weighed more than 1000 g at birth and had received prolonged mechanical ventilation with high pressures and high supplemental oxygen. The investigators proposed that what they would now call BPD was caused by multifactorial injury to the immature lung. They described the *in tandem* clinical and radiographic progression of BPD through four specific stages, with the final stage resulting in the clinical picture of severe respiratory failure associated with the radiographic picture of increased densities secondary to fibrosis and enlarged, emphysematous alveoli adjacent to areas of atelectasis.[3]

Over the ensuing four decades since its original description, the severe clinical and pathologic picture of Northway's BPD has been modified as a result of evolving clinical practices, including widespread administration of antenatal steroids, postnatal surfactant therapy, and a "gentler" approach to mechanical ventilation. In fact, Northway's severe classic presentation of BPD is now infrequently seen. Instead, the

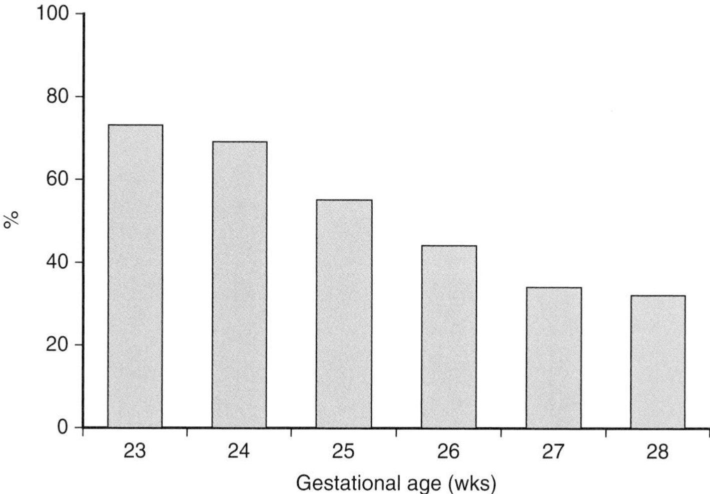

Figure 10-1 Statistics for incidence of bronchopulmonary dysplasia (BPD) by gestational age for inborn premature infants (23-28 weeks) born within the years 2003-2007 at hospitals in the National Institute of Child Health and Human Development (NICHD) Neonatal Network. (w PMA), weeks postmenstrual age. (From Stoll B, Hansen NI, Bell EF, et. al; for the Eunice Kennedy Shriver NICHD Neonatal Research Network. Neonatal outcomes of extremely preterm infants from the NICHD Neonatal Research Network. *Pediatrics.* 2010;126 443-445.)

typical picture of the "new BPD" is one affecting smaller and more immature infants (400-1000 g) than the original study's population (>1000 g). Current infants present with milder lung disease, may start out with only minimal or mild RDS, and, in fact, may receive mechanical ventilation for pneumonia, apnea, or poor respiratory effort. They may require low-pressure ventilatory support with low inspired oxygen concentrations and may already be breathing room air within the first day(s) of life. However, within a few days or weeks after birth, these infants display deteriorating lung function and increased ventilator and/or oxygen requirements. This deterioration in respiratory status may be related to a hemodynamically significant patent ductus arteriosus (PDA), to inflammation caused by bacterial infection or colonization, or to inflammatory processes triggered by oxygen or mechanical ventilation.[6,7] Although infants with "new BPD" may require mechanical ventilation and oxygen for a prolonged period, the majority with this relatively milder form of chronic lung disease are essentially symptom-free by discharge.[1] There remains a small minority of infants with "new BPD" who have more severe lung dysfunction, characterized by progressive respiratory failure that may even be associated with pulmonary hypertension and cor pulmonale, severe airway damage, bronchomalacia, and airway obstruction, and may result in death.[8] If infants with this more severe form of BPD acquire acute bacterial or viral pulmonary infections, their lung damage may be further exacerbated.[9]

New Developments in Understanding of BPD Pathogenesis

When Northway and colleagues[3] originally described BPD, they proposed the following four major factors in its pathogenesis: (1) lung immaturity, (2) respiratory failure, (3) oxygen supplementation, and (4) positive-pressure mechanical ventilation. Beyond these factors, new knowledge suggests additional complex processes involved in the pathogenesis of BPD, including inflammation, aberrations in lung

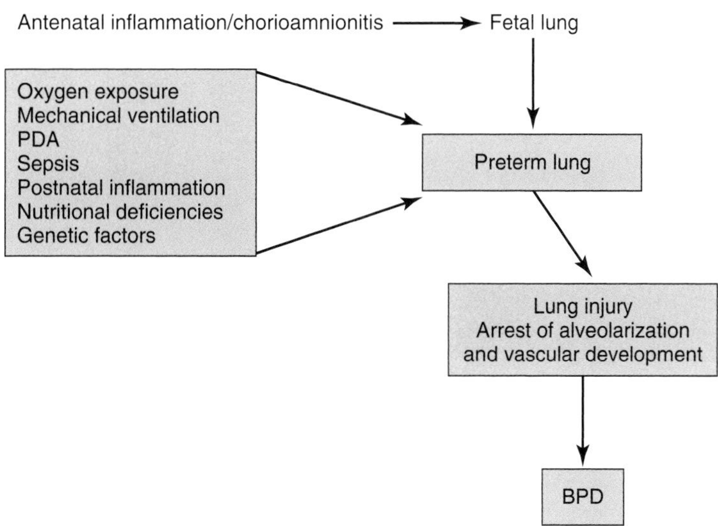

Figure 10-2 Scheme of factors related to pathogenesis of bronchopulmonary dysplasia (BPD). PDA, patent ductus arteriosus.

growth and lung signaling pathways, derangements in transcription factors and growth factors, new evidence related to oxidant lung injury, as well as a broader understanding of the genetics of BPD (Fig. 10-2).

Role of Inflammation in BPD Pathogenesis

Whereas epidemiology has linked infection/inflammation and preterm birth,[10,11] chorioamnionitis, even in its silent form, has been reported in a majority of deliveries occurring before 30 weeks of gestation, with the association of chorioamnionitis and preterm delivery inversely related to gestational age.[12] Evidence suggests that exposure to antenatal inflammation may have a protective effect of reducing the incidence of hyaline membrane disease in premature infants while paradoxically increasing the risk of lung damage and BPD.[13] Correlated with the development of BPD were elevations in amniotic fluid proinflammatory mediators such as interleukin-6 (IL-6), tumor necrosis factor-α (TNF-α), IL-1β, and IL-8 within 5 days of preterm birth.[14,15] Furthermore, in a dose-response fashion, a higher risk for development of BPD was demonstrated in preterm infants exposed to severe histologic chorioamnionitis than in those exposed to mild or no chorioamnionitis.[16] In contrast to these findings linking chorioamnionitis and BPD, Van Marter and associates[17] reported the opposite—that is, a decrease in risk of BPD in a group of preterm infants exposed to chorioamnionitis who did not end up requiring mechanical ventilation or having infection in the postnatal period. Using multivariate logistic regression analysis, Soraisham and coworkers[18] also did not find an increase in BPD associated with clinical chorioamnionitis.

Antenatal inflammatory exposure in the developing fetus may also be related to actual colonization or infection. *Ureaplasma urealyticum* colonization may trigger in utero inflammation, because *Ureaplasma* has been isolated from lungs of many infants who experience BPD.[19] When Kotecha and coworkers[20] used reverse transcriptase polymerase chain reaction (PCR) analysis to study infants with lung inflammation who ultimately had BPD, they found the majority to have *U. urealyticum* in bronchoalveolar lavage fluid at 10 days of age and suggested that antenatal acquisition of this agent may produce early lung inflammation, increasing the likelihood of progression to BPD. However, an attempt to reduce BPD incidence with erythromycin was ineffective in a randomized controlled trial, possibly because the antibiotic may not have successfully eradicated *U. urealyticum* from the trachea.[21] Similarly, a pilot study of prophylactic azithromycin failed to reduce the incidence of BPD, although postnatal steroid use was decreased in the treated infants.[22] Other antenatal infections might also produce inflammation related to BPD, because elevated cord blood immunoglobulin M (IgM) values for adenovirus were found in certain infants who later had BPD.[23]

Whether bacterial or viral postnatal infection in premature infants may also be related to an increased risk of BPD is not clear. For example, premature infants with coagulase-negative staphylococcus sepsis were found to have a significantly higher risk of BPD than uninfected infants.[24] When postnatal infection occurred concomitantly with the presence of PDA, the risk of BPD was increased even further.[6] Both cytomegalovirus and respiratory syncytial virus have been shown to have a negative effect on the preterm lung, with postnatal cytomegalovirus infection being associated with an increased risk of BPD[25] and respiratory syncytial virus infection producing respiratory deterioration in infants with evolving or established BPD.[26] (This topic is discussed in greater detail in the Chapters 3 and 6.]

Inflammation from causes unrelated to infection can also have adverse effects on the preterm lung. In addition to the oxygen free radicals produced by exposure to oxygen, oxidant stress activates inflammatory cells and increases proinflammatory cytokines.[27] High–tidal volume positive-pressure ventilation has also been shown to produce inflammation.[27] Finally, as previously mentioned, a PDA, with increased pulmonary blood flow, can initiate the inflammatory cascade and stimulate neutrophil margination and activation in the lung.[28] Preterm baboons have been shown to demonstrate arrest of alveolar development in the presence of a PDA. When PDA in preterm baboons was treated with early ibuprofen therapy,[29] arrest of alveolarization was partially reversed, possibly owing to PDA closure secondary to ibuprofen and/or to anti-inflammatory effects of ibuprofen; however, PDA closure by ligation failed to reverse alveolarization arrest.[30]

Role of Arrest of Alveolar Development and the Vascular Hypothesis in Pathogenesis of BPD

BPD occurs predominantly in the extremely preterm infant, with an incidence in prematures requiring mechanical ventilation inversely proportional to gestational age and birth weight. As a result, BPD in infants born later than 32 weeks of gestation is extremely rare.[1] At the time of extreme preterm birth, the developing lung is at a highly immature stage of development, which results in greater vulnerability to lung damage. For example, the lung of an infant born at 24 weeks of gestation is only in the canalicular stage, with progression to the saccular stage not occurring until 30 weeks. These extremely immature and vulnerable lungs are easily damaged by postnatal therapies, such as mechanical ventilation and oxygen, and by inflammation and infection, which frequently progress to chronic lung injury.

In addition to actual damage that immature lungs can sustain with preterm birth, exposure to such noxious influences as hyperoxia and inflammation can disrupt the normal progression of lung development, with resultant perturbation or dysregulation of lung morphologic maturation. This dysregulation appears as inhibition of acinar development, causing reduction in alveolar number, reduction in gas exchange surface area, and decreased lung capillaries.[31,32] Because this dysregulation in lung development has been associated with perturbations in angiogenic growth factors, Thébaud and Abman have proposed a "vascular hypothesis" in the pathogenesis of BPD. Whereas normal alveolar development progresses in response to the secretion of angiogenic growth factors, such as vascular endothelial growth factor (VEGF) and nitric oxide (NO), lung angiogenic growth factor expression has been found to be decreased in BPD, a finding that may explain the arrest of vascular growth and impairment of alveolar growth.[33] Multiple studies support this "vascular hypothesis" of BPD, including findings that (1) VEGF signaling disruption reduces alveolarization in the rat,[34] (2) VEGF signaling disruption is produced by hyperoxia in experimental animals,[35,36] and (3) administration of VEGF improves lung structure in experimental models of BPD.[37] In fact, reduced lung VEGF messenger RNA (mRNA) and protein expression, reduction of VEGF receptor, and decreased expression of other endothelial markers, such as platelet/endothelial cell adhesion molecule-1 (PECAM-1) and the cell surface receptor Tie2, were found in human infants dying of BPD.[38] When endothelial colony-forming cells (EPFCs) from preterm infants were exposed to hyperoxia, these cells had decreases in growth, VEGF receptor and endothelial nitric oxide synthase (eNOS) expression, and NO production; growth of the cells was restored by treatment with VEGF or NO.[39] Endoglin, a hypoxia-inducible glycoprotein that is part of the transforming growth factor-β (TGF-β) complex and functions as a regulator of angiogenesis, was found to be upregulated at the mRNA and protein levels in preterm infants needing long-term mechanical ventilation. Findings of reduced mRNA of VEGF, angiopoietin-1, and their receptors, with upregulation of endoglin, suggest a shift from traditional angiogenic growth factors to alternate regulators of angiogenesis as a possible explanation for the impaired microvascularity of BPD.[40]

Role of Alterations in Growth Factors in BPD Pathogenesis

In addition to the major growth factors associated with angiogenesis, other growth factors involved with lung development may have abnormal gene expression in infants in whom BPD develops. Been and coworkers[41] reported not only a decrease in VEGF expression but also a decrease in TGF-α expression and an increase in granulocyte macrophage colony-stimulating factor (GM-CSF) expression in bronchoalveolar lavage fluid from the first day of life in infants who ultimately have BPD.[41] Whereas platelet-derived growth factor (PDGF)-BB concentrations were found to rise in preterm infants receiving mechanical ventilation, those infants in whom BPD developed had higher maximal concentrations of PDGF-BB than those without BPD, suggesting that this growth factor may play a role in the fibrotic component of BPD.[42] Jankov and Tanswell[43] propose complex interactions still to be determined between expression of individual growth factors, including insulin-like growth factor-1 (IGF-1), epithelial growth factor (EGF) and EGF receptor, PDGF, fibroblast growth factor (FGF) and TGF-β, and the development of BPD.[43] Erythropoietin, believed to be functioning as a lung growth factor rather than an antioxidant, was found to have a protective effect, characterized by improved alveolar structure, enhanced vascularity, and decreased fibrosis, on hyperoxia-induced lung injury in experimental animals.[44]

Role of Hyperoxia and Hypoxia in BPD Pathogenesis

Since Northway and associates originally proposed pulmonary oxygen toxicity and lung damage secondary to mechanical ventilation as two major factors in the pathogenesis of BPD, these mechanisms have subsequently been supported by experimental animal models[45-47] and observational and epidemiologic studies.[48-50] As previously mentioned, both oxygen exposure and ventilator-induced lung injury may deleteriously affect the lung via inflammatory pathways. New clinical and experimental data suggest that although hyperoxia alone plays an important role in BPD pathogenesis, intermittent hypoxia occurring during exposure to hyperoxia may actually contribute to exacerbation of BPD through worsening of oxidative lung injury. Most premature infants requiring supplemental oxygen and/or mechanical ventilation have intermittent spells of hypoxia during their acute course, but those infants in whom BPD develops have more frequent episodes of hypoxemia than those without BPD.[51] Experimentally, when newborn mice were exposed to periods of hyperoxia plus intermittent hypoxia, they demonstrated more alveolar growth arrest and lung oxidative stress than mice exposed to hyperoxia alone,[52] suggesting an additive effect of hypoxia plus hyperoxia in the development of BPD. Also using newborn mice, Nwajei and colleagues[53] found that hypoxia worsened hyperoxia-induced lung injury, the worsening manifested as inhibition of alveolarization and decreased vascular density, which was associated with decreased pulmonary antioxidant defenses, specifically, expression of superoxide dismutase (SOD).[53]

Role of Genetics in BPD Pathogenesis

For many years, a genetic predisposition to BPD was thought to exist. However, the actual association of genetic factors with the susceptibility to BPD, through the use of concordance among very LBW twins, was first reported by Parker and coworkers.[54] In a quantitative analysis, Bhandari and his group[55] concluded that genetic factors accounted for 53% of the susceptibility for BPD.[55] In terms of potential specific genes related to the development of BPD, genetic factors associated with abnormal airway reactivity may play a role, in that infants with BPD have a stronger family history of asthma than those without BPD.[56] An extensive list of candidate genes that could play a potential role in pathogenesis of BPD has been proposed; several specific genetic loci linked to the development of BPD include the surfactant protein-B (SP-B) intron 4 deletion (i4del) (which could decrease ability to produce SP-B, particularly in response to injury),[57] polymorphisms of genes coding for VEGF (−460T allele) (which could influence angiogenesis in response to injury),[58] and polymorphisms in the glutathione-S-transferase-P1 gene (which could decrease tolerance to oxidative stress).[59] Italian investigators have now shown that a polymorphism in the macrophage inhibitory factor (MIF) promoter is associated with BPD; specifically, infants with the MIF-173* allele (predisposing to higher MIF production) were shown to have a lower incidence of BPD.[60] Further unraveling of the genetic relationships involved with BPD risk will bring additional understanding of the pathogenesis of this disease. (This issue is discussed in greater detail in Chapter 2.)

New Developments in Prevention and Management of BPD

As noted previously, the pathogenesis of BPD appears to be complex and multifactorial. Therefore, a single modality is unlikely to treat or completely prevent BPD. Using evidence-based data, the following presentation discusses current interventions to prevent or manage BPD that have been found to be effective, those found to be ineffective or inconclusive, and those that are still experimental but promising.

Approach to Oxygen Therapy and BPD Prevention and Management

Although extensive experimental evidence has repeatedly demonstrated the toxicity of oxygen and free radicals to the lung, actual data showing that reduction in supplemental oxygen exposure would actually protect against BPD has been mostly circumstantial. Observational studies showed that those neonatal intensive care units (NICUs) that set goals of lower oxygen saturation levels for premature infants requiring oxygen therapy had less BPD than those using higher oxygen saturation levels.[49,61-63] In fact, Saugstad and Aune,[64] analyzing the composite data from five observational studies comparing the effects of higher and lower oxygen saturation ranges on the development of "BPD and/or lung problems," found a relative risk (RR) for BPD of 0.70 (95% confidence interval [CI] 0.55-0.88) favoring the lower over the higher oxygen saturation groups.

Three randomized trials comparing higher and lower oxygen saturation ranges and analyzing the effect on BPD as an endpoint have now been published.[65-67] Two of these studies initiated the higher or lower oxygen saturation interventions relatively late, when infants were several weeks of age and BPD may already have been evolving.[65,66] Neither of these studies had BPD as the primary outcome. The STOP-ROP trial (Supplemental Therapeutic Oxygen for Prethreshold Retinopathy of Prematurity) did not randomly allocate infants to different treatments until about 35 weeks postmenstrual age (PMA) who met entry criteria for prethreshold ROP. The treatments differed as to oxygen saturation targets, 89% to 94% and 96% to 99%. Secondary outcome analysis revealed a higher incidence of pneumonia and/or exacerbations of BPD (manifested as increased need for oxygen, diuretics, and hospitalization at 3 months corrected age) in infants allocated to higher oxygen saturation therapy (13.2%) than in those receiving lower oxygen saturation therapy (8.5%).[65] The second randomized trial was the BOOST (Benefits of Oxygen Saturation Targeting) trial, which explored the effect of two different oxygen saturation targets (91%-94%) and (95%-98%) initiated in preterm infants at 32 weeks PMA on growth and neurodevelopmental outcome at 12 months corrected age. Secondary analysis found adverse pulmonary outcome (increased death rate and longer duration of supplemental oxygen exposure, with a 40% increase in infants requiring oxygen at 36 weeks PMA and a 70% increase in home oxygen therapy) in infants randomly assigned to the higher oxygen saturation group.[66] The latest randomized clinical trial, SUPPORT (Surfactant Positive Airway Pressure and Pulse Oximetry Trial) was the only study with an *early* intervention, comparing target oxygen saturations of 91% to 95% and 85% to 89% within the first 2 hours of age in 1316 infants born at 24 to 28 weeks of gestation.[67] BPD (oxygen at 36 wk) alone was reduced in the lower oxygen saturation group (RR 0.82; 95% CI 0.72-0.93) but there was no difference in combined outcome of BPD or death by 36 wk (RR 0.91; 95% CI 0.83-1.01). Most alarming, however, was the finding of increased risk of death before discharge (RR 1.27; 95% CI 1.01-1.60) in the lower oxygen saturation group.[67] In all of the studies described here, the ability to maintain oxygen saturations within a tightly prescribed range was difficult. Therefore, it is likely that tools such as automated regulation of inspired oxygen using a "closed loop" system could potentially improve oxygen stability and perhaps become the standard of clinical care of premature infants.[68]

Potential Role for Exogenous Antioxidants in BPD Prevention or Therapy

Because oxygen free radicals have been shown to be toxic to the lung and because preterm experimental animals and human infants are born with immaturity of the pulmonary antioxidant enzyme (AOE) system, investigators have explored whether exogenous administration of antioxidants could have positive effects on BPD prevention and treatment. Animal studies have found a lung-protective effect of exogenously administered AOEs, but human studies have yielded less promising results. The major randomized placebo-controlled trial of the AOE recombinant human copper/zinc SOD (CuZn-SOD) did not demonstrate a reduction in BPD or death in intubated very LBW infants. However, treated infants had a 36% reduction in wheezing episodes requiring bronchodilators, a 55% decrease in emergency room visits, and a 44% decrease in subsequent hospitalizations when followed up at 1 year corrected age.[69]

Not an antioxidant enzyme, glutathione is a major lung antioxidant substance that is deficient in premature infants. Although the amino acid cysteine is a precursor for glutathione, cysteine itself does not cross cell membranes; *N*-acetylcysteine (NAC) does cross to enter cells. Although NAC was theoretically promising in terms of increasing intracellular glutathione and prevention of BPD, a randomized controlled trial of NAC in premature infants failed to show improved pulmonary status in NAC-treated infants. A possible explanation for lack of efficacy of NAC in protection against lung injury was failure of this compound to actually increase intracellular glutathione levels.[70] Allopurinol, an inhibitor of the xanthine oxidase enzyme, which catalyzes reactions generating superoxide radicals, was tested in a randomized controlled trial in premature infants between 24 and 32 weeks of gestation, but its use did not result in a lower incidence of BPD.[71] Although magnesium deficiency could play a possible role in the pathogenesis of BPD on the basis of experimental data showing its association with greater cell susceptibility to peroxidation and worsening inflammatory reactions, administration of magnesium for BPD protection has not yet been subjected to clinical trials.[72] Similarly, deficiency of the trace metal selenium, an essential cofactor for the AOE glutathione peroxidase, could theoretically play a role in the development of BPD,[73] although this possibility was not borne out in a prospective analysis of selenium levels in preterm infants in whom BPD developed[74] or in a randomized trial of selenium supplementation in very LBW infants.[75]

Modalities of Ventilator Support and BPD Prevention and Management

Because of lung immaturity from preterm birth, the majority of premature infants require respiratory assistance to sustain life. As discussed previously, respiratory support can be damaging to the preterm lung, so the therapeutic goal is to provide this lifesaving respiratory support without further compromising the already vulnerable premature lung. As a result of data such as those reported by Avery and colleagues,[76] showing the lowest incidence of BPD in centers with the highest use of continuous positive airway pressure (CPAP) ventilation and avoidance of mechanical ventilation, the early use of CPAP ventilation to avoid mechanical ventilation has been examined in numerous clinical trials and by meta-analysis. Unfortunately, none of these studies has clearly demonstrated that early CPAP ventilation reduces the incidence of BPD.[77-79] As described previously, the SUPPORT trial, enrolled 1316 infants and randomly allocated them to either an "intubation and surfactant treatment" (within 1 hr of birth) group or a "CPAP group," in which CPAP ventilation was initiated in the delivery room with subsequent ventilation only if necessary.[67] No differences were found between groups in composite outcome of death or BPD. Slightly encouraging were findings that those in the "CPAP group" required less postnatal steroid therapy, required fewer days of mechanical ventilation, and were more likely to be alive and off the ventilator by day 7 of age.[80] Another study enrolled 208 infants born at 25 to 28 weeks of gestation who were spontaneously breathing and not in need of intubation at birth, randomly assigning them to either prophylactic surfactant or CPAP ventilation within 30 minutes of age. No differences between the intervention groups, in rate of death or BPD or in the primary endpoint, need for mechanical ventilation in the first 5 days of life, were found.[81]

In an attempt to avoid mechanical ventilation via an endotracheal tube, newer studies have explored the use of nasal intermittent positive-pressure ventilation (NIPPV) as the primary modality of respiratory support. Kugelman and coworkers[82] performed a randomized controlled trial comparing synchronized NIPPV with. CPAP ventilation alone in preterm infants and found a lower rate of BPD in the NIPPV group.[82] Two other studies yielded positive results for rate of BPD with NIPPV. Both the randomized controlled trial comparing synchronized NIPPV after surfactant administration with conventional ventilation and the retrospective analysis of synchronized NIPPV after extubation or for apnea found that use of NIPPV was associated with a lower rate of BPD than management without NIPPV.[83,84] In addition, Meneses and coworkers conducted a randomized controlled trial (n = 200 infants, 100 in each group) comparing the results of early NIPPV and nasal CPAP (NCPAP) on the need for mechanical ventilation in infants with HMD; these investigators found that early NIPPV did not decrease the incidence of BPD or the need for mechanical ventilation.[85] Thus, additional and larger studies will be necessary to definitively determine whether NIPPV rather than CPAP alone or endotracheal ventilation may be a promising approach in protection against BPD.

"Gentle ventilation" is a descriptive term for respiratory support for preterm infants using a low–tidal volume strategy to decrease lung injury, with the acceptance of higher values for $Paco_2$ ("permissive hypercapnia"). However, two randomized controlled trials studying permissive hypercapnia failed to show a reduction in incidence of BPD.[86] High-frequency ventilation, another approach to potentially limit volutrauma, was not found to be consistently protective in preventing or decreasing BPD.[87,88] Several other possible protective modalities of mechanical ventilation, including proportional assist ventilation,[89] volume-controlled ventilation,[90] and the addition of pressure-supported ventilation to synchronized intermittent mandatory ventilation (SIMV),[91] need further study to determine whether any may be efficacious for BPD protection. Another modality of mechanical ventilation, volume-targeted ventilation,[92] was the subject of a Cochrane review in which volume-targeted ventilation was compared with pressure-limited ventilation. Twelve randomized neonatal trials were analyzed, with the results indicating that volume-targeted ventilation resulted in a reduction in combined outcome of death or BPD, pneumothorax, days of mechanical ventilation, and the combined outcome of periventricular leukomalacia (PVL) or grade 3 or 4 intraventricular hemorrhage (IVH).[93]

Inhaled Nitric Oxide and Prevention of BPD

Inhaled nitric oxide (iNO) was originally used in critically ill infants to produce vasodilatation in the treatment of pulmonary hypertension. Since its original clinical application, NO has been extensively investigated in animal models of lung immaturity and lung injury; it has been found to diminish lung inflammation, to reduce lung neutrophil infiltration, and, perhaps more importantly, to enhance lung growth and alveolar development.[94-96] As a result of these promising experimental findings, investigators have questioned whether iNO might play a role in treating and/or protecting against BPD. Multiple randomized controlled trials, enrolling large numbers of infants, have tested whether iNO could have a positive effect on BPD prevention. Two studies yielded positive results for iNO therapy and BPD. Schreiber and coworkers[97] randomly allocated preterm infants born before 34 weeks of gestation to either iNO or placebo early, prior to 72 hours of age, and showed a significantly lower rate of death or BPD for iNO (48.6%, vs. 63.7% for placebo).[97] Randomly allocating subjects at a later time (infants requiring mechanical ventilation at 7-21 days), Ballard and colleagues[98] also found an increase in survival without BPD in the infants receiving iNO.[98] However, two other studies did not find an overall decrease in rate of death or BPD in iNO-treated infants, although after post hoc subgroup analysis, investigators in both studies reported a decrease in BPD or death in the larger infants (>1000 g) treated with iNO.[99,100] Results from the European Union NO trial, in which 800 preterm infants from 36 European centers were randomly assigned within 24 hours of birth to low-dose iNO (5 ppm) or placebo, found no differences in effect of the two treatments on survival without BPD.[101] Finally, upon review of 14 randomized controlled trials and 8 observational studies, investigators did not find a reduction in mortality (RR 0.97; 95% CI 0.82-1.15) or BPD at 36 wks (RR 0.93; 95% CI 0.86-1.003) though there was a modest 7% reduction in risk of composite outcome of death or BPD in premature infants receiving iNO. This group concluded that "there is currently no evidence to support the use of iNO in premature infants outside the context of rigorously conducted randomized controlled trials."[5]

Nutritional Approaches to BPD Treatment and Prevention

Caloric and Protein Nutrition

A frequent problem of extremely premature infants in the first days and weeks after birth, inadequate nutrition often occurs as a result of their critically ill state, fluid restriction, frequent glucose intolerance, and delays in initiation of enteral nutrition. Data from experimental animal studies have shown that ability to handle oxidative lung injury is negatively affected by malnutrition, especially protein malnutrition,[102,103] suggesting that early and rigorous provision of adequate calories and protein to premature infants might potentially improve antioxidant capacity and decrease risk for BPD. No definitive clinical trials have been conducted to test this hypothesis.

Lipid Nutrition

Whereas evidence in newborn experimental animals showed protection against oxygen toxicity with increases in both polyunsaturated fatty acid (PUFA) lipid intake and PUFA content of lung lipid,[104,105] multiple randomized controlled clinical trials in human prematures were unable to affect BPD with early provision of high-PUFA intake in the form of intravenous lipid (Intralipid).[106] This lack of protective effect could be related to the toxicity of lipid hydroperoxide contamination of the lipid preparations used at the time these studies were conducted, which might have obscured or reversed a protective effect for PUFAs. Intralipid manufacturing has now virtually eliminated lipid hydroperoxides, raising the still unresolved question of whether early intravenous lipid free of lipid hydroperoxides might have a preventive effect on BPD.

B

Inositol

Inositol, a carbocyclic polyol compound required for cell growth and survival that is incorporated into lung cell membranes and serves as a precursor for surfactant synthesis, has been reported to be deficient in premature infants. Hallman and associates[107] were the first to conduct a randomized controlled trial of inositol supplementation in prematures, questioning whether inositol supplementation would provide protection against BPD, and found better survival without BPD in inositol-supplemented infants. However, with subgroup analysis, only infants who had not received surfactant derived benefit from inositol, whereas in infants who had received surfactant, no beneficial effect of inositol on BPD prevention was found.[107] Subsequently, inositol was examined in two additional randomized clinical trials. When the three trials were subjected to meta-analysis, results demonstrated a significant reduction in death or BPD in infants who had received inositol, with the writers of this analysis recommending that "a multi-center randomized controlled trial of appropriate size is justified to confirm these findings."[108] However, without further investigation, inositol supplementation has not become part of the standard care of the very LBW infant.

Vitamin A

Vitamin A and retinoic acid play vital roles in differentiation and maintenance of airway epithelial cells and in alveolar development; moreover, similarities have been described between airway epithelial changes seen with BPD and vitamin A deficiency.[109] Preterm infants manifest low vitamin A stores because fetal acquisition of vitamin A occurs largely in the third trimester. Studies by Shenai and colleagues[110] and others have found an association between low serum levels vitamin of A in the first weeks of life and the development of BPD in premature infants.[110] As a result of these experimental and observational findings, multiple double-blind randomized controlled trials of early vitamin A supplementation in preterm infants have been performed, including the National Institute of Child Health and Human Development (NICHD) Neonatal Research Network trial conducted by Tyson and coworkers,[111] which reported a significant reduction (55% vs. 62%) in death or BPD in vitamin A–supplemented infants.[111] When seven randomized controlled trials were subjected to meta-analysis, results demonstrated a significant reduction in death or oxygen requirement at 36 weeks with vitamin A supplementation.[112] Whereas the efficacy of vitamin A in reducing BPD risk is evidence-based, the necessity of delivering vitamin A by repeated intramuscular injections and its relatively modest reduction in BPD have prevented vitamin A from being universally adopted into the standard of care for at-risk premature infants.

BPD Therapies to Reduce Lung Inflammation

Corticosteroids

The anti-inflammatory properties of steroids—including inhibition of prostaglandins, leukotrienes, and cyclooxygenases I and II, decrease of neutrophil recruitment in the lung, reduction in vascular permeability, and improvement of pulmonary edema—make their use an effective postnatal strategy to reduce the risk or severity of BPD.[113] The earliest dexamethasone trials, such as those reported by Avery and coworkers[114] and Mammel and colleagues,[115] were conducted more than 25 years ago; they demonstrated efficacy of postnatal dexamethasone in improving lung function and facilitating both ventilator weaning and extubation. Multiple clinical trials followed, with dexamethasone found to reduce oxygen dependence at 28 days and 36 weeks PMA as well as death or BPD and discharge home on oxygen.

The clinical trials using postnatal dexamethasone in vulnerable preterm infants were designed to explore one of two objectives: whether *early* administration of postnatal dexamethasone (<96 hr of age) could "prevent" BPD and whether *later* therapy could be a treatment modality that could improve BPD status. Although *early* postnatal dexamethasone therapy showed promise in reducing BPD, its short- and long-term complication rates rendered the potential pulmonary benefits untenable.[116] Specifically, infants receiving treatment with postnatal steroids at less than 96 hours of age had a risk for cerebral palsy (CP) that was approximately double that of infants who did not receive steroids. Grier and Halliday[116] concluded that for every 100 babies receiving early postnatal steroids, BPD would be prevented in 10; however, this positive pulmonary effect would be at the expense of an additional 6 infants with gastrointestinal hemorrhage, 12 with CP, and 14 with abnormal neurologic findings on follow-up.

10

In order to examine the effects of postnatal dexamethasone when delivered *later,* after the first week of life, Doyle and colleagues[117] performed meta-analysis of 19 randomized controlled trials of postnatal dexamethasone started after 7 days of age. They found a reduction in BPD both at 28 days and 36 weeks PMA, with decrease in the combined outcome of death or BPD, and additionally a reduction in need for home oxygen therapy and reduced rate of extubation failure. Follow-up data from 12 of the 19 studies (800 infants) indicated that CP and major neurosensory disability were not increased in the dexamethasone-treated infants, although some of the studies did not have school-age follow-up.[117] Follow-up data from the DART (Dexamethasone: A Randomized Trial) study, which assessed the effects of low dose dexamethasone on long-term survival without major neurodevelopmental deficits, did not indicate higher rates of death or major disability at 2 years of age in infants treated with low-dose dexamethasone than in controls.[118] Thus it appears that for maximum pulmonary benefit without increased neurodevelopmental risk, dexamethasone should be given after the first weeks of life and at the lowest possible dose.

Using weighted meta–regression analysis of 20 studies (1721 randomized infants), Doyle and associates[119] found that both the benefits and the long-term complications of steroid treatment were actually related to an infant's risk for BPD. In infants whose risk of BPD was estimated to be less than 35%, postnatal steroid treatment actually increased the risk for CP or death, whereas in infants with a risk of BPD estimated to be greater than 65%, the risk of death or CP was actually found to be reduced.[119] Therefore, if specific high-risk BPD populations can be identified and targeted, postnatal steroid treatment could be potentially beneficial for *both* BPD and also for long term neurodevelopment.

Postnatal hydrocortisone has been less frequently examined for its potential effect on BPD; most studies administered hydrocortisone within the first week of life. When eight randomized controlled trials of postnatal hydrocortisone were studied with meta-analysis, findings indicated that early use of hydrocortisone was not associated with a reduction in mortality, rate of BPD at 36 weeks or the combined outcome of death or BPD or with an increase in rate of CP.[120]

Although inhaled corticosteroids were considered promising in terms of beneficial effects on incidence of BPD with less systemic steroid concentrations and less adverse effects, meta-analysis failed to show reduction in BPD or death at 36 weeks and in fact were associated with longer duration of mechanical ventilation and oxygen dependence, in comparison to systemic steroids.[121]

Methylxanthines and BPD Prevention

Caffeine

Methylxanthines work as phosphodiesterase inhibitors and play an important role in regulating intracellular levels of second messengers cyclic adenosine monophosphate (cAMP) and cyclic guanosine monophosphate (cGMP), and they may have anti-inflammatory properties as well. Caffeine is a medication frequently given to premature infants to reduce apnea and facilitate extubation. To determine the potential effects of caffeine on long-term neurodevelopmental outcome at 18 to 21 months, a randomized placebo-controlled multicenter trial (The CAP trial: Caffeine for Apnea of Prematurity) was performed. Infants were randomly allocated to receive caffeine or placebo if they required therapy for apnea or for facilitation of extubation during the first 10 days of age. Caffeine was found to be associated with better survival without neurodevelopmental disability at 18 to 21 months corrected age, the primary outcome. Post hoc analysis also revealed a significant decrease in BPD (oxygen at 36 weeks PMA) (odds ratio[OR] 0.64; 95% CI (0.52-0.78) in infants who had received caffeine. However, the trial enrolled relatively few extremely LBW infants, those at highest risk for BPD (i.e., those <27 wk gestation), because they tend to remain ventilator-dependent beyond the first 10 days of life and thus were not candidates for enrollment in this trial.[122-124] It will require additional investigation to determine whether early administration of caffeine to these most immature infants would protect them against BPD.[125]

B

Future Directions in Prevention of BPD

Pentoxifylline

Pentoxifylline is a methylxanthine that works as a phosphodiesterase inhibitor. Experimental studies have found that pentoxifylline has a protective effect on hyperoxic lung injury through reduction of inflammation and edema and stimulation of lung antioxidant enzymes and growth factors. Newborn rats treated with pentoxifylline showed improvements in survival in hyperoxia and induction of lung antioxidant enzymes, reduction in fibrin deposition, and reversal of downregulation of VEGF.[126,127] One small pilot trial examined the effect of inhaled pentoxifylline by day 4 of life on incidence of BPD in very LBW infants and found a significant reduction.[128] Because of the properties of pentoxifylline and the results of the studies in rats and preterm infants, this medication deserves testing in randomized controlled trials in human preterms for a potential role in preventing or managing BPD.

Mesenchymal Stem Cells

Bone marrow–derived multipotent mesenchymal stem cells (MSCs) have been found to be efficacious in experimental models of lung injury. In adult animals with either endotoxin- or bleomycin-induced lung injury, MSCs given by either the intravenous or intra-alveolar route decreased lung inflammation and fibrosis and increased survival.[129] In neonatal animals exposed to hyperoxia, the number of MSCs was reduced in lung and blood, suggesting that reduced MSC number could possibly play a role in BPD pathogenesis.[130] MSC therapy was tested in a neonatal rat model of BPD and was found to decrease lung inflammation and improve lung structure, although lung engraftment of the exogenously delivered MSCs was low, suggesting that the protective effect might actually result from substances secreted by the MSCs rather than the cells themselves.[131] Similarly, intravenously administered MSCs in the neonatal mouse had a protective pulmonary effect in hyperoxia-induced lung injury, and more profound lung protection occurred when conditioned medium alone (without the presence of MSCs) was administered. These findings indicate that that the protective function of MSCs may occur through their "secretome" or paracrine release factors, such as macrophage-stimulating factor-1 and osteopontin.[132] These findings, though promising, will require further investigation of the role of MSCs and their "secretome" before being considered for clinical trials investigating a potential role in BPD treatment or prevention. (This subject is discussed in greater detail in Chapter 9.)

Conclusion

It has been more than 40 years since BPD was described and the term bronchopulmonary dysplasia became part of the neonatal lexicon. This period has witnessed an evolution in the clinical picture of BPD and extensive investigation into its pathogenesis, prevention, and treatment. From the greater understanding of the cellular and molecular processes involved in BPD pathogenesis comes the promise of therapies that could reduce the risk or severity of BPD and could have a major effect on the morbidity, mortality, and long-term developmental outcome of premature infants.

References

1. Bancalari E, Claure N, Sosenko IRS. Bronchopulmonary dysplasia: changes in pathogenesis, epidemiology and definition. *Semin Neonatol.* 2003;8:63-71.
2. Stoll B, Hansen NI, Bell EF, et al, for the Eunice Kennedy Shriver NICHD Neonatal Research Network. Neonatal outcomes of extremely preterm infants from the NICHD Neonatal Research Network. *Pediatrics.* 2010;126:443-456.
3. Northway Jr WH, Rosan RC, Porter DY. Pulmonary disease following respiratory therapy of hyaline membrane disease: bronchopulmonary dysplasia. *N Engl J Med.* 1967;276:357-368.
4. SUPPORT Study Group of the Eunice Kennedy Shriver NICHD Neonatal Research Network, Carlo WA, Finer NN, Walsh MC, et al. Target ranges of oxygen saturation in extremely preterm infants. *N Engl J Med.* 2010;362:1959-1969.
5. Allen MC, Donohue P, Gilmore M, et al. Inhaled Nitric Oxide in Preterm Infants. Evidence Report/Technology Assessment No. 195. AHRQ Publication No. 11-E001. <http://www.ahrq.gov/clinic/tp/inoinftp.htm>. 2010;
6. Gonzalez A, Sosenko IRS, Chandar J, et al. Influence of infection on patent ductus arteriosus and chronic lung disease in premature infants weighing 1000 grams or less. *J Pediatr.* 1996;128:470-478.
7. Hyde I, English ER, Williams JA. The changing pattern of chronic lung disease of prematurity. *Arch Dis Child.* 1989;64:448-451.
8. McCubbin M, Frey EE, Wagener JS, et al. Large airway collapse in bronchopulmonary dysplasia. *J Pediatr.* 1989;114:304-307.
9. Groothuis JR, Gutierrez KM, Lauer BA. Respiratory syncytial virus infection in children with bronchopulmonary dysplasia. *Pediatr.* 1988;82:199-203.
10. Wenstrom KD, Andrews WW, Hauth JC, et al. Elevated second trimester amniotic fluid interleukin-6 levels predict preterm delivery. *Am J Obstet Gynecol.* 1998;178:546-550.
11. Watts DH, Krohn MA, Hillier SL, Eschenbach DA. The association of occult amniotic fluid infection with gestational age and neonatal outcome among women in preterm labor. *Obstet Gynecol.* 1992;79:351-357.
12. Goldenberg RL, Hauth JC, Andrews WW. Intrauterine infection and preterm delivery. *N Engl J Med.* 2000;342:1500-1507.
13. Watterberg KL, Demers SM, Scott SM, Murphy S. Chorioamnionitis and early lung inflammation in infants in whom bronchopulmonary dysplasia develops. *Pediatrics.* 1996;97:210-215.
14. Yoon BH, Romero R, Jun JK, et al. Amniotic fluid cytokines (interleukin-6, tumor necrosis factor-a, interleukin-lβ, and interleukin-8) and the risk for the development of bronchopulmonary dysplasia. *Am J Obstet Gynecol.* 1997;177:825-830.
15. Yoon BH, Romero R, Kim CJ, et al. High expression of tumor necrosis factor-α and intereukin-6 in periventricular leukomalacia. *Am J Obstet Gynecol.* 1997;177:406-411.
16. Viscardi RM, Muhumuza CK, Rodriguez A, et al. Inflammatory markers in intrauterine and fetal blood and cerebrospinal fluid compartments are associated with adverse pulmonary and neurological outcomes in preterm infants. *Pediatr Res.* 2004;55:1009-1017.
17. Van Marter LJ, Dammann O, Allred EN, et al. Chorioamnionitis, mechanical ventilation and postnatal sepsis as modulators of chronic lung disease in preterm infants. *J Pediatr.* 2002;140:171-176.
18. Soraisham AS, Singhal N, McMillan DD, et al. A multicenter study on the clinical outcome of chroioamnionitis in preterm infants. *Am J Obstet Gynecol.* 2009;200:372.e1-372.e6.
19. Van Waarde WM, Brus F, Okken A, Kimpen JL. *Ureaplasma urealyticum* colonization, prematurity and bronchopulmonary dysplasia. *Eur Respir J.* 1997;10:886-890.
20. Kotecha S, Hodge R, Schraber JA, et al. Pulmonary *Ureaplasma urealyticum* is associated with the development of acute lung inflammation and chronic lung disease in preterm infants. *Pediatr Res.* 2004;55:61-68.
21. Lyon AJ, McColm J, Middlemist L, et al. Randomized trial of erythromycin on the development of chronic lung disease in preterm infants. *Arch Dis Child Fetal Neonatal Ed.* 1998;78:F10-F14.
22. Ballard HO, Anstead MI, Shook LA. Azithromycin in the extremely low birth weight infant for the prevention of BPD: a pilot study. *Respir Res.* 2007;8:41-49.
23. Couroucli XI, Welty SE, Ramsay PL, et al. Detection of microorganisms in the tracheal aspirates of preterm infants by polymerase chain reaction: association of adenovirus infection with bronchopulmonary dysplasia. *Pediatr Res.* 2000;47:225-232.
24. Liljedahl M, Bodin L, Schollin J. Coagulase negative staphylococcal sepsis as a predictor of bronchopulmonary dysplasia. *Acta Pediatrica.* 2004;93:211-215.
25. Sawyer MH, Edwards DK, Spector SA. Cytomegalovirus infection and bronchopulmonary dysplasia in premature infants. *Am J Dis Child.* 1987;141:303-305.
26. Smith VC, Zupancic JA. McCormick MC, et al. Rehospitalization in the first year of life among infants with bronchopulmonary dysplasia. *J Pediatr.* 2004;144:799-803.

B

27. Kallapur SG, Jobe AH. Contribution of lung inflammation to lung injury and development. *Arch Dis Child Fetal Neonatal Ed*. 2006;91:F132-F135.
28. Varsila E, Hallman M, Venge P, Andersson S. Closure of patent ductus arteriosus decreases pulmonary myeloperoxidase in premature infants with respiratory distress syndrome. *Biol Neonate*. 1995;67:167-171.
29. McCurnin D, Seidner S, Chang LY, et al. Ibuprofen-induced patent ductus arteriosus closure: physiologic, histologic, and biochemical effects on the premature lung. *Pediatrics*. 2008;121:945-956.
30. Chang LY, McCurnin D, Yoder B, et al. Ductus arteriosus ligation and alveolar growth in preterm baboons with patent ductus arteriosus. *Pediatr Res*. 2008;63:299-302.
31. Coalson JJ. Pathology of chronic lung disease of early infancy. In: Bland RJ, Coalson JJ, eds. *Chronic Lung Disease in Early Infancy*. New York: Marcel Dekker; 2002:85-124.
32. Husain AN, Siddiqui NH, Stocker JT. Pathology of arrested acinar development in postsurfactant bronchopulmonary dysplasia. *Human Pathol*. 1998;29:710-717.
33. Thébaud B, Abman SH. Bronchopulmonary dysplasia: Where have all the vessels gone? Roles of angiogenic growth factors in chronic lung disease. *Am J Respir Crit Care Med*. 2007;175: 978-985.
34. Jakkula M, Le Cras TD, Gebb S, et al. Inhibition of angiogenesis decreases alveolarization in the developing rat lung. *Am J Physiol Lung Cell Mol Physiol*. 2000;279:L600-L607.
35. Maniscalco WM, Watkins RH, Chess PR, et al. Hyperoxic injury decreases alveolar epithelial expression of VEGF in neonatal rabbit lung. *Am J Res Cell Mol Biol*. 1997;16:557-567.
36. Klekamp JG, Jarzecka K, Perkett EA. Exposure to hyperoxia decreases the expression of VEGF and its receptors in adult rat lungs. *Am J Pathol*. 1999;154:823-831.
37. Thébaud B, Ladha R, Michelakis ED, et al. VEGF gene therapy increases survival, promotes lung angiogenesis and prevents alveolar damage in hyperoxia induced lung injury. *Circulation*. 2005;112:2477-2486.
38. Bhatt AJ, Pryhuber GS, Huyck H, et al. Disrupted pulmonary vasculature and decreased VEGF, Flt-1, and TIE-2 in human infants dying with BPD. *Am J Resp Crit Care Med*. 2001;164: 1971-1980.
39. Fujinaga H, Baker CD, Ryan SL, et al. Hyperoxia disrupts vascular endothelial growth factor-nitric oxide signaling and decreases growth of endothelial colony forming cells from preterm infants. *Am J Physiol Lung Cell Mol Physiol*. 2009;297:L1160-L1169.
40. DePaepe ME, Patel C, Tsai A, et al. Endoglin (CD105) upregulation in pulmonary microvasculature of ventilated preterm infants. *Am J Respir Crit Care Med*. 2008;178:180-187.
41. Been JA, Debeer A, van Iwaarden JF, et al. Early alternations of growth factor patterns in bronchoalveolar lavage fluid from preterm infants developing BPD. *Pediatr Res*. 2010;67:83-89.
42. Adcock KG, Martin J, Loggins J, et al. Elevated platelet-derived growth factor-BB concentrations in premature infants who develop chronic lung disease. *BMC Pediatrics*. 2004;4:10-20.
43. Jankov RP, Tanswell AK. Growth factors, postnatal lung growth and BPD. *Paediatr Respir Rev*. 2004;5:S265-S275.
44. Ozer EA, Kumral A, Ozer E, et al. Effects of erythropoietin on hyperoxic lung injury in neonatal rats. *Pediatr Res*. 2005;58:38-41.
45. Frank L. Effects of oxygen on the newborn. *Fed Proc*. 1985;44:2328-2334.
46. Deneke SM, Fanburg BL. Normobaric oxygen toxicity of the lung. *N Engl J Med*. 1980;303: 76-86.
47. Gerstmann DR, de Lemos RA, Coalson JJ, et al. Influence of ventilatory technique on pulmonary baroinjury in baboons with hyaline membrane disease. *Pediatr Pulmonol*. 1988;5:82-91.
48. Donn SM, Sinha SK. Minimizing ventilator induced lung injury in preterm infants. *Arch Dis Child Fetal Neonatal Ed*. 2006;91:F226-F230.
49. Tin W, Milligan DW, Pennefather P, Hey E. Pulse oximetry, severe retinopathy, and outcome at one year in babies of less than 28 weeks gestation. *Arch Dis Child Fetal Neonatal Ed*. 2001;84: F106-F110.
50. Finer N, Leone T. Oxygen saturation monitoring for the preterm infant: the evidence basis for current practice. *Pediatr Res*. 2009;65:375-380
51. Bolivar JM, Gerhardt T, Gonzalez A, et al. Mechanisms for episodes of hypoxemia in preterm infants undergoing mechanical ventilation. *J Pediatr*. 1995;127:767-773.
52. Ratner V, Slinko S, Utkina-Sosunova, et al. Hypoxic stress exacerbates hyperoxia-induced lung injury in a neonatal mouse model of bronchopulmonary dysplasia. *Neonatology*. 2009;95: 299-305.
53. Nwajei PO, Young K, Claure N, Ramachandran S, Hehre D, Torres E, Suguihara. Impact of intermittent hypoxia on neonatal hyperoxia-induced lung injury. Society for Pediatric Research E-PAS: 2010 2140.7
54. Parker RA, Lindstrom DP, Cotton RB. Evidence from twin study implies possible genetic susceptibility to bronchopulmonary dysplasia. *Semin Perinatol*. 1996;20:206-209.
55. Bhandari V, Bizzarro MJ, Shetty AH et al. Familial and genetic susceptibility to major neonatal morbidities in preterm twins. *Pediatrics*. 2006;117:1901-1906.
56. Nickerson BG, Taussig LM. Family history of asthma in infants with bronchopulmonary dysplasia. *Pediatrics*. 1980;65:1140-1144.
57. Hallman M, Marttila R, Pertille R, et al. Genes and environment in common neonatal lung disease. *Neonatology*. 2007;91:298-302
58. Przemko K, Miroslaw BM, Zofia M, et al. Genetic risk factors of bronchopulmonary dysplasia. *Pediatr Res*. 2008;114:e243-248.

59. Manar MH, Brown MR, Gauthier TW, et al. Association of glutathione-S-transferase-P1 polymorphisms with bronchopulmonary dysplasia. *J Perinatol.* 2004;24:30-35.
60. Prencipe G, Auriti C, Inglese RD, Ronchetti MP, et al. A polymorphism in the macrophage inhibitor factor promoter is associated with BPD. *Pediatr Res.* 2011;69:142-147.
61. Deulofeut R, Critz A, Adams-Chapman I, Sola A. Avoiding hyperoxia in infants < or =1250 g is associated with improved short and long-term outcomes. *J Perinatol.* 2006;26:700-705.
62. Noori S, Patel D, Friedlich P, et al. Effects of low oxygen saturation limits on the ductus arteriosus in extremely low birth weight infants. *J Perinatol.* 2009;29:553-557.
63. Tokuhiro U, Yoshida T, Nakabayashi Y, Nakauchi S. et al. Reduced oxygen protocol decreases the incidence of threshold ROP in infants of <33 weeks gestation. *Pediatr Int.* 2009;51:804-806.
64. Saugstad OK, Aune D. In search of the optimal oxygen saturation for extremely low birth weight infants: a systematic review and meta-analysis. *Neonatology.* 2011;100:1-8.
65. STOP-ROP Multicenter Study Group. Supplemental therapeutic oxygen for prethreshold retinopathy of prematurity (STOP-ROP), A randomized controlled trial. I: Primary outcomes. *Pediatrics.* 2000;105:295-310.
66. Askie LM, Henderson-Smart DJ, Irwig L, Simpson JM. Oxygen-saturation targets and outcomes in extremely preterm infants. *N Engl J Med.* 2003;349:959-967.
67. Support Study Group of the Eunice Kennedy Shriver NICHD Neonatal Research Network, Carlo WA, Finer NN, Walsh MC, et al. Early CPAP versus surfactant in extremely preterm infants. *N Engl J Med.* 2010;362:1970-1979.
68. Claure N, D'Ugard C, Bancalari E. Automated adjustment of inspired oxygen in preterm infants with frequent fluctuations in oxygenation: A pilot clinical trial. *J Pediatr.* 2009;155:640-645.
69. Davis JM, Parad RB, Michele T, et al. Pulmonary outcome at one year corrected age in premature infants treated at birth with recombinant human CuZn superoxide dismutase. *Pediatrics.* 2003;111:469-476.
70. Sandberg KI, Fellman V, Stigson L, et al. N-Acetylcysteine administration during the first week of life does not improve lung function in extremely low birth weight infants. *Biol Neonate.* 2004;86:275-279.
71. Russell GA, Cooke RW. Randomized controlled trial of allopurinol prophylaxis in very preterm infants. *Arch Dis Child Fetal Neonat Ed.* 1995;73:F27-F31.
72. Caddell JL. Evidence for magnesium deficiency in the pathogenesis of bronchopulmonary dysplasia. *Magnesium Res.* 1996;9:205-216.
73. Falciglia HS, Johnson JR, Sullivan J, et al. Role of antioxidant nutrients and lipid peroxidation in premature infants with respiratory distress syndrome and bronchopulmonary dysplasia. *Am J Perinatol.* 2003;20:97-107.
74. Merz U, Peschgens T, Dott W, Hornchen H. Selenium status and bronchopulmonary dysplasia in premature infants. *Zeit Geburt Neonatol.* 1998;202:203-206.
75. Darlow BA, Inder TE, Sluis KB, et al. Randomized controlled trial of selenium supplementation in New Zealand VLBW infants. *Pediatr Res.* 1998;43:258A.
76. Avery ME, Tooley WH, Keller JB, et al. Is chronic lung disease in low birth weight infants preventable? A survey of 8 centers. *Pediatrics.* 1987;79:26-30.
77. Verder H, Robertson B, Greisen G, et al. Surfactant therapy and nasal continuous positive airway pressure for newborns with respiratory distress syndrome. *N Engl J Med.* 1994;331:1051-1055.
78. Ho JJ, Subramaniam P, Henderson-Smart DJ, et al. Continuous distending airway pressure for respiratory distress syndrome in preterm infants. *Cochrane Database Syst Rev.* 2000;3:CD002271.
79. Morley CJ, Davis PG, Doyle LW, et al. Nasal CPAP or intubation at birth for very preterm infants. *N Engl J Med.* 2008;358:700-708.
80. SUPPORT Study Group of the Eunice Kennedy Shriver NICHD Neonatal Research Network, Finer NN, Carlo WA, Walsh MC. Early CPAP versus surfactant in extremely preterm infants. *N Engl J Med.* 2010;362:1970-1979.
81. Sandri F, Plavka R, Ancora G, Simeoni U, Stranak Z et al. Prophylactic or early selective surfactant combined with nCPAP in very preterm infants. *Pediatrics.* 2010;125:e1402-e1409.
82. Kugelman A, Feferkorn I, Riskin A, et al. Nasal intermittent mandatory ventilation versus nasal continuous positive airway pressure for respiratory distress syndrome: a randomized controlled prospective study. *J Pediatr.* 2007;150:521-526.
83. Bhandari V, Gavino RG, Nedrelow JH, et al. A randomized controlled trial of synchronized nasal intermittent positive pressure ventilation in RDS. *J Perinatol.* 2007;27:697-703.
84. Bhandari V, Finer NN, Ehrenkranz R, et al. Synchronized nasal intermittent positive pressure ventilation and neonatal outcomes. *Pediatrics.* 2009;124:517-526.
85. Meneses J, Bhandari V, Alves J, Hermann D. Noninvasive ventilation for respiratory distress syndrome: A randomized controlled trial. *Pediatrics.* 2011;127:300-307.
86. Woodgate PG, Davies MW. Permissive hypercapnia for the prevention of morbidity and mortality in mechanically ventilated newborn infants. *Cochrane Database Syst Rev.* 2001;2:CD002061.
87. Courtney SE, Durand DJ, Asselin JM, et al. High frequency oscillatory ventilation versus conventional mechanical ventilation for very low birth weight infants. *N Engl J Med.* 2002; 347:643-652.
88. Johnson AH, Peacock JL, Greenough A, et al. High frequency oscillatory ventilation for the prevention of chronic lung disease of prematurity. *N Engl J Med.* 2002;347:633-642.
89. Schulze A, Bancalari E. Proportional assist ventilation in infants. *Clin Perinatol.* 2001;28:561-578.
90. Cheema I, Ahluwalia J. Feasibility of tidal volume-guided ventilation in newborn infants: a randomized crossover trial using the volume guarantee modality. *Pediatrics.* 2001;107:1323-1328.

B

91. Reyes ZC, Claure N, Tauscher MK, et al. Randomized controlled trial comparing synchronized intermittent mandatory ventilation and synchronized intermittent mandatory ventilation plus pressure support in preterm infants. *Pediatrics*. 2006;118:1409-1417.
92. Sinha SK, Donn, SM, Gavey J, et al. Randomized trial of volume controlled versus time cycled, pressure limited ventilation in preterm infants with respiratory distress syndrome. *Arch Dis Child Fetal Neonatal Ed*. 1997;77:F202-F205.
93. Wheeler K, Klingenberg C, McCallion N, Morley CJ, Davis PG. 2010. Volume-targeted versus pressure-limited ventilation in the neonate. Cochrane Database of Systematic Reviews. 11. Art. No.: CD003666.
94. Kinsella JP, Parker TA, Galan H, et al. Effects of inhaled nitric oxide on pulmonary edema and lung neutrophil accumulation in severe experimental hyaline membrane disease. *Pediatr Res*. 1997;41: 457-463.
95. ter Horst SA, Walther FJ, Poorthuis BJ, et al. Inhaled nitric oxide attenuates pulmonary inflammation and fibrin deposition and prolongs survival in neonatal hyperoxic lung injury. *Am J Physiol Lung Cell Mol Physiol*. 2007;293:135-144.
96. Lin YJ, Markham NE. Balasubramaniam V, et al. Inhaled nitric oxide enhances distal lung growth after exposure to hyperoxia in neonatal rats. *Pediatr Res*. 2005;58:22-29.
97. Schreiber MD, Gat-Mestan K, Marks JD, et al. Inhaled nitric oxide in premature infants with respiratory distress syndrome. *N Engl J Med*. 2003;349:2099-2107.
98. Ballard RA, Truog WE, Cnaan A, et al. Inhaled nitric oxide in preterm infants undergoing mechanical ventilation. *N Engl J Med*. 2006;355:343-353.
99. Kinsella JP, Cutter GR, Walsh WF, et al. Early inhaled nitric oxide therapy in premature newborns with respiratory failure. *N Engl J Med*. 2006;355:354-364.
100. Van Meurs KP, Wright LL, Ehrenkranz RA, et al. Inhaled nitric oxide for premature infants with severe respiratory failure. *N Engl J Med*. 2005;353:82-84.
101. Mercier J, Hummler H, Durrmeyer X, et al. for the EUNO Study Group. Inhaled nitric oxide for the prevention of BPD in preterm infants (EUNO): a randomized controlled trial. *Lancet*. 2010;375:346-354.
102. Frank L, Groseclose EE. Oxygen toxicity in newborns: the adverse effects of undernutrition. *J Appl Physiol*. 1982;53:1248-1255.
103. Deneke SM, Gershoff SN, Fanberg BL. Potentiation of oxygen toxicity in rats by dietary protein or amino acid deficiency. *J Appl Physiol*. 1983;54:147-151.
104. Sosenko IRS, Innis SM, Frank. Polyunsaturated fatty acids and protection of newborn rats from oxygen toxicity. *J Pediatr*. 1988;112:630-637.
105. Sosenko IRS, Innis SM, Frank L. Intralipid increases lung polyunsaturated fatty acids and protects newborn rats from oxygen toxicity. *Pediatr Res*. 1991;30:413-417.
106. Sosenko IRS. Polyunsaturated fatty acids: Do they protect against or promote oxidant lung injury? J *Nutrition*. 1995;125:1652-1656.
107. Hallman M, Bry K, Hoppu K, et al. Inositol supplementation in premature infants with respiratory distress syndrome. *N Engl J Med*. 1992;326:1233-1239.
108. Howlett A, Ohlsson A. Inositol for respiratory distress syndrome in preterm infants. *Cochrane Database Syst Rev*. 2003;4;CD000366.
109. Takahashi Y, Miura T, Takahashi K. Vitamin A is involved in maintenance of epithelial cells of the bronchioles and cells in the alveoli of rats. *J Nutr*. 1993;123:634-641.
110. Shenai JP, Chytil F, Stahlman MT. Vitamin A status of neonates with bronchopulmonary dysplasia. *Pediatr Res*. 1985;19:185-189.
111. Tyson JE, Wright LL, Oh W, et al. Vitamin A supplementation for extremely low birth weight infants. *N Engl J Med*. 1999;340:1962-1968.
112. Darlow BA, Graham PJ. Vitamin A supplementation for preventing morbidity and mortality in very low birthweight infants. *Cochrane Database Syst Rev*. 2002;4:CD000501.
113. Rhen T, Cidlowski L. Anti-inflammatory action of glucocorticoids: new mechanisms for old drugs. *N Engl J Med*. 2005;353:1711-1723.
114. Avery GB, Fletcher AB, Kaplan M, Brudno DS. Controlled trial of dexamethasone in respirator-dependent infants with BPD. *Pediatrics*. 1985;75:106-111.
115. Mammel MC, Green TP, Johnson DE, Thompson TR. Controlled trial of dexamethasone therapy in infants with BPD. *Lancet*. 1983;1:1356-1358.
116. Grier DG, Halliday HL. Corticosteroids in the prevention and management of bronchopulmonary dysplasia. *Semin Neonatol*. 2003;8:83-91.
117. Doyle LW, Ehrenhranz RA, Halliday HL. Dexamethasone treatment after the first week of life for BPD in preterm infants: A systematic review. *Neonatology*. 2010;98:289-296.
118. Doyle LW, Davis PG, Morley CJ, et al. Outcome at 2 years of age of infants from the DART study: A multicenter, international, randomized, controlled trial of low-dose dexamethasone. *Pediatrics*. 2007;119:716-721.
119. Doyle LW, Halliday HL, Ehrenkranz RA. Impact of postnatal systemic corticosteroids on mortality and cerebral palsy in preterm infants: effect modification by risk for chronic lung disease. *Pediatrics*. 2005;115:655-661.
120. Doyle LW, Ehrenhranz RA, Halliday HL. Postnatal hydrocortisone for preventing or treating BPD in preterm infants: A systematic review. *Neonatology*. 2010;98:111-117.
121. Shah SS, Ohlsson A, Halliday HL, Shah VS. Inhaled versus systemic corticosteroids for preventing chronic lung disease in ventilated very low birth weight preterm neonates. *Cochrane Database of Syst Rev*. 2003;1:CD002058.

122. Schmidt B, Roberts RS, Davis P, et al. Caffeine therapy for apnea of prematurity. *N Engl J Med.* 2006;354:2112-2121.
123. Bancalari E. Caffeine for apnea of prematurity. *N Engl J Med.* 2006;354:2179-2181.
124. Davis PG, Schmidt B, Roberts RS, et al. Caffeine for apnea of prematurity: benefits may vary in subgroups. *J Pediatr.* 2010;156:382-387.
125. Schmidt B, Roberts R, Millar D, Kirpalani H. Evidence-based neonatal drug therapy for prevention of BPD in very low birth weight infants. *Neonatology.* 2008;93:284-287.
126. ter Horst SA, Wagenaar GT, de Boer E, et al. Pentoxifylline reduces fibrin deposition and prolongs survival in neonatal hyperoxic lung injury. *J Appl Physiol.* 2004;97:2014-2019.
127. Almario B, Wu S, Peng J, Sosenko IRS. Pentoxifylline up-regulates lung vascular endothelial growth factor (VEGF) gene expression and prolongs survival in hyperoxia-exposed newborn rats. *PAS Abstract.* 2006;4132:8.
128. Lauterbach R, Szymura-Oleksiak J, Pawlik D, et al. Nebulized pentoxifylline for prevention of bronchopulmonary dysplasia in very low birth weight infants: a pilot clinical study. *J Matern Fetal Neonatal Med.* 2006;19:433-438 2006.
129. Chem Y, Shao J, Xiang L, et al. Mesenchymal stem cells: a promising candidate in regenerative medicine. *Internat J Biochem Cell Biol.* 2008;40:815-820
130. Van Haaften T, Bryne R, Bonnet S, et al. Airway delivery of mesenchymal stem cells prevents arrested alveolar growth in neonatal lung injury in rats. *Am J Resp Crit Care Med.* 2009;180:1131-1142.
131. Aslam M, Baveja R, Liang OD, et al. Bone marrow stromal cells attenuate lung injury in a murine model of neonatal chronic lung disease. *Am J Resp Crit Care Med.* 2009;180:1122-1130.
132. Abman SH, Matthay MA. Mesenchymal stem cells for the prevention of BPD: delivering the secretome. *Am J Resp Crit Care Med.* 2009;180:1039-1041.

CHAPTER 11

Long-Term Pulmonary Outcome of Preterm Infants

Lex W. Doyle, MD, MSc

11

- Controversies
- What Are the Long-Term Pulmonary Outcomes for Late Preterm Infants?
- What are the Long-Term Pulmonary Outcomes for Very Preterm Infants, and What Is the Effect of Having BPD on These Outcomes?
- What Further Research is Required?
- Summary

Preterm birth is an increasing health problem in the developed world for several reasons. First, the rate of preterm birth is rising, not falling; in the United States it is approaching 13%,[1] and the majority of births are of so-called "late preterm" infants, with gestational ages from 32 to 36 completed weeks. Second, survival rates for preterm neonates, particularly those born very preterm (<32 completed weeks) have increased because of technologic and therapeutic advances, such as antenatal administration of corticosteroids and postnatal exogenous administration of surfactant, combined with a greater willingness to offer intensive care before and after birth. Unfortunately preterm infants are more susceptible to adverse sequelae than are term infants, and the lungs of preterm infants are particularly vulnerable to injury.[2] Despite advances in care, respiratory problems remain the major cause of mortality in extremely preterm (<28 completed weeks) infants in the surfactant era.[3] Of those who survive the neonatal period, some experience bronchopulmonary dysplasia (BPD), both "old"[4] and "new" forms, [2] with prolonged oxygen dependency, occasionally for years. Although most preterm survivors have no ongoing oxygen dependency or respiratory distress in early childhood, their pulmonary outcomes in life must be determined, because they may be more prone to respiratory ill health, in either childhood or adulthood.

Controversies

Some of the controversies regarding pulmonary outcomes of preterm birth are as follows:

What are the pulmonary outcomes for the late preterm infants, who make up the majority of preterm survivors?

What are the pulmonary outcomes for the very preterm infants, including hospital readmissions, respiratory health problems, pulmonary function in childhood and later life, and exercise tolerance?

What are the effects of exogenous surfactant, cigarette smoking, and having had BPD in the newborn period on outcomes in very preterm infants?

This chapter reviews long-term pulmonary outcomes after discharge for preterm infants. If data by gestational age are not available, data by birth weight are substituted, with the assumption that birth weight less than 1500 g is equivalent to gestational age less than 32 weeks, and birth weight less than 1000 g to gestational age less than 28 weeks.

What Are the Long-Term Pulmonary Outcomes for Late Preterm Infants?

Colin and associates[5] reviewed respiratory morbidity for late preterm infants reported between 2000 and 2009. Their search of multiple databases for relevant articles yielded 24, not all of which reported long-term respiratory outcomes. In those studies that did report outcomes after primary hospitalization, there was an emphasis on respiratory morbidity caused by respiratory syncytial virus (RSV) in infancy, with RSV-related readmissions more prevalent in early childhood in late preterm infants than in term controls. In another study of hospital readmissions over the first 6 weeks after discharge in Manitoba, Canada, in infants born 1997 to 2001, preterm birth was a significant risk factor for readmission to hospital: On the basis of birth weights, gestational ages for the majority of the preterm infants in that study (which were not supplied) would have been 32 to 36 weeks.[6] The most common cause for readmission during the 6 weeks was for respiratory illnesses (22%), which was more than twice as common as the next leading cause.

There are relatively few reports of outcomes beyond infancy comparing either respiratory morbidity or pulmonary function in late preterm infants and those born before 32 weeks. With respect to respiratory morbidity, a 2010 cohort study used data from the Third National Health and Nutrition Examination Survey (NHANES III, 1988-1994) linked to U.S. birth certificates to determine whether late preterm birth was associated with a diagnosis of asthma in early childhood.[7] Data were available from 6187 singletons of gestational ages 34 to 41 weeks who were between 2 and 83 months old at the time of the survey; the 537 late preterm (34-36 weeks) children had a slightly higher rate of physician-diagnosed asthma than the 5650 children who were term, but the increase was not statistically significant (adjusted hazard ratio 1.3; 95% confidence interval [CI] 0.8-2.0).

In those few studies with respiratory function data reviewed by Colin and associates,[5] there was more evidence of airway obstruction in late preterm infants compared with controls. One study included in the review was from Brazil, which reported on 26 infants born with a mean gestational age of 32.7 weeks (range 30-34 weeks) who did not have substantial respiratory distress in the neonatal period (received no assisted ventilation or exogenous surfactant, and either no oxygen or oxygen <48 hours [n = 11]); pulmonary function tests performed at a mean age of 10 weeks and repeated at a mean age of 64 weeks showed more airway obstruction compared with 24 term controls, with no evidence of improvement between the two tests.[8] The investigators concluded that preterm birth *per se* resulted in abnormal lung development, but late preterm children clearly need to be reassessed much later in childhood and into adulthood to determine whether lung function abnormalities are permanent. In addition to these studies, Northway and colleagues[9] reported respiratory function at a mean age of 18.3 years of subjects who would have mostly been late preterm; this study is discussed further in the section "Pulmonary Function in Adolescence or Early Adulthood."

What are the Long-Term Pulmonary Outcomes for Very Preterm Infants, and What Is the Effect of Having BPD on These Outcomes?

Hospital Readmissions for Respiratory Illness

Rates of rehospitalization of very preterm infants are several-fold higher than in term controls, and rates of hospital readmission have risen as survival rates of more very preterm infants have increased over time.[10] Overall, respiratory illnesses are the most

Table 11-1 FEATURES AND MAIN FINDINGS OF STUDIES REPORTING PULMONARY FUNCTION TESTS IN CHILDHOOD OF VERY PRETERM CHILDREN IN COMPARISON WITH CONTROLS

Study (Year Published)	Age Studied (yr)	Very Preterm (N) and Definition	Controls (N)	Main Findings
Children Born Prior to the 1990s				
Chan et al[23] (1989)	7	130; <2000 g	120	Airway obstruction
Kitchen et al[24] (1992)	8-9	240; <1000 g or <28 weeks	208	Airway obstruction; worse with BPD
McLeod et al[25] (1996)	8-9	300; <1500 g	590	Airway obstruction with exercise
Kennedy et al[26] (2000)	11	102; <1501 g	82	Airway obstruction and air trapping
Anand et al[27] (2003)	15	128 <1500 g	128	Airway obstruction
Siltanen et al[20] (2004)	10	72; <1501 g	65	Airway obstruction
Children Born After 1990				
Hjalmarson & Sandberg[31] (2002)	Term-corrected age	Mean 32* (range 25-33) weeks	53	Reduced compliance; higher resistance
Korhonen et al[32] (2004)	7-8	34 BPD; 34 no BPD; all <1500 g	34	Airway obstruction
Doyle et al[33] (2006)	8-9	240; <1000 g or <28 weeks	208	Airway obstruction; worse with BPD
Fawke et al[34] (2010)	11	182; <26 weeks	161	Airway obstruction; worse with BPD

BPD, bronchopulmonary dysplasia.
*Minimal neonatal respiratory disease.

common cause of rehospitalization in these early years,[11,12] and they occur more frequently in preterm survivors who had BPD.[11] However, as the rate of hospital readmission declines later in childhood, those who had BPD are no more likely to be readmitted to hospital for respiratory or other reasons.[13]

Respiratory Health Problems

Very preterm children have more ill health than term children over the first few years of life in most areas, but particularly in upper and lower respiratory illnesses,[10,14] and more so in those who had BPD.[10,15-17] Asthma or recurrent wheezing is more prevalent later in life in those born very tiny or preterm than in those not born preterm or very tiny in some[18-20] but not all studies.[13,21] Those who had BPD have even higher rates of asthma than those who did not.[22]

Pulmonary Function in Childhood

Very preterm survivors from the early days of modern neonatal intensive care, prior to widespread treatment with antenatal corticosteroids or exogenous surfactant therapy in the 1990s, had more abnormalities in pulmonary function in childhood, particularly problems with airflow, than term controls, as summarized in Table 11-1.[20,23-27] Very preterm survivors with BPD in the newborn period had even more abnormalities in childhood pulmonary function than did very preterm survivors without BPD.[13,24,28-30]

After 1990, when antenatal corticosteroids and exogenous surfactant were widely used, pulmonary function was still worse in very preterm survivors than in controls[31-34] (see Table 11-1); however, survivors from later eras of neonatal care are on average more immature and lighter at birth than those in earlier eras and hence

Table 11-2 FEV1* FOR STUDIES WITH RESPIRATORY FUNCTION REPORTED IN LATE ADOLESCENCE/EARLY ADULTHOOD

Study (Year Published)	*FEV_1 in Preterm Groups*		FEV_1 in NBW Controls
	BPD	No BPD	
Northway et al[9] (1990)	74.8 (14.5); n = 25†	96.6 (10.2); n = 26	100.4 (10.9); n = 53
Halvorsenet al[18] (2004)	87.8 (13.8); n = 12‡	97.7 (12.9); n = 34	108.1 (13.8); n = 46
Doyle et al[35] (2006)	81.6 (18.7); n = 33†	92.9 (12.8); n = 114	99.4 (9.5); n = 37
Vrijlandt et al[36] (2006)	90.1 (19.8); n = 8§	99.2 (17.9); n = 12§	109.6 (13.4); n = 48
Wong et al[37] (2008)	89.0 (22.6-121.9)¶; n = 21		

BPD, bronchopulmonary dysplasia; FEV_1, forced expiratory volume in 1 second; NBW, normal birth weight.
*Reported as percentage of predicted for age, height, and sex.
†BPD determined by ventilator dependency, oxygen requirement > 28 days, and chest radiograph findings consistent with Northway stage 3 or 4 changes.[4]
‡BPD group had oxygen requirement at 36 weeks of gestation; the remainder of preterm subjects in this study are considered to have no BPD.
§Males only.
¶Range; this study had no controls, either preterm or term.

more at risk for abnormal pulmonary function, so there may have been some improvement in pulmonary function with antenatal corticosteroids and exogenous surfactant that has been offset by the survival of higher-risk survivors. Children who had the "new" BPD[2] in later eras still have the reductions in airflow and increased gas trapping previously observed in the pre–surfactant and antenatal corticosteroid era.[32-34] In the latest of these studies, Fawke and associates[34] measured lung function data with portable devices at 11 years of age in 59% of survivors born before 26 weeks of gestation from the EPICure study of births in the United Kingdom in 1995. They reported large differences in several variables reflecting airway obstruction between these very preterm survivors and term controls. However, the differences reported were wider between preterm survivors and term controls than differences reported in another study of preterm survivors born in the 1990s and evaluated at 8-9 years of age, which measured pulmonary function using standard laboratory tests.[33] It will be important to reassess pulmonary function later in life in such extremely immature infants, particularly to reassess the effects of environmental hazards, such as cigarette smoking.

Pulmonary Function in Adolescence or Early Adulthood

Several studies have reported respiratory function data in the second and third decades of life for very preterm subjects and controls.[9,18,35-38] Results for the forced expired volume in 1 second (FEV_1), reported as percentage of predicted for age, height, and sex, are shown in Table 11-2 for those studies in which data are available separately for preterm subjects with BPD and without BPD as well as for controls. All subjects in these studies were born before exogenous surfactant was available for clinical use.

Northway and colleagues[9] reported respiratory function at a mean age of 18.3 years in 25 subjects born between 1964 and 1973 who had "old" BPD[4]; subjects had required assisted ventilation, were oxygen dependent at 28 days of life, and had chest radiographic evidence of scarring or cystic changes (stages 3 or 4). Data were compared with those from 26 age-matched controls of similar birth weight and gestational age who had not been ventilated as infants, and 53 age-matched normal subjects who were not born preterm. Most of the preterm survivors must have been late preterm because the mean gestational ages were 33.2 and 34.5 weeks for the two preterm groups, respectively. Those with BPD had reductions in variables reflecting airflow and increased gas trapping in comparison with both the preterm controls and the normal controls.

Halvorsen and coworkers[18] reported the pulmonary outcomes for 46 subjects of birth weight less than 1001 g or gestational ages less than 29 weeks at a mean age of 17.7 years from a geographically based cohort of children born between 1982 and 1985 in western Norway. Twelve (26%) of the subjects had moderate or severe BPD (oxygen requirement at postmenstrual age 36 weeks), 24 (52%) had mild BPD (oxygen requirement at 28 days but not 36 weeks), and 10 (22%) had no BPD. In comparison with 46 term controls, the preterm group had reductions in variables reflecting flow, and these variables were lower with increasing severity of BPD.

In a study of 147 survivors of birth weight less than 1501 g born during 1977 through 1982 in the Royal Women's Hospital, Melbourne, Australia, who underwent respiratory function tests at a mean age of 18.9 (SD 1.1) years, the 33 (22%) who had "old" BPD showed substantial reductions in respiratory function variables reflecting airflow; more of the subjects in this group had reductions in airflow in clinically important ranges in comparison with the 114 preterm survivors without BPD.[35] Compared with normal birth weight term controls, the preterm subjects without BPD also had substantially reduced variables reflecting flow.

Vrijlandt and associates[36] studied 42 children at 19 years of age who had been born either before 32 weeks of gestation or at less than 1500 g birth weight in 1983 in The Netherlands, and compared the results with those in 48 nonrandomly selected "healthy" term controls. The respiratory function of the preterm subjects was mostly in the normal range (e.g. FEV_1 mean 95.4% [SD 15.9] predicted) but that in the controls was better than expected (e.g. FEV_1 mean 109.6% [SD 13.4]), so the respiratory data in preterm subjects were significantly lower than in the controls. Results for preterm males with and without BPD were not substantially different (see Table 11-2), but the sample sizes were small and hence the power to detect differences between the groups was low.

Wong and colleagues[37] reported the outcome of 21 survivors with BPD and birth weight <1500 g who had been cared for in one hospital in Western Australia between 1980 and 1987, the subjects being between 18 and 26 years old when they were assessed; two other subjects, ages 17 and 33 years, respectively, referred by respiratory physicians were also included. There were no preterm or term controls in this study, and those who participated represented only 16% (21/133) of all known survivors who required oxygen treatment at 36 weeks' corrected gestational age. Values for FEV_1 were similar to those for BPD subjects in the other studies summarized in Table 11-2. In addition, 19 of the subjects in this study underwent computed tomography of the lungs, which showed changes consistent with emphysema in 16 (84%).

The overall impression from the data in Table 11-2 is that most survivors with BPD have FEV_1 values within the normal range (means >80%), with the exception of the highly selected study by Northway and colleagues,[9] but they are worse than preterm controls without BPD, and even worse relative to term controls.

In contrast with the preceding studies, one study of 58 preterm subjects born in the pre-surfactant era, compared with 48 healthy term controls, found no significant differences in measured z scores for FEV_1, maximum mid-expiratory flow (forced expiratory flow occurring in the middle of the exhaled volume [FEF_{25-75}]) or forced vital capacity (FVC) at 21 years of age.[38] Because the preterm subjects had a median gestational age of 31.5 weeks, the majority of them must have been very preterm (<32 weeks); some, however, must have also been late preterm and even term because the gestational age range was 27 to 37 weeks. In this study, there was a strong positive correlation for z scores for FEV_1 between childhood and adulthood even though the mean z score for FEV_1 fell from childhood to adulthood.[39] In another study, data at 8 years and 18 to 22 years of age in 129 subjects of birth weight less than 1501 g were described; 29 of the 129 subjects had BPD.[35] Compared with respiratory function variables measured at 8 years, the only variable with a statistically significant difference over time in

BPD subjects was a larger drop in FEV_1/FVC between 8 and 18 years of age in comparison with non-BPD preterm subjects (mean reduction 3.4%; 95% CI 0.2%-6.7%).

Exercise Tolerance

Cardiopulmonary limitations may not be evident at rest from standard respiratory function measurements, becoming apparent only when the respiratory and cardiac systems are put under stress during an exercise test. In one study of 10-year-old children born in 1992 through 1994 weighing less than 1000 g and before 32 weeks of gestation, the exercise capacity of the preterm group was approximately one-half that of term controls.[40] Some other studies,[41-43] but not all,[36,44,45] have also reported diminished peak oxygen consumption with exercise testing in preterm children. None of these studies was limited just to very preterm subjects, although one evaluated only infants of less than 801 g birth weight,[43] another selected subjects with less than 32 weeks' gestational age or less than 1500 g birth weight,[36] and the remainder studied just subjects with BPD and not complete cohorts of preterm children.

What Are the Effects of Exogenous Surfactant?

The effect of exogenous surfactant administered soon after birth on later respiratory function on small numbers of children enrolled in clinical trials has been reported to be minimal,[46] or possibly beneficial.[47] Several studies have reported that the effect of BPD in the surfactant era on respiratory function is similar to that before surfactant was available.[32,33] In one study the 34 subjects with BPD had lower FEV_1 at 7 to 8 years of age than 34 very low-birth-weight children without oxygen dependency and 34 term controls.[32] In a geographic study of children born in the state of Victoria, Australia, respiratory function was measured on 81% (240/298) of children born either before 28 weeks of gestation or at less than 1000 g birth weight at a mean age of 8.7 years, and on 79% (208/262) of normal birth weight controls at a mean age of 8.9 years.[33] Most of the preterm children had respiratory function within the expected range. However, some variables reflecting airflow were lower in preterm children with BPD than in both preterm children without BPD and normal birth weight controls, although the differences were not as marked as in the pre-surfactant era. Within this cohort, respiratory function was not substantially different between those preterm subjects who did and those who did not receive surfactant.

What are the Effects of Cigarette Smoking?

Respiratory function in subjects of birth weight less than 1000 g who smoke in early adulthood has been reported to be worse than in those who do not smoke; Doyle and associates[48] reported the results of respiratory function at a mean age of 20.2 years in a cohort of 44 of 60 consecutive survivors born at less than 1000 g birth weight during 1977 through 1980 at the Royal Women's Hospital, Melbourne, Australia. Respiratory function had also been measured in 42 of the 44 subjects at 8 years of age. Respiratory function was compared in the 14 smokers and the 30 nonsmokers. Several respiratory function variables reflecting airflow were significantly diminished in smokers. The proportion with a clinically important reduction in airflow ($FEV_1/FVC < 75\%$) was significantly higher in smokers (64%) than in nonsmokers (20%) ($\chi^2 = 8.3$; $P < 0.01$). There was a significantly larger decrease in the FEV_1/FVC ratio between ages 8 and 20 years in the smokers than in the nonsmokers (mean difference in rate of change: −8.2%; 95% CI −14.1% to −2.4%). Given that the rate of deterioration in respiratory function is more rapid in smokers with less than 1000 g birth weight up to age 20 years and the fact that cigarette smoking is detrimental to respiratory function in all subjects in adulthood,[49,50] preterm-born adults who smoke should undergo respiratory function testing well into adulthood to establish whether chronic obstructive airway disease develops more rapidly and at earlier ages.

What Further Research is Required?

Lower birth weight, and presumably increasing prematurity, is associated with worse respiratory health later in adulthood, including higher death rates from chronic obstructive airways disease and worse respiratory function, as reported in 1991 by Barker and coworkers[51] in a follow-up study of 5718 men born in Hertfordshire, England, from 1911 through 1930. The period of follow-up for preterm survivors of modern perinatal/neonatal intensive care thus far has been only into the third decade and is clearly too short for detection of high rates of chronic obstructive lung disease, which typically occurs much later in life. However, given the higher rates of respiratory ill health and clear reductions in airflow in preterm survivors in comparison with controls up to the third decade, follow-up until much later into adulthood is required.

Summary

- Late preterm (32-36 weeks of gestation) survivors, who greatly outnumber very preterm survivors, have more respiratory ill health in early childhood than controls, and those in whom BPD has developed in the past have worse lung function in late adolescence. However, the duration of follow-up has thus far been very short relative to total life expectancy.
- Very preterm (<32 weeks of gestation) survivors have more readmissions to hospital in early childhood, more upper and lower respiratory tract infections, and more asthma symptoms than controls.
- Very preterm survivors have worse respiratory function than controls, particularly airway obstruction, both in childhood and in adolescence and early adulthood. They also have worse exercise tolerance than controls.
- Exogenous surfactant seems not to have altered long-term respiratory problems for preterm survivors.
- The detrimental effects of cigarette smoking on respiratory function are probably worse in preterm survivors, but more research is required.
- Having had BPD in the newborn period generally exacerbates all of these long-term respiratory problems.
- Respiratory function and respiratory health later in adult life for preterm infants must be determined, because they are more susceptible to earlier onset of chronic obstructive airway disease than controls.

References

1. Goldenberg RL, Culhane JF, Iams JD, Romero R. Epidemiology and causes of preterm birth. *Lancet*. 2008;371:75-84.
2. Jobe AH, Bancalari E. Bronchopulmonary dysplasia. *Am J Respir Crit Care Med*. 2001;163: 1723172-1723179.
3. Doyle LW, Gultom E, Chuang SL, et al. Changing mortality and causes of death in infants 23-27 weeks' gestational age. *J Paediatr Child Health*. 1999;35:255-259.
4. Northway Jr WH, Rosan RC, Porter DY. Pulmonary disease following respirator therapy of hyaline-membrane disease. Bronchopulmonary dysplasia. *N Engl J Med*. 1967;276:357-368.
5. Colin AA, McEvoy C, Castile RG. Respiratory morbidity and lung function in preterm infants of 32 to 36 weeks' gestational age. *Pediatrics*. 2010;126:115-128.
6. Martens PJ, Derksen S, Gupta S. Predictors of hospital readmission of Manitoba newborns within six weeks postbirth discharge: a population-based study. *Pediatrics*. 2004;114:708-713.
7. Abe K, Shapiro-Mendoza CK, Hall LR, Satten GA. Late preterm birth and risk of developing asthma. *J Pediatr*. 2010;157:74-78.
8. Friedrich L, Pitrez PM, Stein RT, et al. Growth rate of lung function in healthy preterm infants. *Am J Respir Crit Care Med*. 2007;176:1269-1273.
9. Northway Jr WH, Moss RB, Carlisle KB, et al. Late pulmonary sequelae of bronchopulmonary dysplasia. *N Engl J Med*. 1990;323:1793-1799.
10. Doyle LW, Ford G, Davis N. Health and hospitalisations after discharge in extremely low birth weight infants. *Semin Neonatol*. 2003;8:137-145.
11. Cunningham CK, McMillan JA, Gross SJ. Rehospitalization for respiratory illness in infants of less than 32 weeks' gestation. *Pediatrics*. 1991;88:527-532.
12. Kitchen WH, Ford GW, Doyle LW, et al. Health and hospital readmissions of very-low-birth-weight and normal-birth-weight children. *Am J Dis Child*. 1990;144:213-218.

B

13. Doyle LW, Cheung MM, Ford GW, et al. Birth weight <1501 g and respiratory health at age 14. *Arch Dis Child.* 2001;84:40-44.
14. O'Callaghan MJ, Burns Y, Gray P, et al. Extremely low birth weight and control infants at 2 years corrected age: a comparison of intellectual abilities, motor performance, growth and health. *Early Hum Dev.* 1995;40:115-128.
15. Yu VY, Orgill AA, Lim SB, et al. Bronchopulmonary dysplasia in very low birthweight infants. *Aust Paediatr J.* 1983;19:233-236.
16. Tammela OK. First-year infections after initial hospitalization in low birth weight infants with and without bronchopulmonary dysplasia. *Scand J Infect Dis.* 1992;24:515-524.
17. Korhonen P, Koivisto AM, Ikonen S, et al. Very low birthweight, bronchopulmonary dysplasia and health in early childhood. *Acta Paediatr.* 1999;88:1385-1391.
18. Halvorsen T, Skadberg BT, Eide GE, et al. Pulmonary outcome in adolescents of extreme preterm birth: a regional cohort study. *Acta Paediatr.* 2004;93:1294-1300.
19. Vrijlandt EJ, Boezen HM, Gerritsen J, et al. Respiratory health in prematurely born preschool children with and without bronchopulmonary dysplasia. *J Pediatr.* 2007;150:256-261.
20. Siltanen M, Savilahti E, Pohjavuori M, Kajosaari M. Respiratory symptoms and lung function in relation to atopy in children born preterm. *Pediatr Pulmonol.* 2004;37:43-49.
21. Steffensen FH, Sorensen HT, Gillman MW, et al. Low birth weight and preterm delivery as risk factors for asthma and atopic dermatitis in young adult males. *Epidemiology.* 2000;11:185-188.
22. Ng DK, Lau WY, Lee SL. Pulmonary sequelae in long-term survivors of bronchopulmonary dysplasia. *Pediatr Int.* 2000;42:603-607.
23. Chan KN, Noble-Jamieson CM, Elliman A, et al. Lung function in children of low birth weight. *Arch Dis Child.* 1989;64:1284-1293.
24. Kitchen WH, Olinsky A, Doyle LW, et al. Respiratory health and lung function in 8-year-old children of very low birth weight: a cohort study. *Pediatrics.* 1992;89:1151-1158.
25. McLeod A, Ross P, Mitchell S, et al. Respiratory health in a total very low birthweight cohort and their classroom controls. *Arch Dis Child.* 1996;74:188-194.
26. Kennedy JD, Edward LJ, Bates DJ, et al. Effects of birthweight and oxygen supplementation on lung function in late childhood in children of very low birth weight. *Pediatr Pulmonol.* 2000; 30:32-40.
27. Anand D, Stevenson CJ, West CR, Pharoah PO. Lung function and respiratory health in adolescents of very low birth weight. *Arch Dis Child.* 2003;88:135-138.
28. Chan KN, Wong YC, Silverman M. Relationship between infant lung mechanics and childhood lung function in children of very low birthweight. *Pediatr Pulmonol.* 1990;8:74-81.
29. Doyle LW, Kitchen WH, Ford GW, et al. Outcome to 8 years of infants less than 1000 g birthweight: relationship with neonatal ventilator and oxygen therapy. *J Paediatr Child Health.* 1991;27: 184-188.
30. Doyle LW, Ford GW, Olinsky A, et al. Bronchopulmonary dysplasia and very low birthweight: lung function at 11 years of age. *J Paediatr Child Health.* 1996;32:339-343.
31. Hjalmarson O, Sandberg K. Abnormal lung function in healthy preterm infants. *Am J Respir Crit Care Med.* 2002;165:83-87.
32. Korhonen P, Laitinen J, Hyodynmaa E, Tammela O. Respiratory outcome in school-aged, very-low-birth-weight children in the surfactant era. *Acta Paediatr.* 2004;93:316-321.
33. Doyle LW; the Victorian Infant Collaborative Study Group. Respiratory function at age 8-9 years in extremely low birthweight/very preterm children born in Victoria in 1991-92. *Pediatr Pulmonol.* 2006;41:570-576.
34. Fawke J, Lum S, Kirkby J, et al. Lung function and respiratory symptoms at 11 years in children born extremely preterm: the EPICure study. *Am J Respir Crit Care Med.* 2010;182:237-245.
35. Doyle LW, Faber B, Callanan C, et al. Bronchopulmonary dysplasia in very low birth weight subjects and lung function in late adolescence. *Pediatrics.* 2006;118:108-113.
36. Vrijlandt EJ, Gerritsen J, Boezen HM, et al. Lung function and exercise capacity in young adults born prematurely. *Am J Respir Crit Care Med.* 2006;173:890-896.
37. Wong PM, Lees AN, Louw J, et al. Emphysema in young adult survivors of moderate-to-severe bronchopulmonary dysplasia. *Eur Respir J.* 2008;32:321-328.
38. Narang I, Rosenthal M, Cremonesini D, et al. Longitudinal evaluation of airway function 21 years after preterm birth. *Am J Respir Crit Care Med.* 2008;178:74-80.
39. Chambers DC. Lung function in ex-preterm adults. *Am J Respir Crit Care Med.* 2009;179:517.
40. Smith LJ, van Asperen PP, McKay KO, et al. Reduced exercise capacity in children born very preterm. *Pediatrics.* 2008;122:e287-e293.
41. Santuz P, Baraldi E, Zaramella P, et al. Factors limiting exercise performance in long-term survivors of bronchopulmonary dysplasia. *Am J Respir Crit Care Med.* 1995;152:1284-1289.
42. Pianosi PT, Fisk M. Cardiopulmonary exercise performance in prematurely born children. *Pediatr Res.* 2000;47:653-658.
43. Kilbride HW, Gelatt MC, Sabath RJ. Pulmonary function and exercise capacity for ELBW survivors in preadolescence: effect of neonatal chronic lung disease. *J Pediatr.* 2003;143:488-493.
44. Bader D, Ramos AD, Lew CD, et al. Childhood sequelae of infant lung disease: exercise and pulmonary function abnormalities after bronchopulmonary dysplasia. *J Pediatr.* 1987;110:693-699.
45. Jacob SV, Lands LC, Coates AL, et al. Exercise ability in survivors of severe bronchopulmonary dysplasia. *Am J Respir Crit Care Med.* 1997;155:1925-1929.
46. Gappa M, Berner MM, Hohenschild S, et al. Pulmonary function at school-age in surfactant-treated preterm infants. *Pediatr Pulmonol.* 1999;27:191-198.

47. Pelkonen AS, Hakulinen AL, Turpeinen M, Hallman M. Effect of neonatal surfactant therapy on lung function at school age in children born very preterm. *Pediatr Pulmonol*. 1998;25:182-190.
48. Doyle LW, Olinsky A, Faber B, Callanan C. Adverse effects of smoking on respiratory function in young adults born weighing less than 1000 grams. *Pediatrics*. 2003;112:565-569.
49. Higgins MW, Enright PL, Kronmal RA, et al. Smoking and lung function in elderly men and women. The Cardiovascular Health Study. *JAMA*. 1993;269:2741-2748.
50. Dockery DW, Speizer FE, Ferris BGJ, et al. Cumulative and reversible effects of lifetime smoking on simple tests of lung function in adults. *Am Rev Respir Dis*. 1988;137:286-292.
51. Barker DJ, Godfrey KM, Fall C, et al. Relation of birth weight and childhood respiratory infection to adult lung function and death from chronic obstructive airways disease. *Brit Med J*. 1991;303:671-675.

SECTION C

Management of Respiratory Failure

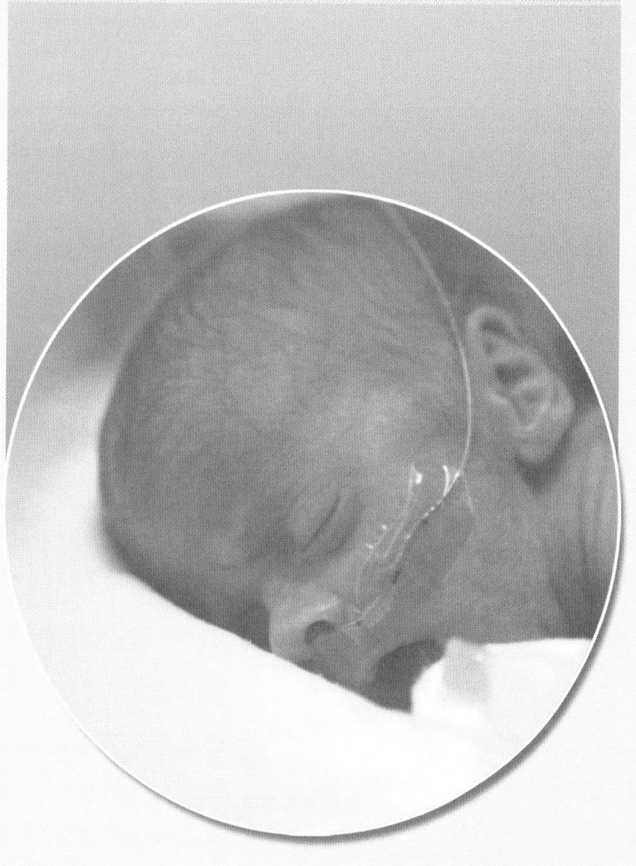

CHAPTER 12

Respiratory and Cardiovascular Support in the Delivery Room

Myra H. Wyckoff, MD

12

- Anticipate the Need for Resuscitation
- Prepare
- Initial Assessment: "The Golden Minute"
- Initial Steps of Resuscitation
- Effective Ventilation: The Key!
- CPAP
- Intubation or Laryngeal Mask Airway
- Oxygenation
- Cardiac Compressions during Delivery Room Resuscitation
- Medications during Delivery Room Resuscitation
- Special Situations

Anticipate the Need for Resuscitation

The majority of newborns successfully transition from in utero to ex utero life without any support; however, approximately 10% will need some form of respiratory support and, on rare occasions, even cardiovascular support at the time of birth.[1] Thus, for every delivery, at least one person trained in neonatal resuscitation should be available to assess the infant and effectively initiate resuscitation at the time of delivery. Asphyxiation is the most common reason that newborns fail to transition successfully. *Asphyxia* is defined as a lack of gas exchange that results in simultaneous hypoxia and carbon dioxide elevation, leading to a mixed metabolic and respiratory acidosis. The asphyxial insult can result from either failure of placental gas exchange before birth or deficient pulmonary gas exchange once the newborn is delivered.[2]

Premature rupture of membranes, fetal hydrops, post-term gestation, multiple gestation, and maternal drug abuse are examples of antenatal risk factors that could inhibit adequate gas exchange prior to delivery. Intrapartum factors that could negatively affect gas exchange include abnormal presentation (breech or transverse position), abnormal fetal heart rate, need for emergency cesarean section, cord compression, placental abruption, placenta previa, meconium-stained amniotic fluid, chorioamnionitis, prolonged ruptured membranes, and maternal pre-eclampsia. Postpartum factors that could impact gas exchange of the newly born include drug-induced respiratory depression (maternal magnesium exposure, opiates, and prolonged maternal general anesthesia), airway obstruction, prematurity, severe lung disease, sepsis, pneumothorax, and congenital malformations of the brain, airway, heart, or lungs. Such risk factors increase the need for resuscitation of the newborn, and when they are present, at least two people with complete neonatal resuscitation skills should be present and prepared. Effective ventilation of the baby's lungs is the most important action in neonatal resuscitation. The following sections describe the necessary steps required to achieve optimal respiratory and cardiovascular stabilization immediately following birth.

Prepare

Prior to delivery, all resuscitation equipment should be identified and checked for working order. The environmental temperature of the delivery room should be optimized to around 25° to 26° C in order to help prevent hypothermia.[1] Hypothermia of the newborn has been associated with hypoglycemia, metabolic acidosis, and increased mortality (particularly for preterm infants).[3] A large cohort study described that for every 1° C decrease in admission temperature, the odds of dying increased by 28% for very low-birth-weight infants.[4] Additional heat loss prevention strategies include use of maximally powered radiant warmers, warm blankets for drying, and other warming aids for preterm infants such as hats,[5] thermal mattresses,[6,7] and polyethylene wrap[8] to cover the body of the preterm infant. There is also evidence from both animal models and preterm infants that using warm, humidified air/oxygen during delivery room stabilization can decrease hypothermia.[9,10] A functional positive-pressure ventilation device (such as a self-inflating bag with pressure manometer and oxygen reservoir, a flow-inflating bag with pressure manometer, or a T-piece device) with the capability for blended oxygen delivery should be available and is the most important piece of equipment needed for newborn resuscitation. Suction devices (bulb syringe as well as wall suction and suction catheters), a functional laryngoscope with appropriate sized blades, appropriate sized endotracheal tubes, and end-tidal CO_2 detectors for confirmation of correct placement of endotracheal tubes should be easily accessible. Note that laryngeal masks are an acceptable alternative advanced airway. Pulse oximetry should be immediately available for all deliveries of preterm infants less than 32 weeks estimated gestational age (EGA) and for any delivery with a significant likelihood of need for resuscitation. In addition, pulse oximetry must be accessible in a timely manner for unanticipated deliveries with need for positive-pressure ventilation (PPV) for more than a few breaths, with persistent cyanosis, or when supplemental oxygen is used.[11] In certain ominous circumstances, an umbilical venous line should be prepared, and epinephrine drawn into a syringe and labeled for potential use.[2]

Initial Assessment: "The Golden Minute"

The vast majority of term newborns respond to birth with good respiratory effort, a rising or stable heart rate greater than 100 beats per minute (bpm), and good tone. Color is of little importance because preductal oxygen saturations increase gradually from a median of near 60% at 1 minute of life to around 90% by 10 minutes of life.[12,13] Clinical judgment of pink color is notoriously difficult.[14] Term babies who respond vigorously to birth with adequate respiratory effort and good heart rate need only routine care such as provision of warmth, clearing of the airway (if needed), and drying, no matter if born through clear fluid or meconium. Such infants can remain with the mother. Infants who respond to birth with poor, gasping, or no respiratory effort, or inadequate heart rate (<100 bpm), and those who are born preterm should be taken to the radiant warmer for further assessment and possible resuscitation interventions (Fig. 12-1). The initial steps, reevaluation, and initiation of PPV when needed are allotted approximately 60 seconds, which has been referred to as "the golden minute." Heart rate should be assessed by listening to the precordium with a stethoscope, because assessment of pulse by palpation is not as accurate.[15,16] Gasping, apnea, and a heart rate less than 100 bpm are signs indicating the need for PPV.

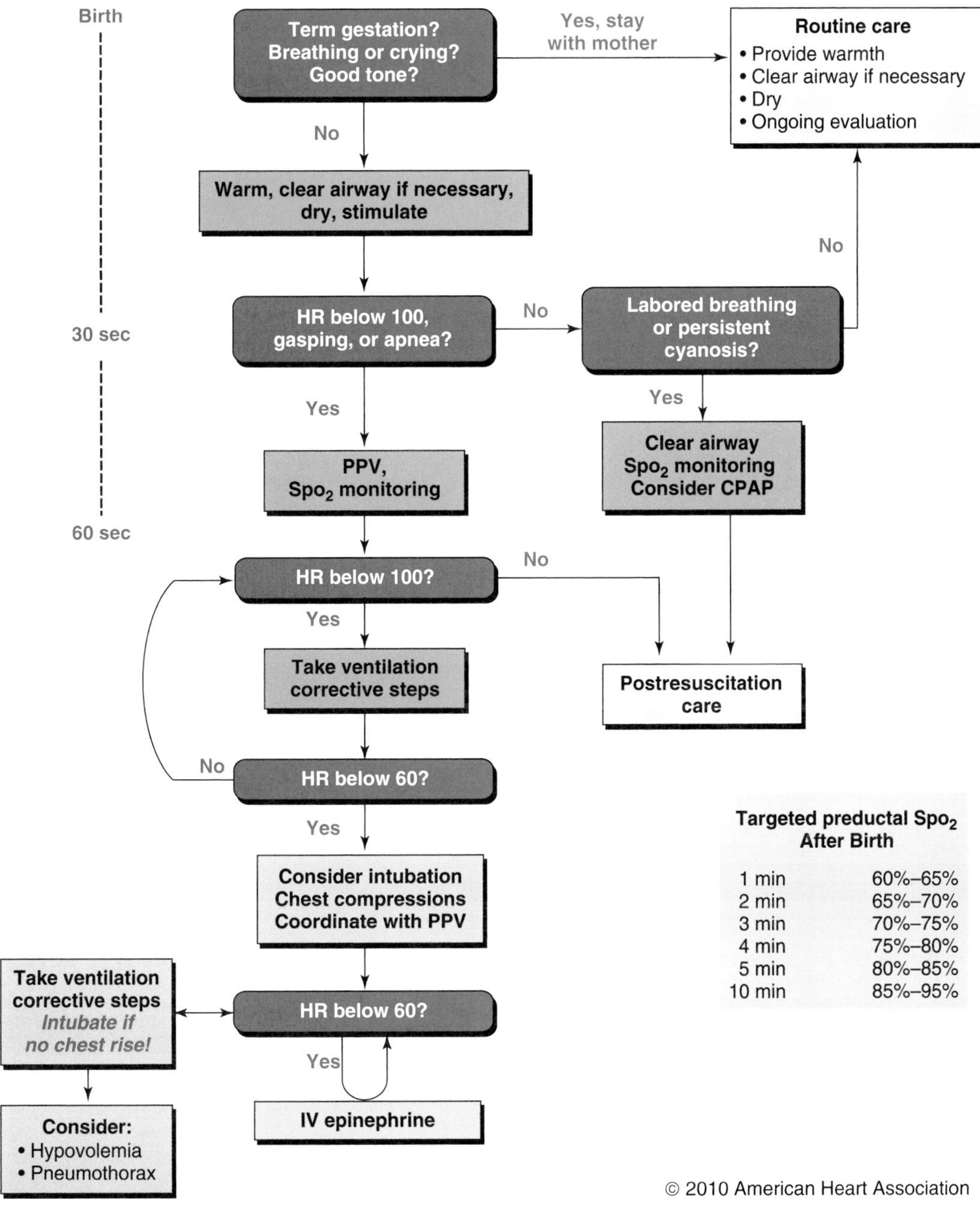

Figure 12-1 Neonatal resuscitation algorithm. CPAP, continuous positive airway pressure; HR, heart rate; IV, intravenous; PPV, positive-pressure ventilation. (Adapted from Kattwinkel J, Perlman JM, Aziz K, et al. Part 15: Neonatal resuscitation: 2010 American Heart Association Guidelines for Cardiopulmonary Resuscitation and Emergency Cardiovascular Care. *Circulation.* 2010;122:S909-S919.)

Initial Steps of Resuscitation

Provide Warmth

Infants who do not qualify for routine care should be received in warm blankets and placed under a preheated radiant warmer set at 100% power. The initial wet receiving blanket should be removed while the infant is dried. Preterm infants can be placed on a chemically activated thermal mattress.[6,7] The infant who is less than 29 weeks estimated gestational age should be immediately placed in a high-diathermancy food-grade polyethylene bag without initial drying up to the level of the shoulders.[3,8] This maneuver allows radiant heat from the warmer to pass through to the infant while essentially stopping evaporative losses. All subsequent resuscitation interventions can be done with the polyethylene wrap in place. It is useful to measure the infant's rectal temperature while in the delivery room to guide further interventions in addition to preventing iatrogenic hyperthermia, which is also detrimental.[17] Perinatal hyperthermia is associated with respiratory depression,[17] and newly born preterm lambs exposed to initial hyperthermia have worse lung injury, acidosis, premature death, pneumothoraces, impaired lung function, and increased inflammatory messenger RNA expression than normothermic animals.[18] The goal is to maintain normothermia and avoid both hypothermia and hyperthermia.

Position

The infant should be placed with the neck in mild extension so that the airway is maximally opened. A shoulder roll can help maintain correct position of the head, especially if there is significant cranial molding.

Clear the Airway (Only If Needed)

For infants born through clear amniotic fluid, initial bulb suctioning should be reserved for those who have respiratory depression or cannot clear secretions on their own. Breaking old habits of routine oral/nasal bulb suctioning immediately following birth may take significant effort for some delivery room providers, who have long embraced the previous mantra "dry, position, suction, stimulate" for every newborn; however, if the infant is crying vigorously, there is no need for routine bulb suctioning.[19] If the infant is apneic or overcome with excessive secretions, a bulb syringe is used to clear the mouth and then the nose. Deep DeLee suctioning is rarely needed, particularly in the early minutes of resuscitation, because it can induce vagal responses that are counterproductive during transition.

Nonvigorous infants born through meconium-stained amniotic fluid may be in secondary apnea and thus may have undergone agonal gasping in utero (Fig. 12-2). This puts them at risk for meconium aspiration syndrome, which can lead to severe respiratory failure and even death. On the basis of physiologic plausibility and expert opinion, it continues to be recommended that nonvigorous meconium-stained infants be immediately intubated for meconium suctioning of the airway before stimulation is provided. There are no randomized clinical trials to support or refute the practice. Much of what was previously routine management of meconium-stained infants has been debunked by well-designed clinical trials over the last decade. Amnioinfusion during labor[20] and routine intrapartum suctioning by the obstetrician make no difference in the outcome of meconium aspiration syndrome or death and are no longer recommended.[21] Vigorous meconium-stained infants are unlikely to have gone through an agonal gasping phase in utero, and intubation and suctioning of such infants made no difference in a large randomized trial.[22] Thus, the vigorous meconium-stained infant should be managed in the same manner as one born through clear fluid and as such can stay with the mother for routine care.

Dry and Stimulate

Once the airway is clear, the infant should be dried thoroughly and briefly stimulated by gently rubbing of the back, trunk, and extremities or flicking of the soles of the feet.

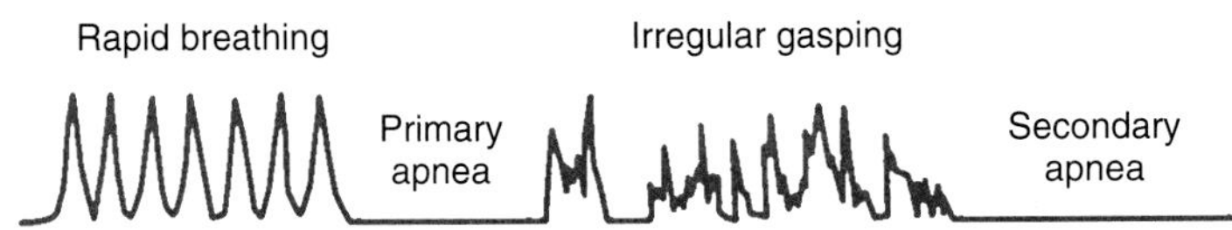

Figure 12-2 Primary apnea and secondary apnea are separated by an irregular gasping phase. (From Kattwinkel J, editor. *Textbook of Neonatal Resuscitation*.6th ed. Elk Grove, IL: American Academy of Pediatrics AHA; 2011.)

Assess

Heart rate and respiratory effort are then assessed. An infant in primary apnea will respond to almost any form of stimulation; however, if the baby remains apneic, is still gasping, or still has an inadequate heart rate, he or she is in secondary apnea, and PPV should be initiated promptly.

Effective Ventilation: The Key!

Effective PPV of the lungs is the most important action to stabilize a newborn infant who is compromised following delivery. Self-inflating bags, flow-inflating bags, and T-piece resuscitators are currently available for ventilation of the newborn at birth. Each device has positive and negative features.[23] Self-inflating bags do not need a compressed gas source and have a pressure-release valve that makes overinflation of the lung less likely. However, a self-inflating bag cannot be used to reliably deliver a sustained inflation, free-flow oxygen, or continuous positive airway pressure (CPAP). Even when outfitted with a special positive end expiratory pressure (PEEP) valve, such bags do not reliably deliver the positive end-expiratory pressure that was set.[24] An oxygen reservoir is needed to provide high concentrations of oxygen. It is now recommended that even self-inflating bags be used with a pressure manometer in order to avoid excessive pressures.[1] The flow-inflating bag can deliver up to 100% oxygen free flow as well as during positive-pressure breaths. It is obvious if the mask seal is inadequate because the bag will not inflate. The disadvantage is that a perfect seal is needed, a gas source is required, and the only safety mechanism to prevent overdistention is to monitor the pressure manometer. It takes a lot more practice to use a flow-inflating bag effectively.[25] T-piece resuscitators more accurately and consistently deliver set inspiratory pressures and positive end-expiratory pressure than the other devices,[26] but they require a compressed gas source and changing the inflation pressures during resuscitation is more difficult.[23] For extremely low-birth-weight infants, one study found the self-inflating bag to be as effective as the T-piece resuscitator in achieving goal oxygen saturation values by 5 minutes of life.[27] When the provider is considering which PPV equipment to use, the important thing is to practice and learn to troubleshoot and to ventilate well with whichever device is available in the delivery area.

Ventilation can be provided via an appropriately sized face mask, endotracheal tube, or laryngeal mask airway. To achieve effective ventilation via face mask, the provider must first check the infant for the open airway "sniffing" position. To achieve a good seal, the mask must rest on the chin and snugly cover the mouth and nose, but not the eyes so as to avoid a deleterious vagal response. Lack of appropriate airway position and inadequate seal are frequent causes of ineffective ventilation. A delivery room study of mask ventilation of premature infants documented that up to 25% of breaths had evidence of airway obstruction and 75% had mask leak.[28] Providers often have difficulty judging the tidal volumes they are delivering or the amount of leak during mask ventilation.[29] Colorimetric end-tidal CO_2 detectors have been used to confirm airway patency during bag-mask ventilation (not just intubation).[30] It has also been suggested that a respiratory function monitor might be helpful in detection of important airway obstruction and mask leak in the delivery room.[28] Providers have a difficult time sensing changes in compliance while providing PPV and, thus, if the compliance suddenly improves, can inadvertently deliver large tidal volumes, which should be avoided.[31] At this time the available positive pressure devices do not measure tidal volume. The respiratory function monitor may be useful in this regard as well.

The best sign that effective ventilation is under way is a rapid rise in heart rate,[32] followed by improvement in oxygen saturation values and tone. If the heart rate has not responded within five to ten breaths and there is poor chest rise, the provider should consider the algorithm **MRSOPA** to achieve effective ventilation, as follows:

Mask—ensure a good seal.
Reposition—ensure the head is in the sniffing position.
Suction—clear the airway of any obstructing secretions.

Open the mouth—and reapply mask.
Pressure—gradually increase the pressure until you hear good breath sounds and see chest rise.
Airway alternative—consider intubation or a laryngeal mask airway.

Ventilation rates of 40 to 60 breaths per minute are recommended.[1] Faster rates must be avoided in order to prevent stacked breaths, which would increase the risk of pneumothorax, and to allow adequate exhalation time for CO_2 removal. Counting out loud in rhythm with the seconds on the radiant warmer's Apgar timer may be helpful.

The optimum inflation pressure, inflation time, and flow rate required to establish an effective functional residual capacity have not been determined.[11] Inflation pressures should be monitored, and thus, even a self-inflating bag should have a pressure manometer. Inflation pressures may initially need to be as high as 30 to 40 cm H_2O but will vary with a goal to provide the minimum inflation required to quickly achieve and maintain a heart rate greater than 100 bpm. Typically the inflation pressure can be lowered quickly once a functional residual capacity is established.[33] In animal models, prolonged initial sustained inflations of 10 to 20 seconds have been shown to achieve functional residual capacity faster and to improve lung function without adverse circulatory effects.[34,35] There is limited clinical data, however, and human trials are needed. Once the heart rate stabilizes and the infant begins to breathe spontaneously, the ventilation rate can be gradually reduced. If there is not adequate improvement, intubation may be required for further support and transport to the neonatal intensive care unit. After 2 minutes of PPV via mask, an orogastric tube should be placed to decompress the stomach to avoid gas distention, which can impede effective ventilation. If the heart rate remains less than 60 bpm despite what would otherwise appear to be effective ventilation with chest rise, cardiac compressions are indicated. It is strongly recommended that chest compressions not be started until an advanced airway is secured.[1]

CPAP

For premature infants, immediate application of CPAP rather than intubation in the delivery room appears to reduce the need for intubation, surfactant, and time on the ventilator but thus far has not been shown to reduce rates of bronchopulmonary dysplasia and death.[36,37] In one study, use of CPAP levels of 8 cm H_2O in the delivery room increased the risk for pneumothorax,[36] but this higher risk was not seen with CPAP levels of 5 cm H_2O in another study.[37] For term babies there is no evidence to support or refute the use of CPAP in the delivery room, but it is frequently employed in the situation of respiratory distress. Although CPAP may help establish and maintain a functional residual capacity in a stiff noncompliant lung, thus improving respiratory distress, it should never be used in place of PPV when respiratory effort is poor or absent.[33] It is also important to remember that flow-inflating bags and T-piece resuscitators are needed in order to deliver CPAP in the delivery room. Self-inflating bags (even those outfitted with a positive end-expiratory pressure valve) cannot deliver CPAP.

Intubation or Laryngeal Mask Airway

Intubation may be performed at various points during a resuscitation and for several different indications, including meconium suctioning of the nonvigorous meconium-exposed infant, inadequate response and/or poor chest rise during mask PPV, need for PPV for more than a few minutes, when chest compressions are needed, for endotracheal delivery of epinephrine if the intravenous route is inaccessible, delivery of prophylactic surfactant, and suspected diaphragmatic hernia. Tube size, laryngoscope blade size, and depth of insertion are based on estimated weight and/or estimated gestational age, as listed in Table 12-1. A stylet may be used with vigilance to ensure that the tip does not protrude beyond the end of the tube, thus preventing accidental trauma.

Table 12-1 LARYNGOSCOPE BLADE SIZE, ENDOTRACHEAL TUBE SIZE & DEPTH OF INSERTION FOR BABIES OF VARIOUS WEIGHTS AND ESTIMATED GESTATIONAL AGE (EGA)

Blade Size (No.)	Tube Size (mm)	Weight (g)	EGA (wks)	Depth of Insertion (cm)
00	2.5	<750	<27	≈6.5
0	2.5	750-1000	27-28	≈7.0
0	3.0	1000-2000	28-34	≈7.0-8.0
1	3.5	2000-3000	34-38	≈8.0-9.0
1	3.5-4.0	>3000	>38	≈9.0-10.0

Adapted from Kattwinkel J. *Textbook of Neonatal Resuscitation. American Academy of Pediatrics.* 6th ed. Elk Grove, IL: American Heart Association AHA; 2011.

12

Intubation is not an easy skill to acquire, and it takes a lot of practice to become proficient.[38,39] The provider places the infant in the open airway position. Holding the laryngoscope in the left hand, the provider opens the infant's mouth and insets the blade gently and gradually into the vallecula (the space between the base of the tongue and epiglottis). The provider gently lifts upward at a 45-degree angle (without rocking, which can put pressure on the alveolar ridge and cause damage) to expose the glottic structures.[33] The cords of a newborn are shaped in an upside-down V and are pink (unlike the adult cords, which are white, as seen in Fig. 12-3). If the cords are closed, the provider waits for them to open, because touching the cords themselves with the tube can cause spasm and a counterproductive vagal response. With the cords open, the provider inserts the endotracheal tube with the right hand in the horizontal plane so that the tube curves from left to right.[1] The tube should not be inserted straight down the barrel of the laryngoscope because the provider's view will be obstructed right at the critical moment of needing to see the tip enter between the cords. The tube is inserted to the level of the vocal cord guide (black hash marks above the tip that are printed on the tube to show were to stop insertion at the level of the cords). The provider double-checks that the insertion depth is reasonable, by using a tip-to-lip estimate of 6 plus the weight in kilograms at the

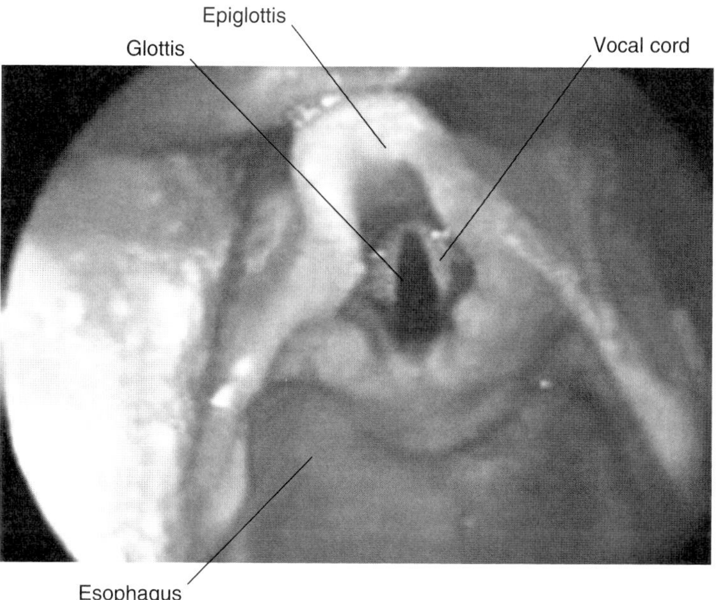

Figure 12-3 Photograph of laryngoscopic view of glottis and surrounding structures. (From Kattwinkel J, editor. *Textbook of Neonatal Resuscitation*. 6th ed. Elk Grove, IL: American Academy of Pediatrics AHA; 2011.)

lip as a guide,[40] and attaches an end-tidal CO_2 ($ETCO_2$) monitor prior to beginning PPV. An increasing heart rate and $ETCO_2$ detection after several breaths are the primary methods of confirming ventilation.[32,41] Secondary confirmatory techniques include seeing chest rise with initiation of PPV through the tube, listening for equal breath sounds, and seeing mist in the tube. Radiographic confirmation of proper tube placement should be obtained as soon as feasible. Incomplete intubation attempts should be interrupted for reapplication of bag mask ventilation if the heart rate starts to fall or remains unstable. Thirty-second intubation attempts have been suggested as a reasonable goal.

C

Laryngeal mask airways are effective for ventilating newborns who are 34 weeks or more estimated gestational age and more than 2000 g in birth weight.[42,43] Use of a laryngeal mask should be considered during resuscitation if face mask ventilation is unsuccessful and intubation is unsuccessful or not feasible.[11] Studies in adult models and patients suggest that placement of a laryngeal mask may be an easier task to learn than endotracheal intubation.[44,45] As with placement of an endotracheal tube, once the device is properly placed, there should be a prompt increase in the baby's heart rate, equal breath sounds, increasing oxygen saturations, chest rise, and a change in color on the colorimetric CO_2 monitor.[1] There is limited data for smaller and younger infants. Laryngeal mask airways have not been evaluated for use with meconium suctioning or during chest compressions or for administration of emergency medications.[11] There are reported case series of surfactant administration via laryngeal mask airway in animal models of respiratory distress syndrome[46] as well as in preterm infants.[47]

Oxygenation

Use of 100% oxygen was routine for newborn resuscitation until changes in resuscitation guidelines.[11,48] In utero oxygen tension values of the fetus are relatively low during development. Pulse oximetry studies of healthy term infants who require no resuscitation at birth demonstrate that preductal oxygen saturation starts at around 60% and takes 5 to 10 minutes to reach 90%.[12,49,50] Percentiles of oxygen saturations per minute of life have been defined.[13,51,52] The goal saturation range per minute of life has been defined as the interquartile range for healthy term infants (Table 12-2), but controversy remains as to whether a lower percentile might be as effective and potentially safer. Clearly, medical providers should not expect infants to be instantaneously pink at birth and should break the habit of routinely exposing infants to oxygen at birth. In fact, clinical judgment of cyanosis is quite poor, and thus it is recommended that use of oxygen be guided by pulse oximetry value rather than clinical judgment alone.[14] The pulse oximeter probe should be placed on the right (preductal) wrist or hand and then connected to the monitor for the quickest, most accurate signal.[53]

Although the optimal starting concentration of oxygen is unknown, the available evidence suggests that 21% O_2 is acceptable as a starting gas concentration for

Table 12-2 TRANSITIONAL GOAL OXYGEN SATURATIONS PER MINUTE OF LIFE

Time after Birth (min)	Goal Oxygen Saturations (Interquartile Range; %)
1	60-65
2	65-70
3	70-75
4	75-80
5	80-85
> 5	85-94

neonatal resuscitation of term infants.[11] Meta-analyses of trials comparing oxygen with room air for newborns during delivery room resuscitation suggest that infants resuscitated with air begin spontaneous breathing faster, reach acceptable oxygen saturation values just as quickly, have less evidence of oxidative damage, and, interestingly, lower mortality.[54-56] Preterm infants are deficient in antioxidant protection and thus face potential adverse effects of oxygen toxicity, such as chronic lung disease, retinopathy of prematurity, and necrotizing enterocolitis. Trials in extremely low-birth-weight infants have also demonstrated that 100% oxygen is rarely needed for successful resuscitation.[50,57] Most preterm infants did need some amount of oxygen supplementation at least transiently. There is growing evidence from animal studies of significant oxidative tissue damage in the lung and brain following asphyxia that is exacerbated by subsequent hyperoxygenation.[58] Several cohort studies reporting an association of delivery oxygen exposure with increased risk for childhood cancer also raise concern about risks of hyperoxygenation in the delivery room.[59-61] This accumulation of data led Sola to write, "Too much oxygen in the blood is a health hazard, and health care providers are the only known cause of neonatal hyperoxemia!"[62]

Current guidelines recommend starting resuscitation with air in term infants. For preterm infants no specific starting oxygen concentration recommendation is made. For all infants, oxygen supplementation should be guided by pulse oximetry and should be adjusted to meet goal saturation values per minute of life. Blended oxygen permits achievement of target saturation faster than either extreme, of air or 100% O_2. Thus, blended oxygen and pulse oximetry should be promptly available at every delivery. The pulse oximeter should be placed on the infant's right hand or wrist whenever resuscitation is anticipated, when PPV is administered for more than a few breaths, when cyanosis is persistent, when supplemental oxygen is administered, and for all preterm infants less than 33 weeks estimated gestational age.[11] If the heart rate remains less than 60 bpm despite effective ventilation, it is recommended that as cardiopulmonary resuscitation (CPR) is started, the oxygen concentration be turned up to 100% until the heart rate is stabilized. Once the heart rate is stabilized, the oxygen concentration should be lowered gradually to meet goal saturation value per minute of life.

Cardiac Compressions during Delivery Room Resuscitation

Effective ventilation will stabilize nearly all newborns in the delivery room regardless of gestational age and thus cardiac compressions are rarely needed in the delivery room.[63] Two reports from a large, urban delivery service with a trained, dedicated neonatal resuscitation team consistently reported the rate of need for cardiac compressions to be around 0.1% of all deliveries,[64,65] although there are reports of increased use in preterm infants.[66] Because effective ventilation is the critical step in newborn resuscitation and chest compressions are likely to interfere with effective ventilation, resuscitation providers are strongly encouraged to optimize assisted ventilation via placement of an advanced airway such as endotracheal tube or laryngeal mask before initiation of chest compressions.[11] The latest Neonatal Resuscitation Program (NRP) guidelines continue to recommend cardiac compressions for a newborn infant with a heart rate less than 60 beats/min despite at least 30 seconds of adequate ventilation.[1] The optimal interval of ventilation prior to initiation of cardiac compressions is unknown. Rationally, there needs to be a balance between ensuring there is adequate ventilation in the hope of avoiding the need for compressions altogether and the risk of additional hypoxic/ischemic injury if circulation is not assisted in a timely enough manner. A study in a neonatal animal model of asphyxia-induced asystole found that under conditions of asystole, there was no advantage or disadvantage in delaying initiation of compressions for 1 minute rather than an initial 30 seconds of room air ventilation; however, when initiation of compressions was delayed for 90 seconds of initial ventilation, fewer animals were successfully resuscitated.[67] Animals that were exposed to 90 seconds of initial ventilation prior to support of the circulation with compressions required more doses of epinephrine to stabilize the heart rate and had lower blood pressures after resuscitation. Whether longer delays in initiation of compressions for bradycardia as opposed to asystole would have the same potential harm is unknown. There is no clinical data to offer guidance.

Two-Thumb Technique

If cardiac compressions are necessary, it is quite likely that the pulse oximeter will no longer provide a reading. It is recommended that at the time of initiation of compressions the oxygen be increased to 100% until recovery of a normal heart rate.[11] Following reestablishment of adequate heart rate and a functional oximeter reading, the oxygen can be titrated down once again. This recommendation is somewhat controversial because asphyxiated infants will be at risk for oxygen free radical damage and hyperoxia should be limited as much as possible. A piglet study of severe asphyxia-induced asystole found that cardiopulmonary resuscitation with room air seemed to be as safe and effective as the use of 100% oxygen.[68] However, in the absence of clinical data, the current recommendation seems like the best compromise to limit both hypoxia and hyperoxia.

Compressions should be centered over the lower third of the sternum rather than the mid-sternum in order to compress most directly over the heart.[69,70] Positioning the thumbs centrally over the sternum is also critical in order to decrease risk of rib fracture, which can lead to a flail chest or pneumothorax (either of which would inhibit effective ventilation) and dislocation of the xiphoid process, which can lead to devastating liver laceration. A compression depth of approximately one third the anterior-posterior (AP) diameter of the chest should be adequate to produce a palpable pulse.[71,72] Although a small case series of 6 infants suggested that a compression depth of half the anterior-posterior diameter of the chest resulted in higher systolic, mean, and systemic perfusion pressures, this greater depth did not result in better diastolic blood pressure than a depth of one third the anterior-posterior diameter.[73] Given that the primary goal of cardiac compressions is to perfuse the heart and brain while awaiting definitive restoration of a cardiac rhythm and that diastolic blood pressure is the critical determinant of coronary perfusion, compression depth should favor one third the anterior-posterior diameter of the chest rather than deeper.

The two-thumb method, in which the provider's hands encircle the newborn chest while the thumbs compress the sternum, should be utilized for neonatal cardiac compressions.[11] A piglet study of asphyxia-induced asystole found that over 2-minute intervals, the two-thumb method produced higher systolic blood pressures than the two-finger method although the diastolic blood pressures were equivalent.[74] When the two techniques were compared over longer (10-minute) compression intervals using a manikin with a customized artificial fixed volume "arterial system," the two-thumb method produced higher mean, systolic, and diastolic blood pressures.[75] Another neonatal manikin study demonstrated that over 2-minute intervals of cardiac compressions, the two-thumb method resulted in improved depth and consistency of compressions as well as less drift away from correct thumb/finger position.[76] Two case reports involving three newborns describe better arterial mean blood pressures and systolic blood pressure with the two-thumb technique than the two-finger technique.[24,25] Higher-level clinical evidence is not available.

In the past, the two-finger technique was used while umbilical access was obtained so that the compressor's arms would be out of the way. Now it is recommended that once the airway is secured (which should have been done before compressions were started anyway), the compressor can move to the head of the bed and continue the two-thumb technique while allowing ample access to the umbilical stump (Fig. 12-4). It is critical that compressions performed from the head of the bed in no way conflict with adequate ventilation and establishment of an advanced airway.

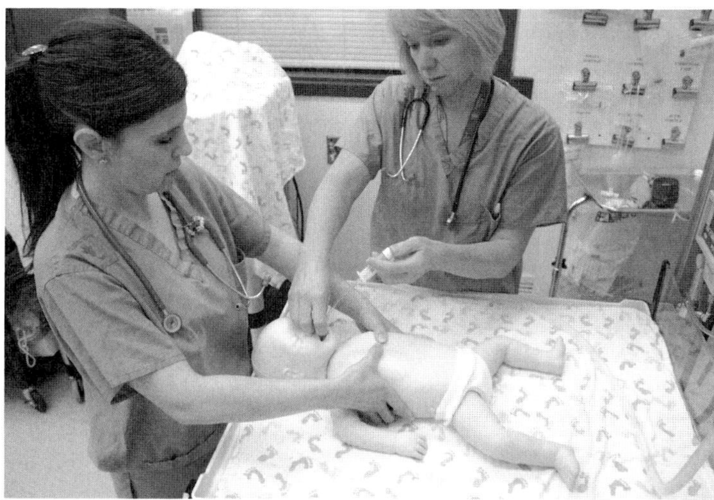

Figure 12-4 Two-thumb technique can be continued from the head of the bed once the airway is secured, leaving ample access to the umbilical stump for emergency placement of an umbilical venous catheter (UVC).

Compression-to-Ventilation Ratio

The ratio of compressions to ventilations that would truly optimize the dual goals of perfusion and ventilation during resuscitation from asphyxia arrest is unknown. What is known is that asphyxiated, asystolic piglets resuscitated with a combination of chest compressions and ventilations have better outcomes than those resuscitated with ventilations or compressions alone,[77,78] especially during prolonged resuscitation.[79] A physiologic mathematical modeling study suggests that higher compression-to-ventilation ratios would result in underventilation of asphyxiated infants.[80] The model predicts that 3 to 5 compressions to 1 ventilation should be most efficient for newborns. A compression-to-ventilation ratio of 3:1, such that 90 compressions and 30 breaths are achieved per minute, is currently recommended in order to optimize ventilation. Later studies have compared 3:1 with 9:3[81] and 3:1 with 15:2 compression-to-ventilation ratios[82] in piglet models of asystole due to asphyxia. Although the 15:2 ratio provided more compressions per minute without compromising $PaCO_2$ and generated statistically higher diastolic blood pressures, the diastolic blood pressure was still inadequate until epinephrine was given, and so there was no difference in time to return of spontaneous circulation. Thus, there is no evidence from quality human, animal, manikin, or mathematical modeling studies to warrant a change from the current 3:1 compression-to-ventilation ratio. Strategies for optimizing the quality of the compressions and ventilations with as few interruptions as possible should be considered. The latest Neonatal Resuscitation Program recommendations have lengthened the interval between auscultation pauses up to at least 1 minute in an effort to decrease interruptions in perfusion.[1]

Coordination of Compressions and Ventilations

Coordination of the compressions and ventilations so that they are not delivered simultaneously is still recommended, but the evidence for this recommendation is quite weak. There is historical concern based on physiologic plausibility that if compressions and ventilations were delivered at the same time, ventilation might be critically compromised. Two cardiac arrest (not asphyxia) animal studies utilized extremely high pressures for the ventilations.[83,84] In both studies, the animals receiving simultaneous compressions and ventilations did have higher PCO_2 values during the resuscitation period, but even so the animals in both groups were considerably overventilated. The simultaneous compressions/ventilations did not enhance cerebral or myocardial perfusion. Given the current lack of evidence of significant benefit and the concern about overventilation, the Neonatal Resuscitation Program continues to recommend coordination of the two activities.[1]

Colorimetric $ETCO_2$ Detectors during Cardiac Compressions

As mentioned in the section on intubation, $ETCO_2$ detection to confirm correct endotracheal intubation is always recommended; however, it is critical that medical providers understand that the colorimetric $ETCO_2$ detector may give a false-negative reading in the situation of an asystolic or severely bradycardic newborn with very poor cardiac output. The reason is that the PPV given prior to intubation may have successfully ventilated off most of the CO_2 present in the lung. With such limited pulmonary blood flow due to the failing pump action of the heart, little subsequent CO_2 is delivered to the lungs, and the $ETCO_2$ detector has negligible CO_2 to detect even if the airway is in the correct position.[85] Removing a correctly placed endotracheal tube because of a false-negative color change on the colorimetric $ETCO_2$ detector wastes valuable time in getting the most effective ventilation started. In this situation, the medical provider will have to judge the success of the intubation on confirmed visualization of the tube passing between the cords, chest rise with positive pressure via the endotracheal tube, mist in the tube, and bilaterally equal and adequate breath sounds.[85]

Capnography during Cardiac Compressions

Frequent repetitive pauses in cardiac compressions and ventilation make it difficult to achieve and maintain adequate coronary perfusion pressure. Use of $ETCO_2$ capnography during CPR may provide a continuous, noninvasive tool to eliminate frequent pauses during CPR to auscultate for heart rate. $ETCO_2$ values reflect a balance among CO_2 production by cellular metabolism, alveolar ventilation, and pulmonary perfusion. During CPR, cellular metabolism and alveolar ventilation are presumed to be at a steady state (provided that PPV is given in a steady manner), so changes in $ETCO_2$ primarily reflect changes in cardiac output.[85] A piglet model of asphyxia-induced asystole has demonstrated that after PPV, $ETCO_2$ falls to near zero with loss of pulmonary blood flow and then increases slightly with initiation of cardiac compressions, reflecting blood being pumped through the lungs by effective CPR. Return of spontaneous circulation correlate with a sudden increase in $ETCO_2$ as the reestablished perfusion brings CO_2-rich blood back to the lungs. In that model, an $ETCO_2$ greater than 15 mm Hg correlated well with return of an audible heart rate higher than 60 bpm.[86] Clinical correlates are needed.

Medications during Delivery Room Resuscitation

When asphyxia is so severe as to result in asystole or agonal bradycardia then the newborn heart has become depleted of energy substrate and can no longer beat effectively.[63] Adequate perfusion of the heart with oxygenated blood must be restored or resuscitation efforts will be unsuccessful. During CPR, coronary blood flow occurs exclusively during diastole, presumably because of increased intramyocardial resistance and increased right atrial pressure during chest compressions.[87] Therefore, coronary perfusion pressure (CPP) is determined by the aortic diastolic blood pressure minus the right atrial diastolic blood pressure. Cardiac compressions plus adequate systemic vascular resistance must generate diastolic blood pressure adequate to achieve return of spontaneous circulation. Given the profound acidemia and resultant vasodilation induced by asphyxia, a vasopressor agent such as epinephrine is frequently required to achieve an adequate aortic diastolic pressure for sufficient coronary perfusion during CPR.

Epinephrine stimulates α-adrenergic receptor–mediated vasoconstriction in order to elevate the diastolic blood pressure and thus the coronary perfusion pressure during CPR (Fig. 12-5). Consequently, if the heart rate remains less than 60 bpm despite 30 seconds of effective PPV and coordinated cardiac compressions and ventilation, then 0.1 to 0.3 mL/kg of 1 : 10,000 epinephrine solution should be given rapidly via the intravenous route followed by 0.5 to 1.0 mL of normal saline

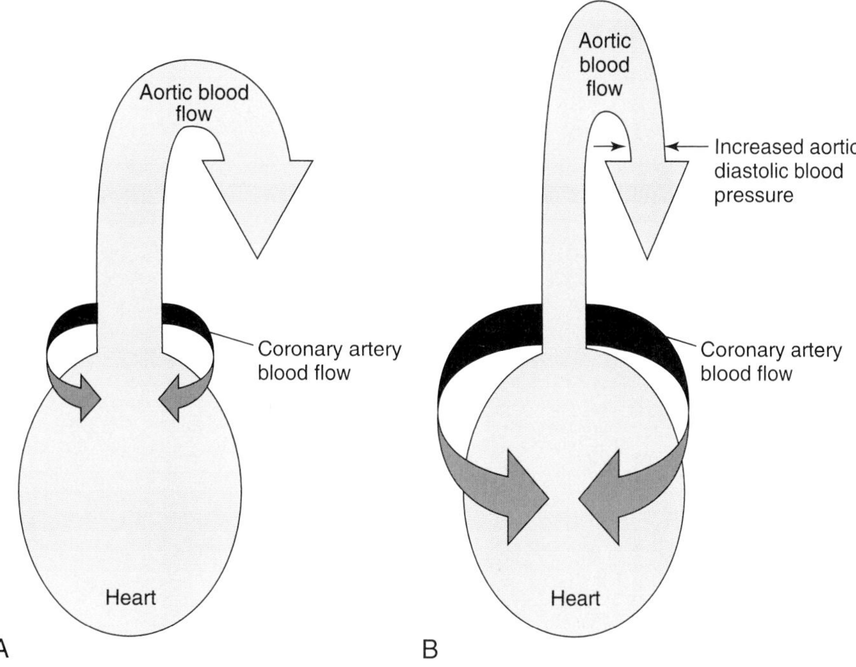

Figure 12-5 The effect of diastolic blood pressure on coronary blood flow during cardiac compressions. **A,** Cardiac compressions with minimal aortic diastolic blood pressure preferentially send the majority of the cardiac output around the aortic arch to the periphery. **B,** Cardiac compressions with improved aortic diastolic blood pressure sends more blood into the coronary arteries to bring oxygenated blood that will help generate adenosine triphosphate to get the heart beating again. (From Wyckoff MH. Neonatal cardiopulmonary resuscitation: critical hemodynamics. *Neoreviews.* 2010;11:e123-e129.)

12

flush.[1] Data regarding efficacious dosing for intravenous epinephrine during delivery room CPR is lacking, other than that this dose is more successful than endotracheal administration of epinephrine. The emphasis on intravenous delivery of epinephrine rather than the endotracheal route mandates that delivery room resuscitation providers be well trained in rapid preparation and placement of umbilical venous catheters.[33] The endotracheal route is no longer considered efficacious or reliable for epinephrine delivery.[88] Newborn transitional physiology does not favor success through the endotracheal route for several reasons. The decreased blood flow may be insufficient to transport drugs from the alveoli to the central circulation, pulmonary vasoconstriction from acidosis could impede drug absorption, unresorbed alveolar fluid may dilute the epinephrine, and potential right to left intracardiac shunts could bypass the pulmonary circulation altogether. However, if the endotracheal route must be used because of persistent lack of intravenous access, a higher dose (0.5-1.0 mL/kg) of 1 : 10,000 epinephrine solution should be used in hopes of improving efficacy.[1] The endotracheal dose should be drawn up in a larger, 3- to 5-mL syringe, to help alert the resuscitation team as to which route the dose is intended, because high doses of epinephrine should not be given intravenously. There is a small case series reporting successful resuscitation of newborns using the intraosseous route for epinephrine delivery. There is no data to support or refute the use of other vasoconstrictor drugs during CPR.[88a]

The vast majority of asphyxiated, severely depressed newborns are not hypovolemic. Volume infusion should be given only if there is a high index of suspicion for blood loss as a cause of shock based on the clinical circumstances surrounding the delivery (cord avulsion, velamentous insertion of the cord, traumatic abruption, etc.) or if the baby appears to be in shock and has not responded to what would otherwise appear to be adequate resuscitation.[33] The best replacement fluid is O-negative blood, but isotonic crystalloid such as normal saline or lactated Ringer's solution is acceptable until blood is available. Volume should be administered in 10-mL/kg aliquots slowly over 5 to 10 minutes with assessment for response. Avoiding a rapid push is important because a poorly functioning asphyxiated, acidemic, neonatal heart will not be able to respond to a sudden increase in preload with a sudden increase in cardiac output. In an asphyxia-induced hypotension and bradycardia model (without hypovolemia), volume infusion during resuscitation increased pulmonary edema, decreased pulmonary dynamic compliance, and did not improve blood pressure either during or after the resuscitation.[89] Thus, volume infusions during delivery room resuscitation may be detrimental and exacerbate poor cardiac output when hypovolemia is not present. They should be reserved for newborns in whom there is a high suspicion of hypovolemia.[33]

There is no evidence to support use of sodium bicarbonate during resuscitation of the newborn. Animal models and adult studies have demonstrated deleterious effects on physiologic end points after administration of sodium bicarbonate during CPR, including depression of myocardial function from the osmolar load with severe acidosis, paradoxical intracellular acidosis, and reduced cerebral blood flow.[33,90] No experimental neonatal animal studies or clinical trials have addressed the specific role of bicarbonate in achieving return of spontaneous circulation in of the patient with severe bradycardia or asystole. The only randomized trial of sodium bicarbonate infusion in neonates requiring PPV in the delivery room showed no benefit on neurologic outcome or survival.[91] Use of sodium bicarbonate should be discouraged during brief CPR. Its use in the newborn should be restricted to post-resuscitation care in the neonatal intensive care unit, which can be guided by results of arterial blood gas measurement or serum chemistry analysis.[92] Sodium bicarbonate should never be given unless there is assurance that adequate ventilation has been achieved, or it will paradoxically worsen acidemia through increased respiratory acidosis.

Special Situations

Other conditions that can lead to severe respiratory depression or distress at birth and that require early resuscitation include bacterial or viral sepsis, pneumothorax, airway obstruction associated with micrognathia (Pierre Robin sequence), choanal atresia, upper airway tumors or webs, massive cardiomegaly, pulmonary hypoplasia, pleural effusions, ascites, and anasarca (hydrops).[33] Many of these conditions interfere with effective ventilation and oxygenation and therefore may require specific management interventions. These conditions are described in more detail elsewhere in this volume and therefore are not within the scope of this section on delivery room resuscitation. If an infant has not responded to what would otherwise appear to be complete and adequate resuscitative measures for more than 10 minutes, resuscitation providers may consider discontinuing their efforts.[11] Current data, from a systematic review conducted by Harrington and colleagues,[93] indicate that after 10 minutes of asystole there are a very few survivors and those infants that do survive are likely to have severe disability. Infants whose 10-minute Apgar scores are 0 but who survived to be admitted to the neonatal intensive care unit and entered into a hypothermia clinical trial had better outcomes than those reported in the systematic review; however, there was significant selection bias.[94]

References

1. Kattwinkel J, ed. *Textbook of Neonatal Resuscitation*. Elk Grove, IL: American Academy of Pediatrics AHA; 2011.
2. Wyckoff MH. Newborn Resuscitation in the Delivery Room. In: Rudolph C, Rudolph R, et al, eds. *Rudolph's Textbook of Pediatrics*. New York: McGraw-Hill; 2011.
3. McCall EM, Alderdice F, Halliday HL, et al. Interventions to prevent hypothermia at birth in preterm and/or low birthweight infants. *Cochrane Database Syst Rev*. 2010;(3):CD004210.
4. Laptook AR, Salhab W, Bhaskar B. Admission temperature of low birth weight infants: predictors and associated morbidities. *Pediatrics*. 2007;119:e643-e649.
5. Trevisanuto D, Doglioni N, Cavallin F, et al. Heat loss prevention in very preterm infants in delivery rooms: a prospective, randomized, controlled trial of polyethylene caps. *J Pediatr*. 2010; 156:914-917.

6. Singh A, Duckett J, Newton T, et al. Improving neonatal unit admission temperatures in preterm babies: exothermic mattresses, polythene bags or a traditional approach? *J Perinatol*. 2010; 30:45-49.
7. Simon P, Dannaway D, Bright B, et al. Thermal defense of extremely low gestational age newborns during resuscitation: exothermic mattresses vs polyethylene wrap. *J Perinatol*. 2011;31:33-37.
8. Vohra S, Roberts RS, Zhang B, et al. Heat Loss Prevention (HeLP) in the delivery room: A randomized controlled trial of polyethylene occlusive skin wrapping in very preterm infants. *J Pediatr*. 2004;145:750-753.
9. Pillow JJ, Hillman NH, Polglase GR, et al. Oxygen, temperature and humidity of inspired gases and their influences on airway and lung tissue in near-term lambs. *Intensive Care Med*. 2009;35:2157-2163.
10. te Pas AB, Lopriore E, Dito I, et al. Humidified and heated air during stabilization at birth improves temperature in preterm infants. *Pediatrics*. 2010;125:e1427-e1432.
11. Kattwinkel J, Perlman JM, Aziz K, et al. Part 15: neonatal resuscitation: 2010 American Heart Association Guidelines for Cardiopulmonary Resuscitation and Emergency Cardiovascular Care. *Circulation*. 2010;122:S909-S919.
12. Kamlin CO, O'Donnell CP, Davis PG, et al. Oxygen saturation in healthy infants immediately after birth. *J Pediatr*. 2006;148:585-589.
13. Dawson JA, Kamlin CO, Vento M, et al. Defining the reference range for oxygen saturation for infants after birth. *Pediatrics*. 2010;125:e1340-e1347.
14. O'Donnell CP, Kamlin CO, Davis PG, et al. Clinical assessment of infant colour at delivery. *Arch Dis Child Fetal Neonatal Ed*. 2007;92:F465-F467.
15. Owen CJ, Wyllie JP. Determination of heart rate in the baby at birth. *Resuscitation*. 2004;60:213-217.
16. Kamlin CO, O'Donnell CP, Everest NJ, et al. Accuracy of clinical assessment of infant heart rate in the delivery room. *Resuscitation*. 2006;71:319-321.
17. Perlman JM. Hyperthermia in the delivery: potential impact on neonatal mortality and morbidity. *Clin Perinatol*. 2006;33:55-63, vi.
18. Ball MK, Hillman NH, Kallapur S, et al. Body temperature effects on lung injury in ventilated preterm lambs. *Resuscitation*. 2010;81:749-754.
19. Gungor S, Kurt E, Teksoz E, et al. Oronasopharyngeal suction versus no suction in normal and term infants delivered by elective cesarean section: a prospective randomized controlled trial. *Gynecol Obstet Invest*. 2006;61:9-14.
20. Fraser WD, Hofmeyr J, Lede R, et al. Amnioinfusion for the prevention of the meconium aspiration syndrome. *N Engl J Med*. 2005;353:909-917.
21. Vain NE, Szyld EG, Prudent LM, et al. Oropharyngeal and nasopharyngeal suctioning of meconium-stained neonates before delivery of their shoulders: multicentre, randomised controlled trial. *Lancet*. 2004;364:597-602.
22. Wiswell TE, Gannon CM, Jacob J, et al. Delivery room management of the apparently vigorous meconium-stained neonate: results of the multicenter, international collaborative trial. *Pediatrics*. 2000;105:1-7.
23. Bennett S, Finer NN, Rich W, et al. A comparison of three neonatal resuscitation devices. *Resuscitation*. 2005;67:113-118.
24. Morley CJ, Dawson JA, Stewart MJ, et al. The effect of a PEEP valve on a Laerdal neonatal self-inflating resuscitation bag. *J Paediatr Child Health*. 2010;46:51-56.
25. Roehr CC, Kelm M, Fischer HS, et al. Manual ventilation devices in neonatal resuscitation: tidal volume and positive pressure-provision. *Resuscitation*. 2010;81:202-205.
26. Dawson JA, Gerber A, Kamlin CO, et al. Providing PEEP during neonatal resuscitation: Which device is best? *J Paediatr Child Health*. 2011;47:698-703.
27. Dawson JA, Schmolzer GM, Kamlin CO, et al. Oxygenation with T-Piece versus Self-Inflating Bag for Ventilation of Extremely Preterm Infants at Birth: A Randomized Controlled Trial. *J Pediatr*. 2011;158:912-918.
28. Schmölzer GM, Dawson JA, Kamlin CO, et al. Airway obstruction and gas leak during mask ventilation of preterm infants in the delivery room. *Archives of Disease in Childhood—Fetal and Neonatal Edition*. 2011;96:F254-F257.
29. Schmolzer GM, Kamlin OC, O'Donnell CP, et al. Assessment of tidal volume and gas leak during mask ventilation of preterm infants in the delivery room. *Arch Dis Child Fetal Neonatal Ed*. 2010;95:F393-F397.
30. Leone TA, Lange A, Rich W, et al. Disposable colorimetric carbon dioxide detector use as an indicator of a patent airway during noninvasive mask ventilation. *Pediatrics*. 2006;118:e202-e204.
31. Kattwinkel J, Stewart C, Walsh B, et al. Responding to Compliance Changes in a Lung Model during Manual Ventilation: Perhaps Volume, Rather Than Pressure, Should be Displayed. *Pediatrics*. 2009;123:e465-e470.
32. Palme-Kilander C, Tunell R. Pulmonary gas exchange during facemask ventilation immediately after birth. *Arch Dis Child*. 1993;68:11-16.
33. Wyckoff MH. Delivery Room Resuscitation. In: Rudolph CD RA, Lister GE, First LR, Gershon AA, ed. *Rudolph's Pediatrics*. 22nd ed. New York, NY: McGraw Hill; 2011:164-170.
34. Sobotka KS, Hooper SB, Allison BJ, et al. An initial sustained inflation improves the respiratory and cardiovascular transition at birth in preterm lambs. *Pediatr Res*. 2011;70:56-60.
35. te Pas AB, Siew M, Wallace MJ, et al. Effect of sustained inflation length on establishing functional residual capacity at birth in ventilated premature rabbits. *Pediatr Res*. 2009;66:295-300.

36. Morley CJ, Davis PG, Doyle LW, et al. Nasal CPAP or intubation at birth for very preterm infants. *N Engl J Med*. 2008;358:700-708.
37. Finer NN, Carlo WA, Walsh MC, et al. Early CPAP versus surfactant in extremely preterm infants. *N Engl J Med*. 2010;362:1970-1979.
38. Leone TA, Rich W, Finer NN. Neonatal intubation: success of pediatric trainees. *J Pediatr*. 2005;146:638-641.
39. Bismilla Z, Breakey VR, Swales J, et al. Prospective evaluation of residents on call: before and after duty-hour reduction. *Pediatrics*. 2011;127:1080-1087.
40. Peterson J, Johnson N, Deakins K, et al. Accuracy of the 7-8-9 Rule for endotracheal tube placement in the neonate. *J Perinatol*. 2006;26:333-336.
41. Wyllie J, Carlo WA. The role of carbon dioxide detectors for confirmation of endotracheal tube position. *Clin Perinatol*. 2006;33:111-119, vii.
42. Trevisanuto D, Micaglio M, Ferrarese P, et al. The laryngeal mask airway: potential applications in neonates. *Arch Dis Child Fetal Neonatal Ed*. 2004;89:F485-F489.
43. Zanardo V, Weiner G, Micaglio M, et al. Delivery room resuscitation of near-term infants: role of the laryngeal mask airway. *Resuscitation*. 2010;81:327-330.
44. Pandit JJ, MacLachlan K, Dravid RM, et al. Comparison of times to achieve tracheal intubation with three techniques using the laryngeal or intubating laryngeal mask airway. *Anaesthesia*. 2002;57:128-132.
45. Ruetzler K, Roessler B, Potura L, et al. Performance and skill retention of intubation by paramedics using seven different airway devices—a manikin study. *Resuscitation*. 2011;82:593-597.
46. Roberts KD, Lampland AL, Meyers PA, et al. Laryngeal mask airway for surfactant administration in a newborn animal model. *Pediatr Res*. 2010;68:414-418.
47. Trevisanuto D, Grazzina N, Ferrarese P, et al. Laryngeal mask airway used as a delivery conduit for the administration of surfactant to preterm infants with respiratory distress syndrome. *Biol Neonate*. 2005;87:217-220.
48. The International Liaison Committee on Resuscitation (ILCOR) consensus on science with treatment recommendations for pediatric and neonatal patients: neonatal resuscitation. *Pediatrics*. 2006;117:e978-e988.
49. Toth B, Becker A, Seelbach-Gobel B. Oxygen saturation in healthy newborn infants immediately after birth measured by pulse oximetry. *Arch Gynecol Obstet*. 2002;266:105-107.
50. Wang CL, Anderson C, Leone TA, et al. Resuscitation of preterm neonates by using room air or 100% oxygen. *Pediatrics*. 2008;121:1083-1089.
51. Rabi Y, Yee W, Chen SY, et al. Oxygen saturation trends immediately after birth. *J Pediatr*. 2006;148:590-594.
52. Altuncu E, Ozek E, Bilgen H, et al. Percentiles of oxygen saturations in healthy term newborns in the first minutes of life. *Eur J Pediatr*. 2008;167:687-688.
53. O'Donnell CP, Kamlin CO, Davis PG, et al. Feasibility of and delay in obtaining pulse oximetry during neonatal resuscitation. *J Pediatr*. 2005;147:698-699.
54. Davis PG, Tan A, O'Donnell CP, et al. Resuscitation of newborn infants with 100% oxygen or air: a systematic review and meta-analysis. *Lancet*. 2004;364:1329-1333.
55. Saugstad OD, Ramji S, Vento M. Resuscitation of depressed newborn infants with ambient air or pure oxygen: a meta-analysis. *Biol Neonate*. 2005;87:27-34.
56. Rabi Y, Rabi D, Yee W. Room air resuscitation of the depressed newborn: a systematic review and meta-analysis. *Resuscitation*. 2007;72:353-363.
57. Escrig R, Arruza L, Izquierdo I, et al. Achievement of targeted saturation values in extremely low gestational age neonates resuscitated with low or high oxygen concentrations: a prospective, randomized trial. *Pediatrics*. 2008;121:875-881.
58. Richmond S, Goldsmith JP. Air or 100% oxygen in neonatal resuscitation? *Clin Perinatol*. 2006;33:11-27, v.
59. Naumburg E, Bellocco R, Cnattingius S, et al. Supplementary oxygen and risk of childhood lymphatic leukaemia. *Acta Paediatr*. 2002;91:1328-1333.
60. Spector LG, Klebanoff MA, Feusner JH, et al. Childhood cancer following neonatal oxygen supplementation. *J Pediatr*. 2005;147:27-31.
61. Cnattingius S, Zack MM, Ekbom A, et al. Prenatal and neonatal risk factors for childhood lymphatic leukemia. *J Natl Cancer Inst*. 1995;87:908-914.
62. Sola A. Oxygen for the preterm newborn: one infant at a time. *Pediatrics*. 2008;121:1257.
63. Wyckoff MH, Berg RA. Optimizing chest compressions during delivery-room resuscitation. *Semin Fetal Neonatal Med*. 2008;13:410-415.
64. Perlman JM, Risser R. Cardiopulmonary resuscitation in the delivery room. Associated clinical events. *Arch Pediatr Adolesc Med*. 1995;149:20-25.
65. Wyckoff MH, Perlman JM, Laptook AR. Use of volume expansion during delivery room resuscitation in near-term and term infants. *Pediatrics*. 2005;115:950-955.
66. Shah PS. Extensive cardiopulmonary resuscitation for VLBW and ELBW infants: a systematic review and meta-analyses. *J Perinatol*. 2009;29:655-661.
67. Dannevig I, Solevag AL, Wyckoff M, et al. Delayed onset of cardiac compressions in cardiopulmonary resuscitation of newborn pigs with asphyctic cardiac arrest. *Neonatology*. 2011;99:153-162.
68. Solevag AL, Dannevig I, Nakstad B, et al. Resuscitation of severely asphyctic newborn pigs with cardiac arrest by using 21% or 100% oxygen. *Neonatology*. 2010;98:64-72.
69. Orlowski JP. Optimum position for external cardiac compression in infants and young children. *Ann Emerg Med*. 1986;15:667-673.

70. Phillips GW, Zideman DA. Relation of infant heart to sternum: its significance in cardiopulmonary resuscitation. *Lancet*. 1986;1:1024-1025.
71. Finholt DA, Kettrick RG, Wagner HR, et al. The heart is under the lower third of the sternum. Implications for external cardiac massage. *Am J Dis Child*. 1986;140:646-649.
72. Braga MS, Dominguez TE, Pollock AN, et al. Estimation of optimal CPR chest compression depth in children by using computer tomography. *Pediatrics*. 2009;124:e69-e74.
73. Maher KO, Berg RA, Lindsey CW, et al. Depth of sternal compression and intra-arterial blood pressure during CPR in infants following cardiac surgery. *Resuscitation*. 2009;80:662-664.
74. Houri PK, Frank LR, Menegazzi JJ, et al. A randomized, controlled trial of two-thumb vs two-finger chest compression in a swine infant model of cardiac arrest [see comment]. *Prehosp Emerg Care*. 1997;1:65-67.
75. Dorfsman ML, Menegazzi JJ, Wadas RJ, et al. Two-thumb vs. two-finger chest compression in an infant model of prolonged cardiopulmonary resuscitation. *Acad Emerg Med*. 2000;7:1077-1082.
76. Christman C, Hemway RJ, Wyckoff MH, et al. The two-thumb is superior to the two-finger method for administering chest compressions in a manikin model of neonatal resuscitation. *Arch Dis Child Fetal Neonatal Ed*. 2011;96:F99-F101.
77. Berg RA, Hilwig RW, Kern KB, et al. Simulated mouth-to-mouth ventilation and chest compressions (bystander cardiopulmonary resuscitation) improves outcome in a swine model of prehospital pediatric asphyxial cardiac arrest. *Crit Care Med*. 1999;27:1893-1899.
78. Berg RA, Hilwig RW, Kern KB, et al. "Bystander" chest compressions and assisted ventilation independently improve outcome from piglet asphyxial pulseless "cardiac arrest." *Circulation*. 2000;101:1743-1748.
79. Dean JM, Koehler RC, Schleien CL, et al. Improved blood flow during prolonged cardiopulmonary resuscitation with 30% duty cycle in infant pigs. *Circulation*. 1991;84:896-904.
80. Babbs CF, Nadkarni V. Optimizing chest compression to rescue ventilation ratios during one-rescuer CPR by professionals and lay persons: children are not just little adults. *Resuscitation*. 2004;61:173-181.
81. Solevag AL, Dannevig I, Wyckoff M, et al. Extended series of cardiac compressions during CPR in a swine model of perinatal asphyxia. *Resuscitation*. 2010;81:1571-1576.
82. Solevag AL, Dannevig I, Wyckoff M, et al. Return of spontaneous circulation with a compression:ventilation ratio of 15:2 versus 3:1 in newborn pigs with cardiac arrest due to asphyxia. *Arch Dis Child Fetal Neonatal Ed*. 2011;96:F417-F421.
83. Berkowitz ID, Chantarojanasiri T, Koehler RC, et al. Blood flow during cardiopulmonary resuscitation with simultaneous compression and ventilation in infant pigs. *Pediatr Res*. 1989;26:558-564.
84. Hou SH, Lue HC, Chu SH. Comparison of conventional and simultaneous compression-ventilation cardiopulmonary resuscitation in piglets. *Jpn Circ J*. 1994;58:426-432.
85. Wyckoff MH. Neonatal Cardiopulmonary Resuscitation: Critical Hemodynamics. *Neoreviews*. 2010;11:e123-e129.
86. Chalak LF, Barber CA, Hynan L, et al. End-tidal CO detection of an audible heart rate during neonatal cardiopulmonary resuscitation after asystole in asphyxiated piglets. *Pediatr Res*. 2011;69:401-405.
87. Kern KB, Hilwig R, Ewy GA. Retrograde coronary blood flow during cardiopulmonary resuscitation in swine: intracoronary Doppler evaluation. *Am Heart J*. 1994;128:490-499.
88. Wyckoff MH, Wyllie J. Endotracheal delivery of medications during neonatal resuscitation. *Clin Perinatol*. 2006;33:153-160, ix.
88a. Ellemunter H, Simma B, Trawoger R, Maurer H. Intraosseous lines in preterm and full term neonates. *Arch Dis Child Fetal Neonatal Ed*. Jan 1999;80(1):F74-75.
89. Wyckoff M, Garcia D, Margraf L, et al. Randomized trial of volume infusion during resuscitation of asphyxiated neonatal piglets. *Pediatr Res*. 2007;61:415-420.
90. Aschner JL, Poland RL. Sodium bicarbonate: basically useless therapy. *Pediatrics*. 2008;122: 831-835.
91. Lokesh L, Kumar P, Murki S, et al. A randomized controlled trial of sodium bicarbonate in neonatal resuscitation-effect on immediate outcome. *Resuscitation*. 2004;60:219-223.
92. Wyckoff MH, Perlman JM. Use of high-dose epinephrine and sodium bicarbonate during neonatal resuscitation: is there proven benefit? *Clin Perinatol*. 2006;33:141-151, viii-ix.
93. Harrington DJ, Redman CW, Moulden M, et al. The long-term outcome in surviving infants with Apgar zero at 10 minutes: a systematic review of the literature and hospital-based cohort. *Am J Obstet Gynecol*. 2007;196:463.e1-5.
94. Laptook AR, Shankaran S, Ambalavanan N, et al. Outcome of term infants using Apgar scores at 10 minutes following hypoxic-ischemic encephalopathy. *Pediatrics*. 2009;124:1619-1626.

CHAPTER 13

Noninvasive Respiratory Support: An Alternative to Mechanical Ventilation in Preterm Infants

Peter G. Davis, MD, FRACP, MBBS, Colin J. Morley, MD, FRACP, FRCPCH, and Brett J. Manley, MBBS, FRACP

- Physiological Principles
- A Brief History of Invasive and Noninvasive Neonatal Ventilation
- NCPAP for Postextubation Care
- Augmenting NCPAP: Nasal Intermittent Positive-Pressure Ventilation
- NCPAP for Babies with RDS or at Risk of Developing RDS
- NCPAP Devices
- How Much Supporting Pressure Should be Used?
- Complications of NCPAP
- When Has NCPAP Failed (i.e., When Should Infants be Intubated)?
- Weaning CPAP
- High-Flow Nasal Cannulae for Respiratory Support
- Conclusions

The primary concern of the clinician making choices about treatment is whether one therapy leads to better outcomes than the alternatives. This chapter draws heavily on evidence from randomized trials found in the neonatal module of the Cochrane Library (http://www.nichd.nih.gov/cochrane/default.cfm). Consistent with presentation in the library, estimates of treatment effect are expressed as relative risk (RR) and the differences are statistically significant if the 95% confidence interval (CI) does not include one. Other levels of evidence, for example, from observational studies, are presented, particularly when no randomized trials exist. In some areas the highest level of available evidence is our own personal experience, which we present cautiously and with humility.

We believe that before the examination of available evidence, summary of the physiologic principles underpinning noninvasive respiratory support usefully informs clinicians and researchers. This chapter focuses on current noninvasive support: nasal continuous positive airway pressure (NCPAP) ventilation, nasal intermittent positive-pressure ventilation (NIPPV), and high-flow nasal cannula (HFNC) ventilation.

Physiological Principles

Why Do Preterm Infants Experience Respiratory Failure and How Can Noninvasive Support Help?

Respiratory Distress Syndrome

Respiratory distress syndrome (RDS) is a disease of newborn infants, increasing in prevalence with decreasing gestational age. It is characterized by immature lung development and inadequate surfactant production. The lungs of affected infants may not expand normally immediately after birth, do not easily maintain a residual volume, and are at risk of atelectasis. Other factors also contribute to a loss of lung volume, including muscle hypotonia, a compliant chest wall, and slow clearance of fetal lung liquid. Repeated lung expansion, followed by atelectasis during expiration, leads to shearing forces that damage the alveolar epithelium and cause leakage of protein-rich fluid from the pulmonary capillaries. This leakage in turn inhibits any endogenous surfactant present.[1] Damage to the lungs is exacerbated by mechanical ventilation and high oxygen concentrations.

Apnea of Prematurity

The pharyngeal airway of the preterm newborn is very compliant. The cartilaginous components are more flexible, and the fat-laden superficial fascia of the neck that stabilizes the upper airway of term infants is not well developed. The intrathoracic airways, including trachea, bronchi, and small airways, are similarly compliant and prone to collapse during expiration.

The breathing patterns of very premature infants are frequently erratic and at times inadequate. The causes of apnea of prematurity include hypoxia due to a reduced functional residual capacity (FRC), particularly in active sleep. Upper airway obstruction, alone or in combination with a central respiratory pause, accompanies most apneic events.

The Role of NCPAP

NCPAP ventilation effectively supports the breathing of preterm infants through a number of mechanisms. It mechanically splints the upper airway, thereby preventing obstruction and reducing apnea.[2] Distension of the airways reduces resistance to air flow and so diminishes work of breathing.[3] NCPAP ventilation aids lung expansion and so reduces ventilation-perfusion mismatch and improves oxygenation. By preventing repeated alveolar collapse and reexpansion, NCPAP reduces protein leak and helps conserve surfactant.

Why Might Noninvasive Support Be Superior to Ventilation via an Endotracheal Tube?

Intermittent positive-pressure ventilation (PPV) via an endotracheal tube (ETT) has been the mainstay of neonatal intensive care almost since its inception. Many lives have been saved by this technique but its adverse effects are well documented, as follows:

- Cardiovascular and cerebrovascular instability during intubation
- Complications of the ETT, including subglottic stenosis and tracheal lesions
- Infections, both pulmonary and systemic
- Acute and chronic lung damage due to large tidal volumes (volutrauma), excessive inflating pressure (barotrauma), and shear stress with each inflation

By avoiding the local mechanical problems of an ETT as well as those of volutrauma, NCPAP ventilation has at least a theoretical advantage over invasive respiratory support.

A Brief History of Invasive and Noninvasive Neonatal Ventilation

The first form of assisted ventilation for neonates was intermittent positive-pressure ventilation provided via an ETT, which became widespread in the late 1960s and early 1970s. George Gregory and associates[4] were the first to describe the use of CPAP in neonates in 1971, a therapy they developed because of the high mortality observed in infants weighing less than 1500 g, particularly those requiring assisted ventilation in the first 24 hours of life. The first series of 20 "severely ill" infants with RDS were treated with CPAP delivered predominantly via an ETT. In an attempt to avoid the complications of endotracheal intubation, other interfaces were developed, including a pressurized plastic bag[5] and a tight-fitting face mask.[6] Two infants in the initial Gregory series were managed in a pressure chamber around the infant's head.[4] In 1976, Ahlström and colleagues[7] described the use of a face chamber providing pressures up to 15 cm H_2O. Rhodes and Hall[8] conducted a controlled trial involving alternate allocation of subjects to CPAP via a tight-fitting face mask or to conventional therapy consisting of warmed humidified oxygen. A trend toward increased survival was noted in the CPAP group, which was statistically significant in the subgroup of infants weighing more than 1500 g.

The local pressure effects of these devices, combined with the problems of accessibility, particularly for suctioning and feeding, led to the development of alternative interfaces for the delivery of CPAP. Novogroder and coworkers[9] described a device composed of two Portex ETTs inserted through the nose and then positioned under direct laryngoscopy in the posterior pharynx, joined by a Y-connector, and attached to a pressure source. Others described shorter binasal devices that were simpler to manufacture and insert.[10,11] An even simpler single nasal prong, made by cutting down an ETT, became widely used.[12] A later development in the field is that of a variable-flow device that uses jet nozzles to assist inspiratory flow while diverting flow away from the patient in expiration.[13] This design is claimed to be superior to conventional CPAP in reducing work of breathing.[14]

It should be noted that of all these trials, only the one conducted by Rhodes and Hall[8] used a control group. Novogroder and coworkers[9] had plans to subject their device to a randomized trial but abandoned them when "the dramatic effect of CPAP (was) observed after a brief period of treatment in all patients." It is likely that other researchers were so convinced of the virtues of endotracheal intubation that trials comparing this therapy with CPAP were considered inappropriate. In an accompanying commentary to the study by Rhodes and Hall, Chernick[15] congratulated the investigators on conducting a "daring controlled study" and suggested that although one or two such studies of CPAP would be welcome, many more "would be foolish."[15] With some notable exceptions it seems researchers heeded his advice. The following sections describe these exceptions.

NCPAP for Postextubation Care

It is generally accepted that early extubation of preterm infants is desirable. The perceived benefits include reducing the risks of infection, local tissue damage, and chronic lung disease. On the other hand, failure of extubation and the need for reintubation is associated with instability and more local trauma. The *Cochrane Systematic Reviews* article on the topic[16] identified nine randomized trials of varying methodologic quality and using different levels of CPAP and devices.[17-25] Pooled analysis showed that NCPAP was associated with a lower rate of respiratory failure (apnea, respiratory acidosis or increased oxygen requirements) after extubation than management in an oxygen hood (RR 0.62; 95% CI, 0.51-0.76) (Fig. 13-1). Four of the studies allowed rescue NCPAP ventilation to be provided for babies in whom the oxygen hood failed. Because rescue treatment with NCPAP ventilation was frequently successful, there was no significant difference in rate of reintubation between the groups RR 0.93 (95% CI, 0.72 -1.19) (Fig. 13-2). A study that directly compared elective with rescue NCPAP ventilation after extubation found no differences in reintubation rates.[26]

Therefore, it can reasonably be concluded that NCPAP ventilation should be used when a very preterm infant is extubated, to prevent the instability associated with possible subsequent respiratory failure and reintubation. However, it appears that reserving the use of NCPAP ventilation for preterm infants in whom respiratory failure is developing after extubation does not lead to increased reintubation.

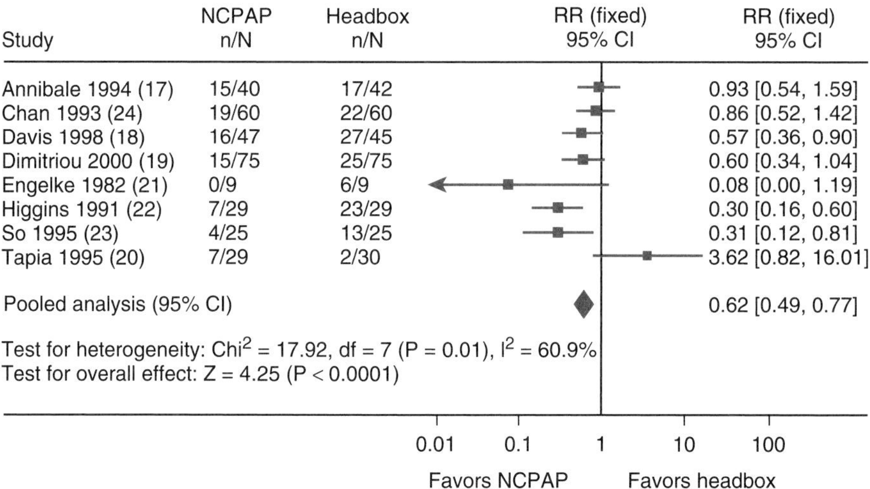

Figure 13-1 NCPAP in comparison with oxygen hood (headbox): effect on rate of extubation failure. See text for details.

Augmenting NCPAP: Nasal Intermittent Positive-Pressure Ventilation

Although NCPAP ventilation is an effective method of postextubation support, researchers have added positive-pressure "inflations" to a background of NCPAP. This technique was used in the 1980s but became unpopular when it was linked to gastrointestinal perforation.[27]

The availability of ventilators that "synchronized" with an infant's inspirations led to studies of NIPPV. Systematic review identified three randomized trials[28-30] that evaluated NIPPV after extubation of preterm infants.[31] Pooled analysis showed

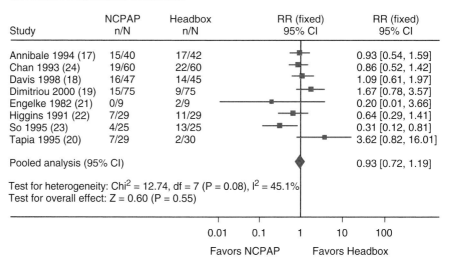

COMPARISON: Nasal CPAP vs Headbox
OUTCOME: Endotracheal reintubation

Study	NCPAP n/N	Headbox n/N	RR (fixed) 95% CI
Annibale 1994 (17)	15/40	17/42	0.93 [0.54, 1.59]
Chan 1993 (24)	19/60	22/60	0.86 [0.52, 1.42]
Davis 1998 (18)	16/47	14/45	1.09 [0.61, 1.97]
Dimitriou 2000 (19)	15/75	9/75	1.67 [0.78, 3.57]
Engelke 1982 (21)	0/9	2/9	0.20 [0.01, 3.66]
Higgins 1991 (22)	7/29	11/29	0.64 [0.29, 1.41]
So 1995 (23)	4/25	13/25	0.31 [0.12, 0.81]
Tapia 1995 (20)	7/29	2/30	3.62 [0.82, 16.01]
Pooled analysis (95% CI)			0.93 [0.72, 1.19]

Test for heterogeneity: $Chi^2 = 12.74$, df = 7 (P = 0.08), $I^2 = 45.1\%$
Test for overall effect: Z = 0.60 (P = 0.55)

0.01 0.1 1 10 100

Favors NCPAP | Favors Headbox

Figure 13-2 NCPAP for extubation in comparison with oxygen hood (headbox): effect on rate of endotracheal reintubation. See text for details.

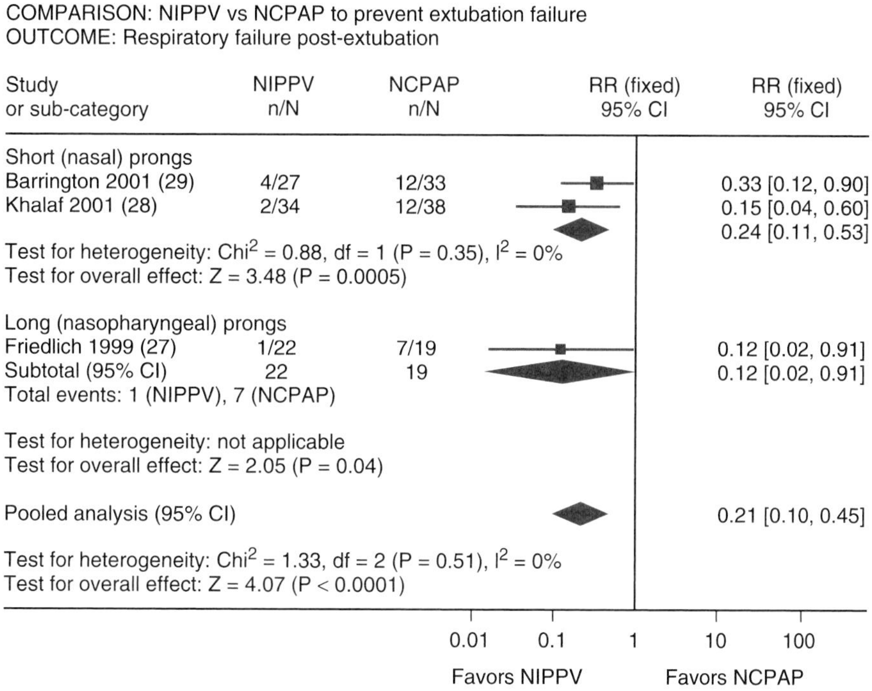

COMPARISON: NIPPV vs NCPAP to prevent extubation failure
OUTCOME: Respiratory failure post-extubation

Study or sub-category	NIPPV n/N	NCPAP n/N	RR (fixed) 95% CI
Short (nasal) prongs			
Barrington 2001 (29)	4/27	12/33	0.33 [0.12, 0.90]
Khalaf 2001 (28)	2/34	12/38	0.15 [0.04, 0.60]
			0.24 [0.11, 0.53]
Test for heterogeneity: $Chi^2 = 0.88$, df = 1 (P = 0.35), $I^2 = 0\%$			
Test for overall effect: Z = 3.48 (P = 0.0005)			
Long (nasopharyngeal) prongs			
Friedlich 1999 (27)	1/22	7/19	0.12 [0.02, 0.91]
Subtotal (95% CI)	22	19	0.12 [0.02, 0.91]
Total events: 1 (NIPPV), 7 (NCPAP)			
Test for heterogeneity: not applicable			
Test for overall effect: Z = 2.05 (P = 0.04)			
Pooled analysis (95% CI)			0.21 [0.10, 0.45]
Test for heterogeneity: $Chi^2 = 1.33$, df = 2 (P = 0.51), $I^2 = 0\%$			
Test for overall effect: Z = 4.07 (P < 0.0001)			

0.01 0.1 1 10 100

Favors NIPPV Favors NCPAP

Figure 13-3 NIPPV in comparison with NCPAP ventilation: effect on rate of extubation failure. See text for details.

NIPPV to be associated with significantly lower risk of respiratory failure (apnea, respiratory acidosis, or increased oxygen requirements) than NCPAP ventilation (RR 0.21; 95% CI, 0.10-0.45) (Fig. 13-3). Two of the studies allowed rescue therapy with NIPPV for infants in whom NCPAP ventilation failed. The effect of NIPPV on rate of reintubation was therefore decreased, although still significant (RR 0.39; 95% CI, 0.180.97) (Fig. 13-4). Reassuringly, there was no significant difference between the two approaches in the rate of abdominal distention, and no infant had gastrointestinal perforation. All three trials in this systematic review used the Infant Star ventilator with a Graseby pneumatic capsule on the abdomen to try to synchronize inflations with inspirations in the infants randomly allocated to NIPPV.

There is little information to help clinicians optimize the NIPPV settings. In the randomized trials the rate of ventilator inflations varied between 10 and 25 per min

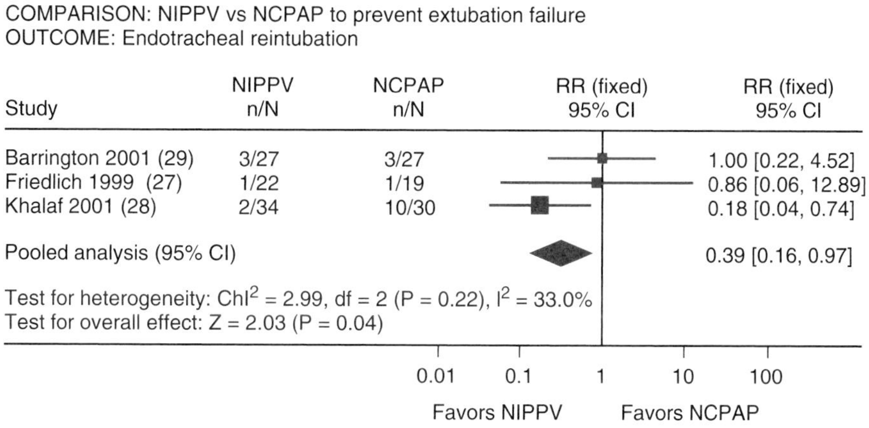

COMPARISON: NIPPV vs NCPAP to prevent extubation failure
OUTCOME: Endotracheal reintubation

Study	NIPPV n/N	NCPAP n/N	RR (fixed) 95% CI
Barrington 2001 (29)	3/27	3/27	1.00 [0.22, 4.52]
Friedlich 1999 (27)	1/22	1/19	0.86 [0.06, 12.89]
Khalaf 2001 (28)	2/34	10/30	0.18 [0.04, 0.74]
Pooled analysis (95% CI)			0.39 [0.16, 0.97]
Test for heterogeneity: $ChI^2 = 2.99$, df = 2 (P = 0.22), $I^2 = 33.0\%$			
Test for overall effect: Z = 2.03 (P = 0.04)			

0.01 0.1 1 10 100

Favors NIPPV Favors NCPAP

Figure 13-4 NIPPV in comparison with NCPAP ventilation: effect on rate of endotracheal reintubation. See text for details.

and the peak inflating pressures (PIPs) were set at or slightly above the PIP used before extubation. The ventilator used in these trials is no longer made. Many neonatal units are now using nonsynchronized NIPPV (NS-NIPPV), and the association with gastrointestinal perforations has not reemerged.

NIPPV is used in other clinical situations. Systematic review of NIPPV for treating apnea of prematurity found only two studies, with a total of 54 infants.[32,33] The pooled analysis showed a modest benefit for NIPPV over NCPAP ventilation and no evidence of harm.[33] It therefore seems reasonable to try NIPPV in infants experiencing troublesome apnea during treatment with NCPAP. Following its success in these situations, some investigators have suggested that NIPPV be used as an initial form of support for preterm infants with respiratory distress. Meneses and colleagues[34] studied NIPPV in this role: 200 preterm infants (26 to 34 weeks of gestation) with RDS were randomly assigned to NIPPV or NCPAP, with surfactant given as a rescue therapy. The rates of reintubation within the first 72 hours of life were no different in the groups (RR 0.71; 95% CI, 0.48-1.14). Observational studies suggest that the use of NIPPV for primary treatment of RDS is worth testing in further randomized trials either alone[35] or in conjunction with prior intubation and exogenous surfactant therapy.[36]

The mechanisms by which NIPPV improves clinical outcomes are uncertain. Owen[37] studied 10 premature infants receiving NS-NIPPV and found that NIPPV pressure peaks resulted in only a small increase in relative tidal volumes when delivered during spontaneous inspiration, and only occasionally led to chest inflations when delivered during apneic periods. Another study in 11 infants demonstrated that during NS-NIPPV, the delivered PIP was variable and frequently lower than the set PIP.[38] Chang and associates[39] compared short-term effects of NS-NIPPV and synchronized NIPPV (S-NIPPV) with NCPAP. Sixteen very preterm infants, 15 ± 14 days old and undergoing treatment with the Infant Star ventilator, were randomly allocated to NCPAP, NS-NIPPV at 20 or 40 inflations/min, and S-NIPPV at 20 or 40 inflations/min for 1 hour each in random order. Tidal volume, minute ventilation, and gas exchange values did not differ significantly among the groups. S-NIPPV resulted in less inspiratory effort than NCPAP ventilation or NS-NIPPV, but NS-NIPPV had no advantage over NCPAP. Active expiratory effort and expiratory duration increased during NS-NIPPV. There were no benefits on gas exchange of either form of nasal ventilation over NCPAP. S-NIPPV reduced breathing effort and resulted in better infant-ventilator interaction than NS-NIPPV.

NIPPV appears to be useful for augmenting NCPAP. Further studies of NIPPV are required to determine the optimal pressure and rate settings, the safety of the nonsynchronized mode, and the role of NIPPV as primary therapy for RDS.

NCPAP for Babies with RDS or at Risk of Developing RDS

The focus of studies on the use of NCPAP ventilation in infants who have or are at risk for RDS has changed over the decades. Questions about the topic are dealt with here in roughly historical order.

Is Prophylactic CPAP Better than No Respiratory Support for Very Preterm Infants?

The rationale for the use of NCPAP ventilation in this context is that it may assist the establishment and maintenance of an FRC and thereby alter the natural history of RDS. Observational studies comparing practices in different centers and in the same centers over time suggested that early use of CPAP leads to a reduction in both the need for PPV and the rate of bronchopulmonary dysplasia (BPD).[40-42] Two randomized trials enrolling 312 preterm infants compared NCPAP ventilation started in the first hours after birth with an oxygen hood.[43,44] Pooled analysis found no significant difference in rates of intubation (Fig. 13-5), BPD, pneumothorax, or

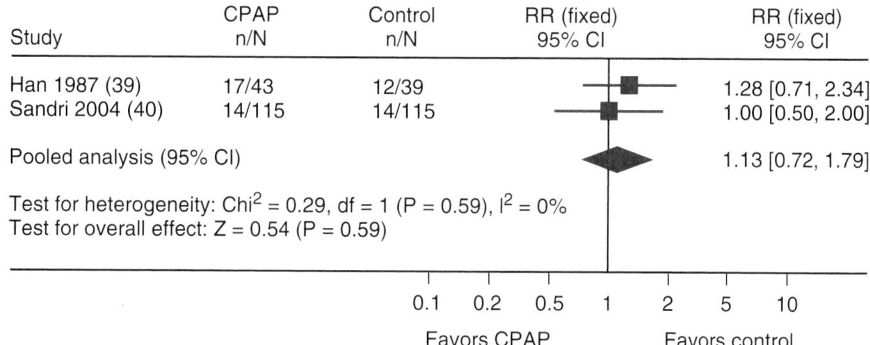

COMPARISON: Prophylactic CPAP vs control
OUTCOME: Endotracheal intubation
Study
CPAP n/N
Control n/N
RR (fixed) 95% CI
RR (fixed) 95% CI
Han 1987 (39) 17/43 12/39 1.28 [0.71, 2.34]
Sandri 2004 (40) 14/115 14/115 1.00 [0.50, 2.00]
Pooled analysis (95% CI) 1.13 [0.72, 1.79]
Test for heterogeneity: Chi² = 0.29, df = 1 (P = 0.59), I² = 0%
Test for overall effect: Z = 0.54 (P = 0.59)
0.1 0.2 0.5 1 2 5 10
Favors CPAP
Favors control

Figure 13-5 Prophylactic NCPAP ventilation: effect on rate of endotracheal intubation. See text for details.

mortality.[45] However, both trials recruited relatively mature infants (up to 32 weeks of gestation) with a low incidence of adverse outcomes.

Is Continuous Distending Pressure (CDP) Better than No CDP for Treatment of RDS?

Continuous distending pressure is the use of any treatment in which a continuous positive airway or negative extrathoracic pressure is applied to the lung. A review of this topic found five studies comparing CDP with no respiratory support, four of which were undertaken in the 1970s.[46] Two used negative-pressure chambers,[47,48] two used face-mask CPAP,[8,49] and one used negative pressure for less severe illness and endotracheal CPAP for severe illness.[50] Pooled analysis of these trials showed that CDP reduced the rate of treatment failure (death or use of assisted ventilation) (RR 0.70; 95% CI, 0.55, 0.88) and mortality (RR 0.53; 95% CI, 0.32-0.87) (Fig. 13-6). However, more pneumothoraces occurred in the patients receiving CDP (RR 2.36; 95% CI, 1.25-5.54) (Fig. 13-7). These studies were conducted before the availability of surfactant, and are of limited relevance in the modern neonatal intensive care era.

COMPARISON: CDP VS STANDARD CARE
OUTCOME: MORTALITY

Study	CDP n/N	Control n/N	RR (fixed) 95% CI
Durbin 1976 (46)	1/12	2/12	0.50 [0.05, 4.81]
Fanaroff 1973 (43)	4/15	6/14	0.62 [0.22, 1.75]
Samuels 1996 (44)	1/26	0/26	3.00 [0.13, 70.42]
Belenky 1976 (45)	4/22	14/29	0.38 [0.14, 0.99]
Rhodes 1973 (8)	6/22	10/19	0.52 [0.23, 1.16]
Pooled analysis (95% CI)			0.52 [0.32, 0.87]

Test for heterogeneity: Chi² = 1.73, df = 4 (P = 0.78), I² = 0%
Test for overall effect: Z = 2.51 (P = 0.01)

0.1 0.2 0.5 1 2 5 10

Favors CDP Favors control

Figure 13-6 Comparison of continuous distending pressure (CDP) and standard care for respiratory distress syndrome RDS: effect on rate of mortality. See text for details.

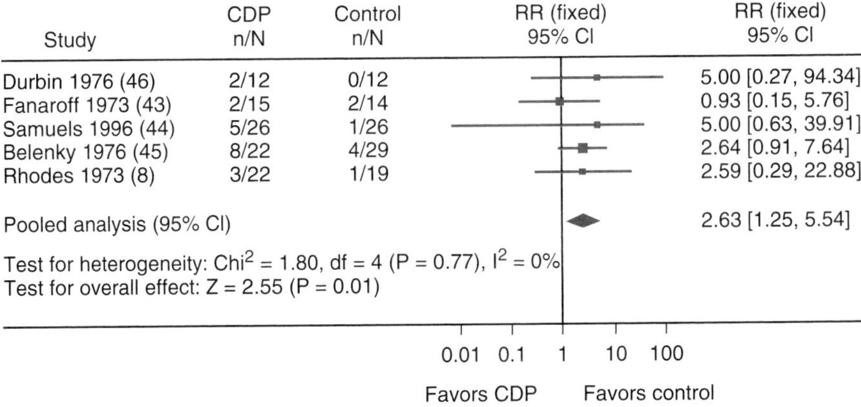

COMPARISON: CDP VS STANDARD CARE
OUTCOME: ANY PNEUMOTHORAX
Study
CDP n/N
Control n/N
RR (fixed) 95% CI
RR (fixed) 95% CI
Durbin 1976 (46) 2/12 0/12 5.00 [0.27, 94.34]
Fanaroff 1973 (43) 2/15 2/14 0.93 [0.15, 5.76]
Samuels 1996 (44) 5/26 1/26 5.00 [0.63, 39.91]
Belenky 1976 (45) 8/22 4/29 2.64 [0.91, 7.64]
Rhodes 1973 (8) 3/22 1/19 2.59 [0.29, 22.88]
Pooled analysis (95% CI) 2.63 [1.25, 5.54]
Test for heterogeneity: Chi2 = 1.80, df = 4 (P = 0.77), I2 = 0%
Test for overall effect: Z = 2.55 (P = 0.01)
0.01 0.1 1 10 100
Favors CDP
Favors control

Figure 13-7 Comparison of continuous distending pressure (CDP) and standard care for respiratory distress syndrome (RDS): effect on rate of pneumothorax. See text for details.

CPAP in the "Surfactant Era"

Surfactant is the most comprehensively evaluated treatment in neonatology. Most of the randomized trials of its use were done over 20 years ago, when early CPAP was not used for very preterm infants, antenatal corticosteroids were given to only 10% of eligible mothers, and neonatal mortality and morbidity were much higher than current rates. Whether given to ventilated babies prophylactically or as treatment, surfactant reduced mortality and the combined outcome of death or chronic lung disease.[51,52] It appeared that surfactant was more beneficial when given early in the course of RDS.[53] Although other methods of administration have been tried,[54] surfactant is usually given via an ETT. It became common practice for all very preterm infants to be intubated in the delivery room for surfactant administration.

Several groups have reported their experience as they have changed policy from early intubation to early NCPAP,[55,56] describing lower mortality and morbidity in the group treated with NCPAP.

Is CPAP an Alternative to Routine Intubation of Very Preterm Infants at Birth?

Several randomized controlled trials have compared intubation in the delivery room with NCPAP ventilation and intubation only if prespecified failure criteria were met. The Nasal CPAP or Intubation at Birth for Very Preterm Infants (COIN) trial[57] randomly assigned 610 breathing infants at 25-29 weeks' gestation to CPAP or intubation and ventilation at 5 minutes after birth. Surfactant was administered to intubated infants at the discretion of the treating clinician. Early NCPAP ventilation did not lead to a significantly lower rate of death or BPD at 36 weeks of gestation than intubation. The benefits of CPAP included halving the intubation rate, a lower risk of the combined outcome of death or the need for oxygen therapy at 28 days, and fewer days of assisted ventilation. However, the CPAP group had a higher rate of pneumothoraces (9%, vs. 3% in the intubated group).

The Surfactant, Positive Pressure, and Oxygenation (SUPPORT) trial[58] enrolled 1316 infants between 24^0 weeks and 27^6 weeks of gestation. The subjects were randomly allocated to intubation and surfactant (within 1 hour after birth) or CPAP in the delivery room. The rates of death or BPD did not differ significantly between the groups after adjustment for gestational age, center, and familial clustering. Although 83.1% of infants in the CPAP group ultimately required intubation and mechanical ventilation, 34.4% were intubated in the delivery room. Overall, infants randomly assigned to CPAP were less likely to be intubated, less likely to receive postnatal corticosteroids, had fewer days of mechanical ventilation, and were more likely to be alive without mechanical ventilation by day 7.

These randomized controlled trials show that NCPAP ventilation can be used from birth in very preterm infants and that nearly half of such infants may not need ventilation or surfactant treatment. The outcomes of the babies treated with CPAP were similar to or better than those of babies intubated and ventilated from birth.

Is CPAP with Early Intubation for Surfactant and Brief Ventilation Better than CPAP Alone?

A systematic review has investigated whether early, brief intubation for surfactant administration followed by extubation to NCPAP ventilation was better than NCPAP ventilation and selective intubation, surfactant, and continued ventilation.[59] Meta-analysis of the six studies identified showed that intubation, ventilation, and early surfactant therapy followed by extubation to NCPAP ventilation was associated with lower incidences of later mechanical ventilation (typical RR 0.67; 95% CI 0.57-0.79), air leak syndromes (typical RR 0.52; 95% CI 0.28-0.96), and BPD (typical RR 0.51; 95% CI 0.26-0.99]. The early surfactant group received about 60% more surfactant. Stratified analysis of FIO_2 at study entry suggested that a lower treatment threshold ($FIO_2 < 0.45$) reduced air leaks and BPD.

Further studies have been published since this review. The Colombian Neonatal Network enrolled infants of 27^0 to 31^6 weeks of gestation, who were receiving oxygen and had increased work of breathing, at 15 to 60 minutes after birth.[60] The infants were treated with bubble NCPAP ventilation at 6 cm H_2O and then randomly allocated to either NCPAP ventilation plus surfactant (n = 141) or NCPAP ventilation alone (n = 137). The primary outcome was the need for PPV started because either the FIO_2 was higher than 0.75 or the $PaCO_2$ higher than 65 mm Hg. The CPAP + surfactant group received two doses of SURVANTA (Abbott Nutrition, Abbott Park, IL), 2 minutes apart, and were then extubated if possible to NCPAP ventilation 6 cm H_2O. The need for PPV was significantly lower in the NCPAP ventilation + surfactant group than in the control group (26% vs. 39%, respectively) although all babies who had received surfactant had been temporarily intubated and ventilated. Mortality, BPD, duration of mechanical ventilation, and oxygen therapy did not differ between the groups. There were fewer air leaks in the group receiving surfactant.

The CURPAP study group randomly assigned 208 infants born at 25^0 to 28^6 weeks of gestation who were not intubated within 30 minutes of birth to either (1) intubation, Curosurf (Cornerstone Therapeutics, Inc., Cary NC) and extubation within an hour (if possible) to NCPAP or (2) NCPAP ventilation with early selective surfactant.[61] PPV was started when FIO_2 exceeded 0.4, the infant had four episodes of apnea per hour, or $PaCO_2$ exceeded 65 mm Hg. There were no significant differences between the groups in rate of PPV at 5 days of life, death or BPD at 36 weeks of gestation, or pneumothoraces.

All these trials show that outcomes in infants stabilized in the delivery room with either NCPAP ventilation or prophylactic surfactant and extubation to NCPAP ventilation appear to be similar to those in infants managed with surfactant followed by ventilation.

Administering Surfactant to Infants Receiving CPAP without the Insertion of an Endotracheal Tube

Techniques of administering surfactant without using an ETT have also been described. Kribs and associates[62] treated extremely premature infants receiving NCPAP ventilation who had ongoing signs of moderate to severe RDS with surfactant given via an intratracheal catheter during spontaneous breathing. Mortality in these infants was lower than in a group of historical controls that were intubated and ventilated prior to surfactant therapy. Dargaville and colleagues[63] have also proposed a method of minimally invasive surfactant therapy to be used in spontaneously breathing preterm infants receiving CPAP. In a feasibility study, unsedated preterm infants on CPAP received surfactant via a 16-gauge vascular catheter under direct vision of the vocal cords. In all cases, surfactant was successfully administered and CPAP was reestablished. These techniques require further evaluation in randomized controlled trials.

NCPAP Devices

Several interfaces have been developed for delivering NCPAP. The nasal prongs may be short, lying 1 to 2 cm inside the nose, or long, with the tip in the nasopharynx (Fig. 13-8). They may be single or binasal. An important determinant of effectiveness of CPAP devices is their ability to transmit the pressure to the airways. This ability depends on the resistance to flow of the device, which in turn depends on the length and diameter of the prongs. In an in vitro comparison of popular devices, short binasal prongs with the largest internal diameters had the lowest resistance.[64]

Since its description by Moa and coworkers[13] in 1988, the variable-flow NCPAP device—Aladdin NCPAP Infant Flow System (now called the Arabella; Hamilton Medical AG, Reno, NV), EME Infant Flow Nasal CPAP (CareFusion, San Francisco), or Infant Flow Driver (Electro Medical Equipment Ltd, Brighton, Sussex, UK)—has become widely used around the world. In vitro studies using models of neonatal ventilation have demonstrated less pressure variation and work of breathing with the variable-flow device.[65] Pandit and colleagues[66] attempted measurement of the work of breathing in preterm infants with the use of respiratory inductance plethysmography and esophageal pressure monitoring. They demonstrated less work of breathing with variable-flow CPAP than with constant-flow CPAP. The same group showed, in a crossover study, that the variable-flow device led to better lung recruitment than either nasal cannulae or constant-flow CPAP.[67]

Having an understanding of the properties of different devices is useful, but for clinicians, the primary question is which one is best at reducing the severity of the respiratory problems and intubation. Head-to-head comparisons of different devices are few. Pooled analysis of the two trials[68,69] comparing single and double nasal prongs after extubation of preterm infants confirms that double prongs are better for preventing extubation failure (RR 0.59; 95% CI 0.41-.85) (Fig. 13-9).[70] Two trials have compared different binasal devices. Stefanescu and associates[71] compared the EME Infant Flow Nasal CPAP with INCA prongs (Ackrad Laboratories Inc, Cranford, New Jersey, USA) and found no difference in rates of extubation failure, death, or BPD. Sun and coworkers[72] reported a lower rate of reintubation using the Infant Flow system than with short binasal prongs.

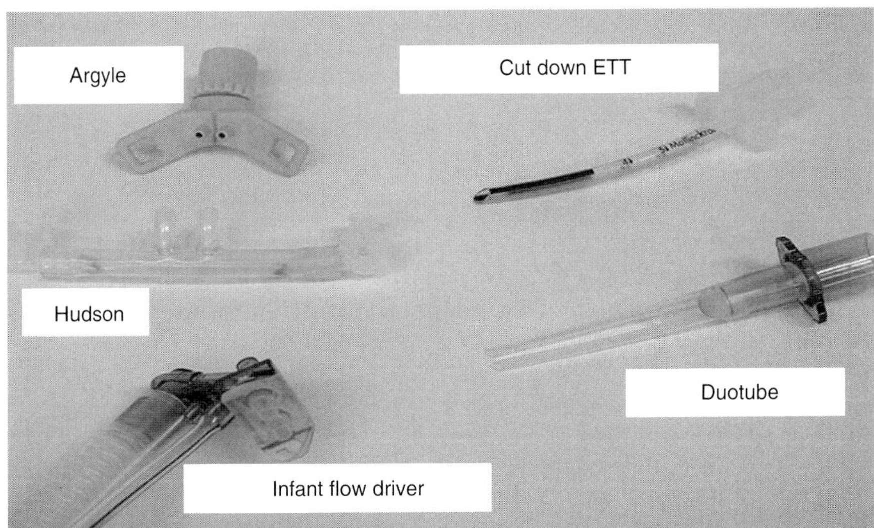

Figure 13-8 NCPAP devices. ETT, endotracheal tube.

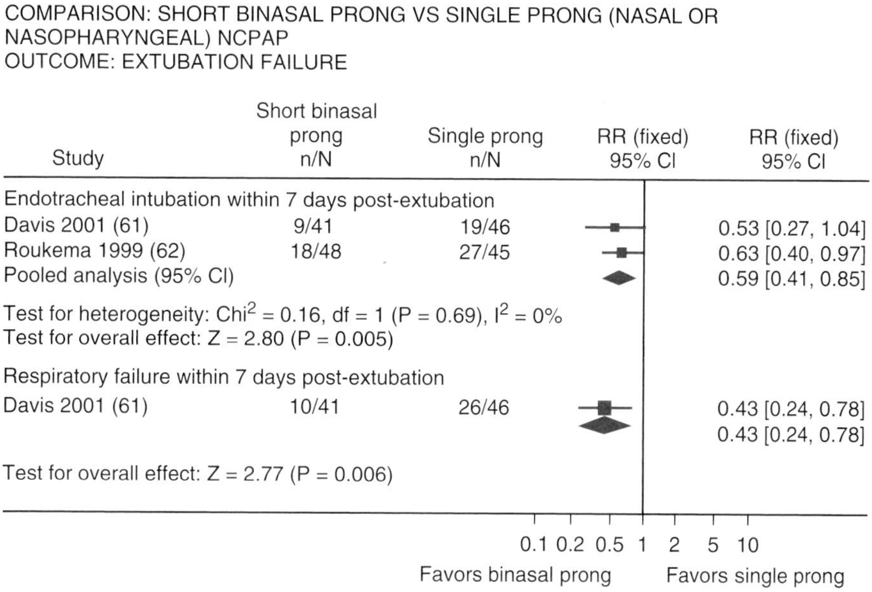

COMPARISON: SHORT BINASAL PRONG VS SINGLE PRONG (NASAL OR NASOPHARYNGEAL) NCPAP
OUTCOME: EXTUBATION FAILURE

Study	Short binasal prong n/N	Single prong n/N	RR (fixed) 95% CI	RR (fixed) 95% CI
Endotracheal intubation within 7 days post-extubation				
Davis 2001 (61)	9/41	19/46		0.53 [0.27, 1.04]
Roukema 1999 (62)	18/48	27/45		0.63 [0.40, 0.97]
Pooled analysis (95% CI)				0.59 [0.41, 0.85]
Test for heterogeneity: $Chi^2 = 0.16$, df = 1 (P = 0.69), $I^2 = 0\%$				
Test for overall effect: Z = 2.80 (P = 0.005)				
Respiratory failure within 7 days post-extubation				
Davis 2001 (61)	10/41	26/46		0.43 [0.24, 0.78]
				0.43 [0.24, 0.78]
Test for overall effect: Z = 2.77 (P = 0.006)				

0.1 0.2 0.5 1 2 5 10

Favors binasal prong Favors single prong

Figure 13-9 Comparison of single-prong (nasal) and double-prong (nasopharyngeal) NCPAP ventilation: effect on extubation failure. See text for details.

Mazzella and associates[73] compared the Infant Flow Driver with a single long nasopharyngeal tube for the treatment of preterm infants with respiratory distress. Although infants randomly assigned to the Infant Flow Driver had lower FIO_2 and respiratory rates, there were no significant differences in the need for ventilation or the duration of CPAP. The lower resistance offered by binasal prongs appears to translate to a clinical advantage for these devices over short or long single nasal prongs.

Gupta and colleagues[74] compared bubble CPAP with the Infant Flow Driver for postextubation management of preterm infants with RDS.[74] The duration of CPAP support was halved in the bubble CPAP group. In the subgroup of infants ventilated for less than 14 days, extubation failed less often in the bubble CPAP group.

How Much Supporting Pressure Should Be Used?

The purpose of nasal CPAP is to deliver a pressure to the airways and lungs. If this purpose is achieved consistently, which device is used may not be important. A pressure of 5 cm H_2O is a traditional starting point. Some neonatal intensive care units hardly vary this pressure and claim good results.[75] There is some evidence from the Cochrane review of NCPAP ventilation for extubation that pressures below 5 cm H_2O are ineffective in this setting (Fig. 13-10).[16] In their landmark publication on CPAP, Gregory and associates[4] used pressures up to 15 mm Hg.[4] A study of infants with mild RDS showed the highest end expiratory lung volume and tidal volume, the lowest respiratory rate, and the least thoracoabdominal asynchrony at a pressure of 8 cm H_2O, which was compared with 0, 2, 4, and 6 cm H_2O.[76]

A baby with RDS, relatively stiff lungs, a high FIO_2 and a chest radiograph showing opaque lungs may need a higher pressure to support lung volume than a baby with a low FIO_2 treated for apneic episodes. If CPAP is to be effective, the pressure may need to be increased to 10 cm H_2O in infants with very low lung compliance.[77] High pressures, if used in a baby with compliant lungs, can interfere with pulmonary blood flow and cause overdistention, leading to CO_2 retention. Judging which pressure is needed remains an art. If an infant shows evidence of lung disease with increasing oxygen requirements and a more opaque chest radiograph, we would increase the pressure in increments of 1 cm H_2O and observe the effect.

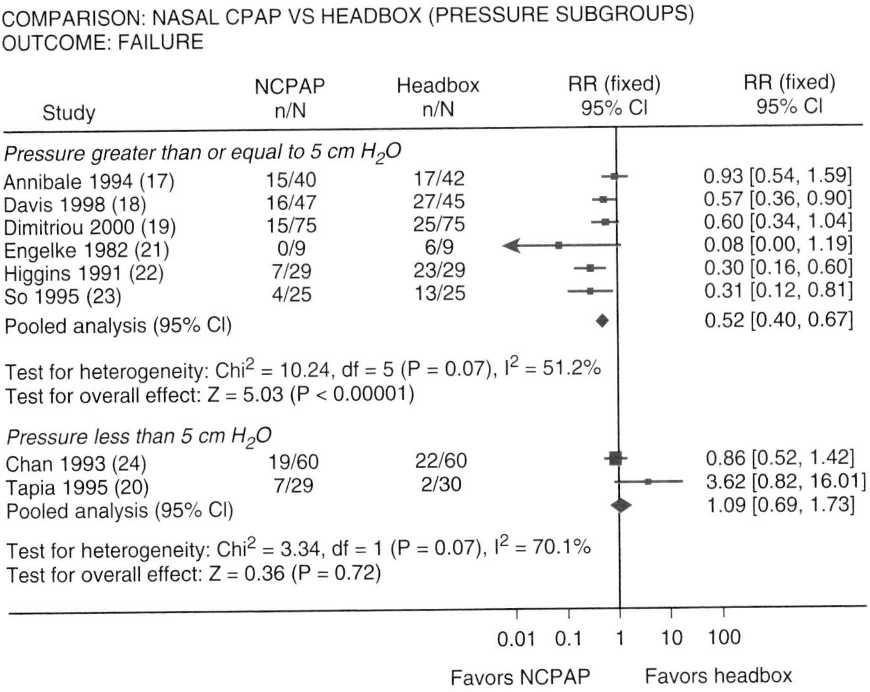

COMPARISON: NASAL CPAP VS HEADBOX (PRESSURE SUBGROUPS)
OUTCOME: FAILURE

Study	NCPAP n/N	Headbox n/N	RR (fixed) 95% CI
Pressure greater than or equal to 5 cm H_2O			
Annibale 1994 (17)	15/40	17/42	0.93 [0.54, 1.59]
Davis 1998 (18)	16/47	27/45	0.57 [0.36, 0.90]
Dimitriou 2000 (19)	15/75	25/75	0.60 [0.34, 1.04]
Engelke 1982 (21)	0/9	6/9	0.08 [0.00, 1.19]
Higgins 1991 (22)	7/29	23/29	0.30 [0.16, 0.60]
So 1995 (23)	4/25	13/25	0.31 [0.12, 0.81]
Pooled analysis (95% CI)			0.52 [0.40, 0.67]
Test for heterogeneity: $Chi^2 = 10.24$, df = 5 ($P = 0.07$), $I^2 = 51.2\%$			
Test for overall effect: $Z = 5.03$ ($P < 0.00001$)			
Pressure less than 5 cm H_2O			
Chan 1993 (24)	19/60	22/60	0.86 [0.52, 1.42]
Tapia 1995 (20)	7/29	2/30	3.62 [0.82, 16.01]
Pooled analysis (95% CI)			1.09 [0.69, 1.73]
Test for heterogeneity: $Chi^2 = 3.34$, df = 1 ($P = 0.07$), $I^2 = 70.1\%$			
Test for overall effect: $Z = 0.36$ ($P = 0.72$)			

0.01 0.1 1 10 100

Favors NCPAP Favors headbox

Figure 13-10 Comparison of NCPAP ventilation with oxygen hood (headbox) for extubation; subgroup analysis by pressure used.

The optimal CPAP pressure is not known and may depend on the condition treated. Future research should evaluate strategies of titrating CPAP pressures to an infant's requirements. In the absence of evidence-based guidelines, we use CPAP pressures in the range 5 to 8 cm H_2O, adjusting them on the basis of oxygen requirements and clinical assessment of work of breathing.

Complications of NCPAP

NCPAP ventilation is a comparatively simple form of respiratory support, yet it is not without complications. The major problems of the early days of CPAP, intracerebellar hemorrhages[78] and hydrocephalus,[79] were solved by alterations in delivery technique. However, nasal trauma may still occur with prongs, ranging in severity from redness and excoriation of the nares to necrosis of the columella and nasal septum requiring surgery. Observational studies suggest that all NCPAP devices may cause trauma[80]; Robertson and coworkers[81] reported a complication rate of 20% in a series of very low-birth-weight babies managed wit the Infant Flow Driver. Techniques to prevent nasal trauma are entirely anecdotal. We try to select a prong with a diameter that is sufficient to snugly fit the infant's nostril (avoiding excessive leak around the device) but which does not cause blanching of the nares. Positioning of binasal prongs so that there is no pressure on the columella is sometimes difficult to achieve but critical. We have observed that supervision by skilled nurses experienced in the technique of securing CPAP prongs has led to a low rate of nasal trauma.

Pneumothoraces occur in preterm infants treated with NCPAP. In the COIN trial,[57] there were significantly more pneumothoraces in the CPAP group than in the ventilated group (9% vs. 3%, respectively), raising concerns in some quarters about the use of early NCPAP. In the previously described Colombian Neonatal Network study, which randomly assigned spontaneously breathing preterm infants on NCPAP ventilation to receive either early surfactant therapy and early extubation to NCPAP or NCPAP alone, the group managed with early surfactant therapy had fewer pneumothoraces (2%, vs. 9% for NCPAP ventilation alone).[60] Conversely, the SUPPORT trial found no difference in rate of pneumothoraces between early CPAP and mechanical ventilation.[58]

When Has NCPAP Failed (i.e., When Should Infants be Intubated)?

There is no universally accepted definition of CPAP failure. Polin and Sahni[82] suggested that "an infant with ventilation that is not improving or inadequate oxygenation with $FIO_2 > 0.6$" should be intubated and given surfactant. Others recommend intubation when oxygen requirements exceed 0.35 to 0.40.[83] We set the following failure criteria for infants randomly allocated to NCPAP ventilation in the COIN trial: FIO_2 more than 0.6 or pH less than 7.25 with a $PaCO_2$ higher than 60 mm Hg or more than one apneic episode per hour requiring stimulation.[57] Whatever threshold is applied, it is important that remediable causes of failure are sought and treated before intubation. They include airway obstruction with secretions and inappropriate (too small) prong size. Treating a large mouth leak and raising the applied pressure may be useful strategies before CPAP is deemed to have failed.

Weaning CPAP

The optimal method of weaning a baby from NCPAP ventilation remains uncertain, and practices vary among units. Robertson and Hamilton[26] randomly allocated 58 premature babies to either a "weaning" strategy or a "rescue" strategy of NCPAP ventilation after extubation. The weaning strategy gradually increased the time "off" CPAP. In the rescue arm, babies were extubated to oxygen hood, and NCPAP ventilation was restarted only if predefined failure criteria were reached; NCPAP ventilation was discontinued after 12 hours and recommenced only if the same failure criteria were met. These investigators found no significant differences between the two groups in ventilator days or days on NCPAP. A randomized trial comparing a strategy of weaning through reducing pressure with one of increasing time "off" NCPAP ventilation showed a significantly shorter duration of weaning with the "pressure" strategy.[84] In a single-centre study, Abdel-Hady[85] randomized 60 preterm infants who were stable on NCPAP 5 cm H_2O with $FIO_2 <0.30$ for at least 24 hours to either ongoing NCPAP with gradual weaning of oxygen then cessation of NCPAP, or to HFNC 2 L/min with gradual weaning of oxygen then flow. The HFNC group had longer duration of oxygen therapy and ventilation, with no difference in success of weaning from NCPAP. The use of HFNC ventilation to facilitate weaning from NCPAP ventilation requires further investigation.

In the absence of good evidence, our practice is to wean infants to a CPAP of 5 cm H_2O, discontinue the NCPAP ventilation when the infant is stable with FIO_2 less than 0.30 and recommence it if oxygen requirements or frequency of apneas increases.

High-Flow Nasal Cannulae for Respiratory Support

Nasal cannulae delivering higher gas flows (i.e., HFNC ventilation) have become a popular form of respiratory support without the intensive scrutiny applied to other modes of assisted ventilation.[86] Definitions of what constitutes "high-flow" vary, but the consensus seems to be flow rates exceeding 1 L/min.[87] HFNC ventilation is being used to treat preterm infants as postextubation support, as initial support for early respiratory distress, or as a "step-down" therapy from NCPAP, with variable flow rate regimens.

Two commercially available HFNC systems are marketed for use in premature and term infants: Vapotherm (VAP, Vapotherm Inc., Stevensville, MD), and Fisher & Paykel Optiflow (F&P; Fisher & Paykel Healthcare, Auckland, NZ). Both are open systems with leaks at the nose and mouth. Gases are heated and humidified, the system allows the blending of oxygen and air, and a range of infant nasal prong sizes (with varying outer diameters and septum widths) is available. The F&P system includes a pressure-relief valve in the circuit, whereas Vapotherm does not. By delivering heated, humidified gases, these systems have gone some way to alleviating earlier concerns about nasal mucosal injury and infection from high flow rates.[88]

How Much Distending Pressure Is Generated by HFNC?

A concern about the use of HFNC ventilation has been the unpredictable pressure generated.[89] This feature contrasts HFNC ventilation with NCPAP ventilation, in which the pressure is set and monitored. Data on pressure generation with HFNC ventilation comes from small observational, crossover, or in vitro studies that have used varying methods and infant populations for pressure measurement. Initially, there were concerns about high airway pressures.[90,91] Locke and associates[90] found that with larger (0.3 cm outer diameter) prongs and a flow rate of 2 L/min, the mean measured esophageal pressure was 9.8 cm H_2O. Data from later studies have been somewhat reassuring, with pressures generated similar to, or less than, those used routinely with NCPAP.[92-94] There have been several attempts to produce a formula to calculate pressure generation at different flow rates on the basis of infant weight, but the formulas available produce dramatically different results.[91,94]

Evidence for the Safety and Efficacy of HFNC Ventilation

There is anecdotal evidence that HFNC ventilation may be a useful and well-tolerated form of respiratory support for preterm infants. It is being advocated as an alternative to NCPAP ventilation in this role. However, there is a paucity of data about its efficacy. Campbell and associates[95] compared HFNC ventilation (in which the air was not heated but was humidified) with the Infant Flow NCPAP device as postextubation support in infants with birth weight less than 1250 g. The HFNC group required reintubation within 7 days at a significantly higher rate than the NCPAP group and also had higher oxygen use and more occurrences of apnea and bradycardia. However, the HFNC flow rates were calculated from the formula developed by Sreenan and colleagues,[91] which resulted in flows in the range of 1.4 to 1.7 L/min. These flow rates are much lower than those in current clinical use. Several retrospective, observational studies have compared heated and humidified HFNC ventilation with NCPAP ventilation in preventing extubation failure of preterm infants, with outcomes that either favor the HFNC method or do not find it inferior to NCPAP.[96-98]

Interpretation of the preceding studies is difficult because of the small sample sizes and differing study designs. Newer systems for delivering HFNC ventilation are heated and humidified, so randomized comparisons of these systems with the current "gold-standard," noninvasive respiratory support (NCPAP ventilation) in a variety of clinical roles would provide the most useful information.

Should HFNC Ventilation Be Used to Treat Preterm Infants?

Despite its increasing popularity, uncertainty remains about the efficacy and safety of HFNC ventilation in the preterm population. Currently this technique should be regarded as promising. There are several randomized controlled trials under way to study HFNC ventilation as postextubation support and as a primary therapy. We await the results of these trials before recommending widespread use.

Conclusions

For Clinicians

On the basis of randomized trials and systematic reviews, the following conclusions can be drawn:

- NCPAP ventilation reduces respiratory instability and the need for extra support after extubation.
- NCPAP ventilation reduces the rate of apnea.

- NIPPV is a useful method for augmenting the benefits of NCPAP ventilation.
- Binasal prongs are superior to single nasal prongs for the delivery of CPAP ventilation.
- It is reasonable to manage very preterm infants on NCPAP ventilation from delivery.

For Researchers

Opportunities to advance knowledge in the field of noninvasive ventilation include studies of the following:

- Alternative techniques of surfactant administration that do not require endotracheal intubation
- Methods available at the bedside to judge optimal levels of CPAP
- NIPPV to determine the best settings in terms of pressures, rates, and synchronization as well as testing its role in the initial management of RDS
- HFNC ventilation to establish safety and efficacy of this technique.

Acknowledgments

PGD is supported by an Australian National Health and Medical Research Council Fellowship. BJM is supported by a postgraduate scholarship from The University of Melbourne, and the Centre for Clinical Research Excellence, Murdoch Childrens Research Institute, Melbourne, Australia.

References

1. Ikegami M, Jacobs H, Jobe A. Surfactant function in respiratory distress syndrome. *J Pediatr*. 1983;102:443-447.
2. Alex CG, Aronson RM, Onal E, Lopata M. Effects of continuous positive airway pressure on upper airway and respiratory muscle activity. *J Appl Physiol*. 1987;62:2026-2030.
3. Saunders RA, Milner AD, Hopkin IE. The effects of continuous positive airway pressure on lung mechanics and lung volumes in the neonate. *Biol Neonate*. 1976;29:178-186.
4. Gregory GA, Kitterman JA, Phibbs RH, et al. Treatment of the idiopathic respiratory-distress syndrome with continuous positive airway pressure. *N Engl J Med*. 1971;284:1333-1340.
5. Barrie H. Simple method of applying continuous positive airway pressure in respiratory-distress syndrome. *Lancet*. 1972;1:776-777.
6. Ackerman BD, Stein MP, Sommer JS, Schumacher M. Continuous positive airway pressure applied by means of a tight-fitting face mask. *J Pediatr*. 1974;85:408-411.
7. Ahlström H, Jonson B, Svenningsen NW. Continuous positive airways pressure treatment by a face chamber in idiopathic respiratory distress syndrome. *Arch Dis Child*. 1976;51:13-21.
8. Rhodes PG, Hall RT. Continuous positive airway pressure delivered by face mask in infants with the idiopathic respiratory distress syndrome: a controlled study. *Pediatrics*. 1973;52:1-5.
9. Novogroder M, MacKuanying N, Eidelman AI, Gartner LM. Nasopharyngeal ventilation in respiratory distress syndrome. A simple and efficient method of delivering continuous positive airway pressure. *J Pediatr*. 1973;82:1059-1062.
10. Wung JT, Driscoll Jr JM, Epstein RA, Hyman AI. A new device for CPAP by nasal route. *Crit Care Med*. 1975;3:76-78.
11. Caliumi-Pellegrini G, Agostino R, Orzalesi M, et al. Twin nasal cannula for administration of continuous positive airway pressure to newborn infants. *Arch Dis Child*. 1974;49:228-230.
12. Field D, Vyas H, Milner AD, Hopkin IE. Continuous positive airway pressure via a single nasal catheter in preterm infants. *Early Hum Dev*. 1985;11:275-280.
13. Moa G, Nilsson K, Zetterstrom H, Jonsson LO. A new device for administration of nasal continuous positive airway pressure in the newborn: an experimental study. *Crit Care Med*. 1988;16:1238-1242.
14. Courtney SE, Aghai ZH, Saslow JG, et al. Changes in lung volume and work of breathing: A comparison of two variable-flow nasal continuous positive airway pressure devices in very low birth weight infants. *Pediatr Pulmonol*. 2003;36:248-252.
15. Chernick V. Continuous distending pressure in hyaline membrane disease: of devices, disadvantages, and a daring study. *Pediatrics*. 1973;52:114-115.
16. Davis PG, Henderson-Smart DJ. Nasal continuous positive airways pressure immediately after extubation for preventing morbidity in preterm infants. *Cochrane Database Syst Rev*. 2003;(1): CD000143.
17. Annibale DJ, Hulsey TC, Engstrom PC, et al. Randomized, controlled trial of nasopharyngeal continuous positive airway pressure in the extubation of very low birth weight infants. *J Pediatr*. 1994;124:455-460.
18. Davis P, Jankov R, Doyle L, Henschke P. Randomised, controlled trial of nasal continuous positive airway pressure in the extubation of infants weighing 600 to 1250 g. *Arch Dis Child Fetal Neonatal Ed*. 1998;79:F54-F57.

19. Dimitriou G, Greenough A, Kavvadia V, et al. Elective use of nasal continuous positive airways pressure following extubation of preterm infants. *Eur J Pediatr*. 2000;159:434-439.
20. Tapia JL, Bancalari A, Gonzalez A, Mercado ME. Does continuous positive airway pressure (CPAP) during weaning from intermittent mandatory ventilation in very low birth weight infants have risks or benefits? A controlled trial. *Pediatr Pulmonol*. 1995;19:269-274.
21. Engelke SC, Roloff DW, Kuhns LR. Postextubation nasal continuous positive airway pressure. A prospective controlled study. *Am J Dis Child*. 1982;136:359-361.
22. Higgins RD, Richter SE, Davis JM. Nasal continuous positive airway pressure facilitates extubation of very low birth weight neonates. *Pediatrics*. 1991;88:999-1003.
23. So BH, Tamura M, Mishina J, et al. Application of nasal continuous positive airway pressure to early extubation in very low birthweight infants. *Arch Dis Child Fetal Neonatal Ed*. 1995;72:F191-F193.
24. Chan V, Greenough A. Randomised trial of methods of extubation in acute and chronic respiratory distress. *Arch Dis Child*. 1993;68(Spec No):570-572.
25. Peake M, Dillon P, Shaw NJ. Randomized trial of continuous positive airways pressure to prevent reventilation in preterm infants. *Pediatr Pulmonol*. 2005;39:247-250.
26. Robertson NJ, Hamilton PA. Randomised trial of elective continuous positive airway pressure (CPAP) compared with rescue CPAP after extubation. *Arch Dis Child Fetal Neonatal Ed*. 1998;79:F58-F60.
27. Garland JS, Nelson DB, Rice T, Neu J. Increased risk of gastrointestinal perforations in neonates mechanically ventilated with either face mask or nasal prongs. *Pediatrics*. 1985;76:406-410.
28. Friedlich P, Lecart C, Posen R, et al. A randomized trial of nasopharyngeal-synchronized intermittent mandatory ventilation versus nasopharyngeal continuous positive airway pressure in very low birth weight infants after extubation. *J Perinatol*. 1999;19:413-418.
29. Khalaf MN, Brodsky N, Hurley J, Bhandari V. A prospective randomized, controlled trial comparing synchronized nasal intermittent positive pressure ventilation versus nasal continuous positive airway pressure as modes of extubation. *Pediatrics*. 2001;108:13-17.
30. Barrington KJ, Bull D, Finer NN. Randomized trial of nasal synchronized intermittent mandatory ventilation compared with continuous positive airway pressure after extubation of very low birth weight infants. *Pediatrics*. 2001;107:638-641.
31. Davis PG, Lemyre B, de Paoli AG. Nasal intermittent positive pressure ventilation (NIPPV) versus nasal continuous positive airway pressure (NCPAP) for preterm neonates after extubation. *Cochrane Database Syst Rev*. 2001;(C3):D003212.
32. Ryan CA, Finer NN, Peters KL. Nasal intermittent positive-pressure ventilation offers no advantages over nasal continuous positive airway pressure in apnea of prematurity. *Am J Dis Child*. 1989;143:1196-1198.
33. Lin CH, Wang ST, Lin YJ, Yeh TF. Efficacy of nasal intermittent positive pressure ventilation in treating apnea of prematurity. *Pediatr Pulmonol*. 1998;26:349-353.
34. Meneses J, Bhandari V, Alves JG, Herrmann D. Noninvasive ventilation for respiratory distress syndrome: a randomized controlled trial. *Pediatrics*. 2011;127:300-307.
35. Manzar S, Nair AK, Pai MG, et al. Use of nasal intermittent positive pressure ventilation to avoid intubation in neonates. *Saudi Med J*. 2004;25:1464-1467.
36. Santin R, Brodsky N, Bhandari V. A prospective observational pilot study of synchronized nasal intermittent positive pressure ventilation (SNIPPV) as a primary mode of ventilation in infants > or = 28 weeks with respiratory distress syndrome (RDS). *J Perinatol*. 2004;24:487-493.
37. Owen LS, Morley CJ, Dawson JA, Davis PG. Effects of non-synchronised nasal intermittent positive pressure ventilation on spontaneous breathing in preterm infants. *Arch Dis Child Fetal Neonatal Ed*. 2011;96(6):F422-8.
38. Owen LS, Morley CJ, Davis PG. Pressure variation during ventilator generated nasal intermittent positive pressure ventilation in preterm infants. *Arch Dis Child Fetal Neonatal Ed*. 2010;95:F359-F364.
39. Chang HY, Claure N, D'Ugard C, et al. Effects of synchronization during nasal ventilation in clinically stable preterm infants. *Pediatr Res*. 2011 Jan;69:84-89.
40. Avery ME, Tooley WH, Keller JB, et al. Is chronic lung disease in low birthweight infants preventable? A survey of 8 centres. *Pediatrics*. 1987;79:26-30.
41. Jacobsen T, Gronvall J, Petersen S, Andersen GE. "Minitouch" treatment of very low-birth-weight infants. *Acta Paediatr*. 1993;82:934-938.
42. Gittermann MK, Fusch C, Gittermann AR, et al. Early nasal continuous positive airway pressure treatment reduces the need for intubation in very low birth weight infants. *Eur J Pediatr*. 1997;156:384-388.
43. Han VK, Beverley DW, Clarson C, et al. Randomized controlled trial of very early continuous distending pressure in the management of preterm infants. *Early Hum Dev*. 1987;15:21-32.
44. Sandri F, Ancora G, Lanzoni A, et al. Prophylactic nasal continuous positive airways pressure in newborns of 28-31 weeks gestation: multicentre randomised controlled clinical trial. *Arch Dis Child Fetal Neonatal Ed*. 2004;89:F394-F398.
45. Subramaniam P, Henderson-Smart D, Davis P. Prophylactic nasal continuous positive airways pressure for preventing morbidity and mortality in very preterm infants. *Cochrane Database Syst Rev*. 2005;(3):CD001243.
46. Ho JJ, Subramaniam P, Henderson-Smart DJ, Davis PG. Continuous distending pressure for respiratory distress syndrome in preterm infants. *Cochrane Database Syst Rev*. 2002;(2):CD002271.
47. Fanaroff AA, Cha CC, Sosa R, et al. Controlled trial of continuous negative external pressure in the treatment of severe respiratory distress syndrome. *J Pediatr*. 1973;82:921-928.

48. Samuels MP, Raine J, Wright T, et al. Continuous negative extrathoracic pressure in neonatal respiratory failure. *Pediatrics*. 1996;98:1154-1160.
49. Belenky DA, Orr RJ, Woodrum DE, Hodson WA. Is continuous transpulmonary pressure better than conventional respiratory management of hyaline membrane disease? A controlled study. *Pediatrics*. 1976;58:800-808.
50. Durbin GM, Hunter NJ, McIntosh N, et al. Controlled trial of continuous inflating pressure for hyaline membrane disease. *Arch Dis Child*. 1976;51:163-169.
51. Soll RF. Prophylactic synthetic surfactant for preventing morbidity and mortality in preterm infants. *Cochrane Database Syst Rev*. 2000;(2):CD001079.
52. Soll RF. Prophylactic natural surfactant extract for preventing morbidity and mortality in preterm infants. *Cochrane Database Syst Rev*. 2000;(2):CD000511.
53. Yost CC, Soll RF. Early versus delayed selective surfactant treatment for neonatal respiratory distress syndrome. *Cochrane Database Syst Rev*. 2000;(2):CD001456.
54. Kattwinkel J, Robinson M, Bloom BT, et al. Technique for intrapartum administration of surfactant without requirement for an endotracheal tube. *J Perinatol*. 2004;24:360-365.
55. Lindner W, Vossbeck S, Hummler H, Pohlandt F. Delivery room management of extremely low birth weight infants: Spontaneous breathing or intubation? *Pediatrics*. 1999;103:961-967.
56. Aly H, Massaro AN, Patel K, El Mohandes AA. Is it safer to intubate premature infants in the delivery room? *Pediatrics*. 2005;115:1660-1665.
57. Morley CJ, Davis PG, Doyle LW, et al; COIN Trial Investigators. Nasal CPAP or intubation at birth for very preterm infants. *N Engl J Med*. 2008;358:700-708.
58. Finer NN, Carlo WA, Walsh MC, et al. Early CPAP versus surfactant in extremely preterm infants. *N Engl J Med*. 2010;362:1970-1979.
59. Stevens TP, Harrington EW, Blennow M, Soll RF. Early surfactant administration with brief ventilation vs. selective surfactant and continued mechanical ventilation for preterm infants with or at risk for respiratory distress syndrome. *Cochrane Database Syst Rev*. 2007;(4):CD003063.
60. Rojas MA, Lozano JM, Rojas MX, et al; Colombian Neonatal Research Network. Very early surfactant without mandatory ventilation in premature infants treated with early continuous positive airway pressure: a randomized, controlled trial. *Pediatrics*. 2009;123:137-142.
61. Sandri F, Plavka R, Ancora G, et al; CURPAP Study Group. Prophylactic or early selective surfactant combined with nCPAP in very preterm infants. *Pediatrics*. 2010;125:e1402-e1409.
62. Kribs A, Pillekamp F, Hunseler C, et al. Early administration of surfactant in spontaneous breathing with nCPAP: feasibility and outcome in extremely premature infants (postmenstrual age </=27 weeks). *Paediatr Anaesth*. 2007;17:364-369.
63. Dargaville PA, Aiyappan A, Cornelius A, et al. Preliminary evaluation of a new technique of minimally invasive surfactant therapy. *Arch Dis Child Fetal Neonatal Ed*. 2010 96:F243-F248..
64. De Paoli AG, Morley CJ, Davis PG, et al. In vitro comparison of nasal continuous positive airway pressure devices for neonates. *Arch Dis Child Fetal Neonatal Ed*. 2002;87:F42-F45.
65. Klausner JF, Lee AY, Hutchison AA. Decreased imposed work with a new nasal continuous positive airway pressure device. *Pediatr Pulmonol*. 1996;22:188-194.
66. Pandit PB, Courtney SE, Pyon KH, et al. Work of breathing during constant- and variable-flow nasal continuous positive airway pressure in preterm neonates. *Pediatrics*. 2001;108:682-685.
67. Courtney SE, Pyon KH, Saslow JG, et al. Lung recruitment and breathing pattern during variable versus continuous flow nasal continuous positive airway pressure in premature infants: an evaluation of three devices. *Pediatrics*. 2001;107:304-308.
68. Davis P, Davies M, Faber B. A randomised controlled trial of two methods of delivering nasal continuous positive airway pressure after extubation to infants weighing less than 1000 g: binasal (Hudson) versus single nasal prongs. *Arch Dis Child Fetal Neonatal Ed*. 2001;85:F82-F85.
69. Roukema H, O'Brine K, Nesbitt Z, Zaw W. A randomized controlled trial of Infant Flow continuous positive airway pressure (CPAP) versus nasopharyngeal CPAP in the extubation of babies ≤1250 g [abstract]. *Pediatr Res*. 1999;45:318A.
70. De Paoli A, Davis P, Faber B, Morley C. Devices and pressure sources for administration of nasal continuous positive airway pressure (NCPAP) in preterm neonates. *Cochrane Database Syst Rev*. 2008;(1):CD002977.
71. Stefanescu BM, Murphy WP, Hansell BJ, et al. A randomized, controlled trial comparing two different continuous positive airway pressure systems for the successful extubation of extremely low birth weight infants. *Pediatrics*. 2003;112:1031-1038.
72. Sun SC, Tien HC. Randomized controlled trial of two methods of nasal CPAP (NCPAP): Flow Driver vs conventional NCPAP. *Ped Res*. 1999;45:322A.
73. Mazzella M, Bellini C, Calevo MG, et al. A randomised control study comparing the Infant Flow Driver with nasal continuous positive airway pressure in preterm infants. *Arch Dis Child Fetal Neonatal Ed*. 2001;85:F86-F90.
74. Gupta S, Sinha SK, Tin W, Donn SM. A randomized controlled trial of post-extubation bubble continuous positive airway pressure versus Infant Flow Driver continuous positive airway pressure in preterm infants with respiratory distress syndrome. *J Pediatr*. 2009;154:645-650.
75. De Klerk AM, De Klerk RK. Nasal continuous positive airway pressure and outcomes of preterm infants. *J Paediatr Child Health*. 2001;37:161-167.
76. Elgellab A, Riou Y, Abbazine A, et al. Effects of nasal continuous positive airway pressure (NCPAP) on breathing pattern in spontaneously breathing premature newborn infants. *Intensive Care Med*. 2001;27:1782-1787.

77. Kamper J, Wulff K, Larsen C, Lindequist S. Early treatment with nasal continuous positive airway pressure in very low-birth-weight infants. *Acta Paediatr*. 1993;82:193-197.
78. Pape KE, Armstrong DL, Fitzhardinge PM. Central nervous system pathology associated with mask ventilation in the very low birthweight infant: a new etiology for intracerebellar hemorrhages. *Pediatrics*. 1976;58:473-483.
79. Vert P, Andre M, Sibout M. Continuous positive airway pressure and hydrocephalus. *Lancet*. 1973;2:319.
80. Buettiker V, Hug MI, Baenziger O, et al. Advantages and disadvantages of different nasal CPAP systems in newborns. *Intensive Care Med*. 2004;30:926-930.
81. Robertson NJ, McCarthy LS, Hamilton PA, et al. Nasal deformities resulting from flow driver continuous positive airway pressure. *Arch Dis Child Fetal Neonatal Ed*. 1996;75:F209-F212.
82. Polin RA, Sahni R. Newer experience with CPAP. *Semin Neonatol*. 2002;7:379-389.
83. Goldbart AD, Gozal D. Non-invasive ventilation in preterm infants. *Pediatr Pulmonol Suppl*. 2004;26:158-161.
84. Bowe L, Smith J, Clarker P, et al. Nasal CPAP weaning of VLBW infants: Is decreasing CPAP pressure or increasing time off the better strategy—results of a randomised controlled trial [Abstract]. Presented to the Pediatric Academic Society Meeting, San Francisco, April 29-May 2, 2006.
85. Abdel-Hady H, Shouman B, Aly H. Early weaning from CPAP to high flow nasal cannula in preterm infants is associated with prolonged oxygen requirement: A randomized controlled trial. *Early Hum Dev*. 2011;87:205-208.
86. Walsh M, Engle W, Laptook A, et al. Oxygen delivery through nasal cannulae to preterm infants: can practice be improved? *Pediatrics*. 2005;116:857-861.
87. Wilkinson D, Andersen C, O'Donnell CPF, De Paoli AG. High flow nasal cannula for respiratory support in preterm infants. *Cochrane Database Syst Rev*. 2011;5:CD006405.
88. Kopelman AE, Holbert D. Use of oxygen cannulas in extremely low birthweight infants is associated with mucosal trauma and bleeding, and possibly with coagulase-negative staphylococcal sepsis. *J Perinatol*. 2003;23:94-97.
89. Finer NN, Mannino FL. High-flow nasal cannula: a kinder, gentler CPAP? *J Pediatr*. 2009;154:160-162.
90. Locke RG, Wolfson MR, Shaffer TH, et al. Inadvertent administration of positive end-distending pressure during nasal cannula flow. *Pediatrics*. 1993;91:135-138.
91. Sreenan C, Lemke RP, Hudson-Mason A, Osiovich H. High-flow nasal cannulae in the management of apnea of prematurity: a comparison with conventional nasal continuous positive airway pressure. *Pediatrics*. 2001;107:1081-1083.
92. Kubicka ZJ, Limauro J, Darnall RA. Heated, humidified high-flow nasal cannula therapy: yet another way to deliver continuous positive airway pressure? *Pediatrics*. 2008;121:82-88.
93. Spence KL, Murphy D, Kilian C, et al. High-flow nasal cannula as a device to provide continuous positive airway pressure in infants. *J Perinatol*. 2007;27:772-775.
94. Wilkinson DJ, Andersen CC, Smith K, Holberton J. Pharyngeal pressure with high-flow nasal cannulae in premature infants. *J Perinatol*. 2008;28:42-47.
95. Campbell DM, Shah PS, Shah V, Kelly EN. Nasal continuous positive airway pressure from high flow cannula versus Infant Flow for Preterm infants. *J Perinatol*. 2006;26:546-549.
96. Shoemaker MT, Pierce MR, Yoder BA, DiGeronimo RJ. High flow nasal cannula versus nasal CPAP for neonatal respiratory disease: a retrospective study. *J Perinatol*. 2007;27:85-91.
97. Holleman-Duray D, Kaupie D, Weiss MG. Heated humidified high-flow nasal cannula: use and a neonatal early extubation protocol. *J Perinatol*. 2007;27:776-781.
98. Saslow JG, Aghai ZH, Nakhla TA, et al. Work of breathing using high-flow nasal cannula in preterm infants. *J Perinatol*. 2006;26:476-480.

CHAPTER 14

Surfactant Replacement: Present and Future

Christian P. Speer, MD, FRCPE, and David Sweet, MD, FRCPCH

- Introduction
- Recommendations for Surfactant Use in 2010
- Which Surfactant Is Best?
- What Dose Should Be Used?
- When Should Surfactant Be Given?
- Should We Use More than One Dose of Surfactant in RDS?
- Surfactant Administration and Ventilation
- Surfactant without Intubation
- Surfactant for Other Neonatal Respiratory Disorders
- The Future

Introduction

Surfactant replacement therapy has revolutionized neonatal respiratory care since its introduction in the 1980s. Along with antenatal steroids, surfactants improve survival for preterm babies, and these agents are now recommended routinely as early in the course of respiratory distress syndrome (RDS) as possible. There have been many randomized controlled trials to determine the best surfactant preparation and the optimal timing of the first and subsequent doses, although it must be borne in mind that many of the studies took place in an era of less antenatal steroid administration and use of continuous positive airways pressure (CPAP) ventilation. Surfactants are licensed only for prophylaxis or treatment of RDS but their use has been explored in other neonatal respiratory disorders. In this chapter we review the evidence to support the current recommendations for surfactant use in RDS and other neonatal pulmonary disorders. We also speculate how surfactant therapy might be used in the future.

Recommendations for Surfactant Use in 2010

Current European and North American recommendations for surfactant therapy for RDS are broadly similar and are summarized in Table 14-1.[1,2] The common theme is that surfactant replacement therapy, if it is going to be used, should be used as early as possible, and at present, natural (animal-derived rather than synthetic) surfactants are the treatments of choice. This statement comes with the caveat that as often as possible we should try to maintain babies without resorting to intubation and mechanical ventilation by maximizing the use of noninvasive respiratory support. It has taken almost 30 years of randomized controlled trials to reach this decision-making algorithm, but even today it is not always clear in individual cases when it is best to intervene with intubation and surfactant therapy.

Table 14-1 SUMMARIES OF CURRENT GUIDELINES FOR THE USE OF SURFACTANT IN NEONATAL RESPIRATORY DISTRESS SYNDROME

	American Academy of Pediatrics Guidelines, 2008	European Consensus Guidelines, 2010
Type of surfactant	Both animal-derived and synthetic surfactants decrease respiratory morbidity and mortality in preterm infants with surfactant deficiency New synthetic surfactants with surfactant protein–like activity are promising new treatments for surfactant deficiency disorders	Babies with or at high risk of RDS should be given *natural* surfactant preparations Poractant alfa in an initial dose of 200 mg/kg is better than 100 mg/kg of poractant alfa or beractant for treatment of moderate to severe RDS
Prophylaxis	Prophylactic surfactant replacement should be considered for extremely preterm infants at high risk of RDS, especially infants who have not been exposed to antenatal steroids	Prophylaxis (within 15 minutes of birth) should be given to almost all babies of < 26 weeks' gestation. Prophylaxis should also be given to all preterm babies with RDS who require intubation for stabilization.
Timing of first dose	Surfactant should be given to infants with RDS as soon as possible after intubation irrespective of exposure to antenatal steroids or gestational age	Early rescue surfactant should be administered to previously untreated babies if there is evidence of RDS Individual units need to develop protocols for when to intervene as RDS progresses depending on gestational age and prior treatment with antenatal steroids
MV vs. CPAP ventilation	CPAP ventilation, with or without exogenous surfactant, may reduce the need for additional surfactant and the incidence of BPD without increased mortality	Consider immediate (or early) extubation to CPAP ventilation or NIPPV following surfactant administration, provided that the baby is otherwise stable The use of CPAP ventilation with early rescue surfactant should be considered in babies with RDS in order to reduce the need for MV
Second and subsequent doses of surfactant	No clear recommendation	A second, and sometimes a third dose of surfactant should be administered if there is ongoing evidence of RDS, such as a persisting oxygen requirement and need for MV

BPD, bronchopulmonary dysplasia; CPAP, nasal continuous positive airway pressure; MV, mechanical ventilation; NIPPV, nasal intermittent positive-pressure ventilation; RDS, respiratory distress syndrome.

The first clinical study of surfactant in humans was published by Fujiwara and associates[3] in 1980. In this study ten babies with severe RDS were given artificial surfactant with subsequent improvement in oxygenation and reduced ventilator settings; eight of them survived. There are now 185 randomized controlled trials of surfactant therapy in the Cochrane Central Register of Controlled Trials, and they have been subjected to 29 *Cochrane Database of Systematic Reviews* studies that looked at various aspects of its use. Twelve types of surfactant have been used in clinical trials,[4] with timing of first administration in trials ranging from immediate prophylaxis in the delivery room to only intervening when babies are 6 to 8 hours old,[5] and the number of doses ranging from one to four.[6] Surfactant therapy is one of the most intensively studied interventions in medicine; nevertheless controversies still exist. In the next section we discuss the journey to the current situation, highlighting some of the controversies, particularly in terms of choosing which

Table 14-2 SURFACTANT PREPARATIONS AND RECOMMENDED DOSES

Generic Name	Trade Name	Source	Producer	Dose (Volume)
Pumactant	ALEC	Synthetic	Britannia (UK)	No longer manufactured
Bovactant	Alveofact	Bovine	Lyomark (Germany)	50 mg/kg/dose (1.2 mL/kg)
Bovine lipid extract surfactant	BLES	Bovine	BLES Biochemicals (Canada)	135 mg/kg/dose (5 mL/kg)
Poractant alfa	Curosurf	Porcine	Chiesi Farmaceutici (Italy)	100-200 mg/kg/ dose (1.25-2.5 mL/kg)
Colfosceril palmitate	Exosurf	Synthetic	GlaxoSmithKline (US)	64 mg/kg/dose (5 mL/kg)
Calfactant	Infasurf	Bovine	ONY Inc. (US)	105 mg/kg/dose (3 mL/kg)
Surfactant-TA	Surfacten	Bovine	Tokyo Tanabe (Japan)	100 mg/kg/dose (3.3 mL/kg)
Lucinactant	Surfaxin	Synthetic	Discovery Labs (US)	Not licensed
Beractant	Survanta	Bovine	Ross Labs (US)	100 mg/kg/dose (4 mL/kg)

14

surfactant, what dose to use, timing and method of administration, and the issue of repeat dosing.

Which Surfactant Is Best?

There are several different types of surfactant preparation licensed for use in babies with RDS. These include synthetic surfactants and natural surfactants (derived from animal lungs). The surfactant preparations available vary in different parts of the world; details of the best-known surfactants are shown in Table 14-2.[7]

The various surfactants were tested in clinical trials in human newborns during the late 1980s and early 1990s, with 13 trials of natural surfactant preparations (human amniotic fluid–derived surfactant, surfactant TA, poractant, and beractant) and 6 of synthetic surfactant (Colfosceril palmitate) being available for Cochrane systematic analysis.[8,9] These metaanalyses confirm that both types of surfactant decrease the risk of pneumothoraces, pulmonary interstitial emphysema, and mortality, with synthetic surfactants having the additional benefit of showing reduction in risk of bronchopulmonary dysplasia, intraventricular hemorrhage, and patent ductus arteriosus, which was not found with the natural surfactants. Natural surfactants contain surfactant proteins that enable them to work more quickly, although it was not initially clear whether this was an advantage. Direct comparative trials of synthetic and natural surfactants took place during the 1990s. These studies mainly compared colfosceril palmitate with calfactant and beractant; there was also one study comparing pumactant with poractant alfa. Eleven comparative trials have been subjected to Cochrane systematic review with the metaanalysis showing improved outcomes if natural surfactants are used.[10] The natural surfactants resulted in fewer pneumothoraces (typical relative risk [RR] 0.63; 95% confidence interval [CI] 0.53-0.75) and a reduction in mortality (typical RR 0.87; 95% CI 0.76-0.98).[10]

Since that time attempts have been made to produce improved synthetic surfactants by the addition of synthetic peptides that mimic the actions of natural surfactant proteins. The rationale for doing so is that synthetic surfactants have highly reproducible compositions and are capable of being produced in large quantities. They may also reduce potential risk for immune reactions to animal proteins or transmission of infections, although to date this theoretical possibility has not been found to be an issue with natural surfactant preparations.[11,12] The synthetic surfactant that has been studied the most is lucinactant. Lucinactant is a surfactant preparation containing phospholipids and a high concentration of a synthetic peptide (sinapultide, formerly known as KL4 peptide) that resembles one of the domains of surfactant protein B.[13] Results of animal studies in primates[14] and pilot studies in newborn babies[15] were promising. Comparative studies of beractant and colfosceril palmitate confirmed that the new synthetic surfactant was better than the older synthetic surfactant,[16] but the study was not large enough, nor designed appropriately, to draw conclusions about equivalence to natural surfactant. Likewise, another study comparing lucinactant with poractant alfa was considered underpowered to draw conclusions about equivalence, and the product has not been licensed for use in newborns.[17] The quest to find a suitable synthetic surfactant preparation therefore continues.[18]

There have also been comparisons made between some of the natural surfactant preparations. Trials comparing the natural bovine surfactants calfactant and beractant showed no differences in outcome when they were given prophylactically or as rescue therapy.[19,20] Trials comparing the porcine poractant alfa and the bovine beractant as rescue therapy individually show more rapid improvements in oxygenation with the former and a trend towards reduced mortality in each trial.[21,22] Overall there is a survival advantage for 200 mg/kg of poractant alfa is over 100 mg/kg of beractant or 100 mg/kg poractant alfa to treat established RDS (RR 0.29; 95% CI 0.10-0.79; number needed to treat [NNT] 14), although this is likely to simply be a dosing effect.[23]

What Dose Should Be Used?

The manufacturers' recommended doses for the various surfactant preparations is shown in Table 14-2. It is clear that there is wide variation in both the recommended dose and the concentration of phospholipid among the various surfactants. The original dosing strategies were derived from animal studies that took place in the 1980s.[24] These studies showed that clinical effects of surfactant were seen with doses as low as around 20 mg/kg; however optimal reduction in surface tension was achieved with a dose of at least 50 mg/kg. These studies did not consider the duration of the observed beneficial effect, but concurred with other estimates of the amount of surfactant needed to cover the alveolar space.[24] The doses we use today come directly from the doses that were chosen for the original surfactant studies, and these doses were usually chosen pragmatically, often on the basis of the volume of surfactant that could be tolerated. The earliest surfactant studies used 100 mg/kg of surfactant TA (3.3 mL/kg),[25] 100 mg/kg of beractant (4 mL/kg),[26] 100 mg/kg or 200 mg/kg of poractant (1.25 or 2.5 mL/kg),[27,28] 50 mg/kg of bovactant (1.2ml/kg)[29] and 64 mg/kg of colfosceril palmitate (5mL/kg).[30]

Early small dose-finding studies suggested better outcomes with higher initial doses of surfactant. Surfactant TA for rescue therapy of RDS at 120 mg/kg was better than 60 mg/kg in terms of a more sustained improvement in oxygenation and a reduction in intraventricular hemorrhage and BPD.[31] Bovactant at 100 mg/kg was also better than 50 mg/kg in terms of sustained improvement in early oxygenation and a reduction in air leaks.[32] In the early 1990s an attempt was made to determine whether higher starting dose (200 mg/kg vs. 100 mg/kg) and maximum allowable cumulative dose (600 mg/kg vs. 300 mg/kg) of poractant alfa would result in any improvement in survival or reduction of BPD.[33] A total of 2168 babies were enrolled from 82 collaborating hospitals from 13 countries. Babies given the high starting dose of 200 mg/kg showed a more rapid and sustained improvement in oxygenation (9% greater reduction in $F\text{IO}_2$ at 12 hours after surfactant administration), and fewer of them required a second dose (69% vs. 77%). However these early improvements did not appear to influence the primary outcome, which was death or oxygen dependency at 28 days (51% each group) and death before discharge (23.5% vs. 25 %). The investigators concluded that the lower-dose regimen was equally effective as the higher and should be employed because it is more cost effective. However it must be borne in mind that this study was conducted in an era when the documented exposure to antenatal steroids was only 17%, the surfactant was given as relatively late rescue therapy, CPAP ventilation was not used, and babies with a mean gestation of 29 weeks were ventilated for a median duration of 6 days.

The issue of dosing has now resurfaced. Nowadays, in the era of noninvasive respiratory support, every effort is made to minimize exposure to sustained mechanical ventilation and supplemental oxygen. The issue of whether different surfactant preparations or doses can influence this has been explored again. Pharmacokinetic studies using carbon 13–labeled poractant alfa have given some insight as to what happens to exogenous surfactant following its administration.[34] The half-life of surfactant can be determined by measuring the decay curve of C 13–labeled diphosphatidyl choline in surfactant. By comparing 21 babies with RDS who had received 200 mg/kg of poractant alfa with 40 similar babies who had received 100 mg/kg, Cogo and associates[35] were able to determine that the higher initial dose of surfactant resulted in a significantly longer half-life of the surfactant (32 ± 19 vs. 15 ± 19 hours; $P < 0.01$). This lengthening of the duration of an effective pool size was mirrored by observed clinical differences, including a lower oxygenation index and less need for subsequent redosing in babies who had received the higher dose. The rate of endogenous surfactant synthesis remained low in both groups, and the observed difference in surfactant half-life is likely to be attributed to recycling of degraded surfactant components. The investigators speculated that the improved effectiveness of the higher dose could potentially lead to earlier extubation, which might in turn result in long-term clinical benefits. Several studies have compared the recommended dose of 200 mg/kg of poractant alfa with the recommended dose of 100 mg/kg of beractant.[21,22,36] Individually the studies are small, but the higher dose of surfactant in each of the trials resulted in more rapid improvement in oxygenation. Meta-analysis of combined survival data from 328 babies in these studies suggest a reduction in mortality favoring 200 mg/kg of poractant alfa (RR 0.29; 95% CI, 0.10-0.79).[23]

When Should Surfactant Be Given?

The issue of the timing of surfactant therapy continues to cause debate among neonatologists. In an ideal world surfactant replacement would be utilized only for babies with surfactant deficiency who require mechanical ventilation. The difficulty comes about because most of the evidence from more than three decades of research has directed clinicians toward the earliest possible administration of surfactant in order to improve survival, but with the caveat that there is no consistently reliable predictive test to determine whether an individual baby was at risk of later severe RDS and that intubation itself may be detrimental. In the next section we describe the current policy of selective prophylaxis for some babies at very high risk for RDS, with very early rescue surfactant for the remainder of extremely preterm babies, and avoidance of intubation for surfactant in the "more mature" preterm babies if it is considered likely that CPAP ventilation will suffice.

The earliest trials of surfactant versus placebo were mainly "rescue" studies in which surfactant was administered to babies with moderately severe established RDS.[9,37] Four randomized trials during the 1990s determined that it was better to treat RDS earlier in its course, rather than waiting until babies were requiring higher amounts of supplemental oxygen.[38] The Cochrane metaanalyses of these studies demonstrated significant reductions in risk of pneumothorax (typical RR 0.70; 95% CI 0.590.82) and of pulmonary interstitial emphysema (typical RR 0.63; 95% CI 0.43-0.93) in infants randomly allocated to early selective surfactant administration. Babies randomly assigned to early selective surfactant administration also demonstrated a decreased risk of neonatal mortality (RR 0.87; 95% CI 0.77-0.99), chronic lung disease (RR 0.70; 95% CI 0.55-0.88), and chronic lung disease or death at 36 weeks (RR 0.84; 95% CI 0.75-0.93).[38]

The next logical step was to determine whether prophylactic administration of surfactant would be superior to rescue therapy. Eight trials conducted during the

1990s using natural surfactants were designed to assess this issue and have been subjected to Cochrane metaanalysis.[39] Metaanalysis supported the use of prophylactic surfactant, with 39% lower neonatal mortality if babies born before 32 weeks of gestation are treated within 15 minutes after birth than if they are treated a few hours later. There was also a reduction in rates of pneumothoraces (RR 0.62; 95% CI 0.42-0.89) and pulmonary interstitial emphysema (RR 0.54; 95% CI 0.36-0.82). However almost 50% more infants received surfactant when being treated prophylactically, suggesting that many of them may not have required surfactant. There was also no reduction in rate of BPD (RR 0.96; 95% CI0.82-1.12) suggesting that the process of intubation and surfactant may have been causing harm in some babies. Of the studies included in the Cochrane metaanalysis, the earliest median time of administration in the rescue surfactant group was 1.5 hours of age. In the study using this time, there were clinical advantages for the babies given prophylaxis.[40] One important study confirmed that it was not essential for babies to receive prophylactic surfactant "before the first breath."[41] In this study of 651 babies there was no difference in clinical outcome between babies given immediate surfactant prophylaxis and those given surfactant prophylaxis at about 10 minutes of age after stabilization and clinical confirmation of correct placement of the endotracheal tube.

It must be borne in mind that the use of antenatal steroids and CPAP ventilation for respiratory support was much lower 20 years ago when these studies were undertaken. Many babies included in these trials would not nowadays be considered eligible for surfactant, particularly if they had received the benefit of antenatal steroids and were managing well on CPAP. Centers that were using more CPAP ventilation and less mechanical ventilation were shown to have similar survival outcomes for very low-birth-weight (VLBW) infants with a lower incidence of BPD, and there was therefore a strong argument to try to determine which babies would require surfactant prophylaxis if antenatal steroids and CPAP ventilation were used.[42] Units adopting policies of more aggressive use of CPAP ventilation seemed to have reduced rates of BPD with no increase in mortality,[43] but only lately has the question of delivery room surfactant in comparison with early initiation of CPAP ventilation has been addressed.

The first of these studies was the COIN (Continuous Positive Airway Pressure or Intubation at Birth) trial.[44] In this study 610 babies born between 25 and 28 weeks of gestation and who were breathing spontaneously but required respiratory support were randomly allocated to either initiation of nasal CPAP ventilation (8 cm H_20) or intubation and mechanical ventilation in the delivery suite. Babies in the CPAP arm were not given surfactant unless they required intubation, the need for which was determined by predefined criteria consisting of apnea, respiratory acidosis, or need for more than 60% oxygen. As this was purely a study of nasal CPAP with mechanical ventilation, surfactant therapy was not mandated in the intubation arm of the trial; 77% of babies who were intubated receiving surfactant, compared with 38% who were started on NCPAP. The primary outcomes of death or BPD were no different in the groups (34% CPAP group vs. 39% intubation group; odds ratio [OR] favoring CPAP, 0.80; 95% CI 0.58- 1.12; P = 0.19). The early NCPAP group had fewer days of mechanical ventilation (median 3 vs. 4 days; $P < 0.001$) but had a higher incidence of pneumothoraces (9% vs. 3%; P < 0.001). This study proved that for a selected population of preterm babies in whom antenatal steroid use was high (94%) and who were breathing after 5 minutes, initiation of early CPAP ventilation would reduce the need for mechanical ventilation and surfactant therapy without any reduction in survival or increase in BPD. There was still some concern, however, that by an attempt to manage babies with RDS without early surfactant might expose them to the increased risk of air leak. Because no protocol requirement for the administration of surfactant was defined, the study does not provide evidence for the superiority of CPAP ventilation over early surfactant.

The second study designed to assess whether prophylactic surfactant was really needed in the era of CPAP was the CURPAP study. This study included 208 babies of 25 to 28 weeks of gestation who did not need intubation for stabilization. Within 30 minutes after birth, babies were either started on NCPAP ventilation or else intubated for prophylactic surfactant followed by immediate extubation to NCPAP ventilation. The number needing subsequent intubation and mechanical ventilation within the first 5 days of life was similar in the two groups (31.4% SURF group vs. 33% NCPAP group; RR 0.95; 95% CI 0.64-1.41). A total of 78.1% of infants in the prophylactic surfactant group and 78.6% in the NCPAP group survived in room air at 36 weeks postmenstrual age.[45] This trial demonstrated that prophylactic surfactant was not superior to NCPAP and early selective surfactant in decreasing the need for mechanical ventilation in the first 5 days of life and the incidence of main morbidities.[45]

The largest study designed to address this issue was SUPPORT (Surfactant Positive Airway Pressure and Pulse Oximetry Randomized Trial).[46] In this multicenter 2-by-2 factorial study (also designed to assess the benefits of high versus low oxygen saturation targeting), a total of 1316 babies born between 24 and 27 weeks of gestation were randomly assigned to receive either intubation and surfactant within 1 hour of birth or early initiation of CPAP ventilation. As the babies had to be recruited before birth, there was a very high rate of successful completion of the full course of antenatal steroids, about 70% in the study population, with more than 95% having had exposure to the benefit of at least one dose of steroid. The intended treatment allocations were largely successful; the surfactant treatment took place 99% of the time in the surfactant group, and initiation of CPAP ventilation in the delivery room 81% of the time, for the CPAP group. Thirty three percent of the CPAP group never received surfactant. The CPAP group had a lower total number of days of mechanical ventilation (mean 25 vs. 28; $P = 0.03$) and a lower incidence of steroid therapy for BPD (7.2% vs. 13.2%; $P < 0.001$), but there was no significant difference between the groups in the combined outcome of death or BPD at 36 weeks postmenstrual age (48% vs. 51%; $P = 0.3$).[47] Post hoc analyses also showed a significant reduction in mortality in the CPAP group in the lower gestational age band, 24 to 25 weeks.[46] This study offers a strong argument against routine intubation for prophylactic surfactant in extremely preterm babies in the current era of CPAP ventilation use. However, one cannot assume that this finding should be generalized to include babies in whom there had been inadequate time for completion of antenatal steroid administration.

Current protocols still include a subgroup of babies deemed to be at very high risk for severe RDS for whom prophylaxis should be considered. For the majority, however, it seems prudent to initiate therapy with CPAP ventilation and intervene with surfactant only when evidence of RDS becomes manifest. The threshold for intervention is also likely to increase with rising gestational and postnatal age.

Should We Use More than One Dose of Surfactant in RDS?

Another issue that lacks clarity is the timing of second and further doses of surfactant. A number of studies have been designed to assess whether multiple doses are more beneficial than a single dose. A large European study showed that in infants with severe respiratory distress, multiple doses of poractant alfa were superior to single doses in reducing the incidence of mortality and pneumothorax.[47] In a study of more mature babies with RDS, repeat dosing with beractant reduced the secondary deterioration in gas exchange.[48] Beyond two doses, there does not appear to be much additional benefit from repeat dosing. The OSIRIS (open study of infants at high risk of or with respiratory insufficiency–the role of surfactant) trial showed no additional benefit of giving four doses over two doses of Colificerol palmitate.[49] A higher cumulative dose of phospholipid, 380 mg/kg over five doses, was not shown to be superior to 242 mg/kg over three doses in the Curosurf 4 trial.[33] A Cochrane review shows that a strategy of allowing multiple doses of natural surfactant rather than a single dose further reduces the risk of pneumothorax (RR 0.51; 95% CI

0.30-0.88) and there is also a trend toward reduction in mortality.[6,50] However, the studies in this review were conducted in the early 1990s, when antenatal steroids were used sparingly, and they also included relatively mature infants. The first dose of surfactant was given comparatively late, about 6 to 12 hours after birth, and the policies at the time would have been to use longer periods of mechanical ventilation rather than CPAP ventilation.

Manufacturers of natural surfactants make specific recommendations regarding re-treatment: Beractant (Survanta) may be repeated within 48 hours at intervals of at least 6 hours for up to 4 doses. Poractant alpha (Curosurf) may be given 12 hours later for two further doses if the infant is still intubated; after prophylaxis may be repeated 6 to 12 hours later and a third dose after further 12 hours. A large trial evaluating 1267 babies who met repeat dosing criteria ($FIO_2 > 0.30$) were randomly assigned to receive a second dose of bovine surfactant either immediately or not until the FIO_2 was more than 0.40.[51] Babies with uncomplicated RDS fared no worse when re-dosed at this higher threshold, although about one quarter were sicker babies with "complicated RDS" (perinatal compromise or sepsis), and this group had lower mortality when re-dosed at the lower threshold.

Extrapolating these data to make recommendations regarding repeat dosing in the current era of increased noninvasive ventilation use is difficult. The 2008 American Academy of Pediatrics guideline makes no clear recommendation for when babies should be re-dosed with surfactant. The 2010 European Guideline is also nonspecific, recommending re-treatment if there is "ongoing evidence of RDS such as the need for mechanical ventilation and supplemental oxygen."[2] A Canadian Guideline from 2005 makes a fairly specific recommendation that babies should be re-treated if they remain in more than 30% oxygen as early as 2 hours after the first dose.[52]

Surfactant Administration and Ventilation

Surfactant preparations are administered via an endotracheal tube usually through a feeding tube that has been cut to an appropriate length to be at a level just above the carina. The peripheral dispersion of surfactant into the terminal airways is facilitated by intermittent positive-pressure ventilation, either manually or using the ventilator. Older synthetic surfactants had to be administered relatively slowly to avoid accumulation and possible obstruction of the endotracheal tube; however, an optimal distribution of natural surfactants can be achieved only when they are given as a bolus, usually in one or two aliquots, depending on the type of surfactant preparation and the volume of fluid needing to be dispersed.[53] Traditionally surfactant administration must therefore always be accompanied by the process of intubation and at least a short period of mechanical ventilation and it is probably these factors, rather than surfactant per se, that cause harm. In animal experiments, slow infusion of natural surfactant over 45 minutes led to a nonhomogeneous distribution in the lungs and markedly reduced effects on pulmonary gas exchange.[53] A randomized trial comparing a bolus with a dual-lumen technique of surfactant application within 1 minute showed a reduced number of desaturations in the group of preterm infants who were not disconnected from the ventilator.[54]

It is now well established that prolonged mechanical ventilation can be avoided in some babies who require surfactant if the INSURE technique is employed (INtubate—SURfactant—Extubate to CPAP). Six studies undertaken during the 1990s and early 2000s comparing early surfactant and CPAP with later surfactant and ventilation have been subjected to Cochrane review.[55] The metaanalysis shows that babies with RDS managed with a policy of earlier surfactant followed by extubation to CPAP results in less need for mechanical ventilation (RR 0.67; 95% CI 0.57-0.79), fewer pneumothoraces (RR 0.52; 95% CI 0.28-0.96) and less BPD (RR 0.51; 95% CI 0.26-0.99). More babies received surfactant and cumulatively more doses per patient were given if the INSURE technique was used. It was also demonstrated that the earlier the decision is made to intervene with INSURE, the greater the chance of avoiding ventilation.[55,56]

Surfactant without Intubation

Avoiding ventilation is one thing, but how important is the actual process of intubation and administration of surfactant? Although it is clear that an experienced team is essential to stabilize a preterm baby, there is now an extensive body of work showing that many extremely preterm babies are not apneic after birth and will manage well if they are supported on CPAP ventilation without resorting to intubation.[44-46] When intubation is attempted, even in the most experienced hands, there is often delay in securing the airway, and there are often multiple attempts at intubation with corresponding episodes of severe desaturation and bradycardia.[57] When this situation occurs, clinicians tend to become anxious and may attempt to "rescue" the situation by administering positive-pressure inflation breaths in order to improve oxygenation and heart rate more quickly. In most delivery room settings, there is no control over the tidal volume delivered with each breath, and it is now clear that even experienced clinicians are not good at judging how much tidal volume is being delivered with each manual breath.[58] Even a few large-volume positive-pressure breaths at initiation of ventilation during resuscitation of the baby may be enough to damage the lungs and set up the inflammatory cascade that leads to BPD.[59-61] An ideal solution would be to find a method of surfactant administration that avoids the process of intubation. Five methods of surfactant administration without intubation have been employed with varying success. These include antenatal intra-amniotic instillation, pharyngeal instillation, laryngeal mask instillation, direct tracheal instillation without intubation, and surfactant nebulization.

14

Intra-amniotic instillation of surfactant in the vicinity of the fetus's mouth and nose was first described in a case series in the 1990s. The surfactant was instilled via an ultrasound-guided needle, and intravenous aminophylline was given to the mothers with the aim of promoting fetal breathing movements. The investigators reported success in a series of six babies with no RDS in four and only mild RDS in the other two.[62] Little more was published on this method until 2004, when a group from China reported their findings in 45 women. Although this study was not a randomized trial, 15 women had been treated with intra-amniotic surfactant, and they were compared with 30 who had not. The treated women had proportionately more babies with biochemically defined lung maturity and less developed RDS.[63] Although it is technically feasible, the risks of this relatively invasive procedure seem to outweigh the benefits, and the quality of the studies cannot be considered suitable for inclusion in a Cochrane metaanalysis.[64]

Nasopharyngeal administration of surfactant has also been described in a feasibility study of 23 babies born at 27 to 30 weeks of gestation. The babies were given surfactant after delivery of the head but before delivery of the body. After birth they were started on CPAP ventilation. Thirteen of 15 vaginally delivered babies required no further intubation, but 5 of 8 babies born by cesarean section required intubation, and 2 received later surfactant.[65] Laryngeal mask instillation of surfactant has also been described in a series of 8 babies undergoing CPAP ventilation.[66] More work is needed before these methods can be recommended.

Surfactant nebulization has also been employed in an attempt to avoid the need for intubation. Surfactants are lipids and therefore relatively difficult to nebulize, although animal studies in the 1990s showed that this approach was technically feasible and resulted in measurable improvements in pulmonary function, albeit at a much slower rate than direct surfactant instillation.[67] Most of the surfactant was deposited in the ventilator tubing, resulting in the need for very large doses for therapeutic effect. A pilot study in 34 preterm babies with RDS who were managed with CPAP ventilation was published in 2000.[68] Babies were randomly allocated to either receive 480 mg of nebulized poractant alfa while undergoing CPAP ventilation or just continued on CPAP ventilation. The results were disappointing, showing absolutely no improvement in oxygenation with the surfactant even though the procedure was well tolerated. No measurable difference in any outcome could be found, and the researchers concluded that further larger studies using this method would not be justified.[68] The concept of nebulization of surfactant has resurfaced with the development of improved methods of aerosolization of surfactant.[69] A small pilot study of aerosolized lucinactant using a vibrating membrane nebulizer has also demonstrated the feasibility of using this method for surfactant treatment of babies who are being managed with CPAP ventilation, but more research is needed before this method can be recommended.[70]

Another method of administering surfactant while avoiding ventilation has been developed in German neonatal units. This technique involves placement of a fine intratracheal catheter while babies keep spontaneously breathing with CPAP. Pilot studies reported that the procedure was tolerated well with good outcomes in comparison with historical controls.[71] Multicenter adaptation of this method enabled comparison of 319 babies with 1222 historical controls, which suggested a reduced need for mechanical ventilation and a lower incidence of BPD.[72] However, whether this method really influences short- and long-term respiratory outcome remains to be proven in a well-designed randomized, controlled trial.

Surfactant for Other Neonatal Respiratory Disorders

Surfactant is used to manage neonatal lung disease other than RDS despite the common paucity of evidence of benefit from randomized trials. Other indications for surfactant include meconium aspiration syndrome (MAS), persistent pulmonary hypertension, pulmonary hemorrhage, and pneumonia. In the following section we review what evidence there is to date to support the use of surfactant therapy in non-RDS pulmonary disorders of the newborn.

Surfactant for Meconium Aspiration

Although MAS is becoming less common in the developed world,[73] on a worldwide basis it remains an important cause of neonatal morbidity and mortality.[74] Meconium aspiration can lead to severe respiratory failure, and some of this may be related to secondary surfactant inactivation.[75,76] Almost as soon as surfactant was introduced into neonatal respiratory care, clinicians wanted to determine whether exogenous surfactant might help in MAS. Case series in newborn infants suggested better oxygenation if surfactant was used,[77] and this finding was confirmed in randomized trials using piglet models of meconium aspiration.[78] Four randomized trials of surfactant therapy in MAS have been included in a Cochrane systematic review that found improved oxygenation and a reduction in need for extracorporeal membrane oxygenation (ECMO) (RR 0.64; 95% CI 0.46-0.91).[79] The studies included in this metaanalysis used a 6-hourly dosing regimen of natural bovine surfactant for up to four doses. Later studies have examined dilute surfactant lavage as a means of removing meconium particles from the lungs.[80] A randomized controlled trial of 66 babies who underwent either lavage with two aliquots of 15 mL/kg of dilute bovine surfactant in addition to standard supportive therapy or standard therapy without surfactant lavage showed that the lavage-treated babies had a reduced combined outcome of death or requirement for ECMO therapy (10% vs. 31%; OR 0.24; 95% CI 0.06-0.97).[81] The lavage resulted in an immediate transient reduction in oxygen saturation, which was followed by a more sustained reduction in mean airway pressure requirements. Future studies may be directed at comparing this method with standard bolus dosing.

Attempts have also been made to formulate surfactant preparations specifically for use in meconium aspiration that are more resistant to inactivation. The addition of polymers such as dextran and polyethylene glycol to surfactants in vitro leads to greater preservation of function in the presence of meconium.[82] Polymyxin B, when added to surfactant, also was found to preserve the surface tension–lowering properties of surfactant in the presence of meconium as well as reduce the growth of gram-negative organisms in an in vitro study.[83] Animal studies in rats with experimental meconium aspiration have shown better preservation of lung function with mixtures of poractant alfa mixed with 5% dextran than with poractant alfa mixed with 5% polyethylene glycol or poractant alfa on its own.[84] A rabbit model of MAS has shown that dilute poractant alfa mixed with dextran was better than dilute poractant alfa alone when used for lung lavage. The surfactant-dextran combination resulted in better recovery of meconium particulate matter in the lavage and improved lung compliance and oxygenation at 60 minutes of age.[85] Further work is under way exploring combinations of polymers and synthetic surfactants as potential therapeutic agents for pulmonary disorders with surfactant inactivation.[86]

Surfactant for Congenital Pneumonia

Group B streptococcal (GBS) pneumonia can closely mimic RDS, and as a result, babies with pneumonia are likely to receive surfactant therapy. Data from babies who were recruited into randomized trials of surfactant therapy and subsequently were diagnosed with GBS pneumonia give some insights into the effects of surfactant in this scenario.[87] Babies with pneumonia were compared with matched controls receiving surfactant for RDS. Surfactant therapy improved gas exchange in the majority of patients with GBS pneumonia. The response to surfactant was slower than in infants with RDS, and repeated surfactant doses were needed more often.[87]

Experimental studies have suggested an additional rationale for using surfactant replacement in the setting of congenital pneumonia, because natural surfactant preparations contain a number of anti-inflammatory properties.[88,89] Studies in rabbits with experimental streptococcal pneumonia show that surfactant reduces inflammation and inhibits bacterial growth.[90] Further experiments on rabbits showed that using surfactant as a vehicle for specific immunoglobulins against GBS resulted in greater reduction in GBS proliferation than surfactant or antibody therapy on its own.[91] In a later study it was shown that the addition of the antimicrobial peptide polymyxin B to surfactant prevents the growth of *Escherichia coli* in experimental rabbits with pneumonia.[92] There was also a significant reduction in lung inflammation and bacterial translocation in these animals. A randomized trial in preterm babies would obviously be ideal but would be extremely difficult to perform, given the problems with the definition of neonatal pneumonia and the normal delay in confirming a microbiologic pathogen.

Surfactant for Pulmonary Hypoplasia

Congenital diaphragmatic hernia leads to pulmonary hypoplasia. The lungs not only are physically small but also may be biochemically immature, with a lower concentration of surfactant per unit lung volume found in animal models. This has been demonstrated in a nitrofen-induced rat model of diaphragmatic hernia[93] and a surgically induced fetal lamb model of diaphragmatic hernia.[94] However, evidence from human babies is conflicting. Studies on bronchoalveolar lavage fluid showed similar concentrations of phospholipids between samples from babies with diaphragmatic hernia and age-matched controls without diaphragmatic hernia.[95,96] Later studies using stable isotopes have shown no differences in surfactant synthesis between babies with and without diaphragmatic hernia, although turnover was faster in babies with diaphragmatic hernia, perhaps suggesting catabolism of surfactant secondary to lung injury from ventilation.[97] Supporting this hypothesis is the demonstration that babies with congenital diaphragmatic hernia and severe lung disease requiring ECMO have lower surfactant synthesis than normal controls.[98]

The role of surfactant therapy in congenital diaphragmatic hernia remains controversial. Animal studies in the fetal sheep model of diaphragmatic hernia show significant improvements in lung function when surfactant is given prophylactically but not when it is given as rescue therapy.[99] A small case series of babies with antenatally diagnosed diaphragmatic hernia and anticipated severe pulmonary hypoplasia who were given prophylactic calfactant and did unexpectedly well suggested a role for this treatment in humans.[100] Surfactant therapy has become accepted practice for stabilization of babies with diaphragmatic hernia; however, there is still no strong evidence to support its use. The Congenital Diaphragmatic Hernia Study Group used registry data from 522 term babies to determine the impact of surfactant therapy on outcome. The 192 babies who had received surfactant were compared with the 322 who had not. The infants appeared to have similar demographic data, although those treated with surfactant appeared to have a higher mortality (43% vs. 30%) and greater need for ECMO (60% vs. 50%).[101] Firm conclusions cannot be drawn from these nonrandomized data, because sicker babies are more likely to have been exposed to more attempts to "rescue" them. However, the findings do enable clinicians to at least remain in equipoise about the benefits of surfactant for congenital diaphragmatic hernia.

Surfactant for Babies with Pulmonary Hemorrhage

Preterm babies with RDS occasionally experience massive pulmonary hemorrhage, particularly in the presence of a large patent ductus arteriosus. Surfactant therapy itself has been implicated as a contributing factor in some instances of pulmonary hemorrhage, particularly in early trials of prophylactic synthetic surfactants, which showed a threefold higher risk (RR 3.28;95% CI 1.50-7.16).[102] Surfactant has also been used to treat massive pulmonary hemorrhage, the rationale being that blood is known to inhibit surfactant function.[103] A case series of 15 babies who received surfactant after pulmonary hemorrhage showed significant improvement in oxygenation, with oxygenation index falling from a mean of 25 before surfactant administration to 8.6 afterwards, although there were no untreated control babies for comparison.[104] Another series from Japan described response to surfactant therapy in 27 babies with hemorrhagic pulmonary edema. A good response to surfactant administration was found in 82% of babies, with the best response being found in those treated sooner after the pulmonary hemorrhage occurred.[105] The researchers in these two reports suggested that further investigation was needed in the form of randomized trials; however such trials have not be constructed to date and are likely to be difficult to organize given the unpredictable nature of pulmonary hemorrhage.[106]

Surfactant for Babies with Severe Respiratory Failure

Apart from the specific indications mentioned previously, surfactant therapy has been considered in term babies in the context of treating severe respiratory failure, particularly babies in whom ECMO is needed or being considered.[107] For babies undergoing ECMO, concomitant surfactant therapy shortened the duration of cannulation for ECMO by 30 hours and reduced the incidence of complications (18% vs. 46%).[108] In a later multicenter trial, 328 babies born after than 36 weeks of gestation who were being considered for ECMO were randomly assigned to receive either four doses of beractant 100 mg/kg or air placebo before ECMO and a further four doses during ECMO if it was initiated. Baseline parameters were similar, but the need for ECMO was reduced in the group receiving surfactant.[109] Introduction of surfactant therapy to the neonatal intensive care unit (NICU) is cited as one of the reasons for the reduction in ECMO utilization that occurred between the early and late 1990s.[110] Surfactant replacement therapy is also increasingly finding a role in the management of older children with severe respiratory failure in the setting of respiratory syncytial viral pneumonitis,[111] HIN1 influenza pneumonia,[112] and drowning.[113]

The Future

Surfactant therapy remains the cornerstone of successful management of premature babies with RDS. In the first decade of this century, the trend initially had been to move to earlier administration of surfactant, with many neonatal units developing protocols for delivery room prophylaxis for the majority of extremely preterm babies. In the light of evidence that this approach may be unnecessary and potentially even harmful, it is likely that in the near future we will see clinicians becoming increasingly comfortable with initiation of early CPAP ventilation in the delivery room for even the smallest infants and reserving intubation and immediate surfactant application for those in whom RDS develops. It is likely that clinicians will continue to work toward methods of delivering surfactant without causing lung injury.

Tests for rapid prediction of RDS might be helpful to enable a policy of selective surfactant prophylaxis for extremely preterm babies for whom surfactant deficiency has been documented. Gastric aspirate analysis for microbubble stability gives a positive predictive value of 62% and negative predictive value of 76%.[114] Combining the stable microbubble test with automated lamellar body counts gives a much better predictive test of surfactant deficiency.[115,116] Unfortunately the time it takes to run the analysis of a tracheal or gastric aspirate sample precluded use of either test for prediction of the need for delivery room surfactant, because symptoms would usually be manifest before the results were available. The main objective of measuring these markers of surfactant deficiency in some cases was to determine the absolute need for surfactant replacement in countries where for economic reasons surfactant was scarce.[115] However, in the current era of "CPAP use and BPD avoidance," there is perhaps an argument for making a stronger case for deciding which babies to intubate solely for surfactant. The predictive tests may become more popular in terms of deciding which babies can be left alone.

Another likely development in the evolution of surfactant therapy will be the production of a synthetic surfactant that can perform as well as natural surfactant. Studies in rabbits using synthetic surfactants with combinations of surfactant protein B and C analogs showed the combinations to be superior to single-peptide surfactants.[117] The mechanism of this effect may be better stabilization of the alveoli at end-expiration, but clinical trials need to be performed before conclusions can be drawn about the ideal composition of synthetic surfactant for RDS.[118] Further work is also likely to continue to develop an ideal surfactant-polymer combination for use in meconium aspiration and other forms of acute lung injury in newborns.[119]

In the future, surfactants may have the potential to be used more extensively to deliver other drugs such as steroids directly to the lungs. A study from Taiwan randomly allocated 116 babies with severe RDS to either standard surfactant therapy with beractant or therapy with beractant mixed with an additional 0.25 mg/kg of budesonide.[120] The babies in the budesonide group had a lower incidence of the combined outcome of death or BPD (19 of 60 vs. 34 of 56) although the babies in budesonide group were less sick to start with.[120] Follow-up did not show a higher incidence of long-term adverse effects in babies treated with topical steroids in this way.[121] A large multicenter trial of this promising new therapy is under way.

References

1. Engle WA; American Academy of Pediatrics Committee on Fetus and Newborn. Surfactant-replacement therapy for respiratory distress in the preterm and term neonate. *Pediatrics*. 2008;121:419-432.
2. Sweet DG, Carnielli V, Greisen G, et al. European Association of Perinatal Medicine. European consensus guidelines on the management of neonatal respiratory distress syndrome in preterm infants—2010 update. *Neonatology*. 2010;97:402-417.
3. Fujiwara T, Maeta H, Chida S, et al. Artificial surfactant therapy in hyaline-membrane disease. *Lancet*. 1980;1:55-59.
4. Halliday HL. History of surfactant from 1980. *Biol Neonate*. 2005;87:317-322.
5. Soll R. Early versus delayed selective surfactant treatment for neonatal respiratory distress syndrome. *Cochrane Database of Systematic Reviews*. 1999;(4):CD001456.
6. Soll R, Özek E. Multiple versus single doses of exogenous surfactant for the prevention or treatment of neonatal respiratory distress syndrome. *Cochrane Database of Systematic Reviews*. 2009;(1):CD000141.
7. Sweet D, Bevilacqua G, Carnielli V, et al; Working Group on Prematurity of the World Association of Perinatal Medicine; European Association of Perinatal Medicine. European consensus guidelines on the management of neonatal respiratory distress syndrome. *J Perinat Med*. 2007;35:175-186.
8. Seger N, Soll R. Animal derived surfactant extract for treatment of respiratory distress syndrome. *Cochrane Database of Systematic Reviews*. 2009;(2):CD007836.
9. Soll R. Synthetic surfactant for respiratory distress syndrome in preterm infants. *Cochrane Database of Systematic Reviews*. 1998;(3):CD001149.
10. Soll R, Blanco F. Natural surfactant extract versus synthetic surfactant for neonatal respiratory distress syndrome. *Cochrane Database of Systematic Reviews*. 2001;(2):CD000144.
11. Strayer DS, Merritt TA, Hallman M. Surfactant replacement: immunological considerations. *Eur Respir J Suppl*. 1989;3:91s-96s.
12. Whitsett JA, Hull WM, Luse S. Failure to detect surfactant protein specific antibodies in sera of premature infants treated with Survanta, a modified bovine surfactant. *Pediatrics*. 1997;87:505-510.
13. Cochrane CG. Surfactant protein B and mimic peptides in the function of pulmonary surfactant. *FEBS Lett*. 1998;430:424-425.

14. Revak SD, Merritt TA, Cochrane CG, et al. Efficacy of synthetic peptide containing surfactant in the treatment of respiratory distress syndrome in preterm infant rhesus monkeys. *Pediatr Res.* 1996;39:715-724.
15. Cochrane CG, Revak SD, Merritt TA, et al. The efficacy and safety of KL4-surfactant in preterm infants with respiratory distress syndrome. *Am J Respir Crit Care Med.* 1996;153:404-410.
16. Moya FR, Gadzinowski J, Bancalari E, et al; International Surfaxin Collaborative Study Group. A multicenter, randomized, masked, comparison trial of lucinactant, colfosceril palmitate, and beractant for the prevention of respiratory distress syndrome among very preterm infants. *Pediatrics.* 2005;115:1018-1029.
17. Sinha SK, Lacaze-Masmonteil T, Valls i Soler A, et al; Surfaxin Therapy Against Respiratory Distress Syndrome Collaborative Group. A multicenter, randomized, controlled trial of lucinactant versus poractant alfa among very premature infants at high risk for respiratory distress syndrome. *Pediatrics.* 2005;115:1030-1038.
18. Kattwinkel J. Synthetic surfactants: the search goes on. *Pediatrics.* 2005;115:1075-1076.
19. Bloom BT, Clark RH; Infasurf Survanta Clinical Trial Group. Comparison of Infasurf (calfactant) and Survanta (beractant) in the prevention and treatment of respiratory distress syndrome. *Pediatrics.* 2005;116:392-399.
20. Bloom BT, Kattwinkel J, Hall RT, et al. Comparison of Infasurf (calf lung surfactant extract) to Survanta (Beractant) in the treatment and prevention of respiratory distress syndrome. *Pediatrics.* 1997;100:31-38.
21. Ramanathan R, Rasmussen MR, Gerstmann DR, et al; North American Study Group. A randomized, multicenter masked comparison trial of poractant alfa (Curosurf) versus beractant (Survanta) in the treatment of respiratory distress syndrome in preterm infants. *Am J Perinatol.* 2004;21:109-119.
22. Speer CP, Gefeller O, Groneck P, et al. Randomized clinical trial of two treatment regimens of natural surfactant preparations in neonatal respiratory distress syndrome. *Arch Dis Child Fetal Neonatal Ed.* 1995;72:F8-F13.
23. Halliday HL. History of surfactant from 1980. *Biol Neonate.* 2005;87:317-322.
24. Ikegami M, Adams FH, Towers B, Osher AB. The quantity of natural surfactant necessary to prevent the respiratory distress syndrome in premature lambs. *Pediatr Res.* 1980;14:1082-1085.
25. Fujiwara T, Konishi M, Chida S, et al. Surfactant replacement therapy with a single postventilatory dose of a reconstituted bovine surfactant in preterm neonates with respiratory distress syndrome: final analysis of a multicenter, double-blind, randomized trial and comparison with similar trials. *Pediatrics.* 1990;86:753-764.
26. Horbar JD, Soll RF, Sutherland JM, et al. A multicenter, randomized, placebo-controlled trial of surfactant therapy for respiratory distress syndrome. *N Engl Jof Med.* 1989;320:959-965.
27. Svenningsen N, Robertson B, Andreason B, et al. Endotracheal administration of surfactant in very low birth weight infants with respiratory distress syndrome. *Critical Care Medicine.* 1987;15:918.
28. Collaborative European Multicenter Study Group. Surfactant replacement therapy for severe neonatal respiratory distress syndrome: an international randomized clinical trial. *Pediatrics.* 1988;82:683-691.
29. Gortner L, Bernsau U, Hellwege HH, et al. A multicenter randomized controlled clinical trial of bovine surfactant for prevention of respiratory distress syndrome. *Lung.* 1990;168(Suppl):864-869.
30. Phibbs RH, Ballard RA, Clements JA, et al. Initial clinical trial of Exosurf, a protein-free synthetic surfactant, for the prophylaxis and early treatment of hyaline membrane disease. *Pediatrics.* 1991;88:1-9.
31. Konishi M, Fujiwara T, Naito T, et al. Surfactant replacement therapy in neonatal respiratory distress syndrome. A multi-centre, randomized clinical trial: comparison of high- versus low-dose of surfactant TA. *Eur J Pediatr.* 1988;147:20-25.
32. Gortner L, Pohlandt F, Bartmann P, et al. High-dose versus low-dose bovine surfactant treatment in very premature infants. *Acta Paediatr.* 1994;83:135-141.
33. Halliday HL, Tarnow-Mordi WO, Corcoran JD, Patterson CC. Multicentre randomized trial comparing high and low dose surfactant regimens for the treatment of respiratory distress syndrome (the Curosurf 4 trial). *Arch Dis Child.* 1993;69:276-280.
34. Torresin M, Zimmermann LJ, Cogo PE, et al. Exogenous surfactant kinetics in infant respiratory distress syndrome: A novel method with stable isotopes. *Am J Respir Crit Care Med.* 2000;161:1584-1589.
35. Cogo PE, Facco M, Simonato M, et al. Dosing of porcine surfactant: effect on kinetics and gas exchange in respiratory distress syndrome. *Pediatrics.* 2009;124:e950-e957.
36. Malloy CA, Nicoski P, Muraskas JK. A randomized trial comparing beractant and poractant treatment in neonatal respiratory distress syndrome. *Acta Paediatr.* 2005;94:779-784.
37. Seger N, Soll R. Animal derived surfactant extract for treatment of respiratory distress syndrome. *Cochrane Database of Systematic Reviews.* 2009;(2):CD007836.
38. Soll R. Early versus delayed selective surfactant treatment for neonatal respiratory distress syndrome. *Cochrane Database of Systematic Reviews.* 1999;(4):CD001456.
39. Soll R, Morley CJ. Prophylactic versus selective use of surfactant in preventing morbidity and mortality in preterm infants. *Cochrane Database of Systematic Reviews.* 2001;1(2):CD000510.
40. Kattwinkel J, Bloom BT, Delmore P, et al. Prophylactic administration of calf lung surfactant extract is more effective than early treatment of respiratory distress syndrome in neonates of 29 through 32 weeks' gestation. *Pediatrics.* 1993;92:90-98.

C

41. Kendig JW, Ryan RM, Sinkin RA, et al. Comparison of two strategies for surfactant prophylaxis in very premature infants: a multicenter randomized trial. *Pediatrics*. 1998;101:1006-1012.
42. Avery ME, Tooley WH, Keller JB, et al. Is chronic lung disease in low birth weight infants preventable? A survey of eight centers. *Pediatrics*. 1987;79:26-30.
43. De Klerk AM, De Klerk RK. Nasal continuous positive airway pressure and outcomes of preterm infants. *J Paediatr Child Health*. 2001;37:161-167.
44. Morley CJ, Davis PG, Doyle LW, et al; COIN Trial Investigators. Nasal CPAP or intubation at birth for very preterm infants. *N Engl J Med*. 2008;358:700-708.
45. Sandri F, Plavka R, Ancora G, et al; CURPAP Study Group. Prophylactic or early selective surfactant combined with nCPAP in very preterm infants. *Pediatrics*. 2010;125:e1402-e1409.
46. SUPPORT Study Group of the Eunice Kennedy Shriver NICHD Neonatal Research Network, Finer NN, Carlo WA, et al. Early CPAP versus surfactant in extremely preterm infants. *N Engl J Med*. 2010;362:1970-1979.
47. Speer CP, Robertson B, Curstedt T, et al. Randomized European multicenter trial of surfactant replacement therapy for severe neonatal respiratory distress syndrome: single versus multiple doses of Curosurf. *Pediatrics*. 1992;89:13-20.
48. Dunn MS, Shennan AT, Possmayer F. Single- versus multiple-dose surfactant replacement therapy in neonates of 30 to 36 weeks' gestation with respiratory distress syndrome. *Pediatrics*. 1990;86:564-571.
49. The OSIRIS Collaborative Group. Early versus delayed neonatal administration of a synthetic surfactant—the judgment of OSIRIS. *Lancet*. 1992;340:1363-1379.
50. Soll RF. Multiple versus single dose natural surfactant extract for severe neonatal respiratory distress syndrome. *Cochrane Database Syst Rev*. 1999;(2):CD000141.
51. Kattwinkel J, Bloom BT, Delmore P, et al. High-versus low-threshold surfactant retreatment for neonatal respiratory distress syndrome. *Pediatrics*. 2000;106:282-288.
52. Fetus and Newborn Committee, Canadian Paediatric Society (CPS). Recommendations for neonatal surfactant therapy. *J Paediatr Child Health*. 2005;10:109-116.
53. Segerer H, van Gelder W, Angenent FW, et al. Pulmonary distribution and efficacy of exogenous surfactant in lung-lavaged rabbits are influenced by the instillation technique. *Pediatr Res*. 1993;34:490-494.
54. Valls-i-Soler A, Fernández-Ruanova B, López-Heredia y Goya J, et al. A randomized comparison of surfactant dosing via a dual-lumen endotracheal tube in respiratory distress syndrome. The Spanish Surfactant Collaborative Group. *Pediatrics*. 1998;101:E4.
55. Stevens TP, Blennow M,Myers EH, Soll R. Early surfactant administration with brief ventilation vs. selective surfactant and continued mechanical ventilation for preterm infants with or at risk for respiratory distress syndrome. *Cochrane Database of Systematic Reviews*. 2007;(4):CD003063.
56. Verder H, Albertsen P, Ebbesen F, et al. Nasal continuous positive airway pressure and early surfactant therapy for respiratory distress syndrome in newborns of less than 30 weeks' gestation. *Pediatrics*. 1999;103:E24.
57. O'Donnell CP, Kamlin CO, Davis PG, Morley CJ. Endotracheal intubation attempts during neonatal resuscitation: success rates, duration, and adverse effects. *Pediatrics*. 2006;117:e16-e21.
58. O'Donnell CP, Davis PG, Lau R, et al. Neonatal resuscitation 2: an evaluation of manual ventilation devices and face masks. *Arch Dis Child Fetal Neonatal Ed*. 2005;90:F392-F396.
59. Hillman NH, Kallapur SG, Pillow JJ, et al. Airway injury from initiating ventilation in preterm sheep. *Pediatr Res*. 2010;67:60-65.
60. Ingimarsson J, Björklund LJ, Curstedt T, et al. Incomplete protection by prophylactic surfactant against the adverse effects of large lung inflations at birth in immature lambs. *Intensive Care Med*. 2004;30:1446-1453.
61. Speer CP. Chorioamniotitis, postnatal factors and proinflammatory response in the pathogenetic sequence of bronchopulmonary dysplasia. *Neonatology*. 2009;95:353-361.
62. Cosmi EV, La Torre R, Piazze JJ, et al. Intraamniotic surfactant for prevention of neonatal respiratory distress syndrome (IRDS): rationale and personal experience. *Eur J Obstet Gynecol Reprod Biol*. 1997;71:135-139.
63. Zhang JP, Wang YL, Wang YH, et al. Prophylaxis of neonatal respiratory distress syndrome by intra-amniotic administration of pulmonary surfactant. *Chin Med J (Engl)*. 2004;117:120-124.
64. Abdel-Latif ME, Osborn DA, Challis D. Intra-amniotic surfactant for women at risk of preterm birth for preventing respiratory distress in newborns. *Cochrane Database of Systematic Reviews*. 2010;(1):CD007916.
65. Kattwinkel J, Robinson M, Bloom BT, et al. Technique for intrapartum administration of surfactant without requirement for an endotracheal tube. *J Perinatol*. 2004;24:360-365.
66. Trevisanuto D, Grazzina N, Ferrarese P, et al. Laryngeal mask airway used as a delivery conduit for the administration of surfactant to preterm infants with respiratory distress syndrome. *Biol Neonate*. 2005;87:217-220.
67. Dijk PH, Heikamp A, Bambang Oetomo S. Surfactant nebulisation prevents the adverse effects of surfactant therapy on blood pressure and cerebral blood flow in rabbits with severe respiratory failure. *Intensive Care Med*. 1997;23:1077-1081.
68. Berggren E, Liljedahl M, Winbladh B, et al. Pilot study of nebulized surfactant therapy for neonatal respiratory distress syndrome. *Acta Paediatr*. 2000;89:460-464.
69. Sun Y, Yang R, Zhong JG, et al. Aerosolised surfactant generated by a novel noninvasive apparatus reduced acute lung injury in rats. *Crit Care*. 2009;13:R31.

70. Finer NN, Merritt TA, Bernstein G, et al. An open label, pilot study of Aerosurf combined with nCPAP to prevent RDS in preterm neonates. *J Aerosol Med Pulm Drug Deliv*. 2010;23:303-309.
71. Kribs A, Pillekamp F, Hünseler C, et al. Early administration of surfactant in spontaneous breathing with nCPAP: feasibility and outcome in extremely premature infants (postmenstrual age </=27 weeks). *Paediatr Anaesth*. 2007;17:364-369.
72. Herting E, Kribs A, Roth B, et al. Surfactant via gastric tube in spontaneously breathing very low birth weight infants on nasal CPAP prevents mechanical ventilation. *Neonatology*. 2010; 97:395.
73. Dargaville PA, Copnell B; Australian and New Zealand Neonatal Network. The epidemiology of meconium aspiration syndrome: incidence, risk factors, therapies, and outcome. *Pediatrics*. 2006;117:1712-1721.
74. Qian L, Liu C, Zhuang W, et al. Neonatal Respiratory Failure: A 12-Month Clinical Epidemiologic Study From 2004 to 2005 in China. *Pediatrics*. 2008;121;e1115-e1124.
75. Wirbelauer J, Speer CP. The role of surfactant treatment in preterm infants and term newborns with acute respiratory distress syndrome. *J Perinatol*. 2009;29(Suppl 2):S18-S22.
76. Moses D, Holm BA, Spitale P, et al. Inhibition of pulmonary surfactant function by meconium. *Am J Obstet Gynecol*. 1991;164:477-481.
77. Auten RL, Notter RH, Kendig JW, et al. Surfactant treatment of full-term newborns with respiratory failure. *Pediatrics*. 1991;87:101-107.
78. Paranka MS, Walsh WF, Stancombe BB. Surfactant lavage in a piglet model of meconium aspiration syndrome. *Pediatr Res*. 1992;31:625-628.
79. El Shahed AI, Dargaville P, Ohlsson A, Soll RF. Surfactant for meconium aspiration syndrome in full term/near term infants. *Cochrane Database Syst Rev*. 2007;(3):CD002054.
80. Dargaville PA, Copnell B, Tingay DG, et al. Refining the method of therapeutic lung lavage in meconium aspiration syndrome. *Neonatology*. 2008;94:160-163.
81. Dargaville PA, Copnell B, Mills JF, et al. Randomized controlled trial of lung lavage with dilute surfactant for meconium aspiration syndrome. *J Pediatr*. 2010;158:383-389.e2.
82. Taeusch HW, Lu KW, Goerke J, Clements JA. Nonionic polymers reverse inactivation of surfactant by meconium and other substances. *Am J Respir Crit Care Med*. 1999;159:1391-1395.
83. Stichtenoth G, Jung P, Walter G, et al. Polymyxin B/pulmonary surfactant mixtures have increased resistance to inactivation by meconium and reduce growth of gram-negative bacteria in vitro. *Pediatr Res*. 2006;59:407-411.
84. Lu KW, Robertson B, Taeusch HW. Dextran or polyethylene glycol added to Curosurf for treatment of meconium lung injury in rats. *Biol Neonate*. 2005;88:46-53.
85. Calkovska A, Mokra D, Drgova A, et al. Bronchoalveolar lavage with pulmonary surfactant/dextran mixture improves meconium clearance and lung functions in experimental meconium aspiration syndrome. *Eur J Pediatr*. 2008;167:851-857.
86. Lu KW, Taeusch HW. Combined effects of polymers and KL(4) peptide on surface activity of pulmonary surfactant lipids. *Biochim Biophys Acta*. 2010;1798:1129-1134.
87. Herting E, Gefeller O, Land M, et al. Surfactant treatment of neonates with respiratory failure and group B streptococcal infection. Members of the Collaborative European Multicenter Study Group. *Pediatrics*. 2000;106:957-964.
88. Speer CP, Robertson B, Halliday HL. Commentary: Randomized trial comparing natural and synthetic surfactant: Increased infection rate after natural surfactant? *Acta Paediatr*. 2000;89: 510-512.
89. Speer CP, Götze B, Robertson B, Curstedt T. Phagocytic functions and TNF secretion of human monocytes exposed to natural porcine surfactant (Curosurf). *Pediatr Res*. 1991;30:69-74.
90. Herting E, Sun B, Jarstrand C, et al. Surfactant improves lung function and mitigates bacterial growth in immature ventilated rabbits with experimentally induced neonatal group B streptococcal pneumonia. *Arch Dis Child Fetal Neonatal Ed*. 1997;76:F3-F8.
91. Herting E, Gan X, Rauprich P, et al. Combined treatment with surfactant and specific immunoglobulin reduces bacterial proliferation in experimental neonatal group B streptococcal pneumonia. *Am J Respir Crit Care Med*. 1999;159:1862-1867.
92. Stichtenoth G, Linderholm B, Björkman MH, et al. Prophylactic intratracheal polymyxin B/surfactant prevents bacterial growth in neonatal E. coli pneumonia of rabbits. *Pediatr Res*. 2010;67: 369-374.
93. Suen HC, Catlin EA, Ryan DP, et al. Biochemical immaturity of lungs in congenital diaphragmatic hernia. *J Pediatr Surg*. 1993;28:471-475.
94. Glick PL, Stannard VA, Leach CL, et al. Pathophysiology of congenital diaphragmatic hernia II: the fetal lamb CDH model is surfactant deficient. *J Pediatr Surg*. 1992;27:382-387.
95. IJsselstijn H, Zimmermann LJ, Bunt JE, et al. Prospective evaluation of surfactant composition in bronchoalveolar lavage fluid of infants with congenital diaphragmatic hernia and of age-matched controls. *Crit Care Med*. 1998;26:573-580.
96. Boucherat O, Benachi A, Chailley-Heu B, et al. Surfactant maturation is not delayed in human fetuses with diaphragmatic hernia. *PLoS Med*. 2007;4:e237.
97. Cogo PE, Zimmermann LJ, Verlato G, et al. A dual stable isotope tracer method for the measurement of surfactant disaturated-phosphatidylcholine net synthesis in infants with congenital diaphragmatic hernia. *Pediatr Res*. 2004;56:184-190.
98. Janssen DJ, Zimmermann LJ, Cogo P, et al. Decreased surfactant phosphatidylcholine synthesis in neonates with congenital diaphragmatic hernia during extracorporeal membrane oxygenation. *Intensive Care Med*. 2009;35:1754-1760.

99. O'Toole SJ, Karamanoukian HL, Sharma A, et al. Surfactant rescue in the fetal lamb model of congenital diaphragmatic hernia. *J Pediatr Surg*. 1996;31:1105-1108.
100. Glick PL, Leach CL, Besner GE, et al. Pathophysiology of congenital diaphragmatic hernia. III: Exogenous surfactant therapy for the high-risk neonate with CDH. *J Pediatr Surg*. 1992;27: 866-869.
101. Van Meurs K; Congenital Diaphragmatic Hernia Study Group. Is surfactant therapy beneficial in the treatment of the term newborn infant with congenital diaphragmatic hernia? *J Pediatr*. 2004;145:312-316.
102. Soll R, Ozek E. Prophylactic protein free synthetic surfactant for preventing morbidity and mortality in preterm infants. *Cochrane Database Syst Rev*. 2010;(1):CD001079.
103. Holm BA, Notter RH. Effects of hemoglobin and cell membrane lipids on pulmonary surfactant activity. *J Appl Physiol*. 1987;63:1434-1442.
104. Pandit PB, Dunn MS, Colucci EA. Surfactant therapy in neonates with respiratory deterioration due to pulmonary hemorrhage. *Pediatrics*. 1995;95:32-36.
105. Amizuka T, Shimizu H, Niida Y, Ogawa Y. Surfactant therapy in neonates with respiratory failure due to haemorrhagic pulmonary oedema. *Eur J Pediatr*. 2003;162:697-702.
106. Aziz A, Ohlsson A. Surfactant for pulmonary hemorrhage in neonates. *Cochrane Database of Systematic Reviews*. 2008;(2):CD005254.
107. Khammash H, Perlman M, Wojtulewicz J, Dunn M. Surfactant therapy in full-term neonates with severe respiratory failure. *Pediatrics*. 1993;92:135-139.
108. Lotze A, Knight GR, Martin GR, et al. Improved pulmonary outcome after exogenous surfactant therapy for respiratory failure in term infants requiring extracorporeal membrane oxygenation. *J Pediatr*. 1993;122:261-268.
109. Lotze A, Mitchell BR, Bulas DI, et al. Multicenter study of surfactant (beractant) use in the treatment of term infants with severe respiratory failure. Survanta in Term Infants Study Group. *J Pediatr*. 1998;132:40-47.
110. Hintz SR, Suttner DM, Sheehan AM, et al. Decreased use of neonatal extracorporeal membrane oxygenation (ECMO): how new treatment modalities have affected ECMO utilization. *Pediatrics*. 2000;106:1339-1343.
111. Luchetti M, Ferrero F, Gallini C, et al. Multicenter, randomized, controlled study of porcine surfactant in severe respiratory syncytial virus-induced respiratory failure. *Pediatr Crit Care Med*. 2002;3:261-268.
112. Busani S, Girardis M, Biagioni E, et al. Surfactant therapy and intravenous zanamivir in severe respiratory failure due to persistent influenza A/H1N1 2009 virus infection. *Am J Respir Crit Care Med*. 2010;182:1334.
113. Varisco BM, Palmatier CM, Alten JA. Reversal of intractable hypoxemia with exogenous surfactant (calfactant) facilitating complete neurological recovery in a pediatric drowning victim. *Pediatr Emerg Care*. 2010;26:571-573.
114. Verder H, Ebbesen F, Linderholm B, et al; Danish-Swedish Multicentre Study Group. Prediction of respiratory distress syndrome by the microbubble stability test on gastric aspirates in newborns of less than 32 weeks' gestation. *Acta Paediatr*. 2003;92:728-733.
115. Daniel IW, Fiori HH, Piva JP, et al. Lamellar body count and stable microbubble test on gastric aspirates from preterm infants for the diagnosis of respiratory distress syndrome. *Neonatology*. 2010;98:150-155.
116. Verder H, Ebbesen F, Brandt J, et al; for the Danish-Swedish Multicenter Study Group for Surfactant Replacement. Lamellar body counts on gastric aspirates for prediction of respiratory distress syndrome. *Acta Paediatr*. 2011;100:175-180.
117. Almlén A, Walther FJ, Waring AJ, et al. Synthetic surfactant based on analogues of SP-B and SP-C is superior to single-peptide surfactants in ventilated premature rabbits. *Neonatology*. 2010;98: 91-99.
118. Curstedt T, Johansson J. Different effects of surfactant proteins B and C—implications for development of synthetic surfactants. *Neonatology*. 2010;97:367-372.
119. Lu KW, Taeusch HW. Combined effects of polymers and KL(4) peptide on surface activity of pulmonary surfactant lipids. *Biochim Biophys Acta*. 2010;1798:1129-1134.
120. Yeh TF, Lin HC, Chang CH, et al. Early intratracheal instillation of budesonide using surfactant as a vehicle to prevent chronic lung disease in preterm infants: a pilot study. *Pediatrics*. 2008; 121:e1310-e1318.
121. Kuo HT, Lin HC, Tsai CH, et al. A follow-up study of preterm infants given budesonide using surfactant as a vehicle to prevent chronic lung disease in preterm infants. *J Pediatr*. 2010; 156:537-541.

CHAPTER 15

Oxygenation Targeting and Outcomes in Preterm Infants: The New Evidence

Win Tin, MD, Waldemar A. Carlo, MD, and
Samir Gupta, MD, FRCPCH

- Historical Perspectives
- Physiologic Considerations
- The Critical Threshold of Fetal Oxygenation
- Oxygenation during Fetal-to-Neonatal Transition
- Oxygen Toxicity in Preterm Infants
- "Normal" Levels of Oxygenation in Newborns
- Optimal Levels of Oxygenation in Preterm Infants: Neonatal Period
- Optimal Levels of Oxygenation in Preterm Infants: Post-Neonatal Period
- Approaches to Oxygen Therapy and Clinical Outcomes
- Controversies in Oxygen Therapy
- Resolving the Uncertainty: The Oxygen Saturation Trials
- New Evidence on Oxygenation Targets in Preterm Infants

Oxygen is the most commonly used therapy in the neonatal nurseries as an integral part of all respiratory support. The goal of oxygen therapy is to achieve adequate delivery of oxygen to the tissue without creating oxygen toxicity and oxidative stress. Oxygen must have been given to more newborn babies than any other medicinal product during the last 70 years. It has been known for more than 50 years that the eyes of preterm infants may be easily damaged by too much oxygen, especially during the first few weeks after birth.[1-3] Although prevention of hyperoxia reduced the rate of retinopathy of prematurity in a large randomized trial,[4] targeting oxygen saturations to the low 90s decreases the risk of death in extremely preterm babies.[5]

Historical Perspectives

Joseph Priestley,[6] Karl Scheele,[7] and Anton Lavoisier[8] all contributed to the discovery that the air we breathe is really a mixture of dephlogisticated or "vital air" and "gas azote." In 1775, Priestley was perceptive enough to write, in his very first description of what we now call oxygen:

> *From the greater strength and vivacity of the flame of a candle, in this pure air, it may be conjectured, that it might be peculiarly salutary to the lungs in certain morbid cases, when the common air would not be sufficient to carry off the phlogistic putrid effluvium fast enough. But, perhaps, we may also infer from these experiments, that though pure dephlogisticated air might be very useful as medicine, it might not be so proper for us in the usual healthy state of the body: for, as a candle burns out much faster in dephlogisticated than in common air, so we*

might, as might be said, live out too fast, and the animal powers be too soon exhausted in this pure kind of air. A moralist, at least, may say, that the air which nature has provided for us is as good as we deserve.

Although the use of oxygen as a medicinal product has a long history,[9] the "routine" use of supplemental oxygen in the care of small or preterm infants had its origins in the 1940s. A report by Wilson and colleagues[10] had a marked influence on this practice, noting that the irregular pattern of periodic breathing commonly seen in babies of short gestation was largely abolished when these babies were given oxygen in a concentration of 70% or more to breathe. These researchers initially commented, "We have no proof that the regular type of respiration which we are accustomed to call normal is better for the premature infant than the periodic type of breathing described. Likewise we have no convincing evidence that an increased oxygen content of arterial blood is beneficial or necessarily of importance. It is evident, however, that these healthy premature babies breathed in a more 'normal' manner in an oxygen enriched atmosphere."[10] However, by 1949, Howard and Bauer[11] were less cautious in their comments, as follows: "Irregular breathing in early infancy should be treated with a mixture of high oxygen even more than at present, as such an atmosphere regularly increases breathing volume and has a steadying effect on the rhythm of respiration. Oxygen is the most valuable single agent available for a premature or full term newborn infant who is showing any evidence of respiratory difficulty, and it should be used early and generously."[11] It was within this climate of opinion that the widespread practice of unrestricted oxygen supplementation for small or sick infants came into force in the early 1950s, and the ensuing epidemic of severe eye disease and blindness is now well known (Fig. 15-1).

The first person to suggest in print that oxygen could be responsible for the rising epidemic of severe retinopathy of prematurity (ROP), or retrolental fibroplasia as it was then known, was Kate Campbell of Melbourne, Australia. She was generous enough to say that news of the idea came to her from colleagues returning from overseas, who made a comparison of the treatment of premature infants in America, where retrolental fibroplasia was a problem and where oxygen was used freely, with the treatment in England, where retrolental fibroplasia was rarely seen and where oxygen was used sparingly. She concluded that the "normal oxygen environment of the newborn full term infant is abnormal for the premature infant."[12] Within a year,

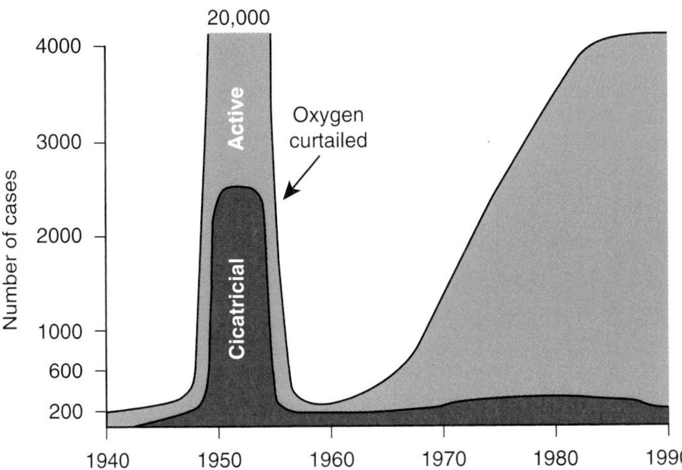

Figure 15-1 Incidence of retinopathy of prematurity (ROP) over time from the 1940s to the 1990s. Note that around 1955, the incidences of cicatricial ROP and active ROP dropped significantly because that is when use of high levels of oxygen for preterms was curtailed. In the late 1960s through the 1990s, survival of very low-birth-weight infants increased along with the incidence of active ROP (*pink area*). Note that the incidence of severe cicatricial ROP (*red area*) has remained relatively low during this period. (From Wright KW, editor: *Textbook of ophthalmology*, Philadelphia, Lippincott Williams & Wilkins 1997, p338.)

Mary Crosse[13] in Birmingham, England, demonstrated more convincing evidence. Additional confirmation came from a randomized trial, started in 1948 by Arnall Patz[1] in the state of Washington, United States, in which babies weighing less than 3.5 pounds were alternately assigned at 24 hours after birth to high oxygen (65%-70% for 4-7 weeks) or less than 40% oxygen for as short a time as possible (1-2 weeks). Seven of the 28 babies nursed in high oxygen experienced stage 3-4 retinopathy, but none of the 37 nursed in as little oxygen as possible did so. The larger Cooperative Trial by Kinsey and colleagues,[2] designed to replicate the Washington trial completed in 1955,[2] was widely interpreted at the time as suggesting that oxygen therapy was safe as long as the inspired oxygen concentration was not more than 40%.[14] The fact that babies in one arm of the trial had not only received more oxygen but also received it for much longer was almost entirely overlooked. So too was the fact that some babies in the restricted-exposure arm still had eye damage. Even more seriously, it took some time for clinicians to realize that a policy of restricting oxygen exposure rather than restricting arterial oxygen levels was almost certainly causing a rise in the number of early neonatal deaths.[15-17]

15

Once it became clear from the Cooperative Trial that although excessive oxygen exposure was at least one of the causes of retinopathy, there was no clarity as to how oxygen administration could be optimized, clinicians started to look for ways of monitoring arterial oxygen levels. Indwelling arterial lines were soon widely used to monitor arterial oxygen tension, but no controlled trial has ever shown that their use reduces the risk of permanent retinal damage.[18] Transcutaneous measurement of the partial pressure of oxygen ($TcPo_2$), a technology developed in the 1970s, appears to approximate actual arterial oxygen levels well in most circumstances.[18] Some nonrandomized studies have claimed a near abolition of retinopathy using $TcPo_2$ monitoring,[19] and others have reported no difference in the incidence or severity of ROP attributable to $TcPo_2$ monitoring.[20] The only randomized trial to date that has examined the effect of transcutaneous monitoring (continuous $TcPo_2$ monitoring versus standard care) on retinopathy suggested a modest improvement in ROP rates for infants with greater than 1000 g birth weight, but no effect on smaller infants, in whom ROP occurs more frequently and more severely. Conversely there was a trend to higher mortality in the group receiving continuous transcutaneous monitoring. The rates of the combined outcome death and ROP were nearly identical in the two groups.[21] Further analyses suggested that retinopathy occurred more often with longer exposure to $TcPo_2$ readings that reached or exceeded 80 mm Hg (10.7 kPa) in the first 4 weeks of life.[22] Oxygen saturation monitoring using pulse oximetry has gained widespread use in neonatal nurseries since the early 1980s[23] because of its ease of use and lack of heat-related side effects, particularly in extremely preterm infants with sensitive skin. The evidence from non randomized studies suggests that pulse oximetry is a reliable measure of oxygenation in infants with chronic lung disease and prolonged oxygen dependency, particularly at lower Pao_2 levels.[24,25] However, the ability of pulse oximeters to reliably detect hyperoxia remains controversial,[26-28] and it has been shown that fractional oxygen saturation values higher than 92% can often be associated with hyperoxia, defined as arterial oxygen tension of more than 80 mm Hg (Fig. 15-2).[29,30]

After the lessons learned from the oxygen-induced blindness epidemic in the 1950s and the ensuing proliferation of oxygen-monitoring devices, many studies over the past 50 years have tried to define what constitutes a safe level of oxygenation for newborn babies. Unfortunately, few studies in this area of medicine have used the methodology known to be the best way of reliably assessing the effects of interventions, the randomized controlled trial.

Physiologic Considerations

Oxyhemoglobin Dissociation Curve

In its basic form, the oxyhemoglobin dissociation curve (Fig. 15-3) describes the relation between the partial pressure of oxygen (*x* axis) and the oxygen saturation (y axis). The hemoglobin's oxygen content increases as Po_2 increases until the

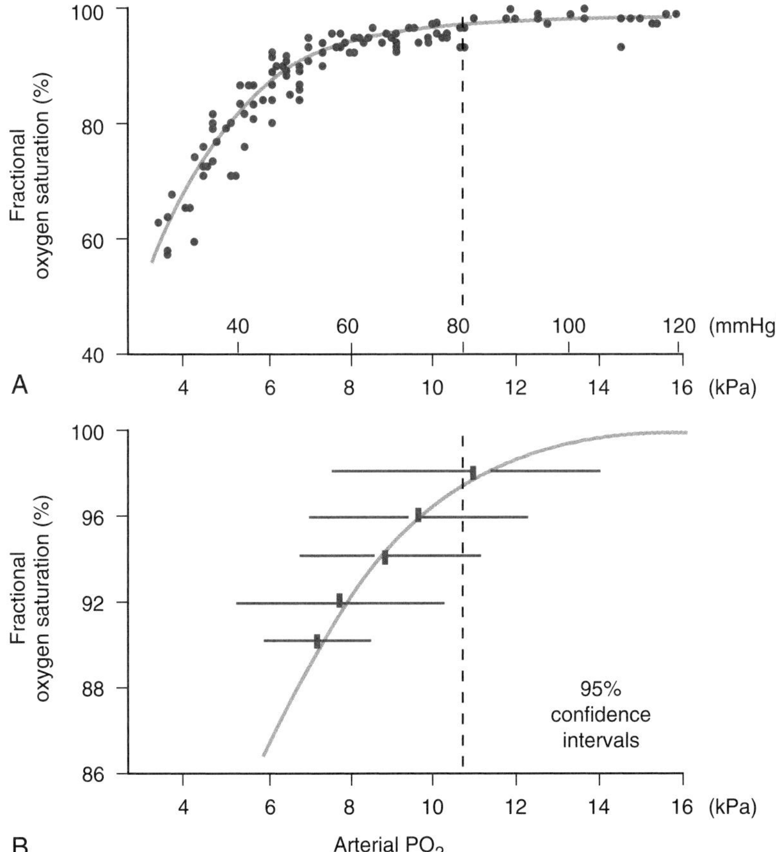

Figure 15-2 **A,** The relation between fractional oxygen saturation, measured with a pulse oximeter, and arterial partial pressure, in mm Hg and kPa. The *dashed line* marks the transcutaneous PO_2 above which there was an increased risk of retinopathy in the study reported by Flynn and associates[21] in 1992. **B,** The *bars* show the range within which 95% of all measures of partial pressure varied when the oximeter read 90%, 92%, 94%, 96%, and 98% in the study reported by Brockway and Hay[29] in 1998. (From Hey E, editor: *Neonatal formulary 4*, London, BMJ Books, 2003, p 187.)

Figure 15-3 Oxyhemoglobin dissociation curve of fetus and mother. The *x*-axis shows the partial pressure of oxygen, PO_2 in mm Hg, and the *y*-axis shows oxyhemoglobin saturation. The points A and B represent fetal and maternal P_{50} values respectively. The *shaded area*—(a-v)O_2—represents the oxygen unloading capacity between given "arterial" and "venous" PO_2 values. (Adapted from Tin W, Wariyar U: Giving small babies oxygen: 50 years of uncertainty. *Semin Neonatol.* 2002; 7:361.)

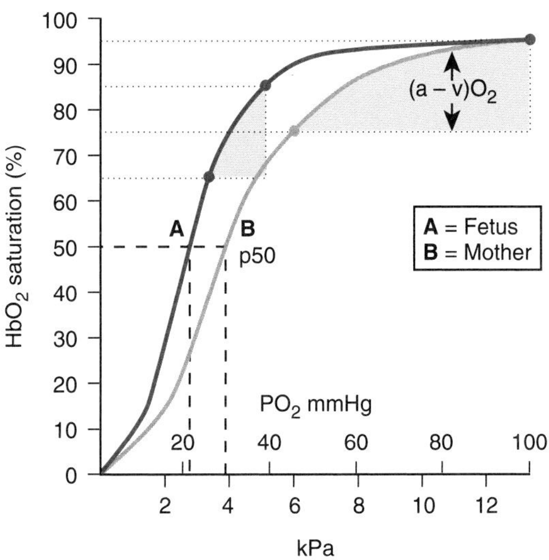

maximum capacity is reached. As this limit is approached, very little additional binding occurs, and the curve levels out as the hemoglobin becomes saturated with oxygen. This makes the curve sigmoid or S-shaped. At pressures above 60 mm Hg, the standard oxyhemoglobin dissociation curve is relatively flat, meaning that the oxygen content of the blood does not change significantly even with large increases in the oxygen partial pressure. To transport more oxygen to the tissue would require either an increase in the hemoglobin content to increase the oxygen-carrying capacity, or supplemental oxygen to increase the oxygen dissolved in plasma.[31]

The partial pressure of oxygen in the blood at which the hemoglobin is 50% saturated at temperature of 37° C and atmospheric pressure is known as the P_{50}. It is a conventional measure of hemoglobin's affinity for oxygen. In the presence of disease or other conditions that change the hemoglobin's oxygen affinity, and consequently shift the curve to the right or left, the P_{50} changes accordingly. An increase in P_{50} indicates a shift of the curve to the right, meaning that a larger partial pressure is necessary to maintain 50% oxygen saturation. This indicates a decreased affinity for oxygen. Conversely, a lower P_{50} indicates a shift to the left, as with fetal hemoglobin (HbF) and a higher affinity of hemoglobin for oxygen. The shift of the oxygen dissociation curve to the right occurs in response to an increase in the partial pressure of carbon dioxide (PCO_2), a decrease in pH, or both, the last of which is known as the Bohr effect. This effect is more pronounced at lower saturations and is less remarkable when blood is depleted of 2,3-diphosphoglycerate (2,3-DPG).[32] The higher oxygen affinity of HbF favors the performance of metabolic functions at the low intrauterine oxygen tensions.

Fetal Oxygenation

The oxygen delivery to the fetus is affected by placental circulation and the oxygen-carrying capacity of the HbF. Due to high oxygen-carrying capacity and increased oxygen affinity of HbF, the oxyhemoglobin saturation and arterial blood oxygen content in the fetus are not much lower than those in the adult despite the lower fetal partial pressure of oxygen (PO_2). In utero the presence of high concentrations of HbF maintains higher affinity for oxygen and thus shifts the dissociation curve to the left. Because of the steeper dissociation curve, oxygen is released more readily even with a small reduction in PO_2 (see Fig. 15-3).

In humans, fetal P_{50} is about 20 mm Hg under standard conditions, and there is a gradual decrease in blood oxygen affinity (increase in P_{50}) during the course of gestation (Fig. 15-4).[33] At the placental level, the high oxygen affinity of HbF favors oxygen uptake by the fetus and adequate oxygen transfer is achieved at relatively low PO_2. In the fetus, the umbilical venous blood has the highest PO_2, which usually

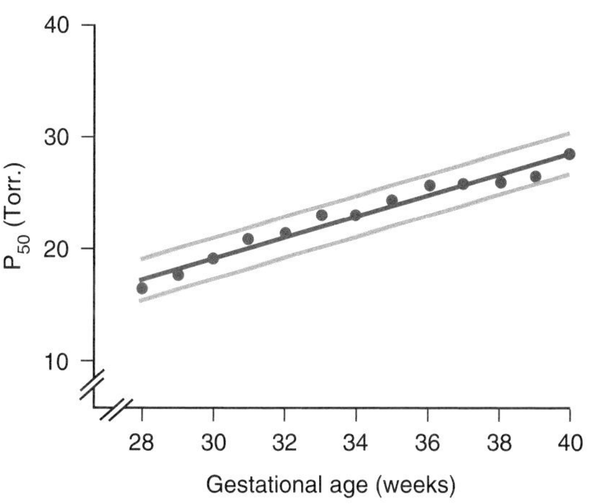

Figure 15-4 Relationship between gestational age and hemoglobin P_{50}. Each *point* represents the mean value for age; outrider *lines* indicate ± 2 SD. (From Polin RA, Fox WF: *Fetal and neonatal physiology*, ed 3, Philadelphia, Elsevier, 2004, p 885.)

does not go much above 30 mm Hg. At this oxygen tension the oxygen saturation of fetal umbilical venous blood is 6% to 8% higher than the oxygen saturation of maternal venous blood.[34]

The Critical Threshold of Fetal Oxygenation

Monitoring of fetal oxygen is technically difficult. Conventional transmission oximeters are unsuitable for fetal use because of the difficulty in accessing fetal parts and the much lower pulse oxygen saturations (SpO_2) values observed in the fetus. With the advances in technology, fetal pulse oximetry is now available either as a stand-alone or integrated with fetal monitoring, but has its inherent limitations. Studies conducted during the first stage of labor have been reported the mean fetal pulse oxygen saturation ($FSpO_2$) to be 49%.[35] The establishment of a clinically useful value below which a fetus is considered to be at risk for hypoxia has been addressed in human studies.[36] Investigators have defined the lower limit of normal $FSpO_2$ (defined as mean − 2SD) to be approximately 30%. Goffinet and associates[37] reported a significant correlation between $FSpO_2$ less than 30% and poor neonatal condition, defined as the presence of at least one of the following: 5-minute Apgar score less than 7, secondary respiratory distress, umbilical artery pH 7.15 or less, transfer to neonatal intensive care unit (NICU), or death. On the basis of animal and relevant human data, several groups have suggested that $FSpO_2$ values greater than or equal to 30% can be considered reassuring in the human fetus.[38,39] Values less than 30% for 10 minutes or longer may require further assessment or intervention.

Fetal pulse oximetry has been compared with other monitoring techniques. The French multicenter study group compared intrapartum $FSpO_2$ with fetal blood analysis (FBA) and reported similar sensitivity and specificity values for the two methods (threshold $FSpO_2$ of 30%) in predicting postpartum umbilical artery pH lower than 7.15.[40] The German multicenter study group, using receiver operator characteristic (ROC) analysis, reported the best predictive range of $FSpO_2$ to be between 30% and 40% and a cutoff at 30% for low scalp pH (<7.20).[38] The researchers reported a sensitivity of 81% and specificity of 100%. These intrapartum data for $FSpO_2$ illustrate that the fetus is capable of maintaining the metabolic function up to the critical value of 30%. However, there are no reported studies correlating the optimal fetal saturation value with clinical outcomes.

Near-infrared spectroscopy (NIRS) has also been used to assess oxygenation of blood and tissue in the fetus. The experimental studies conclude that the interpretation of data from this modality may be more relevant when it is used with other monitoring modalities, such as fetal pulse oximetry, rather than on its own. Studies of near-infrared spectroscopy and color Doppler ultrasound have also shown that fetal hypoxemia (defined as $FSpO_2 < 30\%$) results in an increased cerebral blood volume and flow, which are mediated by greater production of adrenal catecholamines.[41]

Oxygenation during Fetal-to-Neonatal Transition

The birth of a fetus demands postnatal changes to meet the metabolic needs and to adapt to extrauterine life. This process involves pulmonary, circulatory, temperature and metabolic adaptation. The high oxygen affinity of fetal blood has important disadvantages in postnatal life despite being optimally saturated. At the tissue level, the low P_{50} of fetal Hb decreases the driving potential for oxygen delivery and thus limits the rate at which oxygen can be unloaded. However, the newborn needs more oxygen to adapt to postnatal life, and the increase in oxygen consumption in most species is reported to be 100% to 150%.[42] In addition, the stress of a cold environment and muscular activity further increase the infant's metabolic demand for oxygen. Hence, a P_{50} adequate for tissue supply in the fetus may limit the rate of oxygen delivery in the newborn postnatally. This limitation is compensated for in babies born at term gestation by an increase in 2,3-DPG, which shifts the dissociation curve to the right and thus helps in unloading the oxygen at tissue level.

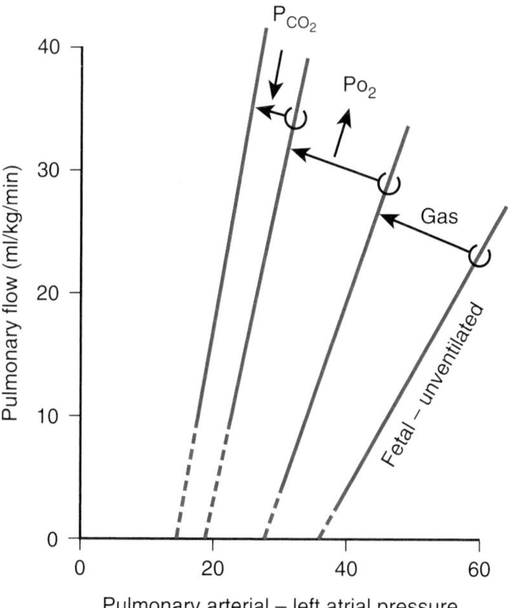

Figure 15-5 Pulmonary vascular conductance increases with the onset of ventilation. Separate curves depict the contributions of gaseous inflation, increased Po_2, and decreased Pco_2. (From Strang LB: The lungs at birth. *Arch Dis Child.* 1965;40:575.)

The physiology of premature infants differs from that of term babies. Preterm infants have higher fetal hemoglobin concentration, lower 2,3-DPG content, and lower P_{50} levels. The functioning fractions of DPG are also significantly lower than those in term infants. Initially, premature infants have less oxygen-unloading capacity than term infants, and this smaller capacity persists during the first 3 months of life.[43] Therefore, premature babies have even higher oxygen saturation (Sao_2) at any given level of arterial Po_2 (Pao_2), and also the oxygen demands of most extremely premature infants can be met by keeping Pao_2 levels just above 50 mm Hg, which will result in saturation levels above 88%.[44]

Although the hemoglobin levels remain high for the first few months and more so in premature infants, the compensatory rise in DPG levels from birth allows the newborn infant to meet the increased oxygen requirements. The low fetal saturations may not be appropriate at birth as the pulmonary, metabolic, and circulatory adaptation takes place. This adaptation requires a drop in the pulmonary vascular resistance with a drop in pulmonary airway resistance after the first breaths and changes associated with the transition from fetal to adult circulation incorporating closure of fetal physiologic shunts (ductus arteriosus, ductus venosus, and foramen ovale). The effect of lung inflation and ventilation on the pulmonary blood flow was studied by Strang,[45] who observed that if the lung is inflated from fetal state and ventilated with gas mixtures that do not change fetal composition of blood gases (i.e., pH 7.35, Pco_2 45 torr, Po_2 25 torr), an increase in pulmonary vascular conductance (decrease in resistance) and in blood flow can be achieved (Fig. 15-5). This increase in conductance was attributed to the expansion of collapsible pulmonary capillaries. In addition, when the blood gas composition was changed by the increase in Po_2 and decrease in Pco_2 similar to ventilation with air, further increases in vascular conductance and blood flow were achieved. These changes, along with the increase in systemic vascular resistance, contribute to circulatory adaptation at birth.

In addition to the reduction in pulmonary vascular resistance, another known important factor that facilitates the closure of the ductus arteriosus is oxygen.[46] The high oxygen saturations would affect closure of physiologic shunts in term babies without causing any adverse effects, but at present there is not enough evidence to suggest that babies born very prematurely and exposed to similar high saturations would have the physiologic transition similar to that in term babies, particularly

C

when the anatomic maturity is far from complete. The saturation value in the fetus critical to preventing adverse metabolic effects has already been discussed. There is a growing interest in addressing the optimal saturations in the early postnatal period in the vulnerable premature babies to minimize the risk of potential oxygen toxicity while maintaining adequate tissue oxygenation during the physiologic transitional changes after birth.

Animal studies have shown that the rise in arterial oxygen tension is the main reason for ductal closure immediately after birth.[47] It is also known that changes in arterial oxygen level have a profound effect on pulmonary vascular tone. The rise in partial pressure of oxygen is one of the three main factors triggering the drop in pulmonary vascular tone[46] and the increase in the pulmonary blood flow seen in the period immediately after birth. The other factors are the expansion and ventilation of the lung and the lower $Pa{CO_2}$ of blood perfusing the lung. The classic experiments of Cassin and associates[48] in exteriorized fetal lambs have shown that raising the oxygen tension in the pulmonary arterial blood from 16 to 34 mm Hg caused an immediate fall in the pulmonary vascular tone. However, Dawes[49] later cautioned that raising the $Pa{O_2}$ from 50 to even as high as 150 mm Hg had virtually no further effect on the pulmonary vascular tone.

Schulze and coworkers[50] studied the effects of arterial oxygenation level on cardiac output, oxygen extraction, and oxygen consumption in low-birth-weight infants receiving mechanical ventilation.[50] The inspired oxygen concentration was adjusted to achieve either low $Sp{O_2}$ (89%-92%) or high $Sp{O_2}$ (93%-96%), and the investigators concluded that there was no mismatch between systemic oxygen delivery and demand in the two groups. Furthermore, the mixed venous oxygen tension decreased with the simultaneous increase in oxygen extraction ratio in the low target range of oxygen saturation. There are limited data on the effects of oxygen on ductus arteriosus in premature fetuses and infants. Rasanen and associates[51] studied the effect of maternal oxygenation on fetal physiology in 40 women, half between 20 and 26 weeks of gestation, and other half between 31 and 36 weeks of gestation. Mothers were randomly assigned to receive either 60% humidified oxygen or room air by face mask, and investigators measured various echocardiographic indices using Doppler ultrasound. They concluded that the reactivity of the human fetal pulmonary circulation increases with advancing gestation. There were no changes during maternal hyperoxygenation in fetuses between 20 and 26 weeks of gestation, but in fetuses between 31 and 36 weeks of gestation, the impedance decreased with a corresponding reduction in the flow in the ductus arteriosus. However, the postnatal data comparing the effect of high and low saturations on ductus arteriosus in preterm babies at different gestations are rather limited. One explanation that has been proposed for why the ductus arteriosus may remain patent in very preterm babies is that they are often not very well oxygenated in the period immediately after birth. Many clinicians are apprehensive that unnecessarily restricting arterial oxygen level in the period after birth for fear of the retinal consequences could result in failure of the ductus arteriosus to close spontaneously, but this concern is not based on hard evidence.

Oxygen Toxicity in Preterm Infants

Oxygen and the Eye

Although the etiopathogenesis of ROP is considered multifactorial, it is primarily affected by the immaturity of the retina itself and levels of retinal arterial oxygenation. The retina is avascular in early fetal life. With the advancement of gestational age, new retinal blood vessels grow outwards from the center around the optic nerve. Retinal vessel development begins at about 16 weeks of gestation.[52] In babies who are born extremely premature, the retina is incompletely vascularized and the avascular part of the retina is most susceptible to injury.

The role of oxygen in the pathogenesis of ROP has been explored by several studies. The chemical signaling by oxygen-regulated vascular endothelial growth

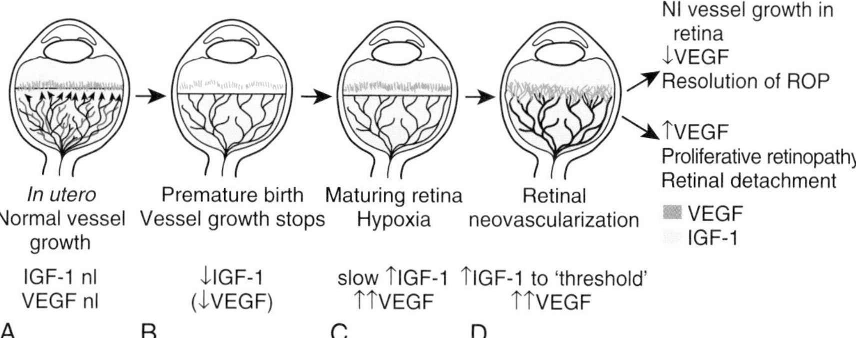

Figure 15-6 Schematic representation of insulin-like growth factor-1 (IGF-1) and vascular endothelial growth factor (VEGF) control of blood vessel development in retinopathy of prematurity (ROP). **A,** In utero, VEGF is found at the growing front of vessels (*arrows*). IGF-1 is sufficient to allow vessel growth. nl, normal levels. **B,** With premature birth, IGF-1 is not maintained at in utero levels, and vascular growth ceases despite the presence of VEGF at the growing front of vessels. Both endothelial cell survival (AKT) and proliferation (MAPK) pathways are compromised. With low IGF-1 and cessation of vessel growth, a demarcation line forms at the vascular front. High oxygen exposure (as occurs in animal models and in some premature infants) may also suppress VEGF, further contributing to inhibition of vessel growth. **C,** As the premature infant matures, the developing but nonvascularized retina becomes hypoxic. VEGF increases in retina and vitreous. With maturation, the IGF-1 level slowly increases. **D,** When the IGF-1 level reaches a threshold at 34 weeks of gestation, with high VEGF levels in the vitreous, endothelial cell survival and proliferation driven by VEGF may proceed. Neovascularization ensues at the demarcation line, growing into the vitreous. If VEGF vitreous levels fall, normal retinal vessel growth can proceed. With normal vascular growth and blood flow, oxygen suppresses VEGF expression so it will no longer be overproduced. If hypoxia (and elevations of VEGF) persists, further neovascularization and fibrosis leading to retinal detachment can occur. (From Smith LEH: Pathogenesis of retinopathy of prematurity. *Semin Neonatol.* 2003; 8:469.)

factor (VEGF) and non–oxygen-regulated insulin-like growth factor-1 (IGF-1) contribute to the development of retinal vasculature. VEGF is upregulated in a hypoxic environment and downregulated by hyperoxia.[53] Low levels of IGF-1 prevent vascular growth.[54] In utero, VEGF is found at the front end of growing vessels, and the levels of IGF-1 are sufficient to allow vessel growth.[55] Under "normal" physiologic conditions, increased oxygen demand from the growing neural retina anterior to the vascularization creates localized hypoxia. The result is increased expression of VEGF and growth of vessels toward this stimulus.

After premature birth, the induction of ROP is characterized by the disruption of normal retinal vascularization process. The pathogenesis of ROP can be described in two phases (Fig. 15-6). The first phase of ROP is related to the exposure to excessive oxygen after premature birth, when the normal retinal vascular growth stops and regression of some already developed vessels ensues. In the relatively hyperoxic environment, vasoconstriction of retinal vessels occurs, leading to arrest of the growth of blood vessels along the border between the vascularized and avascular portions of the retina. Resolution of "normal" in utero hypoxic drive also suppresses VEGF messenger RNA expression[56]; the suppression in turn causes loss of the physiologic wave of VEGF anterior to the growing vascular front. The low levels of IGF-1 due to loss of supply from placenta and amniotic fluid following birth also contribute to impairment of retinal vascular growth.[55] In addition, vascular obliteration may also be caused by apoptosis of vascular endothelial cells.

In contrast, the second phase of ROP is characterized by retinal neovascularization, induced by hypoxia. It is similar to other proliferative retinopathies and occurs at about 32 to 34 weeks postmenstrual age. The magnitude of destruction in the second phase is determined by the extent of damage in the first phase.[54] As the infant matures, the developing but nonvascularized retina becomes hypoxic. This hypoxia stimulates and upregulates the expression of VEGF in the retina and also in the vitreous, a mechanism said to be the critical factor in ocular neovascularization. The levels of VEGF remain high throughout the progression of ROP during this phase. The IGF-1 is also critical to the development of ROP, and the levels increase until ROP reaches the threshold stage. If hypoxia persists, the VEGF levels remain high and may lead to proliferative retinopathy, with or without further complication of retinal detachment.

Oxygen exposure, in terms of fluctuations and concentrations of inspired oxygen around different mean fractional concentration of inspired oxygen (FIO_2) levels, also seems to have an impact on development of ROP. It was observed in animal studies that variations around higher mean FIO_2 levels (mean 24% oxygen) had more severe vascular abnormalities than fluctuations around lower levels (mean 21% oxygen).[57] The studies also showed that breathing higher oxygen concentrations impaired retinal development to the extent of complete vessel ablation in 80% ambient oxygen.[58]

The effect of other biochemical mediators on ROP has also been studied. Increased carbon dioxide tension has been associated with development of ROP, although there have been conflicting reports.[59-61] Hypercarbia in the presence of hyperoxia and variable oxygen levels has been observed to increase the severity of ROP by causing vasodilatation and a resultant increase in blood flow and oxygenation to the retina. This increase leads to downregulation and decreased production of VEGF and a delay in the normal process of retinal vascularization.[62] Blood transfusion and erythropoietin have also been postulated as risk factors for ROP,[63,64] because of the effect on oxygen delivery to tissues and the increase in iron, a known oxidant.

Oxygen and the Brain

The effects of high inspired and arterial oxygen concentrations on immature brain cells and their signaling cascades are not completely understood. It has been known for more than 30 years from an animal study that cerebral vasculature constricts in response to hyperoxia, thus reducing cerebral blood flow.[65] The effects of oxygen on the brain are to some extent similar to those on the retina because the latter is a specialized part of the central nervous system and may share the same pathophysiologic processes. It has been suggested that cerebral damage and retinal damage have a common vasoreactive vascular origin.[66]

Various factors and mechanisms that influence oxygen radical disease of the newborn have been described. These include antioxidants, and the metabolism of glutathione, iron, and nitric oxide. In addition to lipid and protein oxidation, oxygen radicals may also induce neuronal damage through mitochondrial permeability transition and augmentation of the influx of calcium ion into mitochondria,[67] leading to necrosis or apoptosis. Redoxins and peroxiredoxins, which scavenge reactive oxygen species and other free radicals and thus protect from oxidative stress injury, are located in the inner mitochondrial membranes. Glutathione is the most abundant antioxidant and can regenerate other antioxidants.[68] It is also involved in regeneration of oxidized ascorbate and tocopherol, which have been linked with outcome in preterm infants.[69] In preterm babies the availability of glutathione and other antioxidants is limited, giving them a low capacity for detoxification. Nitric oxide (NO) in low concentrations is known to act as an antioxidant, but its reaction with superoxide leads to production of peroxynitrite, which has potential for deleterious effects on immature cellular structures in the neonatal brain.[70]

The effect of exposure to pure oxygen on the brain was described in an animal study as early as 1959. In this historic study, Gyllensten[71] found that rearing mice in pure oxygen for 20 to 30 days had a marked deleterious effect on subsequent cortical vascularization and cellular differentiation. A similar effect was observed on the growth of vessels into the frontal cortex in hamsters.[72] Another animal study also showed that the brain of the newborn rat grew less well when the animal was reared in 70% to 80% oxygen for the first 9 days.[73]

In humans, development of an extensive form of periventricular leukomalacia (PVL) is found to have a strong correlation with sustained hyperoxia.[74] More alarmingly, Ahdab-Barmada and coworkers[75] described pontosubicular lesions in the brains of infants who had PaO_2 values of more than 150 mm Hg in the first few weeks of life.[75] Haynes and colleagues[76] described oxidative damage to premyelinating oligodendrocytes in cerebral white matter as a mechanism of development of periventricular leukomalacia. In a large retrospective study of 1105 low-birth-weight infants by Collins and associates,[77] the risk of disabling cerebral palsy was found to be doubled in those exposed to hyperoxia. The adjusted odds for risk of cerebral palsy was eightfold higher in infants with the highest quintiles than in those with the lowest quintiles of oxygen exposure. Even short exposures to nonphysiologic oxygen levels were observed to trigger apoptotic neurodegeneration in the brain of infant rodents, and the vulnerability to oxygen neurotoxicity in the human was reported to extend from the sixth month of pregnancy to 3 years of age.[78]

Oxygen and the Lung

When bronchopulmonary dysplasia (BPD) was first described in preterm babies receiving mechanical respiratory support, oxygen toxicity was widely believed to be a major contributory factor.[79,80] In early reports the condition was typically seen only in babies exposed to 80% oxygen or higher for at least 6 days. Subsequent studies soon persuaded most people that pressure damage or "barotrauma" from mechanical ventilation was another major factor.[81,82] It was not long before clinicians had come to believe that pressure damage was the main cause.

Independent of mechanical ventilatory support, oxygen can cause lethal damage to the previously normal lung, as shown by an experiment involving 18-week-old lambs.[83] One group of lambs were allowed to breathe air, and another group breathed 100% oxygen. Half of each group were left to breathe spontaneously, and half were anesthetized and ventilated artificially. All the lambs breathing 100% oxygen died within 4 days, and respiratory support neither delayed nor hastened their death. The oxygen in the inspired gas, rather than the oxygen levels in the blood, proved damaging to the lungs in a study in 1970 that showed that cyanosis (created surgically by venoarterial shunt) in dogs failed to protect the lung from the consequence of breathing 100% oxygen at normal barometric pressure for 48 hours,[84] thus implying that oxygen is a direct toxin on the bronchial and alveolar epithelium.

In preterm babies, the effect of high inspired oxygen concentration as an important cause of BPD has been suggested.[85,86] Oxygen can damage the bronchial and alveolar epithelium as well as capillary endothelium, leading to alveolar edema, neutrophil infiltration, proliferation of alveolar cells, and fibrosis.[86] Furthermore, high levels of biochemical markers of oxidative stress have been identified in the pulmonary lavage in the first few days of life in preterm babies who later have BPD.[87]

Newborn infants and especially premature babies are more prone to oxidative stress[87] because they have a higher risk of exposure to high oxygen concentrations, reduced antioxidant defense, and more free iron, leading to production of hydroxyl radicals. The "oxygen radical disease of neonatology" may affect different organs, but the presentations depend on which organ is most vulnerable.[88] It is difficult to control all the pathophysiologic processes underlying oxidative stress injury in preterm infants.

"Normal" Levels of Oxygenation in Newborns

The fetus achieves normal growth in utero with arterial blood that is only about 70% saturated with oxygen (see Fig. 15-3). Children with cyanotic heart disease make the transition to extrauterine life without much difficulty with saturation levels sometimes as low as those in the fetus. However, the practice in neonatal care units over the past four decades has generally been to attempt to keep oxygen levels in "all" newborns in line with those of term and noncompromised preterm infants. Several studies have documented what are often termed "normal" or reference values for arterial oxygen saturation and or PaO_2 levels for both term and well preterm infants.[89-95] These studies demonstrate a relatively narrow range of normal baseline

SpO_2 values during the regular breathing state of the newborn. For preterm and term infants in the neonatal period, the value is 93% to 100%, and for older term infants, between 2 and 6 months of age, 97% to 100%. These data correspond with the few existing studies of arterial partial pressures of oxygen, which have demonstrated a mean PaO_2 of 70 to 76 mm Hg in term infants on days 2 through 7 of life.[96]

What is also known is that preterm infants, in particular those with prolonged dependency on supplemental oxygen, have lower baseline saturation levels,[97] more frequent desaturation episodes,[98] disturbed sleep patterns,[99] greater risk of pulmonary hypertension,[100,101] and higher rates of adverse pulmonary complications than preterm infants without chronic oxygen dependency or infants born at term.[102] What is not known, however, is whether these associations are causal. It remains unclear whether attempts to ameliorate the states previously described by oxygen administration, to reduce desaturation episodes, to decrease PaO_2 variability, or improve sleep, actually make any difference in long-term outcomes such as improving growth and development in infancy, or less serious adverse pulmonary complications, neurologic developmental complications, or death.

Optimal Levels of Oxygenation in Preterm Infants: Neonatal Period

Until recently, there had not been sufficient evidence to determine the optimal oxygen saturation or PaO_2 values to target for preterm infants who receive supplemental oxygen therapy in order to avoid potential oxygen toxicity while ensuring adequate oxygen delivery to tissues.

Three trials published more than 50 years ago clearly demonstrated the effect of unrestricted, high levels of ambient oxygen in causing severe eye disease in premature infants (Fig. 15-7).[1-3] One randomized trial involving 79 infants with "respiratory distress syndrome" was carried out by Usher[103] in Canada, comparing the "high" and "low" oxygen approaches as guided by oxygen tension. The high oxygen approach consisted of providing supplemental oxygen during the first 72 hours of life to maintain oxygen tension values of 70 to 100 mm Hg in arterial or 55 to 70 mm Hg in capillary blood. Such infants often received 60% to 100% oxygen therapy. In contrast, infants randomly allocated to the low oxygen approach received supplemental oxygen only when the arterial tension fell below 40 mm Hg or capillary tension fell below 35 mm Hg. Usher[103] demonstrated that a significantly higher proportion of infants randomly assigned to the "high oxygen approach" had radiologic changes indicating marked pulmonary infiltrates on serial chest radiographs taken during the first 72 hours. However, the combined risk difference in death

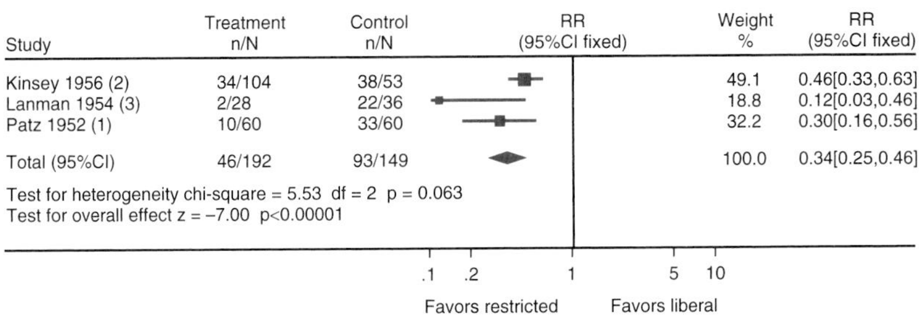

Figure 15-7 Forest plot showing the meta-analysis of three trials included in a 2003 Cochrane review on the use of restricted and liberal oxygen exposure in preterm/low-birth-weight (LBW) infants. CI, confidence interval; RLF, retrolental fibroplasia; RR, relative risk. (From Askie L, Henderson-Smart DJ: Restricted versus liberal oxygen exposure for preventing morbidity and mortality in preterm or low birth weight infants. *Cochrane Database Syst Rev.* 2003;(3):CD001076.)

Table 15-1 SUMMARY OF OBSERVATIONAL STUDIES SHOWING THE POTENTIAL BENEFITS OF LOWER SPO_2 TARGETING

Reference	Study Group	SpO_2 Ranges Compared	Survival	Chronic Lung Disease	ROP (stage 3-4)	ROP (treatment)
Tin et al, 2001[104]	≤27 weeks	Low: 80-90% High: 94-98%	53% 52%	18% 46% $P < 0.01$		6% 27% $P < 0.01$
Sun, 2002[105]	≤1500 g	Low: ≤95% High: >95%	83% 76%	27% 53% $P < 0.01$	10% 29% $P < 0.01$	4% 12% $P < 0.01$
Chow et al, 2003[106]	500-1500 g	Low: 85-93% High: 90-98 %	88% 81%		2.5% 12.5% $P < 0.01$	0-1.3% 4.4% $P < 0.01$
Anderson et al, 2004[107]	≤1500 g, >2 weeks old	Low: ≤92% High: >92%			2.4% 5.5% $P < 0.01$	1.3% 3.3% $P < 0.01$

ROP, retinopathy of prematurity.

15

observed in the early randomized trials from the 1950s was an absolute increase in in-hospital mortality of 49% in the oxygen-restricted groups.[18] In the 1960s, oxygen restriction became a common practice but was estimated to result in an excess of 16 deaths per case of blindness prevented.[17] Bancalari and colleagues,[21] using transcutaneous oxygen monitoring, were able to show that the incidence of ROP in infants who received continuous monitoring to prevent hypoxia and hyperoxia was similar to that in infants who were monitored by intermittent sampling.[21] However, for the subgroup of infants with birth weight more than 1100 g, there was a decrease in the incidence of ROP. There was no long-term follow-up. No randomized trials have been conducted to test the effect of restricting the level of oxygenation in preterm infants from or soon after birth until now (see later).

Evidence from several observational studies suggested that this hypothesis calling for a "restrictive oxygen approach" was worth exploring (Table 15-1).[104-107] A prospective observational study reported by Tin and colleagues[104] in 2001, involving every baby born alive before 28 weeks of gestation to mothers living in the north of England in 1990 through 1994, showed some fairly provocative findings. All the babies were born in or referred to one of five NICUs where the policies on the monitoring of oxygen saturation varied but several other care policies were fairly similar. Two of the five neonatal units had the same oxygen saturation monitoring policy; hence there were four different practices of oxygen monitoring during the study period. Rates of survival and of survivors without evidence of cerebral palsy at 18 months were almost identical in the five units in the 294 of 568 babies of 23 to 27 weeks of gestation (52%) who were still alive a year after birth. In one unit, target fractional oxygen saturation was 80% to 90% (with the lower alarm limit set to operate only if saturation fell below 70%) after the baby was more than 2 to 3 hours old. Such a policy was sustained for all babies thought to need supplemental oxygen until retinal vascularization was complete. In another unit, target functional oxygen saturation was 94% to 98% (with the lower alarm set to operate at 88%). The other three units had intermediate policies. Careful, uniform, ophthalmic review of all the survivors showed that retinopathy severe enough to merit treatment with cryotherapy occurred in 6.3% (95% confidence interval [CI] 1.7%-15.0%) of the babies in the first of these units, and 27.7% (95% CI 17.3%-40.2%) in the latter. No child from the first unit but 4 from the unit where target oxygen saturation was 94% to 98% became blind. The three units employing intermediate policies for target oxygen saturation had threshold retinopathy rates in the middle of this range (Fig. 15-8). In unit with the lower saturation target, half of the 64

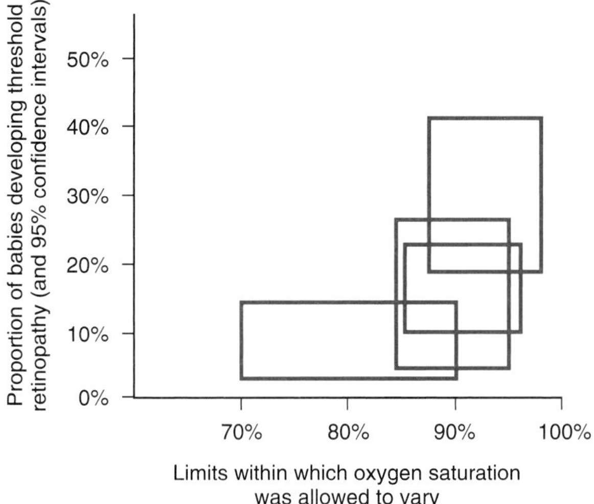

Figure 15-8 The relation between the limits within which oxygen saturation was allowed to vary and the proportion of 1-year survivors so nursed in whom "threshold" ROP later developed; A comparison of four policies. Staff aimed to keep oxygen saturation level in the upper half of the allowed range. (From Tin W, Milligan DWA, Pennefather P, et al: Pulse oximetry, severe retinopathy, and outcome at one year in babies of less than 28 weeks gestation. *Arch Dis Child.* 2001; 84: F106.)

long-term survivors were managed without endotracheal intubation and mechanical ventilation by 7 days and without supplemental oxygen by 30 days. In the unit where target oxygen saturation was 94% to 98%, these milestones were achieved by half the survivors in 21 and 72 days, respectively. There was no evidence that targeting much lower oxygen saturation in these preterm babies had an adverse effect on growth between birth and the time of discharge. In fact growth was curtailed twice as much in the higher oxygen saturation policy unit (possibly because nutritional intake was increased more cautiously in babies still requiring respiratory support). Neurodevelopmental outcomes were similar at 18 months (no child having been lost to follow-up).

Sun[105] collated data from a subset of hospitals that participated in a national evidence-based quality improvement collaborative for neonatology (Vermont Oxford Network), and compared the rates of survival, chronic lung disease, and severe retinopathy of prematurity of 1544 extremely low-birth-weight babies (500-1000 g) who were cared for in units that aimed to keep oxygen saturation at or below 95% and those that intended to keep saturations above 95% while these babies received supplemental oxygen. Sun[105] reported significantly lower incidences of chronic lung disease (27% vs. 53%) as well as stage III/IV ROP (10% vs. 29%) among babies cared for with targeted saturations of 95% or less. Survival rate was marginally higher in the low saturation group, but the difference was not statistically significantly (83% vs. 76%).

Chow and associates[106] reported their observations following the institution in 1993 of a detailed oxygen management policy that included strict guidelines in the practices of increasing and weaning of FIO_2 and the monitoring of oxygen saturation parameters in the delivery room, during inhouse transport of infants to the NICU, and throughout hospitalization. The main objectives were to avoid hyperoxia and repeated episodes of hypoxia-hyperoxia in very low-birth-weight infants. This approach, initiated at birth, included the avoidance of repeated increases and decreases of the FIO_2 and a change in previously used alarm limits. These researchers reported that following the implementation of these new management strategies, the incidence of ROP stage III/IV decreased consistently in a 5-year period from 12.5% in 1997 to 2.5% in 2001 and that the need for ROP laser treatment decreased from 4.5% in 1997 to 0% in the last 3 years. They adopted an SpO_2 range of 85% to 95% for infants born after 32 weeks of gestation at birth and a range of 85% to 93% for infants born before 32 weeks. In addition, some of their faculty members used a range of 83% to 93%. This study did not provide any prospective values of the SpO_2 ranges that were actually achieved in their infants, and thus it is uncertain whether their observed reductions in ROP were related to the altered Spo_2 changes or to overall changes in management over the period of the study. Although these observations are encouraging, the researchers did not report the complete neurodevelopmental outcomes and mortality data for the infants cared for during the period of the new oxygen guidelines, and in the absence of contemporaneous controls, these results cannot be considered as proof that the Spo_2 ranges used by this group are beneficial in terms of significant longer-term neurodevelopmental outcomes and survival.

A national survey of 144 NICU practices reported by Anderson and coworkers[107] in 2004 also showed significantly less stage III/IV ROP (2.4% vs. 5.5%) and retinal surgery (1.3% vs. 3.3%) in babies weighing less than 1501 g at birth in neonatal units where the upper alarm limit of pulse oxygen saturation in babies older than 2 weeks was either 92% or less or more than >92%. The rate of retinal surgery was 5.6% in NICUs using target levels higher than 98%.

In contrast to the report of these observational studies, Poets and associates[108] reported their observation on 891 babies of <30 weeks of gestation and admitted to two neonatal units, using different pulse oxygen saturation alarm limits (80%-92% vs. 92%-97%). Retrospective analysis of their data showed the incidence of ROP (more than stage 2) was significantly higher in the unit that used a lower alarm limit (13% vs. 6%) although no difference was seen in the incidence of ROP that required surgery.

The difficulty with all these observational studies, however, is that the association between target oxygen saturation and outcomes could be deemed causal as the design of the studies lacks the ability to compare groups in which the only difference was the oxygen targeting.

Optimal Levels of Oxygenation in Preterm Infants: Post-neonatal Period

Two randomized trials have been conducted to see whether it is beneficial to keep arterial oxygen saturation high in very preterm babies when they are more than a few weeks old. The Supplemental Therapeutic Oxygen for Prethreshold Retinopathy of Prematurity (STOP-ROP) study,[109] which recruited 649 babies born between 1990 and 1994 with a mean birth gestation of 25.4 weeks and a mean postmenstrual age at trial entry of 35 weeks, showed that keeping fractional oxygen saturation above 95% slightly reduced the number of babies with prethreshold retinopathy who went on to have disease severe enough to require retinal surgery. However, benefit was seen only in those without evidence of "plus disease" (dilated and tortuous vessels in at least two quadrants of the posterior pole) at recruitment (32% vs. 46%). More unexpectedly, targeting the higher oxygen saturation values significantly increased the number of infants who remained in the hospital, receiving supplemental oxygen, and undergoing diuretic therapy at a postmenstrual age of 50 weeks. Significant pulmonary deterioration after recruitment (13.2% vs. 8.5%) was seen only in those with more than average evidence of chronic lung disease at trial entry. The higher oxygenation target did not improve growth or the eventual retinal outcome, as assessed 3 months after the expected date of delivery.

The results of the Benefits of Oxygen Saturation Targeting (BOOST) trial were published in 2003.[110] The aim of this randomized, double-blind study was to see whether maintaining higher oxygen saturations rather than standard levels among oxygen-dependent preterm babies improved their growth and development. This study recruited 358 babies less than 30 weeks of gestation who remained in supplemental oxygen at 32 weeks postmenstrual age. Collaborating units had different policies with regard to optimum oxygenation in the period immediately after birth, but all monitored oxygen saturation using a prespecified Nellcor N-3000 pulse oximeter after recruitment for as long as supplemental oxygen was deemed necessary. Trial oximeters were specially modified (to allow masking) to keep targeted functional saturation in the range of either 91% to 94% or 95% to 98%, depending on allocation at entry, while displaying a targeted figure in the range 93% to 96%. This well-designed study showed no evidence that the growth and developmental outcome of the oxygen-dependent preterm infant was improved by keeping the functional oxygen saturation in the high range. This finding contradicts the substantial body of observational evidence that higher oxygen targeting can improve growth,[111,112] ameliorate sleep pattern abnormalities,[113] and reduce desaturation episodes.[97] In keeping with the observation in the STOP-ROP study, the BOOST trial also showed that infants with the higher oxygen saturation range had greater use of postnatal steroids (58% vs. 50%) and diuretics (52% vs. 44%), more readmissions (54% vs. 48%), and more pulmonary-related deaths (6% vs. 1%).

Although these trials lack the statistical power to assess their results reliably, the consistency of the direction of effect lends weight to the hypothesis that high concentrations of inspired oxygen in preterm infants in their postneonatal life may result in more pulmonary damage.

Approaches to Oxygen Therapy and Clinical Outcomes

Neonatal Mortality and Morbidity Outcomes

The beneficial effect of restricting oxygen therapy on ROP was evident more than 50 years ago. Universal restriction of oxygen therapy, rather than restricting the level of oxygenation in response to this evidence, was believed to be responsible for excessive mortality and morbidity in preterm infants as a result of hypoxic respiratory failure.[15,16] A time-series analysis of first-day infant mortality and still birth rates by Whyte,[114] however, suggested that oxygen restriction could not have been the only reason for the observed increase in mortality during that historical era. Later observational studies[104-107] already described have also suggested that the "restrictive" oxygen therapy compared with the "liberal" approach as guided by noninvasive, continuous pulse oxygen saturation monitoring shortly after birth was associated with significantly lower rates of severe ROP and BPD without the increase in mortality in preterm babies.

Impact of Neonatal Morbidities on Long-Term Outcomes

The prognostic impact of major neonatal morbidities, in particular severe ROP, BPD, and brain injury, is additive, and was shown to be independently correlated to poor outcome at 18 months of age. Schmidt and colleagues[115] reported that preterm babies who were free of these neonatal complications had an 18% risk of death or severe neurosensory impairment at 18 months, compared with a risk of 42% in babies who did have one of these complications, and 62% for those who had two. Babies with all three complications had a poor outcome rate as high as 88%.[115]

The prognostic effect of defined "threshold" ROP on visual outcome should not be underestimated. The ophthalmologic outcome at 10 years of children with birth weights less than 1251 g in whom ROP developed and who were randomly assigned to the Multicenter Trial of Cryotherapy of Prematurity (CRYO-ROP) was reported in 2001.[116] Visual outcome was described as "unfavorable" on the basis of functional outcome (near and distant visual acuity of 20/200 or worse) and structural outcome (posterior retinal folds or worse). Significantly fewer unfavorable outcomes were seen in "treated" than in "control" eyes (44.4% vs. 62.1%) at 10 years of age, and the benefit of cryotherapy for treatment of threshold ROP for both structure and function was maintained until 15 years of age.[117] It is, however, alarming to know that although cryotherapy lowers the risk of unfavorable outcome, more than 40% of infants had long-term visual disability. The results of these CRYO-ROP follow-up studies are likely to be applicable to the current practice of laser treatment for threshold ROP, considering that although a comparative study using historic controls showed that laser photocoagulation resulted in better structural outcome than trans-scleral cryotherapy,[118] a small but well-designed prospective randomized trial did not show any significant difference in visual outcomes at 3 years of age.[119]

Long-Term Outcomes at 18 Months and 10 Years

An observational study by Tin and colleagues[104] is the only published study that has provided data on neurodevelopmental outcome of all surviving children who received early neonatal care under different oxygen-monitoring policies. Findings from the initial follow-up showed that there was no difference in the rate of cerebral palsy (of any type or severity) among 294 survivors. Though important, this fact is still not entirely reassuring, considering that the use of a "restrictive" oxygen therapy approach in early neonatal life may have a negative impact on cognitive and intellectual functions, adaptive skills, and behavior, impairments that will not be apparent at about 18 months of age, when these children were first assessed.

The second follow-up of the same cohort by Bradley and associates[120] involved a total of 124 surviving children who had received early neonatal care under "restrictive" (target saturation 80%-90%) and "liberal" (target saturation 94%-98%) oxygen therapy approaches. Structured assessments were carried out of intellectual and cognitive function (Wechsler Intelligent Scale for Children, 3rd edition),[121] literacy and numeracy skills (Wechsler Objective Reading and Numerical Dimensions),[122] adaptive functioning (Vineland Adaptive Behavior Scale),[123] and behavior (Child Behavior Check List).[124] In addition, information on health (including vision) and education status was also collected. Children were seen at about 10 years of age, and the follow-up rate in this cohort was 96%. The mean score for full-scale IQ of all the 119 children assessed was about one standard deviation below the population mean. More children cared for with the "liberal" approach were found to have cognitive disability than those cared for with the "restrictive" approach (35% vs. 23%), and the mean full-scale IQ of children in the former group was eight points lower than in the latter. The scores varied very widely and showed a skewed distribution, and the difference between the two mean IQ scores was not statistically significant. A similar trend was seen for literacy and numeracy skills. There was also a noticeable but nonsignificant excess of children with very low scores (less than 2nd percentile) on the Vineland Adaptive Behavior Scale in the "liberal" approach group compared with the "restricted" group (34% vs. 20%). These results need to be interpreted with caution because they have not yet been subjected to rigorous scrutiny to see whether any perinatal factors (such as gestation at birth) or socioeconomic factors might be responsible for these observed differences. However, these findings provide reassurance to clinicians that it is highly unlikely that restrictive oxygen therapy, with an aim of keeping functional oxygen saturations between 80% and 90% in babies of less than 28 weeks of gestation until they no longer need supplemental oxygen or their retinal vasculature is fully developed, is associated with any disadvantages in terms of intellectual skills, academic achievements, adaptive functioning, and behavior among long-term survivors. Of 64 surviving children who had "liberal" oxygen therapy in the neonatal period, 5 were registered as blind at 10 years of age, but none of the 60 children in the "restrictive" oxygen therapy group had this degree of visual disability. According to the same definition used in the CRYO-ROP follow-up study,[116] 12.7% of the eyes of children in the "liberal" group had unfavorable visual outcome, compared with only 3% in the "restrictive" group, and this difference is highly significant. Despite cryotherapy, an unfavorable visual outcome was seen in 45% of the eyes that reached threshold ROP, highlighting once again the critical need for well-designed research to find more effective ways of treating ROP[125] and, more importantly, preventing ROP in these preterm babies.

Controversies in Oxygen Therapy

The most historic and arguably the most important of all the questions and controversies on oxygen therapy and monitoring in preterm babies, whether to use a "restrictive" or a "liberal" approach, is the main subject of this chapter. There are some other questions and controversies related to maintenance of oxygenation in preterm infants. Commonly asked questions are discussed in the following sections.

C

Respiratory Support for Convalescent Preterm Infants: CPAP or Oxygen?

The dilemma of using continuous positive airway pressure (CPAP) as an alternative to oxygen therapy in a preterm baby who needs respiratory support is not easy to address because positive airway pressure is also generated with the use of a high-flow nasal cannulas (HFNCs). Locke and associates[126] reported in 1993 that nasal cannulas can inadvertently generate a positive end-distending pressure and that an air-oxygen mixture delivered through nasal cannulas at a flow of 2 L/min can generate a mean pressure of 9.8 cm H_2O. Sreenan and coworkers[127] demonstrated that flow rates between 1.0 and 2.5 L/min given through high-flow nasal cannulas can generate positive distending pressure (measured as end-expiratory esophageal pressure) in management of low-birth-weight infants with apnea of prematurity, comparable to pressures delivered by conventional CPAP devices at 6 cm H_2O. Walsh and colleagues[128] reported a nested cohort study of 187 infants with birth weight less than 1250 g who were receiving oxygen via nasal cannulas. Fifty-two (27.8%) of the study infants were receiving minimal supplemental oxygen with an "effective FIO_2" of less than 30%. When subjected to room air challenge, 87 (46.5%) of study infants were weaned successfully to room air, and this success rate was as high as 72% for infants who were receiving an effective FIO_2 of less than 23% prior to room air challenge.[129] More interestingly, 7 out of 22 infants in this cohort who were receiving only room air with flow rates between 0.13 and 2.0 L/min failed the room air challenge, implying that resultant airway pressure due to the flow, rather than supplemental oxygen, may play an important part in contributing a clinical benefit in some infants perceived to be oxygen-dependent. The use of high-flow nasal cannulas with flow in excess of 1 L/min would demand further evaluation in the smallest infants to ascertain whether their natural airway orifices are capable of acting as intrinsic predictable blow-off valves to prevent the generation of excessive airway pressure.[130] There is no comparative study to answer the question "Is it better to keep a preterm baby on CPAP with room air or off CPAP with supplemental oxygen?" The knowledge of the relationship between flow and airway pressure delivered by high-flow nasal cannulas, the concept of "effective FIO_2,"[131] and the ability to calculate this value in preterm infants should help clinicians rationalize the choice of respiratory support for convalescent preterm infants.

Continuous Noninvasive Monitoring: Oxygen Saturation or Oxygen Tension?

The monitoring of oxygenation in the fetus or newborn demands a reliable way of estimating the oxygen content of blood. Although it is generally accepted that PaO_2 monitoring is the gold standard surrogate of tissue oxygenation in preterm infants, there is no clinical evidence to date to support this perception. Furthermore, PaO_2 monitoring has its inherent limitations, particularly the invasiveness and the risk of iatrogenic complications. Although continuous PaO_2 monitoring is feasible through an indwelling catheter, this method can be used for only a short time, and not throughout the period during which the preterm infant is vulnerable to oxygen toxicity as well as hypoxic damage. Moreover, PaO_2 monitoring provides only intermittent snapshots of oxygenation rather than a continuous trend in most clinical settings. Transcutaneous oxygen monitoring did overcome these limitations, but its clinical use has declined over the past decade for several reasons, including the regular need for calibration and local complications such as skin burns, particularly in extreme preterm babies. Pulse oximetry has become the standard technique for noninvasive oxygen monitoring. Studies have shown a good correlation between blood oxygen saturation and pulse oximeter saturation readings.[132,133] In newborns with high content of HbF, a small reduction of PaO_2 will be magnified into larger reductions in SaO_2 in the steep part of the oxygen-dissociation curve. Moreover, pulse oximeters are highly sensitive in detecting hyperoxia provided that

Box 15-1

$$\text{Functional saturation} = \frac{HbO_2}{HbO_2 + Hb} \times 100$$

$$\text{Fractional saturation} = \frac{HbO_2}{HbO_2 + Hb + CoHb + MetH} \times 100$$

oxyhemoglobin (HbO_2), deoxyhemoglobin (Hb), carboxyhemoglobin (CoHb), and methemoglobin (MetH)

type-specific alarm limits are set (based on whether the oximeter measures functional or fractional saturation) and a low specificity is accepted (Box 15-1).[134] However, pulse oximetry has its own technical limitations (e.g., motion artifacts, electromagnetic interference) and physiologic limitations in clinical situations, including hypotension, hypoperfusion, severe anemia, and dyshemoglobinemias.[135] The flat parts of the sigmoid oxygen-hemoglobin dissociation curve also highlight the lack of accuracy in reflecting true arterial Po_2 when the saturations are very high or very low. Although there is no consensus on whether $TcPo_2$ or Spo_2 is better as noninvasive monitoring, a questionnaire survey of 100 neonatal units in North America in the 1990s showed that 74% of the units were using pulse oximetry as the sole method of continuous monitoring,[136] and it is very likely that this trend will continue.

Optimum Oxygen Saturation in Preterm Infants: Does It Vary with Postnatal Age?

Knowledge of the pathophysiology of ROP often raises the question whether targeting higher oxygen saturation is desirable in preterm infants in whom prethreshold ROP develops. The well-designed randomized STOP-ROP trial, though not conclusive, suggested that "high saturation targeting" may benefit some infants with prethreshold ROP.[109]

Another issue often raised by the clinicians is the effect of blood transfusion or reduction in the content of HbF with advancing postnatal age on optimum oxygen saturations. The effects of HbF and HbA on P_{50} have already been described. The change in P_{50} after blood transfusion in preterm infants has not been thoroughly investigated. However, in one small study of preterm infants with a mean gestational age of 25.3 weeks, it was observed that the HbF content decreased from 92.9% to 43.5% within 2.8 days after transfusion.[137] This decrease was associated with a parallel and significant increase in P_{50} from 18.1 to 21.0 mm Hg. This knowledge of changes in P_{50} could be useful to predict the "optimum oxygen saturation range," but the clinical benefits of attempting to target this range at a different postnatal age or after blood transfusion remains debatable.

Resolving the Uncertainty: The Oxygen Saturation Trials

The lack of knowledge and ongoing uncertainty for more than 50 years about what is "normal" oxygenation for babies making the transition to extrauterine life, particularly when they are born very prematurely, has led on to wide variation of acceptance of what constitutes a safe minimum or maximum level of oxygenation for a small baby in the first few weeks of life. Figure 15-9 shows this variation in policies in the United Kingdom,[138] and the policies in the United States vary just as much.[136] Observational studies over the past 50 years have given us much information, but the only way to resolve the uncertainties and controversies of

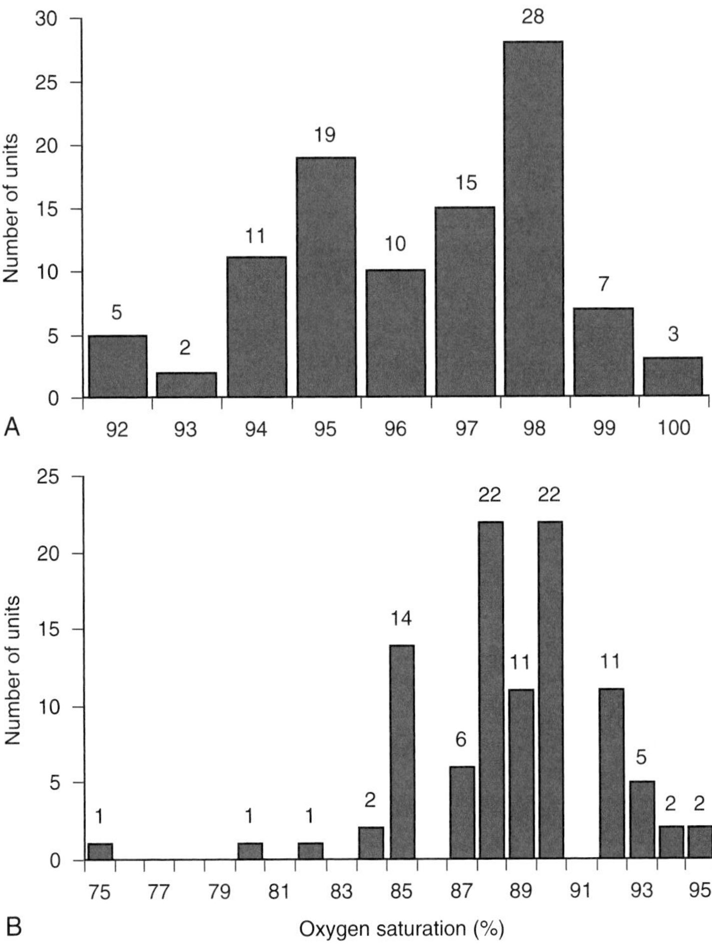

Figure 15-9 Oxygen saturation monitoring policies in the United Kingdom. Results from a telephone survey of 100 units with three or more intensive care cots caring for babies of less than 28 weeks of gestation in 2001. High (**A**) and low (**B**) oximeter alarm settings. (From Tin W, Wariyar U: Giving small babies oxygen: 50 years of uncertainty. *Semin Neonatol.* 2002;7:361.)

oxygen monitoring and therapy is to conduct large, well-designed randomized controlled trials.[139-141]

In response to the growing demand to resolve the controversy on oxygen therapy in very preterm babies, an international collaborative effort has been mounted to conduct large multicenter randomized trials to address the main research question: Does varying the concentration of inspired oxygen to maintain a "low" oxygen saturation range of 85% to 89% versus a "high" range of 91% to 95% in babies of less than 28 weeks of gestation from the day of birth until they are breathing air affect the incidence of (1) death or severe neurosensory disability at corrected age of 2 years; (2) retinal surgery for ROP; (3) the need for supplemental oxygen therapy or respiratory support at 36 weeks postmenstrual age; (4) patent ductus arteriosus requiring treatment (medical or surgical) or necrotizing enterocolitis requiring surgery; and (5) poor growth at 36 weeks postmenstrual age and at 2 years? The oxygen saturation trials across the continents are SUPPORT (The Surfactant Positive Airway Pressure and Pulse Oximetry Trial in Extremely Low Birth Weight Infants), BOOST II (Benefit Of Oxygen Saturation Targeting) trial (Australia), BOOST II trial (New Zealand), BOOST II trial (United Kingdom), and the COT (Canadian Oxygen Trial). All the trials use similar methods. There is a prospective agreement to combine the individual patient data from all the trials in order to increase the ability to detect much smaller differences in the primary outcome, and this controlled trial strategy of prospective meta-analysis[142] is likely to be established for the first time in neonatal medicine from these oxygen trials.

These trials used a design similar to that of SUPPORT.[4] They used masked randomization intervention and assessments. The strategy for blinding shown to be successful in the first Australian BOOST trial[110] helps to minimize co-intervention bias and outcome ascertainment bias. The target oxygen saturation range of the study Masimo Radical Oximeters (with the Signal Extraction Technology) was 88% to 92%, but these trial monitors were adjusted to display the "offset" saturation that is either 3% higher or 3% lower than the actual oxygen saturation, thereby producing two study groups with two different ranges of saturation. The allocated oximeter was used generally as long as oxygen saturation monitoring was required up to 36 weeks of gestation.

Infants of less than 28 weeks gestational age were eligible if they were less than 24 hours old. Inclusion and exclusion criteria were similar. Hospital death/severe ROP was the primary outcome in SUPPORT. The composite of death or major neurosensory disability at 2 years (corrected for prematurity) was the primary outcome in the other trials but will be analyzed in all the trials individually as in the meta-analysis. Uniform definition of major disability included: mental developmental index (MDI) using the Bayley Scales of Infant Development (BSID)[143] of less than 70 (<2 SD below mean), severe visual loss, not walking unaided because of cerebral palsy, and severe hearing loss requiring hearing aids. Other, secondary outcomes were (1) retinal surgery; (2) oxygen dependency at 36 weeks postmenstrual age; the need for supplemental oxygen by physiologic definition[130]; (3) duration of respiratory support (endotracheal intubation, nasal CPAP, supplemental oxygen); (4) patent ductus arteriosus; (5) necrotizing enterocolitis requiring surgery; (6) growth parameters at discharge and at 2 years; (7) hospital readmissions up to 2 years; (8) cerebral palsy; (9) visual impairment; (10) hearing loss; (11) mean MDI on the BSID; and (12) death after 4 weeks chronological age primarily due to pulmonary disease.

New Evidence on Oxygenation Targets in Preterm Infants

To date, SUPPORT Trial is the only one that has been reported in the peer-reviewed literature.[4] This trial enrolled 1316 infants. The baseline characteristics of the two treatment groups were comparable. The median and mean oxygen saturations differed substantially between the two groups. As expected, there was overlap of the achieved oxygen saturations. Furthermore, the duration of oxygen supplementation and the function of oxygen concentration exposure were lower in the lower oxygen saturation target group.

The rates of the composite primary outcome, severe ROP or death before discharge, did not differ significantly between the lower oxygen saturation group and the higher oxygen saturation group (28.3% and 32.1%, respectively; relative risk [RR] with lower oxygen saturation, 0.90; 95% CI, 0.76-1.06; $P = 0.21$) (Table 15-2). Death before discharge occurred in 130 of 654 infants in the lower oxygen saturation group (19.9%), compared with 107 of 662 infants in the higher oxygen saturation group (16.2%) (RR with lower oxygen saturation, 1.27; 95% CI, 1.01-1.60; $P = 0.04$; number needed to harm, 27). The distributions of the major causes of death did not differ significantly between the two groups. Similar results were observed by gestational age strata. The rate of severe ROP among survivors who were discharged or transferred to another facility or who reached the age of 1 year was lower in the lower oxygen saturation group (8.6% vs. 17.9%; RR, 0.52; 95% CI, 0.37-0.73; $P = <0.001$; number needed to treat, 11).

The rate of oxygen use at 36 weeks was less in the lower oxygen saturation group than in the higher oxygen saturation group ($P = 0.002$), but the rates of BPD among survivors, as determined by the physiologic oxygen saturation test at 36 weeks and the composite outcome of BPD or death by 36 weeks, did not differ

Table 15-2 SURFACTANT POSITIVE AIRWAY PRESSURE AND PULSE OXIMETRY TRIAL IN EXTREMELY LOW BIRTH WEIGHT INFANTS (SUPPORT): MAJOR OUTCOMES*

Outcomes	Lower Oxygen Saturations, no./total no. (%) (N = 654)	Higher Oxygen Saturations, no./total no. (%) (N = 662)	Adjusted Relative Risk (95% CI)
Severe retinopathy of prematurity or death before discharge	171/605 (28.3)	198/616 (32.1)	0.90 (0.76-1.06)
Severe retinopathy of prematurity	41/475 (8.6)	91/509 (17.9)	0.52 (0.51-0.73)
Death before discharge	130/654 (19.9)	107/662 (16.2)	1.27 (1.01-1.60)
BPD, physiologic definition, at 36 weeks†	205/504 (38.0)	237/568 (41.7)	0.92 (0.81-1.05)
BPD, physiologic definition, or death by 36 weeks†	319/654 (48.8)	331/662 (50.0)	0.99 (0.90-1.10)
Postnatal corticosteroids for BPD	61/636 (9.6)	69/644 (10.7)	0.91 (0.67-1.24)
Patent ductus arteriosus	307/641 (47.9)	324/648 (50.0)	0.96 (0.86-1.07)
Intraventricular hemorrhage, grade 3 or 4‡	83/630 (13.2)	81/640 (12.7)	1.06 (0.80-1.40)
Intraventricular hemorrhage, grade 3 or 4, or death‡	179/653 (27.4)	156/661 (23.6)	1.18 (0.99-1.42)
Necrotizing enterocolitis, stage ≥ 2§	76/641 (11.9)	70/649 (10.8)	1.11 (0.82-1.51)
Necrotizing enterocolitis, stage ≥ 2,or death§	176/654 (26.9)	155/662 (23.4)	1.18 (0.98-1.43)

BPD, bronchopulmonary dysplasia; CI, confidence interval.
*Values were adjusted for stratification factors (study center and gestational age group) as well as for familial clustering.
†The physiologic definition of BPD includes, as a criterion, the receipt of more than 30% oxygen or the need for positive pressure support at 36 weeks of gestation or, in the case of infants requiring less than 30% oxygen, the need for any oxygen at 36 weeks after an attempt at oxygen withdrawal.
‡There are four grades of intraventricular hemorrhage; higher grades indicate more severe bleeding.
§There are three stages of necrotizing enterocolitis; higher stages indicate more severe necrotizing enterocolitis.
Data from SUPPORT Study Group of the Eunice Kennedy Shriver NICHD Neonatal Research Network, Carlo WA, Finer NN, Walsh MC, et al: Target ranges of oxygen saturation in extremely preterm infants. *N Engl J Med*. 2010;27:362;1959-1969.

significantly between the treatment groups. Other prespecified major outcomes also did not differ significantly between the two groups (see Table 15-2).

The results of SUPPORT were shared confidentially with the data safety and monitoring committees of the other trials, leading to assessment of their results in view of the SUPPORT results. In December 2010, the BOOST-II UK, BOOST-II Australia, and BOOST-II New Zealand trials data were analyzed. The results revealed that preterm babies in whom oxygen was targeted to keep oxygen saturation in the range 91% to 95% were surviving more often than preterm babies in whom their oxygen was targeted to keep the range of 85% to 89%. The difference was so clear that it was extremely unlikely to change if the BOOST II trial continued to the end. For this reason, it was decided that no further babies should be entered into the trial and that babies currently in the trial should not continue in their allocated groups. This decision was communicated immediately to all of the participating neonatal units.

The results of the BOOST II trials and SUPPORT have been pooled and published.[144] The overall results showed that among 3631 infants, those randomly assigned to oxygen saturation targets of 91% to 95% had a higher survival rate than those assigned to oxygen saturation targets of 85% to 89% (mortality 17.3% vs. 14.4%; relative risk for survival associated with high oxygen saturation targets 1.21; 99.73 CI [as pre-specified in the protocol] 0.96 to 1.52; $P = 0.015$).

At present, caution should be exercised regarding the strategy of targeting oxygen saturation levels in the lower ranges used in these trials because it may lead to increased mortality. Until data on long-term outcomes and the prospective meta-analysis are available, it is more prudent to target oxygen saturations of 91% to 95% rather than 85% to 89%. Collaboration across three continents helped Campbell[12] identify the cause of retinopathy in the preterm baby more than 50 years ago. The successful international collaboration to mount the "oxygen saturation trials" and the strategy of prospective meta-analysis will provide further evidence on oxygenation targeting in preterm babies vulnerable to oxygen toxicity. However, clinicians should be aware that the current oxygen trials may not end the questions and controversies on oxygen, a powerful and the most commonly used "drug" in neonatal medicine:

> *The clinician must bear in mind that oxygen is a drug and must be used in accordance with well recognized pharmacologic principles; i.e., since it has certain toxic effects and is not completely harmless (as widely believed in clinical circles) it should be given only in the lowest dosage or concentration required by the particular patient.*
>
> **Julius Comroe (1945)**

15

References

1. Patz A, Hoeck LE, de la Cruz E. Studies on the effect of high oxygen administration in retrolental fibroplasia. 1. Nursery observations. *Am J Ophthalmol.* 1952;35:1248-1253.
2. Kinsey VE, Jacobus JT, Hemphill F. Retrolental fibroplasia: cooperative study of retrolental fibroplasia and the use of oxygen. *Arch Ophthalmol.* 1956;56:481-543.
3. Lanman TJ, Guy LP, Dancis J. Retrolental fibroplasia and oxygen therapy. *JAMA.* 1954;155: 223-226.
4. SUPPORT Study Group of the Eunice Kennedy Shriver NICHD Neonatal Research Network, Carlo WA, Finer NN, Walsh MC, et al. Target ranges of oxygen saturation in extremely preterm infants. *N Engl J Med.* 2010;27:362;1959-1969.
5. Stenson B, Broklehurst P, Tarnow-Mordi W, et al. Interim safety meta-analysis of survival at 36 weeks gestation in studies contributing to the NeOProM oxygen saturation targeting trials collaboration. E-PAS2011; 3123.4.
6. Priestley J. *Experiments and observations on different kinds of air.* London: J Johnson; 1775:101.
7. Scheele KW. Chemische abhandlung von der luft und dem feuer. Upsala and Leipzig, 1777. (See also the English translation: Chemical observations and experiments on air and fire; with an introduction by Torbern Bergman. London: J Johnson; 1780.).
8. Lavoisier A-L. Experiences sur la respiration des animaux. *Mém Soc Sci Paris..* 1777;2:185-194.
9. Tin W, Hey E. The medical use of oxygen: a century of research in animals and humans. *Neo Reviews.* 2003;4:340-349.
10. Wilson JL, Long SB, Howard PJ. Respiration of premature infants: response to variations of oxygen and to increased carbon dioxide in inspired air. *Am J Dis Child.* 1942;63:1080-1085.
11. Howard PJ, Bauer AR. Irregularities of breathing in the newborn period. *Am J Dis Child.* 1949;77:592-609.
12. Campbell K. Intensive oxygen therapy as a possible cause of retrolental fibroplasia: a clinical approach. *Med J Austr.* 1951;ii:48-50.
13. Crosse VM, Evans PJ. Prevention of retrolental fibroplasia. *Arch Ophthalmol.* 1952;48: 83-87.
14. Guy LP, Lanman TJ, Dancis J. The possibility of total elimination of retrolental fibroplasia by oxygen restriction. *Pediatrics.* 1956;17:247-249.
15. Avery ME, Oppenheimer EH. Recent increase in mortality in hyaline membrane disease. *J Pediatr.* 1960;57:553-559.
16. Cross KW. Cost of preventing retrolental fibroplasia? *Lancet.* 1973;2(7835):954-956.
17. Bolton DPG, Cross KW. Further observations on the cost of preventing retrolental fibroplasia. *Lancet.* 1974;1(7855):445-448.
18. Duc G, Sinclair JC. Oxygen administration. In: Sinclair JC, Bracken MB, ed. *Effective care of the newborn infant.* Oxford: Oxford University Press; 1992:178-199.
19. Yamanouchi I, Igarashi I, Ouchi E. Incidence and severity of retinopathy in low birth weight infants monitored by $TCPO_2$. *Adv Exp Med Biol.* 1987;220:105-108.
20. Grylack LJ. Transcutaneous oxygen monitoring and retinopathy of prematurity. *Pediatrics.* 1987; 80:973.
21. Bancalari E, Flynn J, Goldberg RN, et al. Influence of transcutaneous oxygen monitoring on the incidence of retinopathy of prematurity. *Pediatrics.* 1987;79:663-669.

C

22. Flynn JT, Bancalari E, Snyder ES, et al. A cohort study of transcutaneous oxygen tension and the incidence and severity of retinopathy of prematurity. *N Engl J Med*. 1992;326:1050-1054.
23. Hay W. The uses, benefits, and limitations of pulse oximetry in neonatal medicine: consensus on key issues. *J Perinatol*. 1987;7:347-349.
24. Walsh MC, Noble LM, Carlo WA, et al. Relationship of pulse oximetry to arterial oxygen tension in infants. *Crit Care Med*. 1987;15:1102-1105.
25. Southall DP, Bignall S, Stebbens VA, et al. Pulse oximeter and transcutaneous arterial oxygen measurements in neonatal and paediatric intensive care. *Arch Dis Child*. 1987;62:882-888.
26. Bucher HU, Fanconi S, Baeckert P, et al. Hyperoxemia in newborn infants: detection by pulse oximetry. *Pediatrics*. 1989;84:226-230.
27. Poets CF, Wilken M, Seidenberg J, et al. Reliability of a pulse oximeter in the detection of hyperoxemia. *J Pediatr*. 1993;122:87-90.
28. Cochran DP, Shaw NJ. The use of pulse oximetry in the prevention of hyperoxaemia in preterm infants. *Eur J Pediatr*. 1995;154:222-224.
29. Brockway J, Hay WW. Prediction of arterial partial pressure of oxygen with pulse oxygen saturation measurements. *J Pediatr*. 1998;133:63-66.
30. Wasunna A, Whitelaw GL. Pulse oximetry in preterm infants. *Arch Dis Child*. 1987;62:957-958.
31. Blanchette V, Doyle J, Schmidt B, et al. Hematology. In: Avery GB, Fletcher MA, MacDonald MG, ed. *Neonatology, pathophysiology and management of the newborn*. Philadelphia: J.B. Lippincott; 1994:972-973.
32. Hlastala MP, Woodson RD. Saturation dependency of the Bohr effect: interactions among H^+, CO_2 and DPG. *J Appl Physiol*. 1975;38:1126-1131.
33. Barcroft J, Elsden SR. The oxygen consumption of the sheep fetus. *J Physiol*. 1946;105:26.
34. Beer R, Doll E, Wenner J. Shift in oxygen dissociation curve of the blood of infants in the first month of life. *Pflugers Arch*. 1958;265:526-540.
35. East CE, Dunster KR, Colditz PB. Fetal oxygen saturation during maternal breathing down efforts in the second stage of labour. *Am J Perinatol*. 1998;15:121-124.
36. Chua S, Yeong SM, Razvi K, et al. Fetal oxygen saturation during labour. *Br J Obstet Gynaecol*. 1997;104:1080-1083.
37. Goffinet F, Langer B, Carbonne B, et al. Multicenter study on the clinical value of fetal pulse oximetry: I. Methodologic evaluation. *Am J Obstet Gynaecol*. 1997;177:1238-1246.
38. Dildy GA, Clark SL, Garite TJ, et al. Current status of multicenter randomized clinical trial on fetal oxygen saturation monitoring in the United States. *Eur J Obstet Gynaecol Reprod Biol*. 1997;72: S43-S50.
39. Saling E. Fetal Pulse oximetry during labour: issues and recommendations for clinical use. *J Perinat Med*. 1996;24:467-478.
40. East CE, Colditz PB, Dunster KR, et al. Human fetal intrapartum oxygen saturation monitoring: agreement between readings from two sensors on the same fetus. *Am J Obstet Gynaecol*. 1996;174:1594-1598.
41. Nijland R, Jongsma H, Nijhuis J, et al. Arterial oxygen saturation in relation to metabolic acidosis in fetal lambs. *Am J Obstet Gynaecol*. 1995;172:810-819.
42. Avery ME. *The lung and its disorders*. Philadelphia: WB Saunders; 1974.
43. Guyton AC, Grainger HC, Coleman TJ. Autoregulation of the total systemic circulation and its relation to control of cardiac output and arterial pressure. *Circ Res*. 1971;28(Suppl 1):93-97.
44. Dudell G, Cornish JD, Bartlett RH. What constitutes adequate oxygenation? *Pediatrics*. 1990;85: 39-41.
45. Strang LB. The lungs at birth. *Arch Dis Child*. 1965;40:575-582.
46. Moss AJ, Emmanoulides GC, Adams FH, et al. Response of the ductus arteriosus and pulmonary and systemic arterial pressure to changes in oxygen environment in newborn infants. *Pediatrics*. 1964;33:937-944.
47. Born GV, Dawes GS, Mott JC. Oxygen lack and autonomic nervous control of the fetal circulation in the lamb. *J Physiol*. 1956;134:149-166.
48. Cassin S, Dawes GS, Ross BB. Pulmonary blood flow and vascular resistance in immature fetal lambs. *J Physiol*. 1964;171:80-89.
49. Dawes GS. Pulmonary circulation in the fetus and new-born. *Br Med Bull*. 1966;22:61-65.
50. Schulze A, Whyte RK, Way RC, et al. Effect of arterial oxygenation level on cardiac output, oxygen extraction, and oxygen consumption in low birth weight infants receiving mechanical ventilation. *J Pediatr*. 1995;126:777-784.
51. Rasanen J, Wood DC, Debbs RH, et al. Reactivity of the human fetal pulmonary circulation to maternal hyperoxygenation increases during the second half of pregnancy: a randomized study. *Circulation*. 1998;97:257-262.
52. Roth AM. Retinal vascular development in premature infants. *Am J Ophthalmol*. 1977;84:636-640.
53. Shweiki D, Itin A, Soffer D, et al. Vascular endothelial growth factor induced by hypoxia may mediate hypoxia-initiated angiogenesis. *Nature*. 1992;359:843-845.
54. Hellstrom A, Perruzzi C, Ju M, et al. Low IGF-1 suppresses VEGF-survival signaling in retinal endothelial cells: direct correlation with clinical retinopathy of prematurity. *Proc Natl Acad Sci USA*. 2001;98:5804-5808.
55. Smith LE. Pathogenesis of retinopathy of prematurity. *Semin Neonatol*. 2003;8:469-473.
56. Pierce EA, Foley ED, Smith LE. Regulation of vascular endothelial growth factor by oxygen in a model of retinopathy of prematurity [see comments] [published erratum appears in *Arch Ophthalmol*. 1997;115:427]. *Arch Ophthalmol*. 1996;114:1219-1228.

57. McColm JR, Cunningham S, Wade J, et al. Hypoxic oxygen fluctuations produce less severe retinopathy than hyperoxic fluctuations in a rat model of retinopathy of prematurity. *Pediatr Res*. 2004;55:107.
58. Phelps DL, Rosenbaum AL. Effects of marginal hypoxemia on recovery from oxygen induced retinopathy in the kitten model. *Pediatrics*. 1984;73:1-6.
59. Shohat M, Reisner SH, Krikler R, et al. Retinopathy of prematurity: incidence and risk factors. *Pediatrics*. 1983;72:159-163.
60. Tsuchiya S, Tsuyama K. Retinopathy of prematurity: birth weight, gestational age and maximum $PaCO_2$. *Tokai J Exp Clin Med*. 1987;12:39-42.
61. Brown DR, Milley JR, Ripepi UJ, et al. Retinopathy of prematurity. Risk factors in a five year cohort of critically ill premature neonates. *Am J Dis Child*. 1987;141:154-160.
62. Berkowitz BA. Adult and newborn rat inner retinal oxygenation during carbogen and 100% oxygen breathing. *Invest Ophthalmol Vis Sci*. 1996;37:2089-2098.
63. Dani C, Reali MF, Bertini G, et al. The role of blood transfusions and iron intake in retinopathy of prematurity. *Early Hum Dev*. 2001;62:57-63.
64. Romagnoli C, Zecca E, Gallini F, et al. Do recombinant human erythropoietin and iron supplementation increase the risk of retinopathy of prematurity? *Eur J Pediatr*. 2000;159:627-628.
65. Kennedy C, Grave GD, Jehle JW. Effect of hyperoxia on the cerebral circulation of the newborn puppy. *Pediatr Res*. 1971;5:659-667.
66. Fledelius HC. Central nervous system damage and retinopathy of prematurity: an ophthalmic follow-up of prematures born in 1982-84. *Acta Paediatr*. 1996;85:1186-1191.
67. Rybnikova E, Damdimopoulos AE, Gustafsson JA, et al. Expression of novel antioxidant thioredoxin-2 in the rat brain. *Eur J Neurosci*. 2000;12:1669-1678.
68. Nangia S, Saili A, Dutta AK, et al. Free oxygen radicals: predictors of neonatal outcome following perinatal asphyxia. *Indian J Pediatr*. 1998;65:419-427.
69. Silvers KM, Gibson AT, Powers HJ. High plasma vitamin C levels at birth associated with low antioxidant status and poor outcome in premature babies. *Arch Dis Child*. 1994;71:F40-F44.
70. Issa A, Lappalainen U, Kleinman M, et al. Inhaled nitric oxide decreases hyperoxia induced surfactant abnormality in preterm rabbits. *Pediatr Res*. 1999;45:247-254.
71. Gyllensten L. Influence of oxygen exposure on the differentiation of the cerebral cortex of growing mice. *Acta Morphol Neerl Scand*. 1959;2:311-330.
72. Hannah RS, Hannah KJ. Hyperoxia: effects on the vascularisation of the developing central nervous system. *Acta Neuropathol*. 1980;51:141-144.
73. Grave GD, Kennedy C, Sokoloff L. Impairment of growth and development of the rat brain by hyperoxia at atmospheric pressure. *J Neurochem*. 1972;19:187-194.
74. Grunnet ML. Periventricular leukomalacia complex. *Arch Pathol Lab Med*. 1979;103:6-10.
75. Ahdab-Barmada M, Moosy J, Painter M. Pontosubicular necrosis and hyperoxaemia. *Pediatrics*. 1980;65:840-847.
76. Haynes RL, Folkerth RD, Keefe RJ, et al. Nitrosative and oxidative injury to premyelinating oligodendrocytes in periventricular leukomalacia. *J Neuropathol Exp Neurol*. 2003;62:411-450.
77. Collins MP, Lorenz JM, Jetton JR, et al. Hypocapnia and other ventilation related risk factors for cerebral palsy in low birth weight infants. *Pediatr Res*. 2001;50:712-719.
78. Felderhoff MU, Bittigau P, Sifringer M, et al. Oxygen causes cell death in developing brain. *Neurobiol Dis*. 2004;17:273-282.
79. Northway WH, Rosan RC, Porter DY. Pulmonary disease following respirator therapy of hyaline membrane disease: bronchopulmonary dysplasia. *N Engl J Med*. 1967;267:357-368.
80. Anderson WR, Strickland MB, Tsai SH, et al. Light microscopic and ultrastructural study of the adverse effects of oxygen on the neonate lung. *Am J Path*. 1973;73:327-348.
81. Reynolds EOR, Taghizadeh A. Improved prognosis of infants mechanically ventilated for hyaline membrane disease. *Arch Dis Child*. 1974;49:505-515.
82. Taghizadeh A, Reynolds EO. Pathogenesis of bronchopulmonary dysplasia following hyaline membrane disease. *Am J Pathol*. 1976;82:241-2264.
83. deLemos R, Wolfsdorf J, Nachman R, et al. Lung injury from oxygen in lambs. The role of artificial ventilation. *Anesthesiology*. 1969;30:609-618.
84. Miller WM, Waldhausen JA, Rashkind WJ. Comparison of oxygen poisoning of the lung in cyanotic and acyanotic dogs. *N Engl J Med*. 1970;282:943-947.
85. Jobe AH, Bancalari E. Bronchopulmonary dysplasia. *Am J Respir Crit Care Med*. 2001;163: 1723-1729.
86. Weingerger B, Laskin DL, Heck DE, et al. Oxygen toxicity in premature infants. *Toxicol Appl Pharmacol*. 2002;181:60-67.
87. Saugstad OD. Bronchopulmonary dysplasia: oxidative stress and oxidants. *Semin Neonatol*. 2003;8: 39-49.
88. Saugstad OD. Oxidative stress in newborn: a 30 year perspective. *Biol Neonate*. 2005;88:228-236.
89. Poets CF. When do infants need additional inspired oxygen? A review of the current literature. *Pediatr Pulmonol*. 2001;26:424-428.
90. Richard D, Poets CF, Neale S, et al. Arterial oxygen saturation in preterm neonates without respiratory failure. *J Pediatr*. 1993;123:963-968.
91. Poets CF, Stebbens VA, Alexander JR, et al. Arterial oxygen saturation in preterm infants at discharge from the hospital and six weeks later. *J Pediatr*. 1992;120:447-454.
92. Poets CF, Stebbens VA, Lang JA, et al. Arterial oxygen saturation in healthy term neonates. *Eur J Pediatr*. 1996;155:219.

93. Stebbens VA, Poets CF, Alexander JR, et al. Oxygen saturation and breathing patterns in infancy. 1. Full term infants in the second month of life. *Arch Dis Child*. 1991;66:569-573.
94. Poets CF, Stebbens VA, Alexander JR, et al. Oxygen saturation and breathing patterns in infancy. 2: Preterm infants at discharge from special care. *Arch Dis Child*. 1991;66:574-578.
95. Ng A, Subhedar N, Primhak RA, et al. Arterial oxygen saturation profiles in healthy preterm infants. *Arch Dis Child*. 1998;79:F64-F68.
96. Koch G, Wendel H. Adjustment of arterial blood gases and acid base balance in the normal newborn infant during the first week of life. *Biol Neonate*. 1968;12:136-161.
97. Sekar K, Duke JC. Sleep apnoea and hypoxaemia in recently weaned premature infants with and without bronchopulmonary dysplasia. *Pediatr Pulmonol*. 1991;10:112-116.
98. Singer L. Oxygen desaturation complicates feeding in infants with bronchopulmonary dysplasia after discharge. *Pediatrics*. 1992;90:380-384.
99. Fitzgerald D, Van Asperen P, O'Leary P, et al. Sleep, respiratory rate, and growth hormone in chronic neonatal lung disease. *Pediatr Pulmonol*. 1998;26:241-249.
100. Fitzgerald D, Evans N, Van Asperen P, et al. Subclinical persisting pulmonary hypertension in chronic neonatal lung disease. *Arch Dis Child*. 1994;70:F118-F122.
101. Subhedar NV, Shaw NJ. Changes in pulmonary arterial pressure in preterm infants with chronic lung disease. *Arch Dis Child*. 2000;82:F243-F247.
102. Giacoia GP, Venkataraman PS, West-Wilson KI, et al. Follow-up of school-age children with bronchopulmonary dysplasia. *J Pediatr*. 1997;130:400-408.
103. Usher R. Treatment of respiratory distress. In: Winters RW, eds. *Body fluids in pediatrics*. Boston: Little Brown; 1973:303-337.
104. Tin W, Milligan DWA, Pennefather P, et al. Pulse oximetry, severe retinopathy, and outcome at one year in babies of less than 28 weeks gestation. *Arch Dis Child*. 2001;84:F106-F110.
105. Sun SC. Relation of target SpO_2 levels and clinical outcome in ELBW infants on supplemental oxygen. *Pediatr Res*. 2002;51:350.
106. Chow L, Wright KW, Sola S. Can changes in clinical practice decrease the incidence of severe retinopathy in very low birth weight infants? *Pediatrics*. 2003;111:339-345.
107. Anderson CG, Benitz WE, Madan A. Retinopathy of prematurity and pulse oximetry: A national survey of recent practices. *J Perinatol*. 2004;24:164-168.
108. Poets C, Arand J, Hummler H, et al. Retinopathy of prematurity: a comparison between two centers aiming for different pulse oximetry saturation levels. *Biol Neonate*. 2003;84:267.
109. The STOP-ROP Multicenter Study Group. Supplemental Therapeutic Oxygen for Prethreshold Retinopathy of Prematurity (STOP-ROP), a randomized, controlled trial. I. Primary outcomes. *Pediatrics*. 2000;105:295-310.
110. Askie LM, Henderson-Smart DJ, Irwig L, et al. Oxygen-saturation targets and outcomes in extremely preterm infants. *N Engl J Med*. 2003;349:953-961.
111. Groothuis JR, Rosenberg AA. Home oxygen promotes weight gain in infants with bronchopulmonary dysplasia. *Am J Dis Child*. 1987;141:992-995.
112. Hudak BB, Allen MC, Hudak ML, et al. Home oxygen therapy for chronic lung disease in extremely low-birthweight infants. *Am J Dis Child*. 1989;143:357-360.
113. Simakajornboon N, Beckerman RC, Mack C, et al. Effect of supplemental oxygen on sleep architecture and cardiorespiratory events in preterm infants. *Pediatrics*. 2002;110:884-888.
114. Whyte RK. First day neonatal mortality since 1935: re-examination of Cross hypothesis. *BMJ*. 1992;304:343-346.
115. Schmidt B, Asztalos EV, Roberts RS, et al; Trial of Indomethacin Prophylaxis in Preterms (TIPP) Investigators: Impact of bronchopulmonary dysplasia, brain injury, and severe retinopathy on the outcome of extremely low-birth-weight infants at 18 months: results from the trial of indomethacin prophylaxis in preterms. *JAMA*.. 2003;289:1124-1129.
116. Cryotherapy for Retinopathy of Prematurity Cooperative Group. Multicenter Trial of Cryotherapy for Retinopathy of Prematurity: Ophthalmological outcomes at 10 years. *Arch Ophthalmol*. 2001;119:1110-1118.
117. Palmer EA, Hardy RJ, Dobson V, et al; Cryotherapy for Retinopathy of Prematurity Cooperative Group:15-year outcomes following threshold retinopathy of prematurity: final results from the Multicenter Trial of Cryotherapy for Retinopathy of Prematurity. *Arch Ophthalmol*. 2005;123: 311-318.
118. Pearce IA, Pennie FC, Gannon LM, et al. Three year visual outcome for treated stage 3 retinopathy: cryotherapy versus laser. *Br J Ophthalmol*. 1998;82:1254-1259.
119. White JE, Repka MX. Randomised comparison of diode laser photocoagulation versus cryotherapy for threshold retinopathy of prematurity: three year outcome. *J Pediatr Ophthalmol Strabismus*. 1997;34:83-87.
120. Bradley S, Anderson K, Tin W, et al. Early oxygen exposure and outcome at 10 years in babies of less than 28 weeks. *Pediatr Res*. 2004;55:373.
121. Wechsler D. *Intelligence Scale for Children*. San Antonio, Texas: Psychological Corporation; 1991.
122. Wechsler D. *Wechsler Objective Reading Dimension Test*. Sidcup, UK: Psychological Corporation; 1993.
123. Sparrow SS, Balla DA, Cicchetti DV. *Vineland adaptive behavior scales: Interview Edition Survey Forms Manual*. Circle Pines, MN: American Guidance Service; 1984.
124. Achenbach TM, Edelbrock C. *Manual for the child behavior checklist and revised child behavior profile*. Burlington, Vermont: Queen City Printers; 1983.

C

125. Early Treatment for Retinopathy of Prematurity Cooperative Group. Revised indications for the treatment of retinopathy of prematurity: results of the early treatment for retinopathy of prematurity randomized trial. *Arch Ophthalmol.* 2003;121:1684-1696.
126. Locke RG, Wofson MR, Shaffer TH, et al. Inadvertent administration of positive end-distending pressure during nasal cannula flow. *Pediatrics.* 1993;91:135-138.
127. Sreenan C, Lemke RP, Hudson-Mason A, et al. High-flow nasal cannulae in the management of apnea of prematurity: a comparison with conventional nasal continuous positive airway pressure. *Pediatrics.* 2001;107:1081-1083.
128. Walsh M, Engle W, Laptook A, et al. Oxygen delivery through nasal cannulae to preterm infants: can practice be improved? *Pediatrics.* 2005;116:857-861.
129. Walsh MC, Wilson-Costello D, Zadell A, et al. Safety, reliability, and validity of a physiologic definition of bronchopulmonary dysplasia. *J Perinatol.* 2003;23:451-456.
130. Finer NN. Nasal cannula use in the preterm infant: oxygen or pressure? *Pediatrics.* 2005;116: 1216-1217.
131. Benaron DA, Benitz WE. Maximizing the stability of oxygen delivered via nasal cannula. *Arch Pediatr Adolesc Med.* 1994;148:294-300.
132. Major D, Masson M. Estimation of PaO_2 using pulsatile oximetry and the HbO_2 dissociation curve in the premature infant. *Union Med Can.* 1989;118:21-22.
133. Walsh MC, Noble LM, Carlo WA, et al. Relationship of pulse oximetry to arterial oxygen tension in infants. *Crit Care Med.* 1987;15:1102-1105.
134. Bucher H, Fanconi S, Baeckert P, et al. Hyperoxemia in newborn infants: detection by pulse oximetry. *Pediatr.* 1989;84:226-230.
135. Moyle JTB. Limitations. In: Hahn CEW, Adams AP, ed. *Principles and practice series: pulse oximetry.* Plymouth: BMJ Publications; 1998.
136. Vijayakumar E, Ward GJ, Bullock CE, et al. Pulse oximetry in infants <1500 gm at birth on supplemental oxygen: a national survey. *J Perinatol.* 1997;17:341-345.
137. Halleux V, De, Gagnon CG, Bard H. Decreasing oxygen saturation in very early preterm newborn infants after transfusion. *Arch Dis Child.* 2003;88:F163.
138. Tin W, Wariyar U. Giving small babies oxygen: 50 years of uncertainty. *Semin Neonatol.* 2002;7: 361-367.
139. Tin W. Oxygen therapy: 50 years of uncertainty. *Pediatrics.* 2002;110:615-616.
140. Cole CH, Wright KW, Tarnow-Mordi W, et al. Resolving our uncertainty about oxygen therapy. *Pediatrics.* 2003;112:1415-1419.
141. Silverman WA. A cautionary tale about supplemental oxygen: the albatross of neonatal medicine. *Pediatrics.* 2004;113:394-396.
142. Simes RJ. Prospective meta-analysis of cholesterol-lowering studies: the Prospective Pravastatin Pooling (PPP) Project and the Cholesterol Treatment Trialists (CTT) Collaboration. *Am J Cardiol.* 1995;76:122-126.
143. Bayley N. *Manual for the Bayley Scales of Infant Development.* 3rd ed. San Antonio, Texas: Psychological Corporation; 2006.
144. Stenson B, Brocklehurst P, Tarnow-Mordi W. Increased 36-week survival with high oxygen saturation target in extremely preterm infants. *N Engl J Med.* 2011;364:1680-1682.

CHAPTER 16

Hypoxemic Episodes in the Premature Infant: Causes, Consequences, and Management

Nelson Claure, MSc, PhD, and Eduardo Bancalari, MD

- Mechanisms
- Management of Hypoxemia Spells in Ventilated Infants
- Episodes of Hypoxemia after Extubation
- Consequenes of Hypoxemia Episodes in the Premature Infant
- Summary

A large proportion of preterm infants undergoing mechanical ventilation presents with significant respiratory instability. This instability leads to fluctuations in gas exchange that make the preterm infant vulnerable to episodes of hypoxemia and bradycardia and therefore to the short- and long-term consequences of these episodes. The episodes often complicate the management of the premature infant and can prolong the mechanical ventilatory support and oxygen supplementation, both of which are associated with long-term sequelae in preterm infants.

Newer insights on the predisposing factors and mechanisms leading to respiratory instability and spells in mechanically ventilated premature infants continue to emerge from laboratory and clinical research and illustrate their complexity and the difficulties in their management. The mechanisms causing these episodes of hypoxemia, their clinical management, and their possible consequences are discussed in the following sections.

Mechanisms

In contrast to episodes of hypoxemia occurring in spontaneously breathing infants or infants receiving nasal continuous positive airway pressure (CPAP) who present with central or obstructive apnea, the occurrence of spontaneous episodes of hypoxemia in mechanically ventilated infants is often perplexing because these episodes occur in spite of the continued cycling of the ventilator and patency of the airway. The episodes of hypoxemia are characterized by a rapidly declining oxygen saturation (SpO_2) that becomes more frequent in mechanically ventilated infants with evolving or established chronic lung disease who require supplemental oxygen.[1,2]

The mechanisms that trigger these episodes involve an acute decrease in lung volume followed by reduced lung compliance and increased airway resistance, which impair ventilation and consequently lead to a decrease in oxygenation.[3,4] This process is illustrated in Figure 16-1. These acute changes in lung volume and ventilation are caused by a forceful expiratory maneuver. Electromyographic measurements showed that these forceful exhalations are caused by contraction of the abdominal muscles that produces a marked increase in abdominal and intrathoracic pressure.[5] Moreover, repeated and forceful contractions of the abdominal muscles prolong the hypoxemia episodes and increase their severity, as shown in Figure 16-2. In ventilated infants, the endotracheal tube bypasses the glottis and therefore

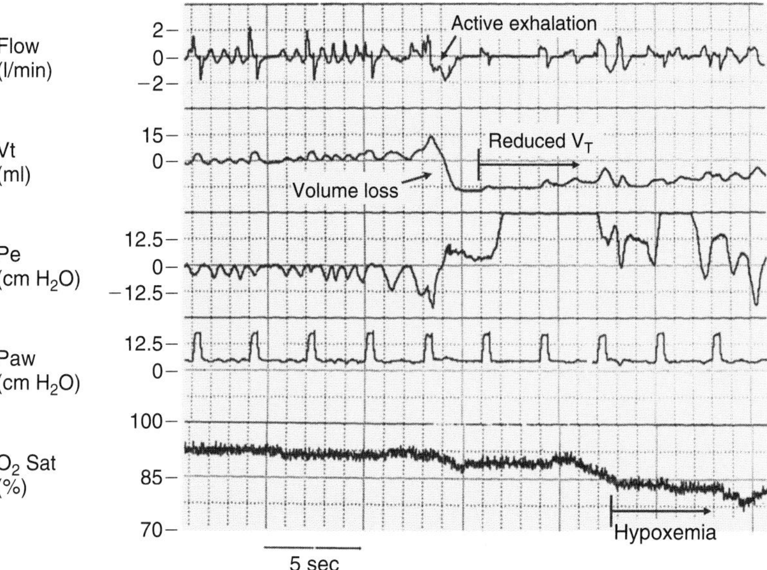

Figure 16-1 Mechanism triggering an episode of hypoxemia in a ventilated infant. Recordings of flow, tidal volume (V_T), esophageal pressure (Pe), airway pressure (Paw), and oxygen saturation (SpO_2) illustrate the mechanism triggering hypoxemia. At first, an active exhalation produces an increase in intrathoracic pressure and a loss in end-expiratory lung volume that is followed by a period of reduced VT in spite of continuous cycling of the ventilator. This results in a decline in SpO_2 and the start of hypoxemia. (From Bolivar JM, Gerhardt T, Gonzalez A, et al: Mechanisms for episodes of hypoxemia in preterm infants undergoing mechanical ventilation. *J Pediatr.* 1995;127:767-773.)

renders useless the upper airway's function to protect lung volume against a rise in intrathoracic pressure.

The reasons that ventilated infants have these forceful exhalations leading to loss in lung volume and hypoventilation are not always clear known. However, the primary trigger of hypoxemia spells in intubated infants seem to be related more to factors that affect the behavior of the infants. Increased body activity, agitation, and squirming are frequently noted in these infants moments prior to the onset of the

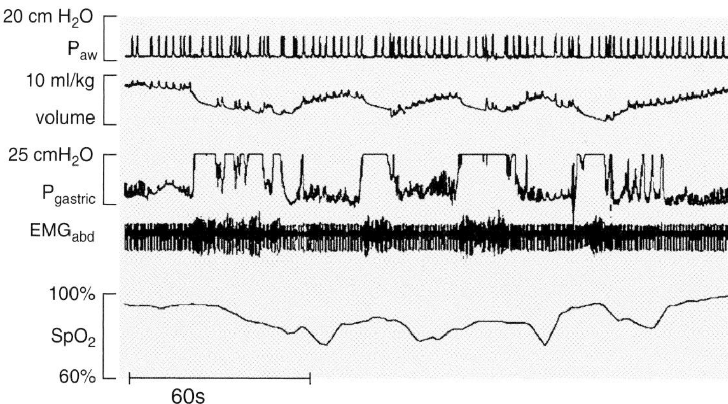

Figure 16-2 Episode of hypoxemia associated with multiple contractions of the abdominal muscles. Recording shows repeated contractions of the abdominal muscles detected by abdominal electromyography(EMG_{abd}) producing increases in gastric pressure ($P_{gastric}$). Each contraction is associated with a decline in end-expiratory lung volume and an acute reduction in tidal volume in spite of continuous cycling of the ventilator that is followed by a progressive decline in oxygen saturation (SpO_2). Paw, airway pressure; s, seconds. (From Esquer C, Claure N, D'Ugard C, et al: Role of abdominal muscles activity on duration and severity of hypoxemia episodes in mechanically ventilated preterm infants. *Neonatology.* 2007;92:182-186.)

hypoxemia spells. Increased body activity accompanied by cardiac acceleration has been reported to precede hypoxemia spells in ventilated infants.[2] More periods of hypoxemia have been observed during awake or indeterminate sleep states than in quiet or active sleep.[6] These findings are important because indeterminate sleep is considered to be the most common sleep state in preterm infants. Prone position has also been associated with fewer spells and shorter duration of hypoxemia than supine position.[7-9]

The combination of increased activity leading to respiratory disturbances and poor lung function due to the underlying lung disease may aggravate the frequency and severity of the hypoxemia episodes. In addition to the bypass of the glottis by the endotracheal tube, the low functional residual capacity and a not fully effective surfactant function characteristic of these infants may increase the likelihood of reaching closing volume in some areas of the lung with even small decreases in lung volume, and the increased surface tension impedes recovery of lung volume.

The decline in $Sp{O_2}$ during these episodes of hypoxemia is more abrupt than what is expected from a decline in ventilation alone, and hypoxemia often persists for some time after minute ventilation has been restored to basal levels.[2] This observation suggests that the initial loss in lung volume and hypoventilation may produce ventilation-perfusion inequalities and some degree of intrapulmonary shunting causing a rapid decline in $Sp{O_2}$. The initial hypoxemia can also provoke an increase in pulmonary vascular resistance and induce right-to-left shunting through extrapulmonary channels. These circulatory changes can explain why these hypoxemia episodes are more commonly observed in infants with some degree of underlying chronic lung disease and increased pulmonary vasculature reactivity. In many of these infants, normoxemia is restored only after the fraction of inspired oxygen ($F{IO_2}$) is increased, a change that may restore oxygenation not only by increasing the alveolar-arterial oxygen gradient but also by attenuating the hypoxia-induced pulmonary vasoconstriction.

Management of Hypoxemia Spells in Ventilated Infants

Ventilatory Strategies

Because the trigger events leading to hypoxemia spells in preterm infants primarily involve changes in lung volume and ventilation, clinicians often resort to higher levels of mechanical ventilatory support in an effort to reduce their frequency or severity. This measure, however, may be of limited efficacy and could carry unwanted consequences. The increase in ventilator settings may involve higher levels of positive end-expiratory pressure (PEEP), ventilator rate, or peak inspiratory pressure (PIP). A higher PEEP may ameliorate the loss in lung volume but it is unlikely to be effective in preventing it because conventional PEEP levels are considerably smaller than the rise in intrathoracic pressure observed during forceful contraction of the abdominal muscles.[3] Higher PIP or ventilator rates can be effective in attenuating the severity of the hypoxemia to a certain extent, but they carry the unwanted effects of providing an excessive support during periods when the infant does not present with episodes of hypoxemia. Avoidance of infant-ventilator asynchrony has been described as effective in reducing hypoxemia in preterm infants, possibly by reducing so-called fighting the ventilator.[10]

Volume-targeted ventilation can automatically adjust the ventilator PIP to maintain a set target tidal volume (V_T). On the basis of this effect, the efficacy of volume-targeted ventilation in attenuating the decreases in V_T and ventilation that precede the episodes of hypoxemia was evaluated in preterm infants. Figure 16-3 shows a typical response of volume-targeted ventilation during an acute decrease in V_T. The automatic rise in PIP during volume-targeted ventilation attenuated the decrease in ventilation, reducing the severity and duration of the episodes of hypoxemia but failing to prevent them.[11,12] This accomplishment, however, required setting a larger target V_T than that delivered by the ventilator during conventional pressure-limited

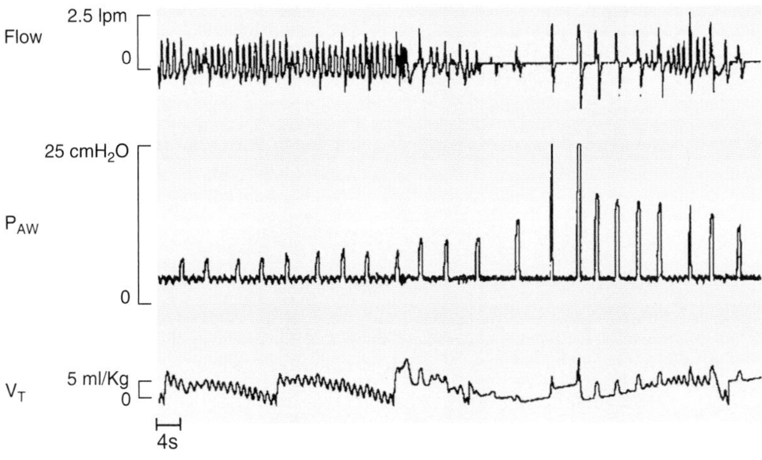

Figure 16-3 Recording of flow, airway pressure (P_{AW}), and tidal volume (V_T) during volume-targeted ventilation shows an automatic increase in peak pressure in response to an acute decline in V_T. This increase was followed by a gradual downward adjustment in pressure as V_T recovered.

ventilation. The larger target exposed the infants to greater V_T and higher PIP during long periods when ventilation was stable.

Automatic adjustment of the ventilator cycling frequency to maintain minute ventilation above a certain level or when Spo_2 declines below a threshold has also been shown effective in reducing the duration of the hypoxemia spells.[13,14] The potential benefit of this strategy is that it involves only a transient increase in ventilator rate. A more effective approach in attenuating the acute changes in ventilation that trigger hypoxemia spells appears to be that of a combined automatic adjustment of PIP and ventilator rate to maintain a target V_T and a minute ventilation level, respectively. The simultaneous increase in ventilator PIP and rate was shown to be more effective in attenuating hypoxemia in an animal model of hypoxemia spells, but this strategy has not been evaluated in infants.[15]

Supplemental Oxygen

The most common response to hypoxemia spells during routine clinical care is a transient increase in Fio_2 until hypoxemia resolves. Frequently, the increase in Fio_2 is excessive or lasts longer than necessary, leading to periods of hyperoxemia. It has been observed that high basal levels of Spo_2 are maintained during routine care to attenuate the frequency or severity of the spells,[16] but this measure is not consistently effective and increases the exposure to high Fio_2, as illustrated in Figure 16-4.

In preterm infants, the respiratory instability that leads to fluctuations in Spo_2 and an often inadequate management of Fio_2 are important limiting factors for the maintenance of Spo_2 within a clinically desired range. The efficacy of the clinical staff in maintaining Spo_2 within the intended range declines with postnatal age[17] as the frequency of episodes of hypoxemia increases.[18] As expected, the efficacy is also influenced by the staff-to-patient ratio.[19]

Systems that automatically adjust Fio_2 have been evaluated in ventilated preterm infants with frequent episodes of hypoxemia.[20-22] In these infants, automatic Fio_2 control is more effective than a fully dedicated nurse and the clinical staff in maintaining Spo_2 within the target range but does not abolish hypoxemia. The reason is that these systems respond only to the hypoxemia and do not prevent the spells, only attenuating their severity and duration. In fact, the frequency of milder episodes of hypoxemia was found to be higher during automatic adjustment of Fio_2 than with routine manual adjustments by the neonatal intensive care unit (NICU) staff. Automatic control was associated with a considerable reduction in hyperoxemia, which illustrates how prevalent the tolerance of high Spo_2 levels is during routine neonatal

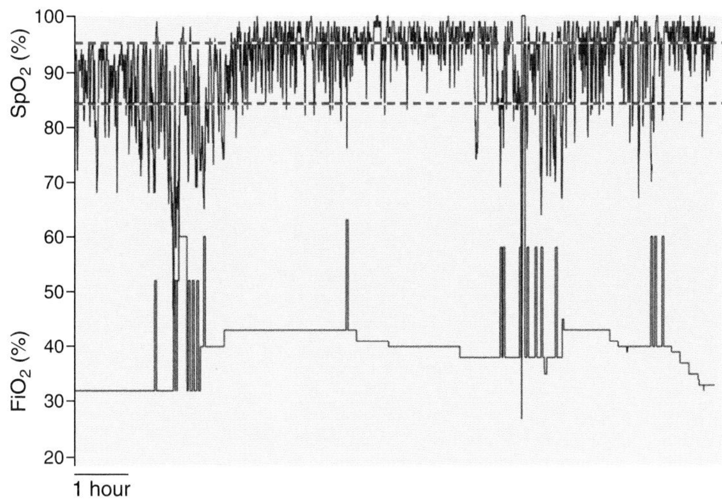

Figure 16-4 Changes in baseline fraction of inspired oxygen (FIO_2) in a ventilated infant with frequent episodes of hypoxemia. Recording from an infant with frequent episodes of hypoxemia shows the response of the caregiver, who first increased FIO_2 transiently when oxygen saturation (SpO_2) decreased into hypoxemia (lower red dashed line). Subsequently, the prolonged increase in the baseline FIO_2 reduced the severity of the fluctuations but also led to hyperoxemia (*upper red dashed line*). Later, the severity of the episodes of hypoxemia increased in spite of the higher baseline FIO_2.

16

intensive care, often inducing severe hyperoxemia in an attempt to prevent hypoxemia spells. However, this strategy is not effective in reducing the frequency and duration of the more severe hypoxemia spells and bradycardia, which are controlled more effectively during automated FIO_2 adjustments.

The data obtained in these studies illustrate the workload involved in maintaining oxygenation in infants with frequent hypoxemia spells. In these infants, a mean of 30 manual adjustments of FIO_2 per hour were conducted by a fully dedicated nurse and 112 adjustments per day by the routine staff in an attempt to keep SpO_2 within the target.

Behavioral Disturbances

None of the strategies mentioned before has been shown effective in preventing the hypoxemia spells. The reason may be the fact that the primary trigger of these spells in the intubated infant is more frequently related to factors that affect the infant's behavior than to pulmonary changes. Observations of less hypoxemia during periods of sleep and with prone position[6-9] suggest the potential benefits of strategies to reduce behavioral disturbances, facilitate sleep, and promote spontaneous respiratory stability in preterm infants who exhibit frequent episodes of hypoxemia.

Episodes of Hypoxemia after Extubation

In some infants, these spontaneous episodes of hypoxemia persist after extubation while the infants are receiving nasal CPAP or breathing spontaneously. These hypoxemia spells were traditionally attributed to central or mixed apnea. However, it has now been shown that spells of hypoxemia in preterm infants after a prolonged course of ventilation are also triggered predominantly by forced exhalation, which causes a decline in lung volume followed by hypoventilation.[23] This mechanism is similar to that observed in intubated infants, as shown in Figure 16-5.

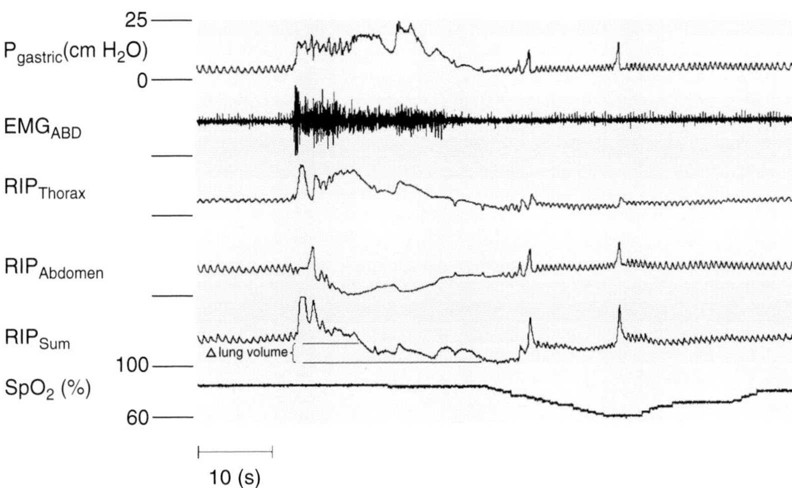

Figure 16-5 Mechanism triggering an episode of hypoxemia in a preterm infant after extubation. Recording from an infant breathing spontaneously shows a contraction of the abdominal muscles (recorded by abdominal electromyography [EMGabd]) that produced an increase in gastric pressure ($P_{gastric}$). This effect was also signified by a decline in the abdominal volume (measured by respiratory inductance plethysmography [$RIP_{Abdomen}$]) that coincided with an initial increase in thoracic volume (RIP_{Thorax}). After these events, a decrease in end-expiratory lung volume was noted in the summary of the thoracic and abdominal RIP bands (RIP_{Sum}) and a brief absence of spontaneous breathing. This was followed by a decline in oxygen saturation (SpO_2) that persisted for some time in spite of resumption of spontaneous breathing. s, seconds. (From Esquer C, Claure N, D'Ugard C, et al: Mechanisms of hypoxemia episodes in spontaneously breathing preterm infants after mechanical ventilation. *Neonatology.* 2008;94:100-104.)

The widespread use of central stimulants, which effectively reduce the occurrence of central apnea, may increase the proportion of episodes that are induced by forced exhalation and decreased lung volume. This possibility is supported by the findings of a trial showing that the administration of caffeine, although effective in treating central apnea, was not effective in reducing the frequency of hypoxemia spells.[24] Preterm infants who undergo a protracted course of ventilation may be more susceptible to lung volume instability because the prolonged presence of the endotracheal tube may affect the upper airway's ability to close and hence to prevent lung volume losses.

Consequences of Hypoxemia Episodes in the Premature Infant

The short- and long-term consequences of episodic hypoxemia in the preterm infant are often subject of debate and controversy. Concerns regarding the deleterious effects of hypoxemia are counterbalanced by the possible side effects of the interventions used for their management.

The changes in brain oxygenation that occur during episodes of hypoxemia are usually transient.[25-27] However, frequent episodes of severe hypoxemia or bradycardia may affect brain tissue oxygenation and possibly induce reoxygenation injury and oxidative damage, effects similar to those observed in animal studies of intermittent hypoxia.[28,29]

The long-term neurologic effects of hypoxemia spells in the preterm infant have not been clearly determined. Mild motor delays and slightly lower mental development quotients have been reported in infants with persistent hypoxemia due to apnea, and even poorer mental and motor development was associated with increasing frequency of apnea and hypoxemia spells.[30-34] The hypoxemia episodes occurring in ventilated infants or immediately after extubation are generally more severe and show a steeper decline in SpO_2 than the hypoxemia spells associated with apnea. Hence, the former are likely to have more striking effects on the central nervous system. However, a cause-and-effect relationship between hypoxemia spells and poor neurologic outcome is difficult to establish because the majority of infants who present with frequent hypoxemia spells also have other morbidities that are independently associated with poor outcome. Hypoxemia spells are more common in preterm infants with underlying lung and central nervous system diseases, and therefore, it is difficult to determine whether the spells are causing brain injury or merely reflect disease conditions associated with poor outcome.

In animal models of retinopathy of prematurity (ROP), fluctuations in oxygenation have been linked to abnormal retinal vasculature development, and more so when fluctuations involved swings into hyperoxia and hypoxia.[35-42] In preterm infants, the frequency of hypoxemia spells increases after the first postnatal week, and infants in whom severe retinopathy of prematurity develops present with more frequent spells especially beyond postnatal week 4.[18] Although this association does not necessarily imply causality, it indicates that further research is needed to confirm the finding.

Persistency of hypoxemia spells over long periods may have deleterious effects on lung growth and function with increased reactivity of the airways and lung vasculature.[43-45] The effects may be compounded by the increased exposure to supplemental oxygen to maintain a higher baseline SpO_2 to reduce episode frequency or when the increase in FIO_2 in response to an episode of hypoxemia is excessive or prolonged. In animal models, intermittent hyperoxia-hypoxia not only led to abnormal development of alveoli and lung vasculature but also impaired the development of the pulmonary antioxidant defenses and surfactant function.[46,47]

Summary

Episodes of hypoxemia are quite prevalent in the ventilated preterm infant, and the hypoxemia spells increase in frequency with postnatal age and chronicity of lung disease. Although there is inconclusive evidence of their effects on the infant's neurologic outcome, these spells cannot be considered benign and reflective only of immaturity and transient respiratory impairment that resolve over time.

These spells need to be evaluated in detail to possibly address their underlying causes and should be managed carefully, in particular when the interventions to control them have inherent risks. Avoidance of specific conditions leading to severe hypoxemia and hypoventilation is recommended. The paucity of data regarding the effects of hypoxemia spells on the preterm infant's developing central nervous system and other major organ systems should encourage more research in this area.

References

1. Garg M, Kurzner SI, Bautista DB, Keens TG. Clinically unsuspected hypoxia during sleep and feeding in infants with bronchopulmonary dysplasia. *Pediatrics*. 1988;81:635-642.
2. Durand M, McEvoy C, MacDonald K. Spontaneous desaturations in intubated very low birth weight infants with acute and chronic lung disease. *Pediatr Pulmonol*. 1992;13:136-142.
3. Bolivar JM, Gerhardt T, Gonzalez A, et al. Mechanisms for episodes of hypoxemia in preterm infants undergoing mechanical ventilation. *J Pediatr*. 1995 Nov;127:767-773.
4. Dimaguila MA, Di Fiore JM, Martin RJ, Miller MJ. Characteristics of hypoxemic episodes in very low birth weight infants on ventilatory support. *J Pediatr*. 1997;130:577-583.
5. Esquer C, Claure N, D'Ugard C, et al. Role of abdominal muscles activity on duration and severity of hypoxemia episodes in mechanically ventilated preterm infants. *Neonatology*. 2007; 92:182-186.
6. Lehtonen L, Johnson MW, Bakdash T, et al. Relation of sleep state to hypoxemic episodes in ventilated extremely-low-birth-weight infants. *J Pediatr*. 2002;141:363-368.
7. McEvoy C, Mendoza ME, Bowling S, et al. Prone positioning decreases episodes of hypoxemia in extremely low birth weight infants (1000 grams or less) with chronic lung disease. *J Pediatr*. 1997;130:305-309.
8. Chang YJ, Anderson GC, Dowling D, Lin CH. Decreased activity and oxygen desaturation in prone ventilated preterm infants during the first postnatal week. *Heart Lung*. 2002;31:34-42.
9. Wells DA, Gillies D, Fitzgerald DA. Positioning for acute respiratory distress in hospitalised infants and children. *Cochrane Database Syst Rev*. 2005;(2):CD003645.

10. Firme SR, McEvoy CT, Alconcel C, et al. Episodes of hypoxemia during synchronized intermittent mandatory ventilation in ventilator-dependent very low birth weight infants. *Pediatr Pulmonol*. 2005;40:9-14.
11. Polimeni V, Claure N, D'Ugard C, Bancalari E. Effects of volume-targeted synchronized intermittent mandatory ventilation on spontaneous episodes of hypoxemia in preterm infants. *Biol Neonate*. 2006;89:50-55.
12. Hummler HD, Engelmann A, Pohlandt F, Franz AR. Volume-controlled intermittent mandatory ventilation in preterm infants with hypoxemic episodes. *Intensive Care Med*. 2006;32:577-584.
13. Claure N, Gerhardt T, Hummler H, et al. Computer controlled minute ventilation in preterm infants undergoing mechanical ventilation. *J Pediatr*. 1997;131:910-913.
14. Herber-Jonat S, Rieger-Fackeldey E, Hummler H, Schulze A. Adaptive mechanical backup ventilation for preterm infants on respiratory assist modes—a pilot study. *Int Care Med*. 2006;32:302-308.
15. Claure N, Suguihara C, Peng J, et al. Targeted minute ventilation and tidal volume in an animal model of acute changes in lung mechanics and episodes of hypoxemia. *Neonatology*. 2009;95:132-140.
16. McEvoy C, Durand M, Hewlett V. Episodes of spontaneous desaturations in infants with chronic lung disease at two different levels of oxygenation. *Pediatr Pulmonol*. 1993;15:140-144.
17. Hagadorn JI, Furey AM, Nghiem TH, et al. Achieved versus intended pulse oximeter saturation in infants born less than 28 weeks' gestation: the AVIOx study. *Pediatrics*. 2006;118:1574-1582.
18. Di Fiore JM, Bloom JN, Orge F, et al. A higher incidence of intermittent hypoxemic episodes is associated with severe retinopathy of prematurity. *J Pediatr*. 2010; 157:69-73.
19. Sink DW, Hope SA, Hagadorn JI. Nurse:patient ratio and achievement of oxygen saturation goals in premature infants. *Arch Dis Child Fetal Neonatal Ed*. 2011;96:F93-F98.
20. Claure N, Gerhardt T, Everett R, et al. Closed-loop controlled inspired oxygen concentration for mechanically ventilated very low birth weight infants with frequent episodes of hypoxemia. *Pediatrics*. 2001;107:1120-1124.
21. Claure N, D'Ugard C, Bancalari E. Automated adjustment of inspired oxygen in preterm infants with frequent fluctuations in oxygenation: a pilot clinical trial. *J Pediatr*. 2009;155:640-645.
22. Claure N, Bancalari E, D'Ugard C, et al. Multicenter crossover study of automated adjustment of inspired oxygen in mechanically ventilated preterm infants. *Pediatrics*. 2011;127:e76-e83.
23. Esquer C, Claure N, D'Ugard C, et al. Mechanisms of hypoxemia episodes in spontaneously breathing preterm infants after mechanical ventilation. *Neonatology*. 2008;94:100-104.
24. Bucher HU, Duc G. Does caffeine prevent hypoxaemic episodes in premature infants? A randomized controlled trial. *Eur J Pediatr*. 1988;147:288-291.
25. Livera LN, Spencer SA, Thorniley MS, et al. Effects of hypoxaemia and bradycardia on neonatal haemodynamics. *Arch Dis Childhood*. 1991;66:376-380.
26. Claure N, Sanchez V, D'Ugard C, Bancalari E. Changes in cerebral oxygenation during spontaneous episodes of hypoxemia in mechanically ventilated preterm infants. Pediatric Academic Societies' 2000-2010 Archive Abstracts2View™, http://www.abstracts2view.com/pasall/, E-PAS2003:2529.
27. Esquer C, Claure N, Capasso C, et al. Effect of spontaneous episodes of hypoxemia on brain oxygenation and brain-stem function in preterm infants. Pediatric Academic Societies' 2000-2010 Archive Abstracts2View™, http://www.abstracts2view.com/pasall/, E-PAS2005:2625.
28. Ratner V, Kishkurno SV, Slinko SK, et al. The contribution of intermittent hypoxemia to late neurological handicap in mice with hyperoxia-induced lung injury. *Neonatology*. 2007;92:50-58.
29. Row BW, Liu R, Xu W, et al. Intermittent hypoxia is associated with oxidative stress and spatial learning deficits in the rat. *Am J Resp Crit Care Med*. 2003;167:1548-1553.
30. Koons AH, Mojica N, Jadeja N, et al. Neurodevelopmental outcome of infants with apnea of infancy. *Am J Perinatol*. 1993;10:208-211.
31. Levitt GA, Mushin A, Bellman S, Harvey DR. Outcome of preterm infants who suffered neonatal apnoeic attacks. *Early Hum Dev*. 1998;16:235-243.
32. Cheung P, Barrington KJ, Finer NN, Robertson CMT. Early childhood neurodevelopment in very low birth weight infants with predischarge apnea. *Pediatr Pulmonol*. 1999;27:14-20.
33. Pillenkamp F, Hermann C, Keller T, et al. Factors influencing apnea and bradycardia of prematurity-Implications for neurodevelopment. *Neonatology*. 2007;91:155-161.
34. Janvier A, Khairy M, Kokkotis A, et al. Apnea is associated with neurodevelopmental impairment in very low birth weight infants. *J Perinatol*. 2004;24:763-768.
35. Penn JS, Henry MM, Tolman BL. Exposure to alternating hypoxia and hyperoxia causes severe proliferative retinopathy in the newborn rat. *Pediatr Res*. 1994;36:724-731.
36. Saito Y, Omoto T, Cho Y, et al. The progression of retinopathy of prematurity and fluctuation in blood gas tension. *Graefes Arch Clin Exp Ophthalmol*. 1993;231:151-156.
37. Reynaud X, Dorey CK. Extraretinal neovascularization induced by hypoxic episodes in the neonatal rat. *Invest Ophthalmol Vis Sci*. 1994;35:3169-3177.
38. Phelps DL, Rosenbaum A. Effects of marginal hypoxemia on recovery from oxygen-induced retinopathy in the kitten model. *Pediatrics*. 1984;73:1-6.
39. Cunningham S, McColm JR, Wade J, et al. A novel model of retinopathy of prematurity simulating preterm oxygen variability in the rat. *Invest Ophthalmol Vis Sci*. 2000;41:4275-4280.
40. Coleman RJ, Beharry KD, Brock RS, et al. Effects of brief, clustered versus dispersed hypoxic episodes on systemic and ocular growth factors in a rat model of oxygen-induced retinopathy. *Pediatr Res*. 2008;64:50-55.

41. McColm JR, Cunningham S, Wade J, et al. Hypoxic oxygen fluctuations produce less severe retinopathy than hyperoxic fluctuations in a rat model of retinopathy of prematurity. *Pediatric Res.* 2004;55:107-113.
42. McColm JR, Greisen P, Hartnett ME. VEGF isoforms and their expression after a single episode of hypoxia or repeated fluctuations between hyperoxia and hypoxia: relevance to clinical ROP. *Mol Vis.* 2004;10:512-520.
43. Tay-Uyboco JS, Kwiatkowski K, Cates DB, et al. Hypoxic airway constriction in infants of very low birth weight recovering from moderate to severe bronchopulmonary dysplasia. *J Pediatr.* 1989;115:456-459.
44. Unger M, Atkins M, Briscoe WA, King TK. Potentiation of pulmonary vasoconstrictor response with repeated intermittent hypoxia. *J Appl Physiol.* 1977;43:662-667.
45. Custer JR, Hales CA. Influence of alveolar oxygen on pulmonary vasoconstriction in newborn lambs versus sheep. *Am Rev Respir Dis.* 1985;132: 326-331.
46. Ratner V, Slinko S, Utkina-Sosunova I, et al. Hypoxic stress exacerbates hyperoxia-induced lung injury in a neonatal mouse model of bronchopulmonary dysplasia. *Neonatology.* 2009;95:299-305.
47. Nwajei PO, Young K, Claure N, et al. Impact of intermittent hypoxia on neonatal hyperoxia-induced lung injury. Pediatric Academic Societies' 2000-2010 Archive Abstracts2View™, http://www.abstracts2view.com/pasall/, E-PAS2010: 2140.7.

CHAPTER 17

Patient-Ventilator Interaction

Eduardo Bancalari, MD, and Nelson Claure, MSc, PhD

- Conventional Mechanical Ventilation
- Synchronized Mechanical Ventilation
- Infant-Ventilator Interaction During Noninvasive Ventilation
- Summary

Mechanical ventilation is an important tool in the management of premature infants with severe respiratory distress syndrome (RDS). In spite of a continuing trend toward a reduced use of mechanical ventilation, a large proportion of preterm infants require intubation and mechanical ventilation. However, mechanical ventilation has been associated with an increased risk of acute and chronic lung injury and other associated morbidities in the premature infant.

The earlier association between mechanical ventilation and the risk for lung injury was primarily believed to be due to aggressive use of the ventilator, which produced injurious lung expansion. Since then, neonatal ventilatory support has evolved, and gentler strategies have been implemented to ameliorate lung injury. These strategies involve careful management to minimize the support to avoid volume injury and shorten the duration of mechanical ventilation. As a result, the ventilatory support provided to the premature infant in respiratory failure has changed from a strategy to fully control ventilation with the target of normal blood gas values to a less invasive approach in which the ventilator is used as a tool to supplement the infant's spontaneous respiratory effort.

During the course of the mechanical ventilatory support, there is continuous interaction between infant and the ventilator. Some of these interactions can have negative effects on the infant's spontaneous breathing effort and affect ventilation. This chapter describes these interactions, details their effects, and discusses alternatives to avoid or minimize them.

Conventional Mechanical Ventilation

The interaction between the patient and the ventilator can be extremely complex and is influenced by many factors, including the patient's respiratory drive, various respiratory reflexes, the mechanical characteristics of the respiratory system, and the timing, flow, and pressure characteristics of the mechanical breaths. In part because of this complex interaction and because of the limitations of the older ventilators, clinicians for years elected to impose a respiratory pattern on their patients, taking over their ventilation completely. Patients were sedated, were paralyzed, or, worse, were hyperventilated to suppress their spontaneous respiratory drive. These approaches were associated with many problems that led to prolonged ventilator dependence and higher rates of complications. The patient who does not exerce the respiratory pump for long periods is less likely to be successfully weaned from mechanical ventilation. The likelihood of hyperventilation and hypoventilation is

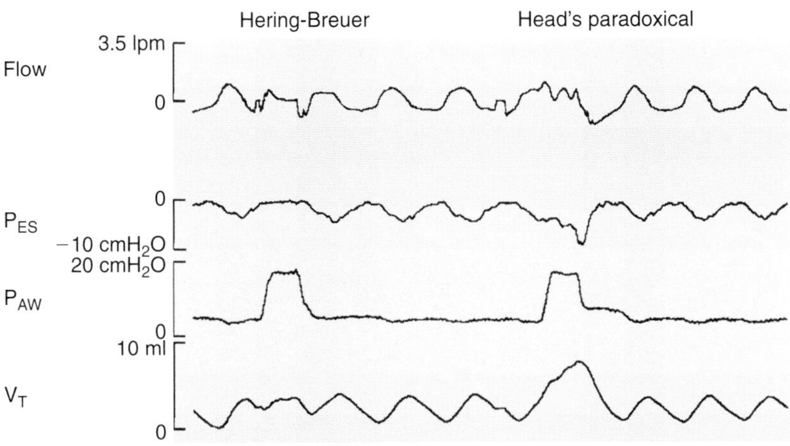

Figure 17-1 Recordings of flow (measured in liters per minute [lpm]), esophageal pressure (P_{ES}), airway pressure (P_{AW}), and tidal volume (V_T) illustrate the activation of the Hering-Breuer inhibitory reflex by a ventilator cycle that delays the initiation of the next spontaneous inspiration. The following ventilator cycle elicits an increase in inspiratory effort (greater negative deflection in P_{ES}) within the same spontaneous inspiration that results in a greater V_T in a pattern characteristic of the Head's paradoxic reflex.

higher during controlled ventilation because the settings must be constantly adjusted to match the metabolic demands and changing mechanical conditions of the respiratory system.

Infant-Ventilator Asynchrony

Asynchrony between the infant and the ventilator occurs frequently during intermittent mandatory ventilation (IMV) because the timing of mechanical breaths delivered at fixed intervals and duration does not coincide with the infant's spontaneous inspiration. Asynchronous mechanical cycles can interact in various ways with the infant's spontaneous breathing and reflex activity. The effects vary, depending on the timing and volume of the spontaneous inspiration or positive pressure.[1-3] Respiratory reflexes influence the infant's spontaneous respiratory rhythm. Activation of the Hering-Breuer vagal inhibitory reflex by lung inflation can shorten neural inspiration, whereas its activation by lung inflation during neural expiration will delay the onset of the next spontaneous inspiration. Also active in the newborn, Head's paradoxical reflex can be activated by a rapid lung inflation and elicit a greater inspiratory effort. This process can lead to a higher transpulmonary pressure, larger tidal volume (V_T), and, possibly, higher risk of alveolar rupture. These interactions are illustrated in Figure 17-1.

Inspiratory asynchrony occurs when the mechanical breath is delivered toward the end of the spontaneous inspiration and extends beyond the end of inspiration. Figure 17-2 shows an example of asynchrony during the spontaneous inspiratory phase. The resulting inspiratory hold can affect the spontaneous respiratory rate, and the additional lung inflation may also increase the risk of volutrauma.

Expiratory asynchrony occurs when the mechanical breath is delivered during exhalation and prolongs the spontaneous expiratory phase, in turn affecting the spontaneous breathing frequency, as shown in Figure 17-3. Sometimes this asynchrony can also elicit active exhalation against an elevated pressure at the airway, producing a rise in intrathoracic pressure.

Asynchrony can affect gas exchange and has been associated with air leaks.[4,5] Concerns also exist regarding its effects on brain blood flow and possible risk of intraventricular hemorrhage (IVH).[6] Earlier reports of the elimination of asynchrony by neuromuscular paralysis also suggested a reduction in intraventricular

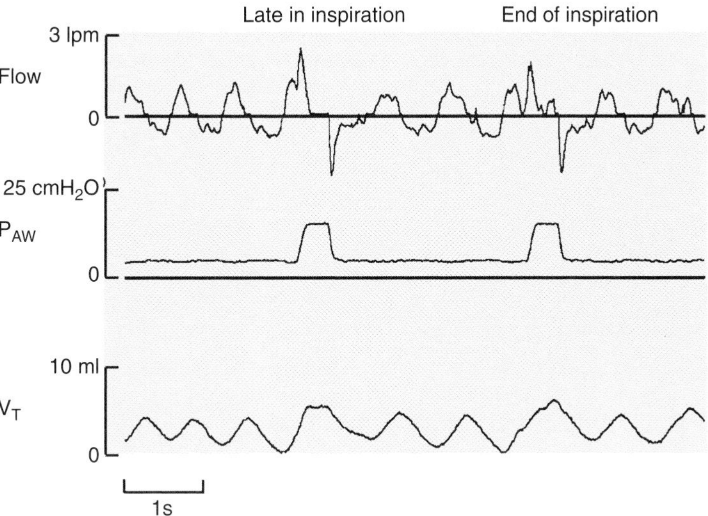

Figure 17-2 Tracings of flow (measured in liters per minute [lpm]), airway pressure (P_{AW}), and tidal volume (V_T) show intermittent mandatory ventilation (IMV) cycles delivered toward the second half or at the end of the infant's spontaneous inspiratory phase. These asynchronous cycles produce a volume plateau or a larger V_T that delays the onset of the next spontaneous inspiration. s, second.

hemorrhage and air leaks with this approach.[7,8] Manipulation of the IMV settings can decrease asynchrony,[9,10] but this method requires continuous fine tuning of inspiratory and expiratory times. The use of high ventilator rates was suggested as a way to prevent asynchrony and reduce the need for paralysis.[11] However, it may not be the most adequate alternative in preterm infant because of the risk of hypocapnia and its association with central nervous system and lung injury.

Asynchrony was common in the earlier IMV devices. Monitoring was limited to visual assessment of chest expansion and breathing rate, with no ability to detect

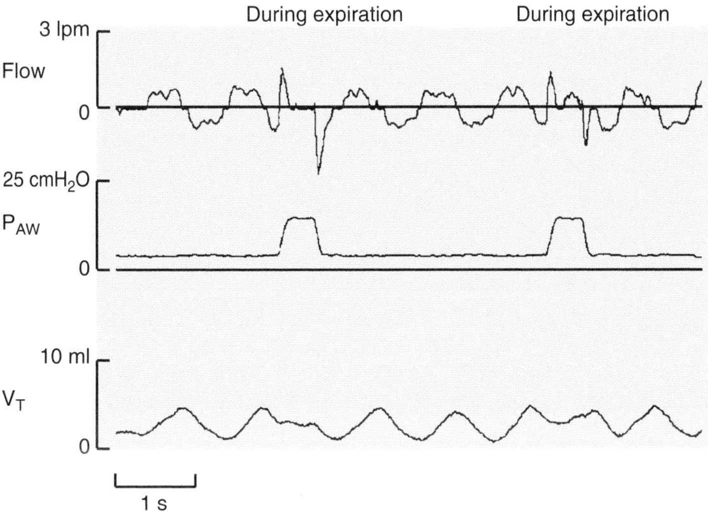

Figure 17-3 Tracings of flow, airway pressure (P_{AW}), and tidal volume (V_T) show intermittent mandatory ventilation (IMV) cycles delivered during the spontaneous expiratory phase. These asynchronous cycles prolong the expiration and affect the spontaneous breathing frequency by delaying the next spontaneous inspiration. lpm, liters per minute; s, second.

asynchrony as well as inadequate or excessive lung inflation. Because of lack of ventilation monitoring in older IMV devices, prolonged periods of asynchrony and excessive or insufficient ventilation could go undetected.

Because of the serious drawbacks of controlled ventilation, in the last two decades there has been a significant shift toward using ventilators to supplement the patient's inspiratory effort instead of taking over and controlling their ventilation. This approach offers many advantages and has improved the outcome of such infants. Their spontaneous respiratory activity is not inhibited, so infants are more likely to be weaned sooner from mechanical ventilation because their respiratory muscles remain fit and can cope with the increased work of breathing during the weaning process. Because the ventilator is used only to supplement the baby's respiratory effort, lower positive pressures are needed to maintain adequate minute ventilation. The likelihood of hyperventilation or hypoventilation is also reduced by allowing the infant to determine the total minute ventilation. To effectively deliver assisted ventilation, one must use a system that can respond on a timely basis to the demands of the infant. This can be best accomplished by using some of the devices that are now available for synchronized or patient-triggered ventilation even in the smallest infants.

Synchronized Mechanical Ventilation

Incorporation of sensors and microprocessors for monitoring and control of different functions has made possible the development of ventilators that respond to the demands of even the smallest preterm infants. Ventilatory modalities in which the ventilator cycle is synchronized with the infant's spontaneous inspiration are now available.

The main objective of synchronized ventilation is to avoid or minimize the unwanted effects when asynchrony develops between the infant's spontaneous breathing and the ventilator. This objective may be more relevant today because ventilatory management has changed from mandatory ventilation to a more gentle assistance of the spontaneous effort and preservation of the infant's breathing rhythm. Synchrony offers the benefits of supporting the infant's breathing and ensuring ventilation without disturbing the infant's respiratory drive. Cycling of the ventilator shortly after the onset of the spontaneous inspiration and the addition of the positive-pressure cycle to the negative pressure generated by the contraction of the diaphragm raises the transpulmonary pressure and produces a larger V_T than that generated by the infant or the ventilator alone, as illustrated in Figure 17-4. This positive interaction explains the better gas exchange and ventilation with more consistent V_T during synchronized than during conventional ventilation.[12-21]

Synchronous ventilation has been shown to reduce the stress response and fluctuations in blood pressure and oxygenation in preterm infants.[17,20,22-24] Synchronized ventilation has also been demonstrated to reduce breathing effort and work of breathing,[20,21] but it is not clear whether synchrony reduces the metabolic demands of respiration.[25] One of the most consistent and important advantages of patient-triggered ventilation is that by preserving spontaneous respiration, the method can facilitate weaning from the ventilator and shorten the duration of mechanical ventilation.[26] This advantage may explain the improved respiratory outcome and reduction in BPD among the smaller infants assisted with synchronized ventilation.[27]

Methods of Synchronization

Synchronization of the ventilator cycle with spontaneous inspiration is achieved by using different methods to detect inspiratory activity. Their efficacy and reliability vary and can significantly influence the interaction between the ventilator and the infant's spontaneous inspiratory effort.

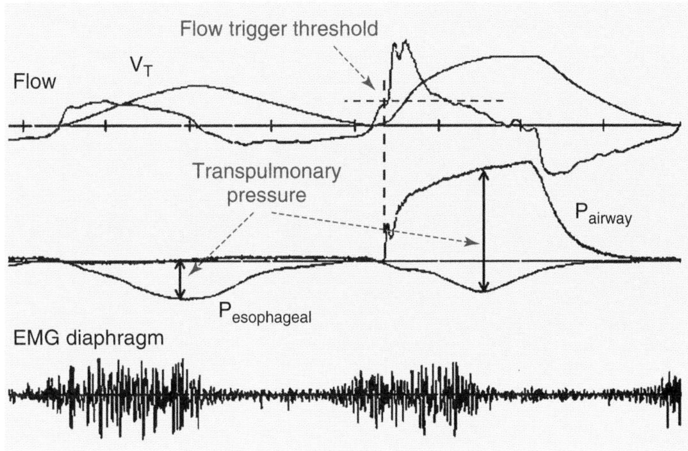

Figure 17-4 Tracings of flow (measured in liters per minute [lpm]), tidal volume (V_T), airway pressure (P_{airway}), esophageal pressure ($P_{esophageal}$) and electrical activity of the diaphragm obtained from a preterm infant to illustrate how the contraction of the diaphragm (measured by electromyography [EMG]) generates the negative pressure responsible for the inspiratory flow. Timely triggering of the ventilator cycle shortly after the onset of the inspiratory flow increases the transpulmonary pressure, and a larger V_T is achieved than in the preceding, nonassisted spontaneous inspiration.

17

Flow Sensors

Mainstream (proximal) or internal flow sensors are used in neonatal ventilators to detect the inspiratory flow generated by the infant's spontaneous inspiratory effort. The ventilator is triggered when the inspiratory flow exceeds a set threshold (see Fig. 17-4). Flow triggering has been shown to be more sensitive and specific than other methods,[28-30] and the ability to use low flow thresholds for triggering make this method appealing for use in the sicker and more immature infants.

Flow sensors are also used to monitor V_T and ventilation. In some ventilators, internal sensors are used in lieu of mainstream sensors. It is unknown whether internal sensors differ in their efficacy for synchrony, but there are concerns about the accuracy for V_T monitoring in small infants because the range of V_T measurements in this group is much smaller than the gas volume compressed in the ventilator circuit.[31,32]

Flow triggering is limited by the presence of gas leaks around the endotracheal tube. Leaking gas travels through the flow sensor in the same direction as the inspiratory flow, and the synchronization algorithm of the ventilator confuses the leaking gas with the onset of spontaneous inspiratory effort. Although mainstream flow sensors are usually small, they increase the instrumental dead space and affect carbon dioxide (CO_2) elimination, particularly in the smaller infants.[33-35]

Graseby Pressure Capsule

Outward motion of the abdomen during inspiration is pronounced in the newborn and even more in preterm infants. This outward motion is detected by the Graseby pressure capsule when it is applied on the abdominal surface. The use of this device for ventilator triggering is relatively simple but requires individualized sensitivity adjustment to avoid autocycling during patient activity, because outward motion of the abdomen is not specific to inspiration.

Airway Pressure

The transmission of the negative pressure changes produced by spontaneous inspiration to the airway can also be used for triggering. However, because of their respiratory disease and relatively weak respiratory pump, preterm infants do not consistently produce the pressure changes at the airway required for triggering, resulting in low

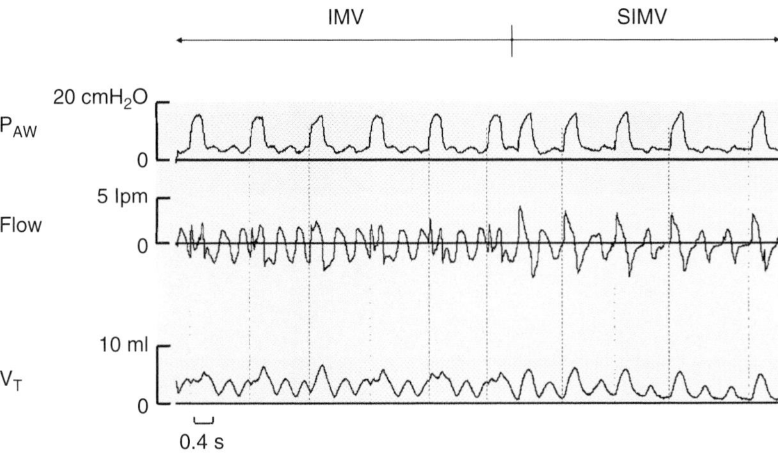

Figure 17-5 Tracings of airway pressure (P_{AW}), flow (measured in liters per minute [lpm]), and tidal volume (V_T) during transition intermittent mandatory ventilation (IMV) and synchronized IMV (SIMV) show how IMV cycles delivered at fixed intervals occur during different phases of the spontaneous breath. In contrast, synchronous ventilator cycles during SIMV achieve a more consistent V_T and do not disturb the respiratory rhythm of the infant. Note that the interval between ventilator cycles is variable during SIMV to accommodate the infant's spontaneous breathing. s, seconds.

sensitivity and triggering delays when airway pressure is used for synchronized ventilation in such patients.[36-38]

Modalities of Synchronized Ventilation

Synchronized Intermittent Mandatory Ventilation

Synchronized IMV (SIMV) is similar to conventional IMV, but with synchronous delivery of ventilator cycles. In both IMV and SIMV, the number of ventilator cycles delivered every minute is set by the clinician but the interval between cycles (expiratory duration, Te), which is constant in IMV, is variable in SIMV. Figure 17-5 illustrates how synchrony is achieved during SIMV and compares the effects of synchrony and IMV.

Assist/Control Ventilation

In assist/control (A/C) ventilation, every spontaneous inspiratory effort is assisted with a mechanical breath, which, because of the synchrony, reduces spontaneous inspiratory effort and improves V_T, as illustrated in Figure 17-6. Most preterm infants have an inconsistent respiratory drive. Hence, in A/C ventilation, a backup IMV rate is set by the clinician to avoid hypoventilation if the infant stops breathing. Backup ventilator cycles delivered during apnea may not always prevent hypoventilation if the rate is insufficient. On the other hand, a backup rate near the infant's breathing frequency may lead to ventilator takeover if it provides all the required minute ventilation.

In some neonatal ventilators, the duration of inspiration (Ti) in A/C ventilation is fixed, and in others, the ventilator cycle can be automatically terminated in synchrony with the declining inspiratory flow at the end of inspiration. This latter arrangement is also known as *flow cycling*. Automatic termination of the cycle in A/C ventilation allows the preterm infant to increase breathing frequency without shortening Te and affecting V_T, unlike A/C ventilation with a fixed Ti.[38]

Pressure-Support Ventilation

Pressure-support ventilation (PSV) is a flow-cycled modality in which, as in A/C ventilation, every breath is assisted and the positive pressure is automatically terminated at the end of inspiration. This modality gives the infant complete control of

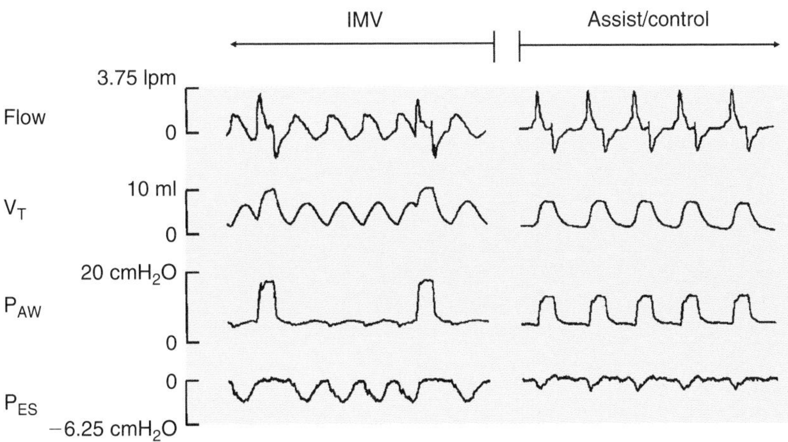

Figure 17-6 Tracings of flow (measured in liters per minute [lpm]), tidal volume (V_T), airway pressure (P_{AW}), and esophageal pressure (P_{ES}) during intermittent mandatory ventilation (IMV) and assist/control ventilation illustrate how the delivery of synchronous positive-pressure cycles triggered by every spontaneous breath reduces the inspiratory effort and avoids the disturbances to the infant's breathing rate observed when IMV cycles are delivered during exhalation.

17

the frequency and duration of inspiration. The synchronous "support" pressure is aimed at compensating for the loads induced by the disease and instruments—reduced lung compliance and increased endotracheal tube resistance.[16,39]

A consistent respiratory drive is needed to ensure maintenance of ventilation in PSV, but if apnea occurs, a backup IMV rate prevents hypoventilation. In some ventilators PSV can be combined with SIMV and spontaneous breaths are pressure-supported. Because the aim of PSV is mainly to boost the spontaneous effort, the pressure-supported breaths are usually assisted with lower pressures and result in smaller volumes than those breaths assisted with SIMV.

The addition of PSV to SIMV in preterm infants is aimed at boosting the spontaneous breaths and thus reducing the reliance on the larger SIMV breaths. PSV used with SIMV has been shown to reduce breathing effort and increase V_T in proportion to the support pressure used.[40-42] The combined use of SIMV and PSV has been found to enable earlier weaning in preterm infants than SIMV alone, preferentially in infants weighing more than 700 g at birth.[43] This advantage is likely due to these babies' more consistent respiratory drive, which ensures effective triggering of the ventilator.

Limitations and Potential Negative Infant-Ventilator Interaction with Synchronized Ventilation

Although the goal of synchronized ventilation is to provide some degree of unloading to the respiratory muscles by sharing the respiratory workload, the opposite occurs when there is maladaptation between the patient and the ventilator and the infant fights the ventilator. This lack of adaptation can be due to inadequate function of the synchronization mechanism, which leads to delayed triggering or trigger failure, autocycling, end-inspiratory asynchrony, or flow starvation. These problems may vary among ventilators, according to their triggering methods and other characteristics, but there is also great variability during routine clinical practice, depending on the infant population, the underlying lung disease, and the ventilator settings.

Long Inspiration Time and End-Inspiratory Asynchrony

End-inspiratory asynchrony occurs when the Ti of the ventilator cycle exceeds the patient's neural inspiration or there is delayed triggering and the mechanical cycle starts late during spontaneous inspiration. Continuation of mechanical inflation into

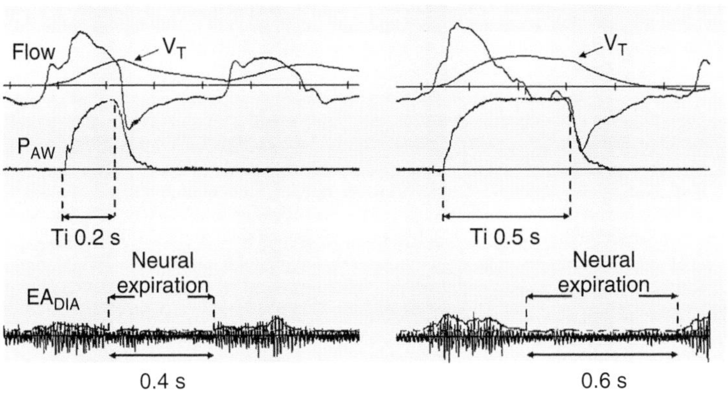

Figure 17-7 Tracings of flow, tidal volume (V_T), airway pressure (P_{AW}), and electromyographic activity of the diaphragm (EA_{DIA}) illustrate the effects of a ventilator cycle with a prolonged inspiratory time (Ti) on the neural respiratory activity in a preterm infant. The prolonged volume plateau extends beyond the inspiratory activity and prolongs the neural expiratory phase, delaying the start of the following spontaneous inspiration. s, second(s).

neural expiration results in a prolonged inspiratory plateau similar to an inspiratory hold and decreases the time for unopposed exhalation. In some cases it can elicit active exhalation efforts against the positive pressure. The effect of an excessively long Ti on the infant's breathing rhythm is mediated by the Hering-Breuer inhibitory reflex. The long Ti produces a prolonged volume plateau that keeps the lung distended and delays the initiation of the next spontaneous inspiration. It is illustrated in Figure 17-7.

In A/C ventilation, an excessive Ti may also result in an inverse inspiration-to-expiration ratio and gas trapping, if the spontaneous breathing frequency increases (Fig. 17-8). This development can limit breathing frequency and disrupt the neural breathing pattern.[44,45] Reports indicate that in preterm infants a large proportion of mechanical breaths extend beyond the end of spontaneous inspiration.[38,46] To avoid

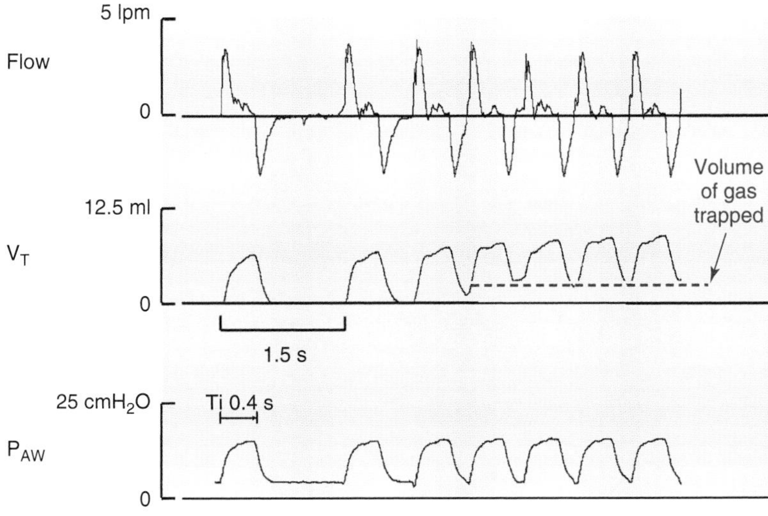

Figure 17-8 Tracings of flow (measured in liters per minute [lpm]), tidal volume (V_T), and airway pressure (P_{AW}) during assist/control ventilation with a constant inspiratory time (Ti) that exceeds the duration required to complete inspiration. Note the prolonged periods near zero flow and volume plateau. An increase in the spontaneous frequency produces an inverse inspiration-to-expiration (I:E) ratio that produces gas trapping because of insufficient time to complete exhalation. s, seconds.

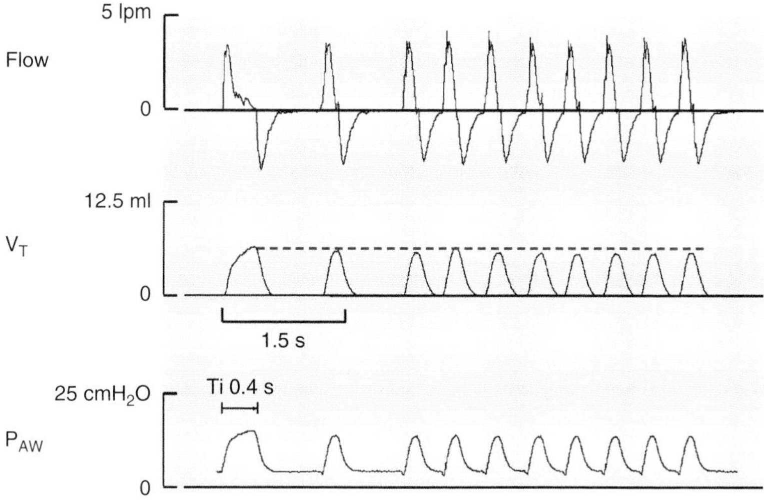

Figure 17-9 Tracings of flow (measured in liters per minute [lpm]), tidal volume (V_T), and airway pressure (P_{AW}) during assist/control ventilation with automatic termination of the ventilator cycle. The variable inspiratory time (Ti) permits the infant to have a higher spontaneous breathing frequency, and the resulting V_T is comparable to that achieved with the long Ti of the first breath. s, seconds.

this problem, mechanical breaths can be terminated automatically at the end of inflation or the spontaneous inspiration based on the decline of the inspiratory flow below a set level. Figure 17-9 shows an example of automatic termination of Ti. This automatic termination of mechanical inspiration may not work properly when a large gas leak around the endotracheal tube is present, because the leak can maintain the measured inspiratory flow above the threshold used to end inspiration. In this situation the cycling-off will occur later during the patient's neural expiration, and the infant may terminate the mechanical breath with active expiratory efforts. When automatic termination is not available, the adjustment of Ti can be achieved manually by observing the inspiratory flow and V_T waveforms to determine the set Ti necessary to complete inspiration. Mechanical breaths shorter that the infant's spontaneous Ti also occur frequently, but the consequences, other than reducing the peak transpulmonary pressure and tidal volume, are not known.

Delayed Triggering:

Delayed triggering can increase breathing effort[47] and produce a prolonged inspiratory hold. The effects are similar to those observed in IMV cycles occurring late in inspiration. The effects may be also similar to those of long Ti, described previously, and may be more relevant in A/C ventilation than in SIMV. Asynchronous or delayed triggering is usually due to a relatively low trigger sensitivity setting in relation to the inspiratory effort generated by the patient.

Trigger Failure

Trigger failure occurs because of trigger malfunction or low trigger sensitivity. As a result, the infant will be supported only by the IMV or AC ventilation backup rate in a nonsynchronized mode.

Autocycling

Autocycling is one of the most common problems with patient-triggered ventilation. It occurs when the ventilator cycles at a high uncontrolled rate rather than in response to the patient's inspiratory effort. The consequences are more serious in

A/C ventilation or PSV because none of the currently available neonatal ventilators offers the option to limit the cycling frequency. Autocycling at a high ventilator rate can induce hyperventilation, hypocapnia, and gas trapping. If the autocycling persists, it is likely to blunt the spontaneous respiratory drive through hyperventilation. In contrast, the effects of autocycling in SIMV are limited because the autocycling rate is limited by the ventilator rate set by the clinician, and therefore the ventilator behaves as if were in the IMV mode instead of SIMV.

The most common causes of autocycling are gas leaks around the endotracheal tube and water condensation in the ventilator circuit, both of which produce changes in gas flow that are detected by the flow sensor as the beginning of a spontaneous inspiration.[48] Leaks around the endotracheal tube are common among infants who remain ventilated for long periods because they frequently outgrow the tube size. Small leaks can be compensated for by an increase in the flow trigger threshold, and some ventilators have systems for automatic compensation of leaks. However, when the leaks are too large or variable, leak compensation becomes less effective and some times the endotracheal tube can be replaced to reduce the leak.

Excessive or Insufficient Circuit Flow

Flow starvation occurs when the flow through the ventilator circuit is lower than the peak inspiratory flow generated by the patient through inspiratory effort. In older patients flow starvation produces a sensation of air hunger and anxiety. In infants it can be a cause of agitation and maladaptation to the ventilator, because there is not enough fresh gas for the infant's spontaneous breaths between ventilator cycles. Some ventilator modes have the capacity to automatically increase the flow to match the patient demand, but if this feature is not available, it is critical that the ventilator flow be adjusted to meet the demands of the patient. Flow starvation can be recognized when the patient struggles during inspiration. When the circulating flow in the ventilator circuit is insufficient, the ventilator does not consistently reach the peak pressures set by the operator. It is important to recognize this condition because the infant is receiving less ventilatory support than intended, and it is frequently associated with agitation. On the other hand, high circuit flows modify the pressure profile of the ventilator cycle, resulting in a rapid increase to the PIP. This change accelerates the inspiratory flow rate and results in rapid lung inflation rates that are not observed during normal spontaneous breathing.

Peak Inspiratory Pressure

As explained before, ventilator cycles triggered by the onset of the infant's inspiration generally deliver a greater V_T than that produced by the spontaneous effort alone. Although not occurring in a consistent manner, the larger lung inflation produced by triggered ventilator cycles with high PIP can inhibit the infant's neural inspiration through activation of the stretch inhibitory reflex, as illustrated in Figure 17-10. The conditions that influence the sensitivity to inhibition of the neural inspiratory activity by lung inflation in preterm infants have not been clearly defined. In addition to the magnitude of the inflation, the sensitivity of the infant's respiratory center to stretch receptor activity is likely modulated by the chemical respiratory drive and possibly by the rate of lung inflation.

Although, the possible impact of inhibition of the infant's inspiratory effort on the development of consistent spontaneous breathing is unknown, the occurrence of such inhibition in a persistent manner over time may have unwanted consequences. On the other hand, it can be postulated that inhibition of spontaneous inspiration when V_T is excessive is a protective mechanism. Hence, an inconsistent or decreased sensitivity to stretch receptor activity may increase the infant's risk for lung injury when PIP is excessive during synchronized ventilation. The conditions that lead to increased or decreased sensitivity to stretch-related inspiratory inhibition during synchronized ventilation and their consequences need to be defined.

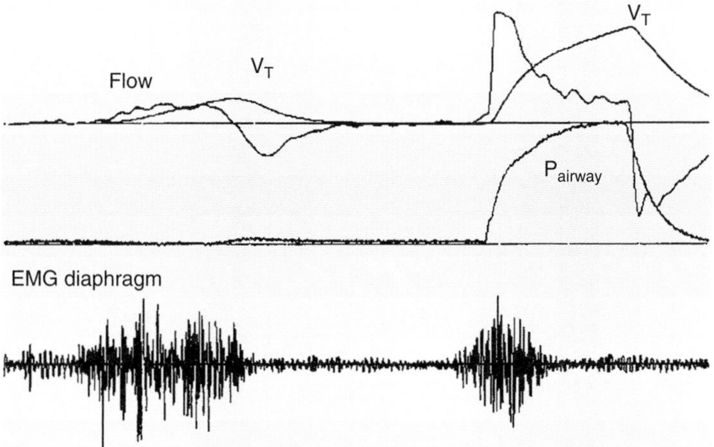

Figure 17-10 Recordings of flow (measured in liters per minute [lpm]), tidal volume (V_T), airway pressure (P_{airway}), and electromyographic activity (EMG) of the diaphragm during spontaneous intermittent mandatory ventilation (SIMV) show inhibition of the infant's inspiration by a synchronous ventilator cycle that produces a V_T that is considerable greater than the V_T produced by the preceding spontaneous inspiration.

17

Excessive Positive End-Expiratory Pressure

The positive effect of PEEP on oxygenation was demonstrated long ago[49] and is due to resolution of areas of atelectasis and decreased pulmonary shunting. However, excessive levels of PEEP can produce a rise in CO_2 owing to greater anatomic dead space resulting from distention of airways and decreased ventilation due to overdistension and reduced lung compliance.[50-53] The reduction in compliance is caused by a rise in lung volume to the flatter portion of the pressure-volume relationship. It is important to note that because of alveolar recruitment, an increase in PEEP achieve a greater gain in lung volume than the gain in V_T achieved by an increase in PIP of the same magnitude.[54]

In small preterm infants, increasing PEEP does not produce a compensatory increase in diaphragmatic activity to keep ventilation unchanged.[53] The reason may be activation of inhibitory stretch receptors at higher lung volumes.[55] The inability to maintain ventilation at rising PEEP levels may also be affected by decreased contractility and tension generation when the diaphragm is displaced downward at higher lung volumes.[56] On the other hand, PEEP levels that produce excessive lung volumes can elicit activation of expiratory muscles to actively exhale against the pressure generated by the ventilator,[57] as illustrated in Figure 17-11.

Although the optimal PEEP level in preterm infants is difficult to determine, it is clear that insufficient or excessive PEEP can lead to negative infant-ventilator interactions.

Infant-Ventilator Interaction during Noninvasive Ventilation

Noninvasive ventilation was one of the earliest forms of support used in neonates, but only recently has it been used increasingly to reduce the need for intubation or facilitate weaning from invasive ventilatory support in preterm neonates. Noninvasive ventilation is commonly provided with the same ventilators used for conventional mechanical ventilation, but functionally noninvasive ventilation may be more similar to continuous positive airway pressure (CPAP) than to invasive ventilation. In contrast to invasive ventilation, in which the endotracheal tube bypasses the infant's upper airway and guarantees to a large extent the transmission of the positive pressure to the infant's airways, pressure transmission during noninvasive ventilation

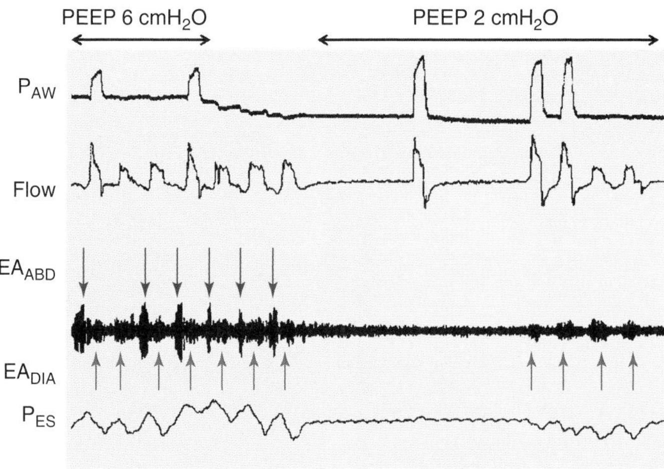

Figure 17-11 Tracings of airway pressure (P_{AW}), flow (measured in liters per minute [lpm]), electrical activity of the abdominal (EA_{ABD}, *red arrows*), and diaphragmatic (EA_{DIA}, *grey arrows*) muscles, and esophageal pressure (P_{ES}) during a decrease in positive end-expiratory pressure (PEEP) from 6 to 2 cm H_2O in a preterm infant. Contractions of the abdominal muscles during every expiration accelerate the expiratory flow rate at high PEEP but disappear when PEEP is reduced.

depends on the patency and resistance of the upper airway and on the large leaks present in an open system. The complexity of the mechanisms that determine upper airway patency and modulate its resistance makes it difficult to predict the degree of transmission of the positive pressure applied on the nose to the infant's distal airways.[58-63]

Sufficient transmission of the positive pressure during apnea is particularly important, because nasal ventilation is often used in infants with an immature respiratory control. The efficacy of nasal ventilation during apnea is not consistent, and it is inadequate if the infant's upper airway is not patent, as shown in Figure 17-12.

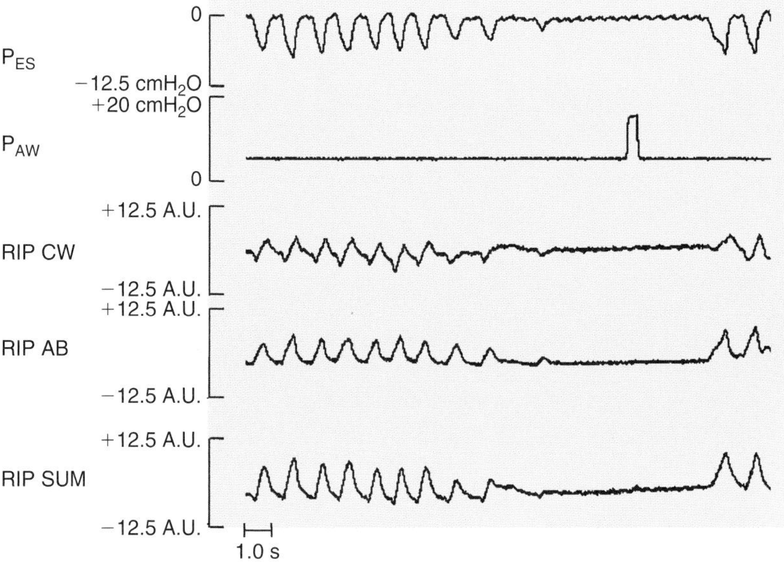

Figure 17-12 Tracings of esophageal pressure (P_{ES}), airway pressure (P_{AW}), and chest wall (RIP CW) and abdominal (RIP AB) expansion by respiratory inductance plethysmography and their sum (RIP SUM) show that a single nasal positive-pressure cycle delivered during a brief apneic pause does not produce transmission of the pressure to the chest. A.U., arbitrary units. s, seconds.

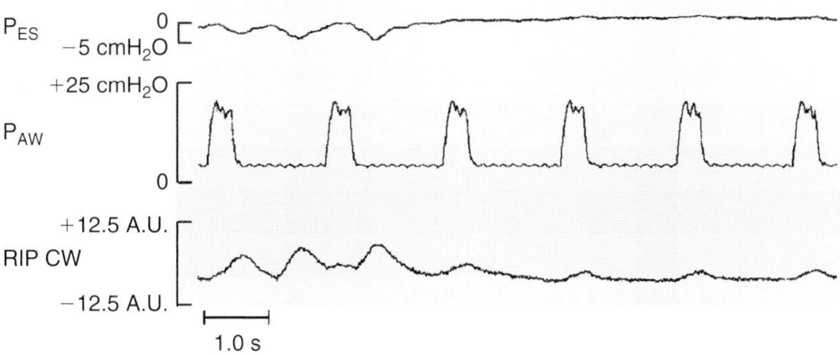

Figure 17-13 Tracings of esophageal pressure (P_{ES}), airway pressure (P_{AW}), and chest expansion by respiratory inductance plethysmography (RIP CW) show that pressure transmission of nasal intermittent positive-pressure ventilation (IPPV) cycles delivered when the infant was apneic produced some expansions of the chest, although these were smaller than with the preceding spontaneous breaths. A.U., arbitrary units. s, seconds.

In some instances, however, when the airway is open and leaks are not excessive, the positive pressure cycles produce lung inflation (Fig. 17-13).

Adequate transmission of the positive pressure during nasal synchronized ventilation can increase V_T,[64] but this process appears to be more effective in infants with greater ventilatory demands who cannot achieve sufficient ventilation.[65] Another important benefit of synchronized delivery of the positive-pressure cycle is that of unloading the respiratory pump, which is primarily reflected in a lesser inspiratory effort than with continuous positive airway pressure alone.[65-67]

In stable preterm infants, the reduction in breathing effort appears to be mediated by inhibitory reflexes rather than by decreased central drive, as illustrated by a significant attenuation in inspiratory effort during synchronous nasal IMV cycles (Fig. 17-14). In contrast, nonsynchronized ventilator cycles during nasal IMV do not increase ventilation or reduce breathing effort; instead, they appear to negatively affect the infant's respiratory rhythm, as is observed with invasive IMV (Fig. 17-15).[67]

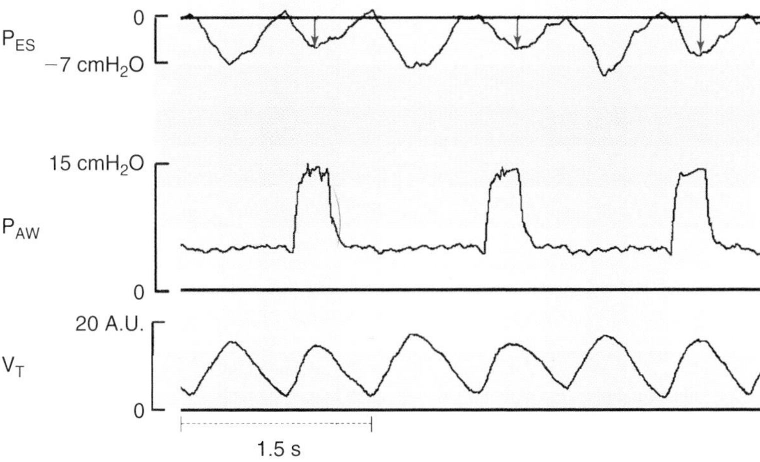

Figure 17-14 Tracings of esophageal pressure (P_{ES}), airway pressure (P_{AW}), and tidal volume (V_T) during synchronized nasal spontaneous intermittent mandatory ventilation (SIMV) illustrate the reduction in the infant's spontaneous inspiratory effort with each synchronized cycle of the ventilator. *Red arrows* mark the smaller negative deflections in P_{ES} during inspiration. s, second. A.U., arbitrary units. (From Chang HY, Claure N, D'Ugard C, et al: Effects of synchronization during nasal ventilation in clinically stable preterm infants. *Pediatr Res.* 2011;69: 84-89.)

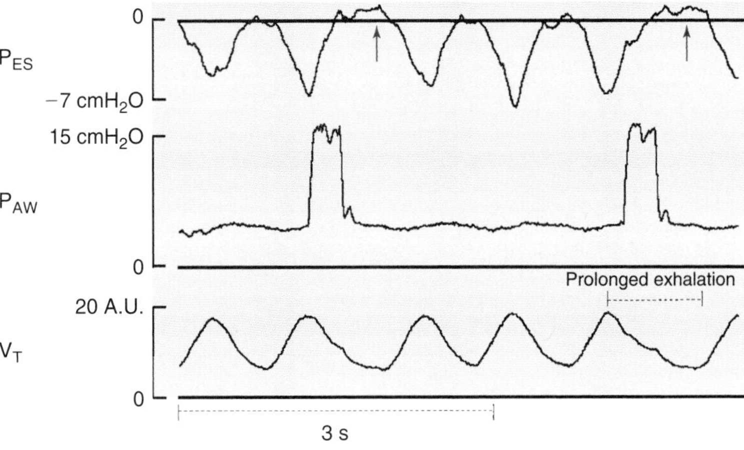

Figure 17-15 Tracings of esophageal pressure (P_{ES}), airway pressure (P_{AW}), and tidal volume (V_T) during nonsynchronized nasal spontaneous intermittent mandatory ventilation (SIMV) illustrate prolongation of the exhalation and active expiratory effort (marked by *red arrows*) with asynchronous ventilator cycles delivered toward the end of the infant's inspiration or during exhalation. A.U., arbitrary units. s, seconds. (From Chang HY, Claure N, D'Ugard C, et al: Effects of synchronization during nasal ventilation in clinically stable preterm infants. *Pediatr Res.* 2011;69:84-89.)

Summary

Important interactions between the infant and the ventilator occur routinely during invasive and noninvasive ventilatory support. Some of these interactions can have significant effects on ventilation and gas exchange, but the extent to which the interactions affect long-term respiratory or neurologic outcome is unknown. Nonetheless, they may play an important indirect role by prolonging respiratory support and disturbing the development of a stable and consistent respiratory rhythm in the preterm infant.

References

1. Greenough A, Morley C, Davis J. Interaction of spontaneous respiration with artificial ventilation in preterm babies. *J Pediatr*. 1983;103:769-773.
2. Greenough A, Morley CJ, Davis JA. Respiratory reflexes in ventilated premature babies. *Early Human Dev*. 1983;8:65-75.
3. Greenough A, Morley CJ, Davis JA. Provoked augmented inspirations in ventilated premature babies. *Early Human Dev*. 1984;9:111-117.
4. Stark AR, Bascom R, Frantz 3rd ID. Muscle relaxation in mechanically ventilated infants. *J Pediatr*. 1979;94:439-443.
5. Greenough A, Morley CJ. Pneumothorax in infants who fight ventilators. *Lancet*. 1984;1(8378):689.
6. Perlman JM, McMenamin JB, Volpe JJ. Fluctuating cerebral blood-flow velocity in respiratory-distress syndrome. Relation to the development of intraventricular hemorrhage. *N Engl J Med*. 1983;309:204-209.
7. Perlman JM, Goodman S, Kreusser KL, et al. Reduction in intraventricular hemorrhage by elimination of fluctuating cerebral blood-flow velocity in preterm infants with respiratory distress syndrome. *N Engl J Med*. 1985;312:1353-1357.
8. Greenough A, Wood S, Morley CJ, et al. Pancuronium prevents pneumothoraces in ventilated premature babies who actively expire against positive pressure inflation. *Lancet*. 1984;1(8367):1-3.
9. Field D, Milner AD, Hopkin IE. Manipulation of ventilator settings to prevent active expiration against positive pressure inflation. *Arch Dis Child*. 1985;60:1036-1040.
10. South M, Morley CJ. Synchronous mechanical ventilation of the neonate. *Arch Dis Child*. 1986;61:1190-1195.
11. Greenough A, Morley CJ, Pool J. Fighting the ventilator—are fast rates an effective alternative to paralysis? *Early Human Dev*. 1986;13:189-194.
12. Greenough A, Hird MF, Chan V. Airway pressure triggered ventilation for preterm neonates. *J Perinat Med*. 1991;19:471-476.
13. Greenough A, Pool J. Neonatal patient triggered ventilation. *Arch Dis Child*. 1988;63:394-397.
14. Hird MF, Greenough A. Patient triggered ventilation using a flow triggered system. *Arch Dis Child*. 1991;66:1140-1142.

15. Servant GM, Nicks JJ, Donn SM, et al. Feasibility of applying flow-synchronized ventilation to very low birth weight infants. *Respir Care*. 1992;37:249-253.
16. Brochard L, Rua F, Lorina H, et al. Inspiratory pressure support compensates for the additional work of breathing caused by the endotracheal tube. *Anesthesiology*. 1991;75:739-745.
17. Amitay M, Etches PC, Finer NN, et al. Synchronous mechanical ventilation of the neonate with respiratory disease. *Crit Care Med*. 1993;21:118-124.
18. Bernstein G, Heldt GP, Mannino FL. Increased and more consistent tidal volumes during synchronized intermittent mandatory ventilation in newborn infants. *Am J Respir Crit Care Med*. 1994:1444-1448.
19. Cleary JP, Bernstein G, Mannino FL, et al. Improved oxygenation during synchronized intermittent mandatory ventilation in neonates with respiratory distress syndrome: a randomized, crossover study. *J Pediatr*. 1995;126:407-411.
20. Hummler H, Gerhardt T, Gonzalez A, et al. Influence of different methods of synchronized mechanical ventilation on ventilation, gas exchange, patient effort and blood pressure fluctuations in premature neonates. *Pediatr Pulmonol*. 1996;22:305-313.
21. Jarreau PH, Moriette G, Mussat P, et al. Patient-triggered ventilation decreases the work of breathing in neonates. *Am J Respir Crit Care Med*. 1996;153:1176-1181.
22. Quinn MW, de Boer RC, Ansari N, et al. Stress response and mode of ventilation in preterm infants. *Arch Dis Child Fetal Neonatal Ed*. 1998;78:F195-F198.
23. Schulze A, Gerhardt T, Musante G, et al. Proportional assist ventilation in low birth weight infants with acute respiratory disease: A comparison to assist/control and conventional mechanical ventilation. *J Pediatr*. 1999;135:339-344.
24. Firme SR, McEvoy CT, Alconcel C, et al. Episodes of hypoxemia during synchronized intermittent mandatory ventilation in ventilator-dependent very low birth weight infants. *Pediatr Pulmonol*. 2005; 40:9-14.
25. Roze JC, Liet JM, Gournay V, et al. Oxygen cost of breathing and weaning process in newborn infants. *Eur Respir J*. 1997;10:2583-2585.
26. Greenough A. Update on patient-triggered ventilation. *Clin Perinatol*. 2001;28:533-546.
27. Bernstein G, Mannino FL, Heldt GP, et al. Randomized multicenter trial comparing synchronized and conventional intermittent mandatory ventilation in neonates. *J Pediatr*. 1996;128:453-463.
28. John J, Bjorklund LJ, Svenningsen NW, et al. Airway and body surface sensors for triggering in neonatal ventilation. *Acta Paediatr*. 1994;83:903-909.
29. Hummler H, Gerhardt T, Gonzalez A, et al. Patient triggered ventilation in neonates: comparison of a flow/volume and an impedance-triggered system. *Am J Resp Crit Care Med*. 1996;145: 1049-1054.
30. Dimitriou G, Greenough A, Cherian S. Comparison of airway pressure and airflow triggering systems using a single type of neonatal ventilator. *Acta Paediatr*. 2001;90:445-447.
31. Cannon ML, Cornell J, Tripp-Hammel DS, et al. Tidal volumes for ventilated infants should be determined with a pneumotachometer placed at the endotracheal tube. *Am J Respir Crit Care Med*. 2000;162:2109-2112.
32. Chow LC, Vanderhal A, Raber J, et al. Are tidal volume measurements in neonatal pressure-controlled ventilation accurate? *Pediatr Pulmonol*. 2002;34:196-202.
33. Figueras J, Rodriguez-Miguelez JM, Botet F, et al. Changes in $TcPCO_2$ regarding pulmonary mechanics due to pneumotachometer dead space in ventilated newborns. *J Perinat Med*. 1997;25:333-339.
34. Claure N, D'Ugard C, Bancalari E. Elimination of ventilator dead space during synchronized ventilation in premature infants. *J Pediatr*. 2003;143:315-320.
35. Estay A, Claure N, D'Ugard C, et al. Effects of instrumental dead space reduction during weaning from synchronized ventilation in preterm infants. *J Perinatol*. 2010;30:479-483.
36. Laubscher B, Greenough A, Kavadia V. Comparison of body surface and airway triggered ventilation in extremely premature infants. *Acta Paediatr*. 1997;86:102-104.
37. Dimitriou G, Greenough A, Cherian S. Comparison of airway pressure and airflow triggering systems using a single type of neonatal ventilator. *Acta Paediatr*. 2001;90:445-447.
38. Dimitriou G, Greenough A, Laubscher B, et al. Comparison of airway pressure-triggered and airflow-triggered ventilation in very immature infants. *Acta Paediatr*. 1998;87:1256-1260.
39. Brochard L, Harf A, Lorino H, Lemaire F. Inspiratory pressure support prevents diaphragmatic fatigue during weaning from mechanical ventilation. *Am Rev Respir Dis*. 1989;139:513-521.
40. Osorio W, Claure N, D'Ugard C, et al. Effects of pressure support during an acute reduction of synchronized intermittent mandatory ventilation in preterm infants. *J Perinatol*. 2005;25: 412-416.
41. Gupta S, Sinha SK, Donn SM. The effect of two levels of pressure support ventilation on tidal volume delivery and minute ventilation in preterm infants. *Arch Dis Child Fetal Neonatal Ed*. 2009;94: F80-F83.
42. Patel DS, Rafferty GF, Lee S, et al. Work of breathing during SIMV with and without pressure support. *Arch Dis Child*. 2009;94:434-436.
43. Reyes Z, Claure N, Tauscher M, et al. Randomized controlled trial comparing synchronized intermittent mandatory ventilation (SIMV) and SIMV plus pressure support (SIMV+PS) in preterm infants. *Pediatrics*. 2006;118:1409-1417.
44. Upton CJ, Milner AD, Stokes GM. The effect of changes in inspiratory time on neonatal triggered ventilation. *Eur J Pediatr*. 1990;149:648-650.
45. Beck J, Tucci M, Emeriaud G, et al. Prolonged neural expiratory time induced by mechanical ventilation in infants. *Pediatr Res*. 2004;55:747-754.

46. De Luca D, Conti G, Piastra M, Paolillo PM. Flow-cycled versus time-cycled sIPPV in preterm babies with RDS: a breath-to-breath randomised cross-over trial. *Arch Dis Child Fetal Neonatal Ed.* 2009;94:F397-F401.
47. Lorino H, Moriette G, Mariette C, et al. Inspiratory work of breathing in ventilated preterm infants. *Pediatr Pulmonol.* 1996;21:323-327.
48. Bernstein G, Knodel E, Heldt GP. Airway leak size in neonates and autocycling of three flow-triggered ventilators. *Crit Care Med.* 1995;23:1739-1744.
49. DeLemos RA, McLaughlin GW, Robison EJ, et al. Continuous positive airway pressure as an adjunct to mechanical ventilation in the newborn with respiratory distress syndrome. *Anesth Analg.* 1973;52:328-332.
50. Dinger J, Topfer A, Schaller P, Schwarze R. Effect of positive end expiratory pressure on functional residual capacity and compliance in surfactant-treated preterm infants. *J Perinat Med.* 2001;29:137-143.
51. Dimitriou G, Greenough A, Laubscher B. Appropriate positive end expiratory pressure level in surfactant-treated preterm infants. *Eur J Pediatr.* 1999;158:888-891.
52. Consolo L, Palhares D, Consolo L. Assessment of pulmonary function of preterm newborn infants with respiratory distress syndrome at different positive end expiratory pressure levels. *J Pediatr (Rio J).* 2002;78:403-408.
53. Alegría X, Claure N, Wada Y, et al. Acute effects of PEEP on tidal volume and respiratory center output during synchronized ventilation in preterm infants. *Pediatr Pulmonol.* 2006;41:759-764.
54. Bartholomew KM, Brownlee KG, Snowden S, Dear PR. To PEEP or not to PEEP? *Arch Dis Childhood.* 1994;70:F209-F212.
55. Hassan A, Gossage J, Ingram D, et al. Volume of activation of the Hering-Breuer inflation reflex in the newborn infant. *J Appl Physiol.* 2001;90:763-769.
56. Smith J, Bellemare F. Effect of lung volume on in vivo contraction characteristics of human diaphragm. *J Appl Physiol.* 1987;62:1893-1900.
57. South M, Morley CJ, Hughes G. Expiratory muscle activity in preterm babies. *Arch Dis Child.* 1987;62:825-829.
58. Carlo WA, Martin RJ, Bruce EN, et al. Alae nasi activation (nasal flaring) decreases nasal resistance in preterm infants. *Pediatrics.* 1983;72:338-343.
59. Carlo WA, Kosch PC, Bruce EN, et al. Control of laryngeal muscle activity in preterm infants. *Pediatr Research.* 1987;22:87-91.
60. Eichenwald EC, Howell 3rd RG, Kosch PC, et al. Developmental changes in sequential activation of laryngeal abductor muscle and diaphragm in infants. *J Appl Physiol.* 1992;73:1425-1431.
61. Carlo WA, Miller MJ, Martin RJ. Differential response of respiratory muscles to airway occlusion in infants. *J Appl Physiol.* 1985;59:847-852.
62. Duara S, Silva Neto G, Claure N, et al. Effect of maturation on the extrathoracic airway stability of infants. *J Appl Physiol.* 1992;73:2368-2372.
63. Duara S, Silva Neto G, Claure N. Role of respiratory muscles in upper airway narrowing induced by inspiratory loading in preterm infants. *J Appl Physiol.* 1994;77:30-36.
64. Moretti C, Gizzi C, Papoff P, et al. Comparing the effects of nasal synchronized intermittent positive pressure ventilation (nSIPPV) and nasal continuous positive airway pressure (nCPAP) after extubation in very low birth weight infants. *Early Hum Dev.* 1999;56:167-177.
65. Ali N, Claure N, Alegria X, et al. Effects of non-invasive pressure support ventilation (NI-PSV) on ventilation and respiratory effort in very low birth weight infants. *Pediatr Pulmonol.* 2007;42:704-710.
66. Aghai ZH, Saslow JG, Nakhla T, et al. Synchronized nasal intermittent positive pressure ventilation (SNIPPV) decreases work of breathing (WOB) in premature infants with respiratory distress syndrome (RDS) compared to nasal continuous positive airway pressure (N-CPAP). *Pediatr Pulmonol.* 2006;41:875-881.
67. Chang HY, Claure N, D'Ugard C, et al. Effects of synchronization during nasal ventilation in clinically stable preterm infants. *Pediatr Res.* 2011;69:84-89.

C

CHAPTER 18

Strategies for Limiting the Duration of Mechanical Ventilation

Eduardo Bancalari, MD, and Nelson Claure, MSc, PhD

18

- Weaning Ventilator Settings
- Modes of Ventilation and Weaning
- Prediction of Successful Extubation
- Automatic Weaning
- Conclusion

Mechanical respiratory support is necessary for the survival of most extremely premature and other infants with severe respiratory failure. However, mechanical ventilation is associated with many acute complications and long-term sequelae.[1,2] For this reason it is important to avoid or limit as much as possible the duration of invasive respiratory support in any patient but most especially in the newborn. Although this goal is easy to achieve in the larger infants, it is difficult in the very immature infant because of their more severe lung disease, inconsistent respiratory drive, and weak respiratory pump. This makes the very immature infant extremely prone to become ventilator-dependent for long periods and to enter into a vicious circle in which the longer the infant remains ventilator-dependent the more damaged the lungs are and the more difficult it is to wean the infant from mechanical support.

For many years infants were ventilated by controlling their respiration with sedation, hyperventilation, and even muscle relaxation and providing most of their minute ventilation with the machine. This approach has been changed to strategies that use ventilators preferentially to assist and complement the patient's respiratory effort in achieving the necessary ventilation and gas exchange. This change has been an important step in reducing the duration of mechanical ventilation and some of its complications; it has been made possible by the introduction of ventilators that can synchronize the mechanical cycle with the infant's inspiratory effort.

Weaning Ventilator Settings

The risk of complications increases the longer the patient is on mechanical respiratory support. Therefore the first decision that must be taken is when to start weaning from mechanical ventilation and what parameters to reduce first. The aim should always be to try to wean the infant as soon as possible, and therefore, weaning should begin as soon as respiratory function is stabilized. This effort should persist until the infant is successfully extubated and breathing spontaneously with no mechanical respiratory support.

The decision regarding which parameters the infant must be weaned from first should take into consideration the cause of the respiratory failure and the association of the individual parameter with a greater risk of complications. For example, in an infant with severe pulmonary interstitial emphysema (PIE), the first step should be to reduce the pressures and tidal volume (V_T) to avoid the progression of the PIE.

C

In an infant with compromised hemodynamic function, however, reductions in positive end-expiratory pressure (PEEP) and mean airway pressure (MAP) may be the most appropriate first step.

Although the main goal of the weaning process is extubation, minimizing exposure to high ventilator settings may have as much relevance. This is particularly important in the most immature infants until their lungs are sufficiently developed and healed from the initial respiratory illness and their respiratory center is sufficiently mature. Weaning from the ventilator settings has been facilitated by the availability of tools to continuously monitor ventilation and gas exchange.

One of the most important parameters from which to wean an infant is the peak inspiratory pressure (PIP) to avoid the risk of overdistention. This is easier now that it is possible to measure V_T, allowing the weaning from PIP as lung compliance and spontaneous inspiratory effort improve. The PIP selected is generally chosen to achieve adequate V_T values in the range of 3 to 5 mL per kg body weight and is also determined by the levels of $PaCO_2$ in the arterial blood. When V_T measurement is not available, reduction in PIP must be based on observed chest movement, degree of aeration on chest radiograph and $PaCO_2$ levels. Monitoring V_T during weaning from PIP is also helpful for detecting hypoventilation if the reduction in PIP was too large. This is important to prevent a gradual alveolar collapse and the risk of lung injury during reopening.

PEEP is key in the maintenance of the end-expiratory lung volume required to improve oxygenation and to avoid ventilation near the closing lung volume. The level of PEEP required depends on the type and severity of the underlying lung disease, and the value chosen is frequently guided by the requirement for supplemental oxygen and radiographic picture. PEEP is usually kept between 4 and 8 cm H_2O to maintain an adequate end-expiratory volume and can be decreased gradually as oxygenation improves until a pressure of 4 to 5 cm H_2O, is reached. Thereafter, this level is maintained until extubation to avoid lung collapse.

The adjustment of ventilator rate depends on the modality of ventilation being used. When modalities in which the infant determines the mechanical rate, such as assist/control (A/C) ventilation and pressure-support ventilation (PSV), the set ventilator rate will only take over as a backup when the rate in the patient falls below that setting. Therefore it is relevant only when the infant becomes apneic or hypoventilates. With intermittent mandatory ventilation (IMV) or synchronized IMV (SIMV), the rate is gradually reduced as spontaneous breathing contributes to the total minute ventilation more consistently and as long as $PaCO_2$ remains within an acceptable range. Monitoring of ventilation is important if the reduction in ventilator rate is hasty and requires a large compensatory increase in spontaneous effort. Inadvertent periods with ventilation below adequate levels not only may affect CO_2 elimination but also may lead to lung collapse and hypoxemia. When the infant's ventilation is controlled the ventilator rate is adjusted by the clinician, and the chosen rate is generally based on $PaCO_2$.

The fraction of the inspired oxygen (FIO_2) is lowered according to arterial oxygen tension or, more frequently, according to oxygen saturation measured by pulse oximetry (SpO_2). The aim is to avoid hyperoxemia and reduce the exposure of the lung tissue to high oxygen levels. In infants with lung disease, continuous monitoring of SpO_2 is helpful to balance lowering FIO_2 against the risk of hypoxemia. The optimal ranges for oxygenation targets for preterm infants are still not well defined, but until more definitive data become available, the goal of most clinicians is to maintain SpO_2 above a minimum level, usually defined as between 87% and 90%, but without exceeding an upper limit that is usually defined as between 93% and 95%.

When weaning an infant from the ventilator, it is always advisable to make gradual changes, reducing one setting at a time, to evaluate the response of the infant to each change. The availability of continuous oxygen and carbon dioxide monitoring has expedited weaning considerably. Now it is not necessary to wait for arterial blood gas measurements before changing ventilator settings, and weaning can proceed at a considerably faster pace.

During weaning from respiratory support, as respiratory system mechanics improves and the spontaneous respiratory effort becomes stronger, tidal volume and minute ventilation increase. Continuous monitoring of V_T can therefore be used to lower PIP as patient condition improves. Measuring V_T can also facilitate detection of pulmonary overdistention and consequently avoid associated complications such as air leaks and intraventricular hemorrhage.[3,4] Automatic weaning from PIP settings the basis of generated tidal volumes is the base for targeted-volume ventilation, which is discussed later.

Permissive Hypercapnia

Following the experience in adults with chronic respiratory failure, it has been suggested that the same strategy of tolerating higher arterial CO_2 levels could be applied in the premature infant as a way of facilitating weaning from mechanical support and thus reducing the risk of ventilator-induced lung damage. Several clinical trials have been conducted to explore this strategy in this population, but the results have been inconsistent. Although some studies have shown a reduction in the duration of mechanical ventilation with such tolerance, they have not shown a clear reduction in lung damage or bronchopulmonary dysplasia (BPD) is not consistent.[5,6] A later trial showed no benefit in terms of duration of ventilation but there was a possible increase in mortality and neurologic impairment in infants in the minimal ventilation group.[7] These results have prompted a serious caution against tolerating high CO_2 levels in premature infants during their acute respiratory course. However, it is very difficult, if not impossible, to wean infants with chronic respiratory failure from ventilator settings unless some degree of hypercapnia is tolerated. In infants with severe BPD and chronic CO_2 retention, it is common to observe metabolic alkalosis that persists for long periods. This problem is frequently aggravated by long-term diuretic therapy. What $Pa{CO_2}$ can be tolerated under these conditions is not clear and should be decided on an individual base.

Respiratory Center Stimulants

Aminophylline and caffeine are both effective respiratory stimulants that improve central respiratory drive in preterm infants and reduce the incidence of apneic episodes. For this reason, these drugs also increase the chance of successful weaning from mechanical ventilation and decrease the need for reintubation. Although the two drugs are similarly effective in reducing apnea, caffeine is generally preferred because of a longer half-life, broader therapeutic range, and fewer side effects. Concerns regarding the risks of prolonged caffeine administration in preterm infants have been put to rest by a large multicenter randomized trial showing that its use resulted in better pulmonary outcome and improved long-term neurologic outcome than placebo, without detectable side effects.[8,9] On the basis of this evidence, most preterm infants receive a loading dose of caffeine or aminophylline before extubation and then receive maintenance therapy using one of these stimulants for at least the first few days after extubation while they also receive nasal continuous positive airway pressure (CPAP) or nasal ventilation.[10]

Postnatal Steroids

There is clear evidence that systemic administration of steroids to ventilator-dependent infants produces a rapid improvement in lung function, facilitating weaning from the ventilator and reducing the incidence of bronchopulmonary dysplasia.[11]

Steroids can improve lung function through several mechanisms: enhanced production of surfactant and antioxidant enzymes, decreased bronchospasm, decreased pulmonary and bronchial edema and fibrosis, improved vitamin A status, and decrease in the response of inflammatory cells and mediators in the injured lung.

On the other hand, systemic steroid administration is associated with a number of complications, such as masking of the signs of infection, arterial hypertension, hyperglycemia, increased proteolysis, adrenocortical suppression, somatic and lung growth suppression, and hypertrophic myocardiopathy.

Of greater concern is the fact that findings of many long-term follow-up studies have suggested that infants who received prolonged steroid therapy have worse neurologic outcome, including a higher incidence of cerebral palsy.[12] Because of the seriousness of the neurologic side effects, specifically, when systemic steroids are used early after birth and for prolonged periods, the use of systemic steroids should be considered only after the first 2 weeks of life in infants who show clear evidence of severe and progressive pulmonary damage and who remain oxygen- and ventilator-dependent. The duration of steroid therapy must be limited to the minimum necessary to achieve the desired effects, usually 5 to 7 days, and according to the recommendation of the American Academy of Pediatrics, the potential benefits and risks should be discussed with the family before this therapy is initiated.

Steroids can also be administered by nebulization to ventilator-dependent infants. Inhaled steroids may reduce the need for systemic steroids, reducing the side effects associated with prolonged systemic therapy, although data on effectiveness of topical steroids are not conclusive enough to recommend their routine use.[13]

Dead Space Reduction

Because the anatomic dead space in a preterm infant is relatively large,[14] any additional instrumental dead space reduces alveolar ventilation[15] and can contribute to respiratory failure and delay weaning from the ventilator.

This problem has been addressed by continuous tracheal gas insufflation (CTGI), whereby gas is pumped through small capillaries built in the wall of the endotracheal tube to produce a continuous washout of the tube lumen. This modality of ventilation was shown to reduce arterial CO_2 with the same ventilator settings or to maintain similar CO_2 levels with less support,[16] and in a randomized trial, continuous tracheal gas insufflation shortened the process of weaning from mechanical ventilation.[17] Because this method requires a special ventilator and endotracheal tube, it has not gained wide acceptance.

Proximal flow sensors used for synchronization and volume measurement have small dead space but they can induce CO_2 rebreathing in the smaller infants who are forced to increase their spontaneous ventilation to compensate for the larger dead space. This problem is minimized when there are leaks around the endotracheal tube, which allow flow through the lumen driven by the PEEP during expiration. A simple method consisting of a continuous gas leak in the endotracheal tube connector that washes the sensor and connector reducing rebreathing in small infants has also been described.[18,19]

Extubation from Intermittent or Continuous Positive Airway Pressure

For many years infants receiving mechanical ventilation were extubated only after they had tolerated several hours of CPAP applied through the endotracheal tube and were able to maintain acceptable arterial blood gas levels. This approach was changed after a small trial showed that infants extubated after receiving a low IMV frequency had higher success rates than those undergoing CPAP for 6 hours before extubation.[20] Maintenance of a low ventilator rate probably avoids exhausting the infant before extubation and thus preserves the infant's breathing effort for the challenging period that follows extubation.

Modes of Ventilation and Weaning

Synchronized or Patient-Triggered Ventilation

As mentioned earlier, because ventilators are used now more to assist the patient's respiratory effort that to control ventilation, synchronized ventilation, or patient-triggered ventilation (PTV), has become a standard practice in neonatal respiratory care. Almost every randomized trial comparing patient-triggered ventilation with nonsynchronized ventilation has shown a shorter duration of mechanical ventilation in infants treated with synchronized modes than in those treated with conventional, nonsynchronized ventilation.[21] This advantage of patient-triggered ventilation is most likely due to the fact that during it allows the infant to retain most of the control on ventilation and to continue to "exercise" the respiratory pump. Also the effectiveness of the mechanical and spontaneous breaths in generating V_T is increased by the simultaneous action of the positive pressure and the inspiratory effort generated by the infant.

SIMV, PSV, and A/C ventilation are the most common modes of synchronized mechanical ventilation used in neonates. Studies have not indicated consistent differences in weaning from mechanical ventilation between A/C ventilation and SIMV in premature infants.[22,23] Assisting each spontaneous inspiration during A/C ventilation may avoid respiratory fatigue and allow faster weaning. The same can be achieved by using PSV, which also provides some degree of unloading for each breath. During IMV or SIMV, the weaning is accomplished by gradual reduction of the mechanical rate, allowing the patient to increase his or her contribution to minute ventilation. The rate reduction depends on the tolerance of each infant and is assessed by monitoring the stability of blood gases and frequency of apnea or hypoxemia episodes. During A/C ventilation, the reduction of the ventilator rate does not have any effect except for reducing the backup rate when the infant stops breathing or slows down spontaneous breathing frequency to below that set in the ventilator.

The only randomized trial comparing PSV with SIMV in preterm infants also revealed faster weaning and shorter duration of ventilation in infants who were treated with SIMV in combination with PSV than in those treated with SIMV alone.[24] The addition of PSV allowed faster weaning from the larger SIMV breaths; this effect may make it possible to reduce volume damage to the lung and increase spontaneous respiratory drive, accelerating weaning, as shown in the example in Figure 18-1. With this strategy, the proportion of ventilator-dependent infants during the first 28 days was lower in infants treated with SIMV plus PS. and they were weaned from mechanical ventilation earlier than infants supported by SIMV alone (Fig. 18-2). Infants with birth weights between 700 and 1000 grams who were treated with SIMV plus PS also spent less time on supplemental oxygen than those managed with SIMV alone.

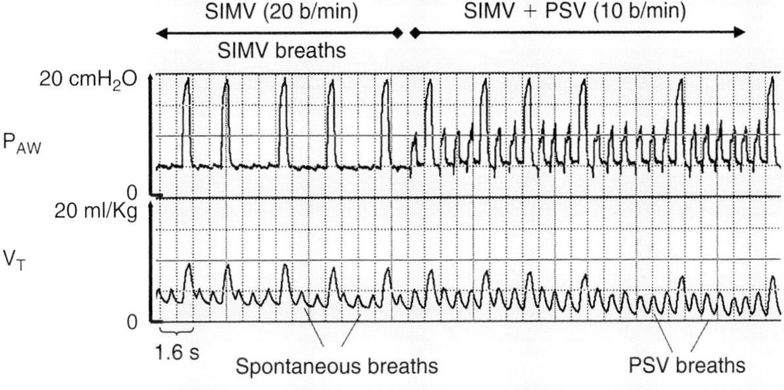

Figure 18-1 Recordings of airway pressure (PAW) and tidal volume (V_T) during a reduction of the spontaneous intermittent mandatory ventilation (SIMV) rate from 20 to 10 breaths per minute (b/m) while combined with pressure-support ventilation (SIMV + PSV). V_T in spontaneous breaths assisted with PSV is higher than with nonassisted spontaneous breaths. s, seconds.

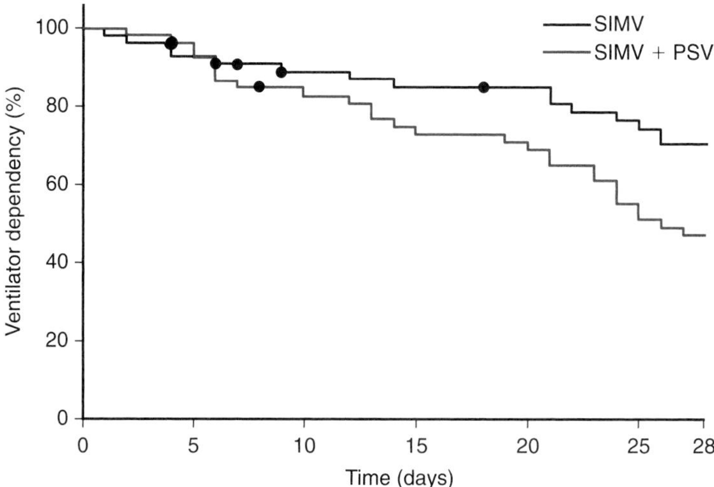

Figure 18-2 Ventilator dependency until postnatal day 28 in infants weaned with spontaneous intermittent mandatory ventilation (SIMV) and SIMV plus pressure-support ventilation (SIMV + PSV). Infants supported by the combined SIMV + PSV modality were weaned from mechanical ventilation earlier than infants supported by SIMV alone. (From Reyes ZC, Claure N, Tauscher MK, et al: Randomized, controlled trial comparing synchronized intermittent mandatory ventilation and synchronized intermittent mandatory ventilation plus pressure support in preterm infants. *Pediatrics.* 2006;118:1409-1417.)

Nasal Continuous Positive Airway Pressure after Extubation

Owing to a number of impediments facing infants after extubation, failure of extubation is very common, requiring reintubation and resumption of mechanical ventilation. This is especially true for smaller infants. The impediments to a successful extubation include upper airway damage and retained secretions leading to obstruction and atelectasis, loss of lung volume due to poor respiratory effort, and a highly compliant chest wall. It has been shown that the application of CPAP through the nose can significantly reduce the deterioration that frequently occurs in smaller infants after extubation. Surprisingly, despite this improvement in respiratory function associated with nasal CPAP, the need for reintubation has not been consistently reduced by the use of nasal CPAP.[25]

Nasal Ventilation after Extubation

Nasal ventilation has been used for many years in premature infants as a substitute for invasive ventilation. It has now been reintroduced as an effective alternative to respiratory support after extubation. In comparison with nasal CPAP, the use of nasal synchronized ventilation after extubation has been shown to significantly reduce both respiratory failure after extubation and the need for reintubation.[26] Although the studies with these findings have included small numbers of infants and the techniques used for nasal ventilation have varied considerably, the effects have been consistently positive. Nasal ventilation has been shown to decrease apnea, inspiratory effort, and chest wall distortion and, in some studies, to improve tidal volume.[27-31] Despite the possible advantages of synchronization, it is not clear at this point whether the use of synchronization during nasal ventilation improves its effectiveness or not,[31] and at this time there are no ventilators available in the United States to provide synchronization during noninvasive ventilation.

The settings used during nasal ventilation have varied considerably, and there are no studies comparing their effectiveness. In general the settings used during noninvasive ventilation are similar to those used during the final stages of weaning from invasive ventilation. They include rates of 10 to 40 cycles per minute with peak pressures of 12 to 18 cm H_2O, inspiratory times of 0.25 to 0.35 seconds, and a PEEP of 4 to 6 cm H_2O. Because during nasal ventilation there are considerable leaks in the upper airway, it is frequently necessary to use relatively high gas flows, 10 to 15 liters per minute, to generate the desired pressures.

Nasal ventilation is a promising alternative to invasive ventilation that has been proven effective in reducing extubation failure but needs further evaluation and the development of suitable equipment to provide noninvasive respiratory support in premature infants.

Weaning from High-Frequency Ventilation

In most occasions infants ventilated with high-frequency ventilation (HFV) are switched to conventional ventilation prior to extubation but this is not always necessary. It is possible to wean and extubate infants from high-frequency ventilation and this can be accomplished following steps that are similar to those used during weaning from conventional ventilation. Reduction in MAP is accomplished following oxygenation and lung expansion estimated by chest radiographs while inspired oxygen concentration (FIO_2) is adjusted to maintain the desired levels of arterial oxygenation. Weaning of the pressure amplitude is done gradually following the levels of $PaCO_2$. When MAP is weaned to low levels before the infant has spontaneous respiratory effort, there can be a gradual loss of lung volume and atelectasis compromising gas exchange. In order to avoid this it is advisable to lower first the pressure amplitude to allow the CO_2 to increase and stimulate spontaneous breathing before MAP is lowered below 10 or 8 cm H_2O. Like with conventional ventilation the use of respiratory stimulants should also be considered before weaning from high frequency ventilation.

18

Prediction of Successful Extubation

Although the indications for initiating ventilation are relatively standardized, the decision to wean an infant from the ventilator is much more difficult to achieve. For this reason, many infants remain intubated for longer than they really need to be. This problem is illustrated by the fact that many infants who are accidentally extubated, if given the opportunity, are able to breathe spontaneously without the need for further respiratory support. Many studies have evaluated different tools that could help predict successful extubation. They have included measurements of lung mechanics, inspiratory strength, ability to cope with mechanical loads, lung volume levels before and after extubation, and the ability of spontaneous ventilation to maintain gas exchange during a period when ventilator cycling is stopped.[31-34] For instance, a simple test is the "spontaneous breathing test," in which the ventilator cycling is turned off and the infant is observed for 3 minutes while receiving CPAP. If no hypoxia or bradycardia is observed during this period, the infant has a good chance of tolerating extubation.[34] Although some of these tools predict successful extubation with some accuracy, none has been widely accepted in clinical practice.

The decision to remove an infant from mechanical ventilation is usually based on the level of inspired oxygen and ventilator support that the infant is requiring to maintain acceptable arterial blood gas levels. Most clinicians attempt extubation when an infant is receiving less than 30% or 40% oxygen, the ventilator rate is less than 15 or 20 breaths per minute, peak pressures are below 15 or 16 cm H_2O, and blood gas levels are acceptable. The lower the gestational age, the higher the rate of failure and the need for reintubation and mechanical ventilation. In most cases this failure is due to poor respiratory effort or severe apneic episodes, although in others it is due to loss of lung volume with growing distress and rising oxygen requirement after extubation. Upper airway damage and obstruction due to edema or retained secretions can also be a cause of respiratory failure after extubation. Table 18-1 lists the factors and interventions aimed at facilitating the weaning process.

Because there is frequently some inertia or concern about weaning infants from mechanical ventilation, it is useful to have written criteria to guide extubation and weaning from the ventilator as soon as the infant has a reasonable chance to remain extubated. In order to achieve adherence, the extubation guideline should be

Table 18-1 STRATEGIES TO MINIMIZE DURATION OF MECHANICAL VENTILATION

- Optimize lung function: Maintenance of lung volume and airway patency, avoid fluid overload and closure of symptomatic patent ductus arteriosus (PDA).
- Avoid conditions leading to respiratory depression (e.g., metabolic alkalosis, drugs, infections).
- Patient-triggered ventilation: Preserve spontaneous breathing.
- Volume-targeted ventilation: Manually or ventilator-adjusted.
- Permissive hypercapnia in infants with chronic ventilator dependency.
- Avoid routine reintubation after self-extubation.
- Respiratory stimulants.
- Post-extubation nasal continuous positive airway pressure (N-CPAP) and nasal intermittent positive-pressure ventilation (N-IPPV).
- Adherence to preestablished extubation criteria.

relatively simple and should provide sufficient flexibility to the clinician for decision making. An example of extubation criteria is included in Table 18-2.

Automatic Weaning

Volume-Targeted Ventilation

With volume-targeted ventilation, the clinician sets the desired V_T value and the ventilator automatically adjusts the PIP to deliver the set V_T. As the mechanical characteristics of the lung improve and the contribution of spontaneous breathing effort increases, the ventilator delivers lower pressures.[35] Thus, volume-targeted ventilation achieves automatic weaning from the PIP independent of the clinician, who only has to decide what V_T is delivered by the ventilator in combination with the infant's effort. There is evidence from randomized trials and a meta-analysis that volume-targeting strategies can achieve faster weaning from mechanical ventilation and possibly reduce the incidence of bronchopulmonary dysplasia.[36-38]

Targeted Minute Ventilation

Most preterm infants show significant fluctuations in spontaneous ventilation as a result of inconsistent respiratory drive and acute changes in respiratory mechanics. In order to avoid hypoventilation and hypoxemia during these fluctuations, clinicians usually set higher ventilator rates or PIP values to provide sufficient ventilation at all times, a policy that delays the weaning process.

In *targeted minute ventilation* the mechanical rate is adjusted automatically to maintain a target minute ventilation level. During periods when the infant has consistent spontaneous breathing and minute ventilation is above the target level, the ventilator rate is automatically reduced to a minimum, whereas during periods when ventilation drops below the target, the rate is increased to restore ventilation toward the set target. In a study of preterm infants recovering from respiratory distress

Table 18-2 EXTUBATION CRITERIA

Ventilator Settings	To Consistently Maintain
$F_{IO_2} \leq 0.30$-0.40 PEEP ≤ 5 cm H_2O	$Sp_{O_2} \geq 88\%$
PIP ≤ 15-16 cm H_2O PSV < 8-10 cmH_2O Mandatory rate ≤ 15-20 bpm	$Pa_{CO_2} \leq 65$ mm Hg, pH ≥ 7.25

bpm, breaths per minute; PEEP, positive end-expiratory pressure; PIP, peak inspiratory pressure; PSV, pressure-support ventilation.

syndrome (RDS), targeted minute ventilation reduced the ventilator rate to half that in SIMV. The lower mechanical rate was compensated by greater spontaneous minute ventilation, and arterial blood gas values remained unchanged.[38] Targeted minute ventilation and volume-targeted ventilation have been combined experimentally to achieve automated adjustments of rate and PIP simultaneously. The application of this combined mode in an animal model of hypoxemic episodes resulted in weaning from support during periods of stable breathing and also improved stability of ventilation and gas exchange during periods of apnea or impaired lung mechanics.[39]

Mandatory minute ventilation is a weaning mode that has been used in adults and now is also available for infants. In this mode the ventilator rate is turned off if minute ventilation exceeds a set level or otherwise delivers volume-controlled breaths at a preset rate. A study using this mode in a group of near-term infants without lung disease also achieved a reduction in ventilatory support.[40]

Computer-Assisted Weaning

Patients undergoing mechanical ventilation require frequent adjustments of ventilator settings to maintain desirable gas exchange and blood gas values. To achieve this goal on a more consistent basis, a number of algorithms for ventilator management have been proposed. One of these algorithms based on input from blood gas values and ventilator settings was developed for infants with respiratory distress syndrome; its use resulted in improvements in gas exchange and avoided unnecessary increases in ventilator settings.[41] This experience illustrated to some degree the relative inertia about weaning from ventilator settings and supplemental oxygen during routine care with more effective responses to correct the occurrence of hypoxemia and hypercapnia than hyperoxia or hypocapnia. In contrast, computer-assisted weaning was similarly effective in responding to both situations. Algorithms for computer-assisted ventilation may play an important role in expediting weaning in clinical settings, where different teams are responsible for patient care decisions, or in teaching institutions, where less experienced individuals may be responsible for ventilator management decisions.

Automatic Weaning from Supplemental Oxygen

Most ventilated infants need supplemental oxygen, which increases the risk for lung and retinal injury, particularly when exposure to high FIO_2 is prolonged. In these infants hyperoxemia is frequently induced by an excessive FIO_2 value, which should be avoided with appropriate weaning. However, because many of these infants have frequent spontaneous fluctuations in oxygenation, they can spend prolonged periods with arterial oxygen saturation values above the recommended levels.[42] Pulse oximeter alarms are often ignored or set above the recommended range,[43] and FIO_2 is often set too high to prevent or ameliorate the episodes of hypoxemia.[44] Automated FIO_2 control has been shown to be more effective in keeping oxygenation within a desired range than manual adjustments by the clinical staff during routine care. This was in large part accomplished by avoidance of hyperoxemia resulting from the automatic reduction of FIO_2.[45,46]

Conclusion

Many strategies can be used to expedite weaning of infants from mechanical respiratory support and reduce exposure to invasive ventilation and its complications. Automation of ventilator settings can make this task more consistent and less demanding on staff. Whether automation will improve long-term outcome still needs to be determined.

References

1. Walsh MC, Morris BH, Wrage LA, et al. Extremely low birthweight neonates with protracted ventilation: mortality and 18-month neurodevelopmental outcomes. *J Pediatr*. 2005;146:798-804.
2. Doyle LW, Anderson PJ. Long-term outcomes of bronchopulmonary dysplasia. *Semin Fetal Neonatal Med*. 2009;14:391-395.

3. Fisher JB, Mammel MC, Coleman JM, et al. Identifying lung overdistention during mechanical ventilation by using volume-pressure loops. *Pediatr Pulmonol*. 1988;5:10-14.
4. Rosen WC, Mammel MC, Fisher JB, et al. The effects of bedside pulmonary mechanics testing during infant mechanical ventilation: a retrospective analysis. *Pediatr Pulmonol*. 1993;16:147-152.
5. Mariani G, Cifuentes J, Carlo WA. Randomized trial of permissive hypercapnia in preterm infants. *Pediatrics*. 1999;104:1082-1088.
6. Carlo WA, Stark AR, Wright LL, et al. Minimal ventilation to prevent bronchopulmonary dysplasia in extremely-low-birth-weight infants. *J Pediatr*. 2002;141:370-374.
7. Thome UH, Carroll W, Wu TJ, et al. Outcome of extremely preterm infants randomized at birth to different PaCO2 targets during the first seven days of life. *Biol Neonate*. 2006;90:218-225.
8. Schmidt B, Roberts RS, Davis P, et al. Caffeine therapy for apnea of prematurity. *N Engl J Med*. 2006;354:2112-2121.
9. Schmidt B, Roberts RS, Davis P, et al. Long-term effects of caffeine therapy for apnea of prematurity. *N Engl J Med*. 2007;357:1893-1902.
10. Henderson-Smart DJ, Davis PG. Prophylactic methylxanthines for endotracheal extubation in preterm infants. *Cochrane Database Syst Rev*. 2010;(12):CD000139.
11. Halliday HL, Ehrenkranz RA, Doyle LW. Late (>7 days) postnatal corticosteroids for chronic lung disease in preterm infants. *Cochrane Database Syst Rev*. 2009;(1):CD001145.
12. Doyle LW, Ehrenkranz RA, Halliday HL. Dexamethasone treatment after the first week of life for bronchopulmonary dysplasia in preterm infants: a systematic review. *Neonatology*. 2010;98:289-296.
13. Cole CH, Colton T, Shah BL, et al. Early inhaled glucocorticoid therapy to prevent bronchopulmonary dysplasia. *N Engl J Med*. 1999;340:1005-1010.
14. Numa AH, Newth CJ. Anatomic dead space in infants and children. *J Appl Physiol*. 1996;80:1485-1489.
15. Figueras J, Rodriguez-Miguélez JM, Botet F, et al. Changes in $TcPCO_2$ regarding pulmonary mechanics due to pneumotachometer dead space in ventilated newborns. *J Perinat Med*. 1997;25:333-339.
16. Danan C, Dassieu G, Janaud JC, Brochard L: Efficacy of dead-space washout in mechanically ventilated premature newborns. *Am J Respir Crit Care Med*. 1996;153:1571-1576.
17. Dassieu G, Brochard L, Benani M, et al. Continuous tracheal gas insufflation in preterm infants with hyaline membrane disease. A prospective randomized trial. *Am J Respir Crit Care Med*. 2000;162:826-831.
18. Claure N, D'Ugard C, Bancalari E. Elimination of ventilator dead space during synchronized ventilation in premature infants. *J Pediatr*. 2003;143:315-320.
19. Estay A, Claure N, D'Ugard C, et al. Effects of instrumental dead space reduction during weaning from synchronized ventilation in preterm infants. *J Perinatol*. 2010;30:479-483.
20. Kim EH, Boutwell WC. Successful direct extubation of very low birth weight infants from low intermittent mandatory ventilation rate. *Pediatrics*. 1987;80:409-414.
21. Greenough A. Update on patient-triggered ventilation. *Clin Perinatol*. 2001;28:533-546.
22. Chan V, Greenough A. Comparison of weaning by patient triggered ventilation or synchronous mandatory intermittent ventilation. *Acta Paediatr*. 1994;83:335-337.
23. Dimitriou G, Greenough A, Griffin F, Chan V. Synchronous intermittent mandatory ventilation modes versus patient triggered ventilation during weaning. *Arch Dis Child*. 1995;72:F188-F190.
24. Reyes ZC, Claure N, Tauscher MK, et al. Randomized, controlled trial comparing synchronized intermittent mandatory ventilation and synchronized intermittent mandatory ventilation plus pressure support in preterm infants. *Pediatrics*. 2006;118:1409-1417.
25. Davis PG, Henderson-Smart DJ. Nasal continuous positive airways pressure immediately after extubation for preventing morbidity in preterm infants. *Cochrane Database Syst Rev*. 2003;(2):CD000143.
26. De Paoli AG, Davis PG, Lemyre B: Nasal continuous positive airway pressure versus nasal intermittent positive pressure ventilation for preterm neonates: a systematic review and meta-analysis. *Acta Paediatr*. 2003;92:70-75.
27. Lin CH, Wang ST, Lin YJ, et al. Efficacy of nasal intermittent positive pressure ventilation in treating apnea of prematurity. *Pediatr Pulmonol*. 1998;26:349-533.
28. Moretti C, Gizzi C, Papoff P, et al. Comparing the effects of nasal synchronized intermittent positive pressure ventilation (nSIPPV) and nasal continuous positive airway pressure (N-CPAP) after extubation in very low birth weight infants. *Early Hum Dev*. 1999;56:167-177.
29. Ali N, Claure N, Alegria X, et al. Effects of non-invasive pressure support ventilation (NI-PSV) on ventilation and respiratory effort in very low birth weight infants. *Pediatr Pulmonol*. 2007;42:704-710.
30. Kiciman NM, Andreasson B, Bernstein G, et al. Thoracoabdominal motion in newborns during ventilation delivered by endotracheal tube or nasal prongs. *Pediatr Pulmonol*. 1998;25:175-181.
31. Chang HY, Claure N, D'Ugard C, et al. Effects of synchronization during nasal ventilation in clinically stable preterm infants. *Pediatr Res*. 2011;69:84-89.
32. Vento G, Tortorolo L, Zecca E, et al. Spontaneous minute ventilation is a predictor of extubation failure in extremely-low-birth-weight infants. *J Matern Fetal Neonatal Med*. 2004;15:147-154.
33. Gillespie LM, White SD, Sinha SK, Donn SM. Usefulness of the minute ventilation test in predicting successful extubation in newborn infants: a randomized controlled trial. *J Perinatol*. 2003;23:205-207.
34. Kamlin CO, Davis PG, Morley CJ. Predicting successful extubation of very low birthweight infants. *Arch Dis Child Fetal Neonatal Ed*. 2006;91:F180-F183.

35. Herrera CM, Gerhardt T, Claure N, et al. Effects of volume-guaranteed synchronized intermittent mandatory ventilation in preterm infants recovering from respiratory failure. *Pediatrics*. 2002;110: 529-533.
36. Sinha SK, Donn SM, Gavey J, McCarty M. Randomised trial of volume controlled versus time cycled, pressure limited ventilation in preterm infants with respiratory distress syndrome. *Arch Dis Child Fetal Neonatal Ed*. 1997;77:F202-F205.
37. Singh J, Sinha SK, Clarke P, et al. Mechanical ventilation of very low birth weight infants: Is volume or pressure a better target variable? *J Pediatr*. 2006;149:308-313.
38. Claure N, Gerhardt T, Hummler H, et al. Computer-controlled minute ventilation in preterm infants undergoing mechanical ventilation. *J Pediatr*. 1997;131:910-913.
39. Claure N, Suguihara C, Peng J, et al. Targeted minute ventilation and tidal volume in an animal model of acute changes in lung mechanics and episodes of hypoxemia. *Neonatology*. 2009;95: 132-140.
40. Guthrie SO, Lynn C, Lafleur BJ, et al. A crossover analysis of mandatory minute ventilation compared to synchronized intermittent mandatory ventilation in neonates. *J Perinatol*. 2005;25:643-646.
41. Carlo WA, Pacifico L, Chatburn RL, Fanaroff AA. Efficacy of computer-assisted management of respiratory failure in neonates. *Pediatrics*. 1986;78:139-143.
42. Hagadorn JI, Furey AM, Nghiem TH, et al. AVIOx Study Group: Achieved versus intended pulse oximeter saturation in infants born less than 28 weeks' gestation: the AVIOx study. *Pediatrics*. 2006;118:1574-1582.
43. Clucas L, Doyle LW, Dawson J, et al. Compliance with alarm limits for pulse oximetry in very preterm infants. *Pediatrics*. 2007;119:1056-1060.
44. McEvoy C, Durand M, Hewlett V. Episodes of spontaneous desaturations in infants with chronic lung disease at two different levels of oxygenation. *Pediatr Pulmonol*. 1993;15:140-144.
45. Claure N, D'Ugard C, Bancalari E. Automated adjustment of inspired oxygen in preterm infants with frequent fluctuations in oxygenation: a pilot clinical trial. *J Pediatr*. 2009;155:640-645.
46. Claure N, Bancalari E, D'Ugard C, et al. Multicenter crossover study of automated adjustment of inspired oxygen in mechanically ventilated preterm infants. *Pediatrics*. 2011;127:e76-e83.

CHAPTER 19

Automation of Respiratory Support

Nelson Claure, MSc, PhD, and Eduardo Bancalari, MD

19

- Automation of Mechanical Ventilatory Support
- Volume Targeted Ventilation
- Targeted Minute Ventilation
- Proportional Assist Ventilation
- Neurally Adjusted Ventilatory Assist
- Automated Adjustment of Supplemental Oxygen
- Summary

An important proportion of premature infants with respiratory distress require mechanical ventilatory support and supplemental oxygen. However, these forms of respiratory support increase the risk for lung injury particularly when provided for a prolonged time. Oxygen supplementation is also associated with greater risk for eye injury as well as oxidative damage to the central nervous system and other organs. More importantly, these neonatal morbidities have been associated with long-term respiratory impairment and poor neurodevelopmental outcome.[1-5] During routine neonatal intensive care, caregivers are required to make frequent adjustments in respiratory support on the basis of monitored parameters of ventilation and oxygenation to minimize the risk of those unwanted side effects. Nonetheless, the respiratory support often exceeds what is actually needed by the infant or at the time is insufficient. This problem is due to the intrinsic respiratory instability of the preterm infant and to limitations of neonatal intensive care unit (NICU) staff that do not allow minute-to-minute adaptation of the level of respiratory support to the infant's needs.

Newer forms of neonatal respiratory support have been introduced or are currently being evaluated. Development of these forms of support, largely facilitated by the use of newer technology in neonatal ventilators, improved sensing devices and automation techniques, is aimed primarily at tailoring the level of respiratory support on the basis of monitored physiologic parameters. These newer forms of neonatal respiratory support offer potential improvements in patient care by adapting the mechanical respiratory support to the changing needs of preterm infants. This chapter describes these forms of support, presents the existing evidence obtained from their application in clinical studies, and discusses their possible advantages and shortcomings.

Automation of Mechanical Ventilatory Support

In spite of continuous efforts to reduce the use of mechanical ventilation during the acute phase of respiratory distress syndrome (RDS) by means of noninvasive forms of respiratory support, a considerable proportion of preterm infants require intubation and mechanical ventilation. As the initial respiratory failure improves, two divergent patterns are commonly observed. In some infants, the weaning process proceeds rapidly, but in others, weaning is difficult and they remain on prolonged mechanical ventilatory support.

In addition to the various degrees of lung disease, factors that prolong the mechanical ventilatory support in preterm infants include immaturity of the respiratory center, variability in lung compliance or airway resistance, instability of lung volume due to a very compliant chest wall, and ineffective surfactant function. These conditions increase the respiratory instability and variability in gas exchange, which, compounded with an inconsistent weaning management and staff limitations, lead to protracted ventilation and increased risk for lung injury.

Common modes of neonatal ventilation, such as intermittent mandatory ventilation (IMV), synchronized IMV (SIMV), and assist/control (A/C) ventilation, provide a constant ventilatory support whereby the peak inspiratory pressure (PIP), ventilator cycling frequency, or both are constant and cannot adapt to the changing needs of the preterm infants without manual adjustment by a caregiver. In these modes, as the ventilator frequency and PIP are reduced, spontaneous inspiratory effort plays a greater role in generating the tidal volume (V_T) as well as in maintaining minute ventilation. However, minute ventilation can be affected by the infant's inconsistent respiratory drive because of frequent reductions in or cessation of spontaneous breathing effort and by acute changes in lung mechanics that reduce the V_T produced by the ventilator and the spontaneous inspiratory effort. In order to maintain adequate ventilation at all times, clinicians often provide higher ventilator frequencies or PIP. On the other hand, when lung mechanics improve, the set PIP and ventilator frequency may exceed the infant's needs and provide excessive V_T and minute ventilation, raising the risk of volutrauma and hypocapnia. In order to overcome these limitations, new automated modes have been developed to maintain different ventilatory parameters at a desired target level.

Volume Targeted Ventilation

In volume-targeted ventilation, the ventilator peak pressure or inspiratory duration is automatically adjusted from one cycle to the next or within the cycle to maintain the V_T of the mechanical cycle at a set target level. The advantages of volume-targeted ventilation are based on a more effective maintenance of a stable V_T, which can prevent excessive lung inflation or lung volume loss due to insufficient V_T and lead to a more stable gas exchange during changes in lung mechanics and spontaneous respiratory effort. Figure 19-1 shows typical adjustments in peak pressure to changes in spontaneous respiratory effort during volume-targeted ventilation.

Although the general concept is similar, there are multiple systems for the implementation of volume-targeted ventilation. These may differ in the volume parameter being controlled, that is, the volume delivered to the patient during inspiration, the volume returning from the patient during the expiratory phase, or the volume delivered by the ventilator to the circuit and patient.

A number of modalities of volume-targeted ventilation have become available. However, only a few of them have been evaluated clinically in preterm infants. The next sections present an overview and discussion of the modalities of volume-targeted ventilation that have been examined in preterm infants.

Volume guarantee (VG) ventilation is a modality in which PIP is adjusted from one cycle to the next to maintain a target V_T. The measured exhaled V_T from previous cycles is compared with the target, and a built-in algorithm adjusts the PIP of the subsequent cycle on the basis of the comparison. Because the positive pressure during the inspiratory phase often produces gas leakage around the endotracheal tube, which leads to overestimation of V_T, VG ventilation is based on the V_T measured during expiration. The clinician is responsible for setting the target V_T and the maximal inspiratory pressure that determines the working range for the automatic adjustments of PIP. VG ventilation can be used in combination with A/C ventilation, pressure support ventilation (PSV), SIMV, and IMV.

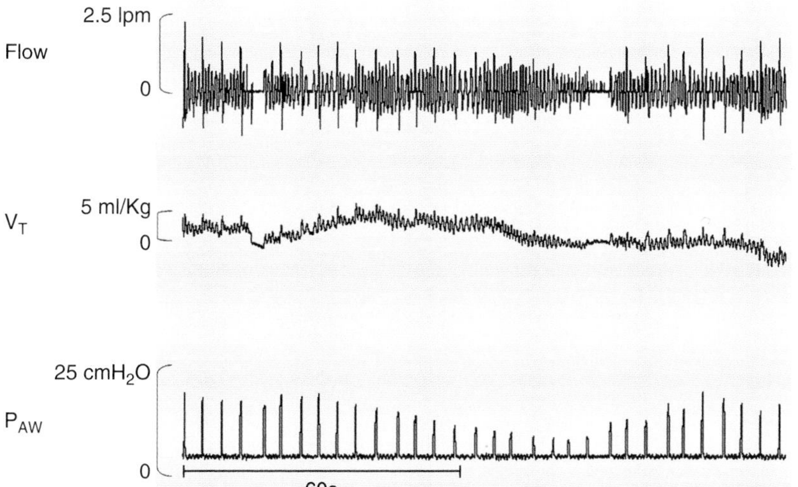

Figure 19-1 Automatic adjustments in peak pressure in response to changes in spontaneous breathing effort during volume-targeted ventilation. Flow (measured in liters per minute [lpm]), tidal volume (V_T), and airway pressure (P_{AW}) tracings during volume-targeted ventilation show automatic downward adjustments in peak pressure as the infant's contribution to V_T increased. They are followed by upward adjustments in peak pressure when V_T decreased. s, second.

Pressure-regulated–volume-controlled (PRVC) ventilation is a modality in which, after an initial diagnostic cycle to determine the respiratory system compliance, PIP is subsequently adjusted from cycle to cycle to deliver a target volume. The measured volume can be that delivered by the ventilator to the circuit or the estimated infant's inspiratory V_T after the volume compressed in the circuit is compensated for. Measurements during the inspiratory phase may considerably overestimate V_T in the presence of gas leaks around the endotracheal tube.

In *volume-controlled (VC) ventilation,* a set volume of gas is delivered to the infant and the inspiratory phase ends when this volume is delivered. In some ventilators the volume targeted is that delivered to the circuit, which is much larger than the preterm infant's V_T. Because V_T is only a fraction of the volume delivered to the ventilator circuit, compensation for the volume compressed in the circuit is required in VC ventilation to estimate the actual V_T delivered to the infant. Volume-controlled breaths can be used in combination with A/C ventilation, SIMV or IMV. Alternatively, some ventilators offer a volume-limiting function as a safeguard against volutrauma during conventional pressure-controlled ventilation.

Clinical studies in infants with RDS showed VG can reduce the variability in V_T, the number of ventilator cycles delivering too large or small V_T, and the occurrence of hypocapnia in comparison with conventional pressure-limited ventilation.[6-10] Also, the automatic increase in PIP can attenuate the hypoventilation that leads to episodes of hypoxemia.[11] This effect reduces the duration of the hypoxemia spells but does not prevent their occurrence.[12,13]

One of the proposed advantages of volume-targeted ventilation is that of achieving an automatic reduction of the peak pressure as the infant's lung function improves or the contribution of the spontaneous inspiratory effort to V_T increases. In several studies in infants with RDS, VG ventilation achieved only a slight reduction in PIP compared with conventional pressure-limited ventilation.[7-10,14] This was likely because the targeted V_T in those studies was comparable to that observed during pressure-limited ventilation. It is possible that a more striking automatic weaning could be achieved in centers that are less attentive in adjusting PIP to maintain V_T within the goal range.

During volume-targeted ventilation, the reduction of PIP proceeds as long as V_T remains above the target level, and further weaning is not achieved unless the

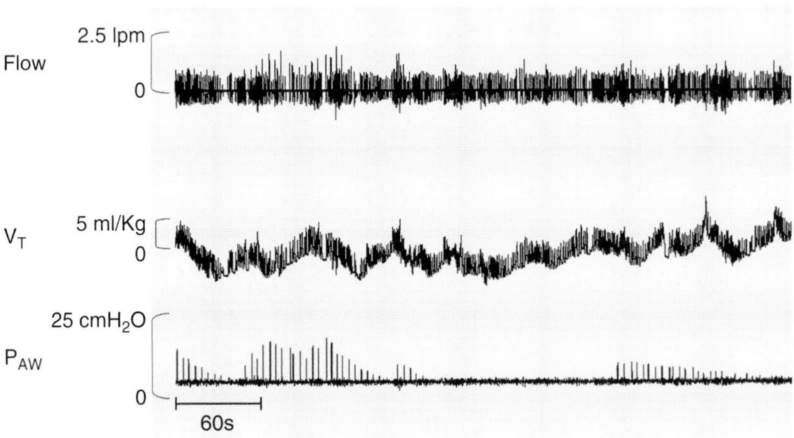

Figure 19-2 Automatic reduction in peak pressure during volume-targeted ventilation with a low target tidal volume (V_T). Tracings of flow (measured in liters per minute [lpm]), V_T, and airway pressure (P_{AW}) during volume-targeted ventilation show a declining peak pressure as the infant maintained V_T above the target V_T. This resulted in periods when the infant was left receiving only positive end-expiratory pressure (PEEP). s, seconds.

measured V_T increases as a result of a greater spontaneous effort or an improvement in lung mechanics. A possible alternative to achieve further weaning is targeting a smaller V_T. This approach, however, would rely on the infant's respiratory drive to consistently maintain ventilation while the ventilator would only ensure a minimal V_T to avoid a severe hypoventilation. In one study, targeting of relatively low V_T in the range typically observed in unassisted spontaneous breaths did indeed achieve a more striking weaning from PIP but required a compensatory rise in spontaneous breathing effort or resulted in higher transcutaneous $P\text{CO}_2$ levels in infants whose spontaneous ventilation was insufficient.[7] A target V_T that is too low and can be easily exceeded by the spontaneous breathing effort can result in periods when the peak pressure is reduced to very low levels or can even result in periods when the infant does not receive any support and is left only receiving positive end-expiratory pressure (PEEP), as shown in Figure 19-2.

Randomized clinical trials in preterm infants with RDS, showed volume-targeted ventilation has more striking effects on weaning in the smaller premature infants, although reports from individual trials are not entirely consistent. In two studies in infants with birth weight less than 1000 g, PRVC ventilation in the A/C mode decreased the duration of ventilation in comparison with IMV only but not in comparison with SIMV.[15,16] In infants with birth weight of 1200 g or less, two studies found that weaning was faster with VC ventilation than with pressure-limited ventilation, and this difference was even more striking in infants of birth weight less than 1000 g.[17,18]

It has also been proposed that by reducing exposure to excessive lung inflation, volume-targeted ventilation could avert lung injury and the concomitant inflammatory process. Infants with RDS who were ventilated with VG had lower levels of inflammatory cytokines in bronchoalveolar fluid during the first week than infants ventilated with the conventional pressure-limited mode.[19] However, inflammatory markers were actually increased in infants with RDS ventilated with VG at a smaller volume target.[20] This second finding suggests that avoidance of a too low V_T value may be as relevant as avoiding overinflation. The selection of the target V_T should be aimed at balancing effective weaning and maintenance of adequate blood gas values against the risk of hypoventilation leading to atelectasis or an excessive increase in respiratory effort.

In spite of the faster weaning and shorter duration of ventilation shown in the randomized trials, bronchopulmonary dysplasia (BPD) and the rates of acute adverse events such as air leaks or other morbidities were not consistently improved.

However, a meta-analysis showed that the combined outcome death or bronchopulmonary dysplasia was improved by volume-targeted ventilation.[20] Although a greater improvement in respiratory outcome could have been expected, the increased awareness of the need to avoid excessive ventilator pressures during conventional ventilation concurrent with the introduction of volume-targeted ventilation may have attenuated the differences. Hence, benefits of volume-targeted ventilation are likely to be relative to the conventional management used in individual centers. Although the different modalities of volume-targeted ventilation have similar aims, their relative efficacies have not been evaluated.

The clinician is responsible for setting the target V_T, but at present there is a profound paucity of data on the most appropriate V_T for the different phases of lung disease in preterm infants and on the most effective target V_T to be used with different ventilator modes. Therefore, caution should be exercised in selecting the target V_T and, more importantly, in setting the limits to PIP and inspiratory time.

Targeted Minute Ventilation

Targeted minute ventilation describes various modalities of ventilatory support in which the ventilator frequency is automatically adjusted to maintain a set level of minute ventilation. The primary objective is to achieve a reduction in ventilatory support in the form of fewer ventilatory breaths while maintaining adequate minute ventilation. This is primarily accomplished by reducing the ventilator rate when the infant is capable of maintaining most of the minute ventilation or by increasing it as needed to avoid hypoventilation.

An experimental modality of targeted minute ventilation consists of automatic adjustments of the ventilator rate in an inverse proportion to the difference between measured and target minute ventilation values. The clinician sets the target minute ventilation and the range of ventilator rates the algorithm is allowed to operate within. If minute ventilation exceeds the set target, ventilator rate is automatically reduced stepwise to the lower limit. If minute ventilation declines below the target or even if it is above target with a declining trend in minute ventilation, the ventilator rate is increased.

Our group compared this modality of targeted minute ventilation with SIMV in preterm infants recovering from RDS.[20] There was an automatic reduction in ventilator rate to one half of the SIMV rate, and the infants were able to compensate and maintain the total minute ventilation and stable gas exchange. In this study, there were also transient automatic increases in ventilator rate that at times exceeded the SIMV rate to prevent hypoventilation during periods of central apnea or reduced V_T. Typical adjustments of the ventilator rate during targeted minute ventilation are shown in Figure 19-3. In the same study, the ventilator contributed approximately 40% of the total minute ventilation in SIMV mode. In contrast, the ventilator's contribution to total minute ventilation was consistently reduced, but total minute ventilation remained within the same range, as illustrated in Figure 19-4. The effects of different target levels of minute ventilation have not been assessed. The level of minute ventilation targeted in this study was a fraction of the infant's total minute ventilation. Maintenance of minute ventilation at or above this level was assumed to be adequate for gas exchange. On the other hand, a target level near the infant's total minute ventilation, which may be more effective in preventing hypoventilation, would not achieve weaning from the ventilator rate unless the infant maintains spontaneous ventilation above this level to elicit a decrease in ventilator rate. A high minute ventilation target level could also lead to the ventilator's taking over if the ventilation required by the infant is provided in its entirety by the ventilator.

An alternative form of targeted minute ventilation to adjust the ventilator's rate and PIP simultaneously for maintenance of a target minute ventilation and V_T, respectively, has been developed by our group. The objective of this combined approach is to achieve automated weaning of the ventilator rate and pressure as well as to maintain better ventilation stability during periods of apnea or worsened lung

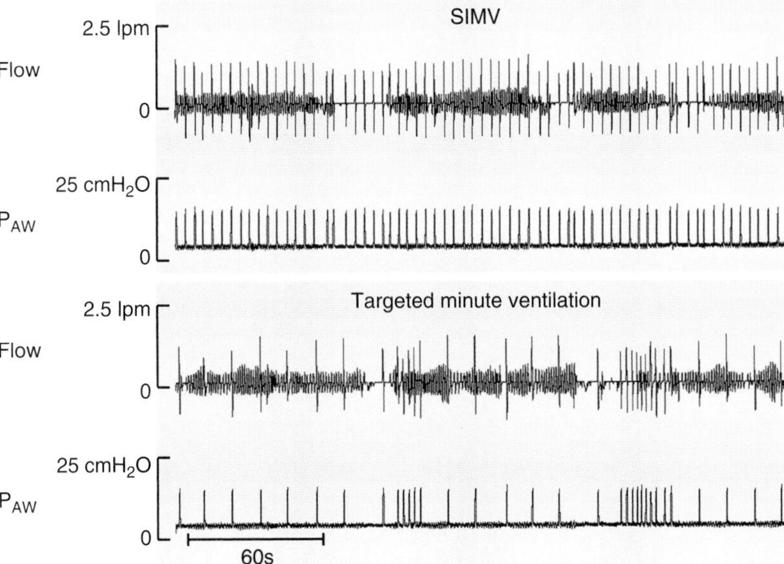

Figure 19-3 Automatic adjustments in ventilator rate during SIMV (*top*) and targeted minute ventilation (*bottom*). Tracings of flow and airway pressure (P_{AW}) show a considerable reduction in ventilator rate during targeted minute ventilation when the infant's spontaneous ventilation was sufficient. Transient automatic increases in ventilator rate to preserve ventilation during periods of apnea were also observed during targeted minute ventilation. lpm, liters per minute; s, seconds; SIMV, spontaneous intermittent mandatory ventilation.

mechanics, as shown in Figure 19-5. In an animal model replicating the mechanisms leading to hypoxemia in preterm infants, automatic increases in ventilator rate or PIP were individually effective in attenuating the severity of hypoxemia and the simultaneous adjustment further improved ventilation stability and attenuated hypoxemia.[21] This strategy has not been evaluated in infants.

Mandatory minute ventilation (MMV) is a modality in which the measured minute ventilation is continuously compared with a set target level. Ventilator mandatory breaths stop when this target level is exceeded, and minute ventilation is maintained by unassisted spontaneous breaths or by spontaneous breaths assisted with pressure support. If minute ventilation declines below the target level, the ventilator delivers volume-targeted cycles at a constant rate to keep minute ventilation at the set target. In near-term infants without lung disease, MMV was found to be associated with a lower ventilator rate than SIMV while spontaneous breaths were assisted by PSV.[22] This mode has not been yet evaluated in premature infants with lung disease.

Apnea backup ventilation is a modality of support available in newer neonatal ventilators that is used in combination with PSV. In this modality, spontaneous breaths are assisted by pressure support, and upon the occurrence of apnea, the ventilator initiates mechanical breaths at a constant rate and PIP set by the clinician. This modality differs from A/C ventilation in that the backup cycles can be set at a different peak pressure than pressure support. The clinical effects of this modality have not yet been evaluated in preterm infants.

Adaptive mechanical backup ventilation is a new modality in which, in addition to the spontaneous breathing, the ventilator monitors the arterial oxygen saturation (SpO_2). Upon the occurrence of apnea or hypoxemia, the ventilator provides a backup rate until the episode is resolved. In preterm infants recovering from RDS, adaptive backup ventilation using SpO_2 was found to attenuate the frequency and duration of episodes of hypoxemia in comparison with conventional backup ventilation set to respond to apnea alone.[23] These results suggest a role for hybrid ventilatory modes to improve the maintenance of gas exchange stability.

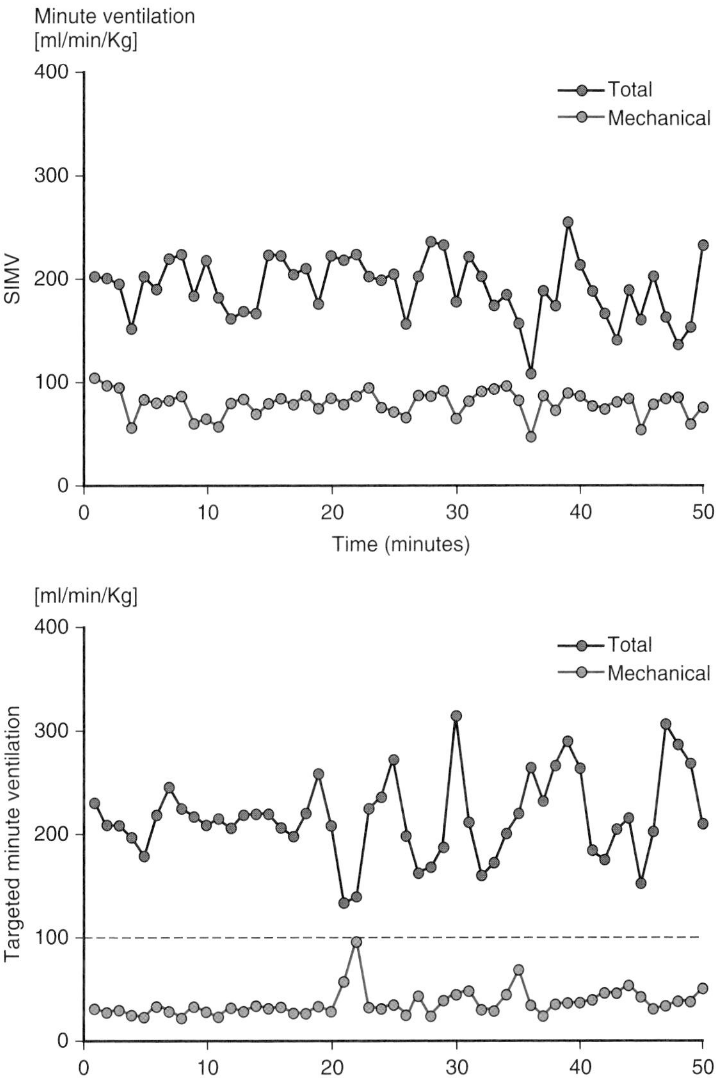

19

Figure 19-4 Minute ventilation over time during spontaneous intermittent mandatory ventilation (SIMV; *top*) and targeted minute ventilation (*bottom*). Minute-to-minute values of minute ventilation show that the contribution of the ventilator during SIMV represented approximately 40% of the total minute ventilation. During targeted minute ventilation, the contribution of the ventilation was considerably smaller except during a brief period when the ventilator rate was increased in response to a declining trend in total minute ventilation toward the target level (*dotted line*).

Proportional Assist Ventilation

The respiratory pump of the ventilated preterm infant has to overcome mechanical impediments to generate an adequate V_T. These loads are induced by obstructive or restrictive conditions resulting from the underlying lung disease. Application of positive pressure to the airway in synchrony with the infant's spontaneous inspiration helps overcome such loads. New modalities of mechanical ventilation in which the positive pressure applied to the airway is enslaved to the timing and to the magnitude of the inspiratory effort are now available.

Proportional assist ventilation (PAV) is a modality whereby the ventilator pressure is automatically adjusted in proportion to the volume, flow, or both, generated by the respiratory pump. This arrangement enhances the infant's volume- or

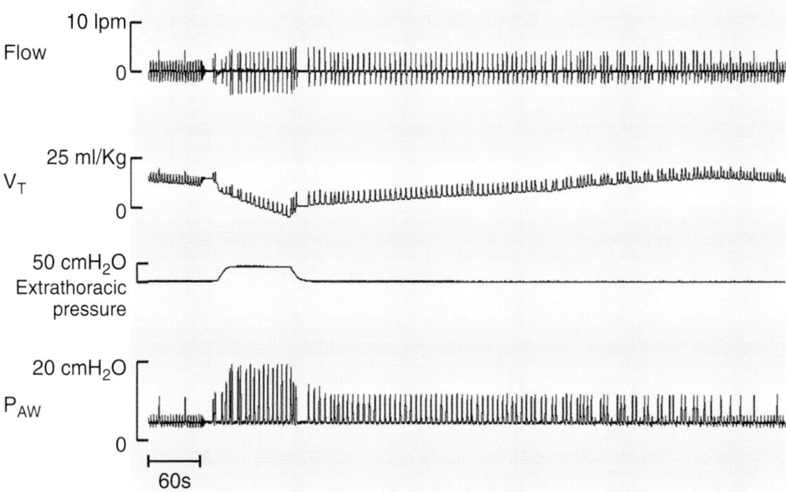

Figure 19-5 Automatic adjustments of ventilator rate and peak pressure. Recordings of flow (measured in liters per minute [lpm]), tidal volume (V_T), extrathoracic pressure, and airway pressure (P_{AW}) illustrate simultaneous adjustments of ventilator rate and peak inspiratory pressure (PIP) in response to a reduction in respiratory system compliance produced by compression of the chest and the induction of apnea by a bolus of propofol in an experimental animal. PIP returned to baseline as soon as compliance improved, and the initial increase in ventilator rate was followed by a gradual reduction as the animal's spontaneous breathing resumed.

flow-generating ability and results in a perceived reduction in the impediments to breathe. PAV is intrinsically different from synchronized pressure or volume modalities, and its management is quite different. In PAV, the user determines the degree of mechanical unloading by setting the elastic (volume-proportional) and resistive (flow-proportional) gains in pressure. These gains must be suited to each infant and require estimation of the respiratory compliance and/or airway resistance. Higher gains result in larger increases in airway pressure per unit of volume or flow generated by the infant. An elastic gain that exceeds the elastic recoil of the lungs can lead to a runaway increase in pressure, whereas a resistive gain that compensates beyond the airway resistance can lead to pressure oscillations.

PAV may at first seem counterintuitive and opposite to what happens during conventional IPPV, in which the positive pressure is reduced when V_T or the inspiratory effort increases. However, adjustment of the PAV gains to maintain adequate ventilation is not strikingly different from adjustments during PSV or A/C ventilation, in which the peak pressure is increased when V_T is not sufficient, or reduced when V_T is excessive. The positive airway pressure is automatically adjusted by the ventilator during PAV but the clinician is responsible for setting appropriate limits for peak pressure, delivered volume, and inspiratory time. The use of PAV in preterm infants also requires backup mandatory breaths during apnea.

The acute physiologic and short-term clinical effects of PAV in preterm infants include reduced breathing effort and improvements in ventilation and gas exchange with lower peak airway pressures in comparison with IMV, A/C ventilation, and SIMV during the weaning phase of RDS and in the evolving phases of chronic lung disease.[24-26] These data suggest short-term benefits, but further research is needed to identify the population or lung disease stage that could benefit most from PAV and to determine the modality's role in improving long-term pulmonary outcome.

Neurally Adjusted Ventilatory Assist

Neurally adjusted ventilatory assist (NAVA) is a modality in which the positive pressure applied to the airway is proportional to the electrical activity of the crural diaphragm. NAVA is being proposed as an improvement over standard methods used for synchronization, which may be limited by inadequate coupling of the force generated by the diaphragm and the components of the respiratory system that do not accurately reflect the timing and magnitude of the respiratory center's neural output. During NAVA, much as in PAV, the airway pressure is greater as the infant's inspiratory effort increases. The clinician is responsible for setting the gain that determines the amplitude of the airway pressure per microvolt of diaphragmatic activity, the peak inspiratory pressure limit, and the backup support in the event of apnea.

In NAVA, increasing the proportionality gain can produce an increase in V_T, a reduction in diaphragmatic activity, or both. V_T and the electrical activity of the diaphragm are monitored continuously and are used to adjust the NAVA gain. However, data on the relation between the electrical activity of the diaphragm and inspiratory effort or volume generation, and the variability between or within patients are scant for preterm infants.

19

In one study, NAVA was shown to maintain ventilation and gas exchange similarly to conventional PSV and PSV with VG in preterm infants. This was accompanied by a slower neural respiratory rhythm, but there were no striking effects on the activity of the diaphragm as an indicator of effort with the gain used in this study.[27] The application of NAVA for nasal ventilation, also described in this study, represents a promising alternative for noninvasive ventilatory support in neonates. In a study of term neonates and pediatric patients, NAVA maintained gas exchange with a slightly lower peak pressures than PSV.[28]

The use of NAVA requires insertion of a special esophageal catheter to measure the electrical activity of the diaphragm. Although this maneuver may seem slightly invasive, the catheter is dual-purpose similar to catheters used routinely for feeding or gastric gas decompression. The position of the catheter for an optimum diaphragmatic signal quality is important. The practicality and reliability of NAVA in the busy NICU environment have not been established. Until now, NAVA has been shown to be well tolerated, but further research is needed to assess its physiologic and clinical effects in premature infants.

Automated Adjustment of Supplemental Oxygen

Most preterm infants with lung disease and respiratory insufficiency require supplemental oxygen to maintain adequate oxygenation. However, the concentration of inspired oxygen may at times be excessive. The exposure to high levels of inspired oxygen and the resulting hyperoxemia are associated with increased risk for chronic lung injury, eye damage, and oxidative stress in other organs, including the central nervous system.[29-32] In order to reduce the associated risks, arterial oxygen saturation is continuously monitored by pulse oximetry (SpO_2), and the fraction of inspired oxygen (FIO_2) is adjusted to keep oxygen exposure at a minimum and avoid the extreme ranges of SpO_2. However, observational multicenter data revealed that in preterm infants receiving supplemental oxygen, SpO_2 is within the range of oxygenation intended by the clinician only about half the time, is above the range one third of the time, and is below the range one fifth of the time.[33,34] These data also showed that maintenance of the intended range of oxygenation worsens over time and is only slightly improved by the use of alarms set at or just outside the intended range of SpO_2.[35] Maintenance of oxygenation within the intended range has been shown to be largely influenced by the nurse-to-patient ratio.[36]

During routine care, FIO_2 should be gradually reduced to avoid high SpO_2 levels and also should be adjusted if SpO_2 decreases below the intended range so as to avoid tissue hypoxia. Maintenance of the intended range of SpO_2 worsens over time because most preterm infants present with more frequent fluctuations in SpO_2.[37,38] These fluctuations exacerbate the difficulty of keeping oxygenation within the desired range and increase the demand for staff effort. Data suggest these fluctuations may be associated with retinal injury,[38,39] more particularly when they involve hyperoxemia.[40,41] The fluctuations may also have negative effects on airway function, lung vasculature, and other organs.[42-45] Standard conditions in the NICU do not permit a fully dedicated caregiver's attention for each patient. Frequently, the response to the finding of SpO_2 outside the intended range is not optimal, and SpO_2 levels above the intended range are often tolerated.

Systems that automatically adjust FIO_2 to maintain SpO_2 within a target range or at set level have been evaluated in preterm infants. These systems conduct the time-consuming and repetitive adjustments of FIO_2 required of nursing staff in the maintenance of SpO_2 within a desired range in preterm infants with the goal of reducing periods of hyperoxemia and hypoxemia and the exposure to high levels of FIO_2.

C

Effects on Oxygenation, Inspired Oxygen Concentration, and Workload

The feasibility of several systems for automated adjustment of FIO_2 in infants has been explored.[46-53] These studies found that automated control maintained oxygenation within the desired range better than manual adjustments made by the infant's caregivers and showed efficacy comparable to or better than a fully dedicated research nurse.

Evaluating automatic FIO_2 control for the maintenance of oxygenation stability and oxygen exposure during routine clinical conditions is particularly important because it provides a true measure of effect and provides insight into potential safety issues and interaction with the routine care in the NICU. Studies conducted under routine clinical NICU conditions documented improved maintenance of SpO_2 within the desired range as well as significant reductions in hyperoxemia and inspired oxygen concentration with use of automatic FIO_2 control.[54,55] These issues are particularly important in infants who present with frequent fluctuations in oxygenation and offer a significant challenge to the clinical staff.

Data obtained in these studies showed that in an attempt to attenuate the frequency of hypoxemia episodes, the clinical staff tolerates high SpO_2 levels, which often exceed target or alarm ranges. This tendency results in exposure to higher FIO_2, as illustrated in Figure 19-6. In these studies the reduction in hyperoxemia during automated FIO_2 control was accompanied by more frequent but milder fluctuations in SpO_2, just below the target range, than with routine manual adjustment, as illustrated in Figure 19-7. To what extent these relatively mild episodes may raise the risks of adverse effects and offset the benefits of avoiding hyperoxemia is not known.

An important goal of automatic FIO_2 control is reducing the concentration of oxygen in the inspired gas with the aim of reducing oxygen radical injury in the lung. FIO_2 has been consistently reduced by automatic FIO_2 control.[54,55] This reduction is primarily the result of the avoidance of high SpO_2 levels and is therefore largely relative to the efficacy of manual FIO_2 control under routine conditions.

Reducing the need for manual adjustments of FIO_2 by automated FIO_2 control is being proposed as a way to reduce workload. Studies have documented manual FIO_2 adjustments at intervals ranging from 7 to 120 minutes during routine care to every 2 minutes by a fully dedicated nurse.[47,48,54-55] Although the interval between adjustments is largely determined by the frequency or severity of the fluctuations in SpO_2, maintenance of SpO_2 within a desired range improves with more attentive care.[40,43,44] Figure 19-8 illustrates how demanding the task is for the staff to maintain SpO_2 with manual FIO_2 adjustments. In infants with frequent episodes of hypoxemia, caregivers manually adjusted FIO_2 a mean of 112 times in 24 hours, compared with only 10 times during automated FIO_2 control.[55]

Possible Limitations of Automated FIO_2 Control

Automated FIO_2 control could lead to a reduction in caregiver attentiveness to the patient. For instance, an automatic increase in FIO_2 could mask a condition (e.g., hypoventilation) that could otherwise result in hypoxemia and call the caregiver's attention. To avoid this situation, built-in warnings should alert the caregiver not

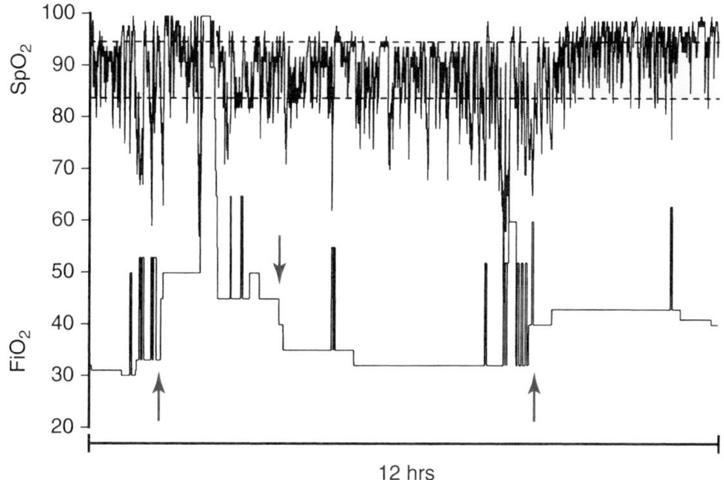

Figure 19-6 Manual adjustments of fractional inspired oxygen (FIO_2) during episodes of hypoxemia. Twelve-hour recordings of oxygen saturation (SpO_2) and FIO_2 from a preterm infant with frequent fluctuations in oxygenation show typical adjustments in response to hypoxemia spells during routine care. These adjustments consisted of multiple transient increases in FIO_2 in response to episodes with SpO_2 declining into hypoxemia (*below bottom dotted line*) and changes in the baseline FIO_2 level (*red arrows*). Increases in basal FIO_2 attenuated the severity of the hypoxemia spells but increased both the periods with SPO_2 in hyperoxemia (*above top dotted line*) and the exposure to higher concentrations of inspired oxygen.

only when SpO_2 decreases but also when FIO_2 is consistently increased. On the other hand, the more rapid automatic response could be beneficial by preventing the detrimental effects of worsened hypoxemia until the proper corrective actions take place.

Pulse oximetry is the most common method of oxygenation monitoring in the NICU and is the preferred choice for automated FIO_2 control because it is

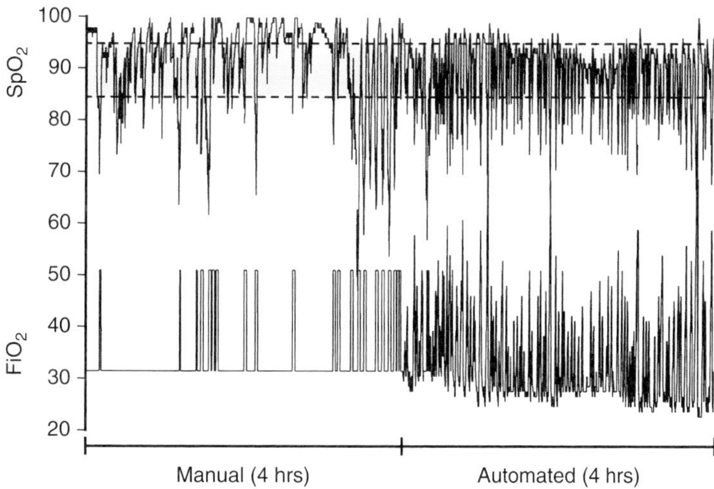

Figure 19-7 Manual and automatic adjustments to fractional inspired oxygen (FIO_2) during episodes of hypoxemia. Recordings of oxygen saturation (SpO_2) and FIO_2 from a preterm infant with episodic hypoxemia show frequent manual increases in FIO_2 in response to episodes of hypoxemia (SpO_2 declining below bottom dotted line) while the basal FIO_2 was kept unchanged during routine manual care. The continuously high basal FIO_2 led to periods of hyperoxemia (SpO_2 above top dotted line). During automated control, a gradual weaning of the basal FIO_2 prevented hyperoxemia, but it was accompanied by more frequent and milder episodes of hypoxemia.

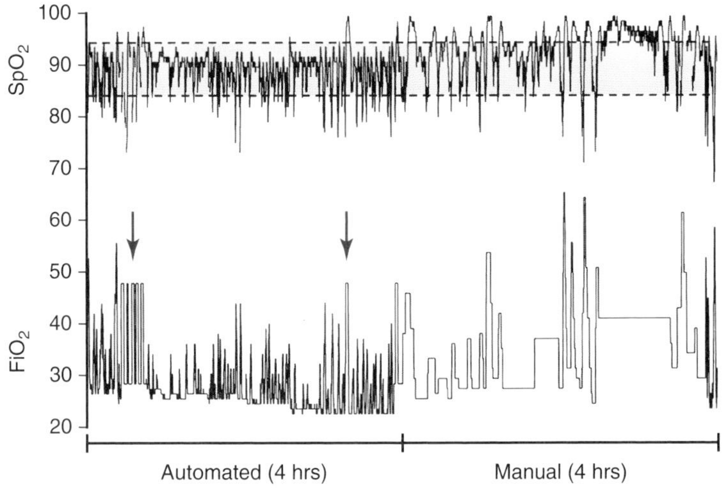

Figure 19-8 Manual adjustments to fractional inspired oxygen (F_{IO_2}) in response to hypoxemic spells. Representative recordings of oxygen saturation (Sp_{O_2}) and F_{IO_2} are illustrative of the difficult and intense task of maintaining Sp_{O_2} within a desired range indicated by the dotted lines with manual adjustments of F_{IO_2} during routine care. In contrast, fewer manual adjustments were needed during automated F_{IO_2} control, and these occurred mostly during care procedures (*red arrows*).

noninvasive nature and continuous availability in preterm infants. Although pulse oximetry has improved considerably over the years, its reliability in preterm infants can be affected by motion, poor perfusion, and inadequate probe placement.[56-59] Poor Sp_{O_2} reliability during automated F_{IO_2} control can lead to hyperoxemia if hypoxemia is erroneously detected. This problem is not exclusive to automated F_{IO_2} control; it may also occur during routine care. When certain conditions affect Sp_{O_2} reliability, the clinician can elect not to consider Sp_{O_2} readings in the patient management. Stricter criteria should be applied when the use of Sp_{O_2}-targeted automated F_{IO_2} control is considered.

One of the most important considerations before automatic F_{IO_2} control is used clinically in preterm infants is that the clinician is responsible for setting the target range. This issue is particularly relevant because the optimal range of oxygenation for preterm infants has not been defined. There may be important physiologic effects of specific target ranges of Sp_{O_2} that could become apparent when such ranges are more effectively maintained. Hence, caution is recommended in the selection of the Sp_{O_2} range to be set as target for an automatic F_{IO_2} controller.

Summary

Most of the currently available ventilatory modalities do not adapt to the frequently changing needs of the preterm infant. However, newer and experimental modes becoming available could potentially address some of these limitations. Initial evidence suggests some beneficial effects of automation in ventilation of preterm infants, and further evidence of their effects is being gathered. The effects of these modalities of mechanical ventilation on long-term outcomes have not been explored.

Supplemental oxygen is commonly administered to preterm infants. However, it has significant side effects, in part due to the limitations in the way it is conventionally managed. Automatic F_{IO_2} controllers are being proposed as means to improve the maintenance of adequate oxygenation while reducing exposure to extreme ranges of oxygenation and inspired oxygen. Currently available evidence from short-term evaluations indicates benefits of automatic control, but only large clinical trials will determine its effects on long-term respiratory, ophthalmic, and neurodevelopmental outcomes in preterm infants.

References

1. Stoll BJ, Hansen NI, Bell EF, et al. Neonatal outcomes of extremely preterm infants from the NICHD Neonatal Research Network. *Pediatrics*. 2010;126:443-456.
2. Ehrenkranz RA, Walsh MC, Vohr BR, et al. Validation of the National Institutes of Health consensus definition of bronchopulmonary dysplasia. *Pediatrics*. 2005;116:1353-1360.
3. Walsh MC, Morris BH, Wrage LA, et al. National Institutes of Child Health and Human Development Neonatal Research Network. Extremely low birth weight neonates with protracted ventilation: mortality and 18-month neurodevelopmental outcomes. *J Pediatr*. 2005;146:798-804.
4. Lifschitz MH, Seilheimer DK, Wilson GS, et al. Neurodevelopmental status of low birth weight infants with bronchopulmonary dysplasia requiring prolonged oxygen supplementation. *J Perinatol*. 1987; 7:127-132.
5. Schmidt B, Asztalos EV, Roberts RS, et al. Impact of bronchopulmonary dysplasia, brain injury, and severe retinopathy on the outcome of extremely low-birth-weight infants at 18 months: results from the trial of indomethacin prophylaxis in preterms. *JAMA*. 2003;289:1124-1129.
6. Abubakar KM, Keszler M. Patient-ventilator interactions in new modes of patient-triggered ventilation. *Pediatr Pulmonol*. 2001;32:71-75.
7. Herrera CM, Gerhardt T, Claure N, et al. Effects of volume-guaranteed synchronized intermittent mandatory ventilation in preterm infants recovering from respiratory failure. *Pediatrics*. 2002;110: 529-533.
8. Keszler M, Abubakar K. Volume guarantee: stability of tidal volume and incidence of hypocarbia. *Pediatr Pulmonol*. 2004;38:240-245.
9. Cheema IU, Sinha AK, Kempley ST, Ahluwalia JS. Impact of volume guarantee ventilation on arterial carbon dioxide tension in newborn infants: A randomized controlled trial. *Early Hum Dev*. 2007;83:183-189.
10. Dawson C, Davies MW. Volume-targeted ventilation and arterial carbon dioxide in neonates. *J Paediatr Child Health*. 2005;41:518-521.
11. Polimeni V, Claure N, D'Ugard C, et al. Effects of volume-targeted synchronized intermittent mandatory ventilation on spontaneous episodes of hypoxemia in preterm infants. *Biol Neonate*. 2006;89:50-55.
12. Bolivar JM, Gerhardt T, Gonzalez A, et al. Mechanisms for episodes of hypoxemia in preterm infants undergoing mechanical ventilation. *J Pediatr*. 1995;127:767-773.
13. Dimaguila MA, DiFiore JA, Martin R, et al. Characteristics of hypoxemic episodes in very low birth weight infants on ventilatory support. *J Pediatr*. 1997;130:577-583.
14. Cheema IU, Ahluwalia JS. Feasibility of tidal volume-guided ventilation in newborn infants: a randomized, crossover trial using the volume guarantee modality. *Pediatrics*. 2001;107:1323-1328.
15. Piotrowski A, Sobala W, Kawczynski P. Patient-initiated, pressure-regulated, volume-controlled ventilation compared with intermittent mandatory ventilation in neonates: a prospective, randomised study. *Intensive Care Med*. 1997;23:975-981.
16. D'Angio CT, Chess PR, Kovacs SJ, et al. Pressure-regulated volume control ventilation vs synchronized intermittent mandatory ventilation for very low-birth-weight infants: a randomized controlled trial. *Arch Pediatr Adolesc Med*. 2005;159:868-875.
17. Sinha SK, Donn SM, Gavey J, et al. Randomised trial of volume controlled versus time cycled, pressure limited ventilation in preterm infants with respiratory distress syndrome. *Arch Dis Child Fetal Neonatal Ed*. 1997;77:F202-F205.
18. Singh J, Sinha SK, Donn SM, et al. Mechanical ventilation of very low birth weight infants: Is volume or pressure a better target variable? *J Pediatr*. 2006;149:308-313.
19. Wheeler K, Klingenberg C, McCallion N, et al. Volume-targeted versus pressure-limited ventilation in the neonate. *Cochrane Database Syst Rev*. 2010;(11):CD003666.
20. Claure N, Gerhardt T, Hummler H, et al. Computer controlled minute ventilation in preterm infants undergoing mechanical ventilation. *J Pediatr*. 1997;131:910-913.
21. Claure N, Suguihara C, Peng J, et al. Targeted minute ventilation and tidal volume in an animal model of acute changes in lung mechanics and episodes of hypoxemia. *Neonatology*. 2009;95: 132-140.
22. Guthrie SO, Lynn C, Lafleur BJ, et al. A crossover analysis of mandatory minute ventilation compared to synchronized intermittent mandatory ventilation in neonates. *J Perinatol*. 2005;25:643-646.
23. Herber-Jonat S, Rieger-Fackeldey E, Hummler H, Schulze A. Adaptive mechanical backup ventilation for preterm infants on respiratory assist modes—a pilot study. *Int Care Med*. 2006;32:302-308.
24. Musante G, Schulze A, Gerhardt T, et al. Proportional assist ventilation decreases thoracoabdominal asynchrony and chest wall distortion in preterm infants. *Pediatr Res*. 2001;49:175-180.
25. Schulze A, Rieger-Fackeldey E, Gerhardt T, et al. Randomized crossover comparison of proportional assist ventilation and patient triggered ventilation in extremely low birth weight infants with evolving chronic lung disease. *Neonatology*. 2007;92:1-7.
26. Schulze A, Gerhardt T, Musante G, et al. Proportional assist ventilation in low birth weight infants with acute respiratory disease: A comparison to assist/control and conventional mechanical ventilation. *J Pediatr*. 1999;135:339-344.
27. Beck J, Reilly M, Grasselli G, et al. Patient-ventilator interaction during neurally adjusted ventilatory assist in low birth weight infants. *Pediatr Res*. 2009;65:663-668.
28. Breatnach C, Conlon NP, Stack M, et al. A prospective crossover comparison of neurally adjusted ventilatory assist and pressure-support ventilation in a pediatric and neonatal intensive care unit population. *Pediatr Crit Care Med*. 2010;11:7-11.

29. Flynn JT, Bancalari E, Snyder ES, et al. A cohort study of transcutaneous oxygen tension and the incidence and severity of retinopathy of prematurity. *N Engl J Med*. 1992;326:1050-1054.
30. Supplemental therapeutic oxygen for prethreshold retinopathy of prematurity (STOP-ROP), a randomized, controlled trial. I: primary outcomes. *Pediatrics*. 2000;105:295-310.
31. Askie LM, Henderson-Smart DJ, Irwig L, Simpson JM. Oxygen-saturation targets and outcomes in extremely preterm infants. *N Engl J Med*. 2003;349:959-967.
32. Collins MP, Lorenz JM, Jetton JR, Paneth N. Hypocapnia and other ventilation-related risk factors for cerebral palsy in low birth weight infants. *Pediatr Res*. 2001;50:712-719.
33. Hagadorn JI, Furey AM, Nghiem TH, et al. AVIOx Study Group. Achieved versus intended pulse oximeter saturation in infants born less than 28 weeks' gestation: the AVIOx study. *Pediatrics*. 2006;118:1574-1582.
34. Laptook AR, Salhab W, Allen J, et al. Pulse oximetry in very low birth weight infants: can oxygen saturation be maintained in the desired range? *J Perinatol*. 2006;26:337-341.
35. Clucas L, Doyle LW, Dawson J, et al. Compliance with alarm limits for pulse oximetry in very preterm infants. *Pediatrics*. 2007;119:1056-1060.
36. Sink DW, Hope SA, Hagadorn JI. Nurse:patient ratio and achievement of oxygen saturation goals in premature infants. *Arch Dis Child Fetal Neonatal Ed*. 2011;96:F93-F98.
37. Garg M, Kurzner SI, Bautista DB, Keens TG. Clinically unsuspected hypoxia during sleep and feeding in infants with bronchopulmonary dysplasia. *Pediatrics*. 1988;81:635-642.
38. Cunningham S, McColm JR, Wade J, et al. A novel model of retinopathy of prematurity simulating preterm oxygen variability in the rat. *Invest Ophthalmol Vis Sci*. 2000;41:4275-4280.
39. Di Fiore JM, Bloom JN, Orge F, et al. A higher incidence of intermittent hypoxemic episodes is associated with severe retinopathy of prematurity. *J Pediatr*. 2010;157:69-73.
40. Penn JS, Henry MM, Tolman BL. Exposure to alternating hypoxia and hyperoxia causes severe proliferative retinopathy in the newborn rat. *Pediatr Res*. 1994;36:724-731.
41. McColm JR, Cunningham S, Wade J, et al. Hypoxic oxygen fluctuations produce less severe retinopathy than hyperoxic fluctuations in a rat model of retinopathy of prematurity. *Pediatric Res*. 2004;55:107-113.
42. Tay-Uyboco JS, Kwiatkowski K, Cates DB, et al. Hypoxic airway constriction in infants of very low birth weight recovering from moderate to severe bronchopulmonary dysplasia. *J Pediatr*. 1989;115: 456-459.
43. Unger M, Atkins M, Briscoe WA, King TK. Potentiation of pulmonary vasoconstrictor response with repeated intermittent hypoxia. *J Appl Physiol*. 1977;43:662-667.
44. Custer JR, Hales CA. Influence of alveolar oxygen on pulmonary vasoconstriction in newborn lambs versus sheep. *Am Rev Respir Dis*. 1985;132:326-331.
45. Barlow B, Santulli T. Importance of multiple episodes of hypoxia or cold stress on the development of enterocolitis in an animal model. *Surgery*. 1975;77:687-690.
46. Beddis JR, Collins P, Levy NM, et al. New Technique for servo-control of arterial oxygen tension in preterm infants. *Arch Dis Child*. 1979;54:278-280.
47. Dugdale RE, Cameron RG, Lealman GT. Closed-loop control of the partial pressure of arterial oxygen in neonates. *Clin Physics Physiol Meas*. 1988;9:291-305.
48. Bhutani VK, Taube JC, Antunes MJ, Delivoria-Papadopoulos M. Adaptive control of the inspired oxygen delivery to the neonate. *Pediatr Pulmonol*. 1992;14:110-117.
49. Morozoff PE, Evans RW. Closed-loop control of SaO2 in the neonate. *Biomed Instrum Technol*. 1992;26;117-123.
50. Sun Y, Kohane IS, Stark AR. Computer-assisted adjustment of inspired oxygen concentration improves control of oxygen saturation in newborn infants requiring mechanical ventilation. *J Pediatr*. 1997;131:754-756.
51. Morozoff EP, Smyth JA. Evaluation of three automatic oxygen therapy control algorithms on ventilated low birth weight neonates. *Conf Proc IEEE Eng Med Biol Soc*. 2009;2009:3079-3082.
52. Claure N, Gerhardt T, Everett R, et al. Closed-loop controlled inspired oxygen concentration for mechanically ventilated very low birth weight infants with frequent episodes of hypoxemia. *Pediatrics*. 2001;107:1120-1124.
53. Urschitz MS, Horn W, Seyfang A, et al. Automatic control of the inspired oxygen fraction in preterm infants: a randomized crossover trial. *Am J Respir Crit Care Med*. 2004;170:1095-1100.
54. Claure N, D'Ugard C, Bancalari E. Automated adjustment of inspired oxygen in preterm infants with frequent fluctuations in oxygenation: a pilot clinical trial. *J Pediatr*. 2009;155:640-645.
55. Claure N, Bancalari E, D'Ugard C, et al. Multicenter crossover study of automated adjustment of inspired oxygen in mechanically ventilated preterm infants. *Pediatrics*. 2011;127:e76-e83.
56. Hay Jr WW, Rodden DJ, Collins SM, et al. Reliability of conventional and new pulse oximetry in neonatal patients. *J Perinatol*. 2002;22:360-366.
57. Bohnhorst B, Peter CS, Poets CF. Pulse oximeters' reliability in detecting hypoxemia and bradycardia: comparison between a conventional and two new generation oximeters. *Crit Care Med*. 2000;28: 1565-1568.
58. Bohnhorst B, Peter CS, Poets CF. Detection of hyperoxaemia in neonates: data from three new pulse oximeters. *Arch Dis Child Fetal Neonatal Ed*. 2002;87:F217-F219.
59. Bucher HU, Keel M, Wolf M, et al. Artifactual pulse-oximetry estimation in neonates. *Lancet*. 1994;343:1135-1136.

CHAPTER 20

Management of the Infant with Congenital Diaphragmatic Hernia

Roberta L. Keller, MD

20

- The Pathophysiology of Congenital Diaphragmatic Hernia
- Acute Respiratory Management in the Patient with CDH
- Assessment and Management of Pulmonary Hypertension
- Approach to Patients with Congenital Heart Disease
- Longer-Term Issues in Survivors of CDH
- Antenatal Therapies

The Pathophysiology of Congenital Diaphragmatic Hernia

Congenital diaphragmatic hernia (CDH) is a developmental abnormality of the lung, the pulmonary vascular bed, and the diaphragm. The initiating event is failure of development and fusion of the embryonic elements of the diaphragm, which should occur by 8 weeks of gestation. Subsequently, abdominal contents herniate into the thorax, with the volume of the hernia contents depending on the size of the diaphragmatic defect. Bilateral major airway and vessel branching to the level of the terminal bronchioles (completed in the pseudoglandular stage, by 16-17 weeks of gestation) are deficient.[1-4] The mechanisms for these abnormalities and the resultant lung and vascular hypoplasia are not known. Both transpulmonary pressure and fetal breathing movements, critical for normal lung development, are deranged in fetal CDH[5-9]; thus abnormal tonic and phasic stretch likely contribute to this arrest of development.

Intra-acinar alveolar numbers are preserved, but because acinar numbers are decreased, the total number of alveoli at birth is reduced (6 million at term in one morphometric study, compared with a mean of approximately 50 million in non-affected newborns).[1,2,10] Alveolar maldevelopment results in low lung compliance and decreases in both ventilation and surface area for gas exchange.[11-13] Oxygenation is thus impaired, further exacerbated by the diminished cross-sectional area of the vascular bed,[1,2] which increases pulmonary vascular resistance, potentially reducing pulmonary blood flow. The muscular structure of the resistance arteries is also abnormal, with its origins in the fetus. In fetuses with lung hypoplasia, there are fewer vessels after 20 weeks of gestation and higher smooth muscle actin content after 22 weeks of gestation.[14] Vessels are smaller in CDH, the muscle media layer is hypertrophied, and there is abnormal distal extension of the muscle in some infants.[1-3,15] Increased medial muscle mass is present both ipsilateral and contralateral to the hernia, and in one series, pulmonary artery muscle mass was inversely proportional to the extent of lung hypoplasia.[3,16]

Lung hypoplasia and its consequences have implications for survival as well as for lung function in infants who survive to tracheal extubation.[12,17,18] Ipsilateral diaphragmatic function remains abnormal, even after primary repair of the diaphragm, possibly contributing to ongoing respiratory difficulties after endotracheal extubation in the newborn.[19,20] Fetal and neonatal factors therefore influence the early management of cardiorespiratory support in this patient population, yet supportive therapies may cause further impairment of lung and vascular development and of recovery. Given the chronic nature of illness and anatomic and physiologic abnormalities in CDH, management strategies in the newborn should focus on optimizing the potential for long-term lung and vascular growth and function while monitoring for adequate tissue oxygen delivery and minimizing the potential for complications of neonatal intensive care.

Acute Respiratory Management in the Patient with CDH

Approach to Mechanical Ventilation

Most of the literature pertaining to newborns and survivors of CDH includes reports on infants presenting with respiratory distress at less than 6 to 24 hours of age, or (in later reports) with a prenatal diagnosis of the anomaly. Infants and older children presenting later, usually with either mild respiratory distress or intestinal obstruction, and those with Morgagni (anterior) hernias (who generally have mild lung hypoplasia), are not the focus of the following discussion. This chapter is oriented toward management of more severely affected newborns requiring respiratory support from birth, with Bochdalek (posterior-lateral) hernias.

For many years, CDH was considered a surgical emergency, because the reduction of intrathoracic hernia contents was thought to be critical to improving lung function. Clinicians subsequently moved toward a strategy of preoperative stabilization, often in concert with the availability of extracorporeal membrane oxygenation (ECMO) support. Much attention was paid to maintaining decompression of herniated intestines from the time of birth, with wide use of pharmacologic sedation and paralysis. The only aspect of this strategy studied by a randomized trial is delayed (defined as >24 hours) versus immediate (<24 hours) repair of the diaphragmatic defect, which was evaluated in two small studies in the 1990s.[21] Although there is no definitive answer as to which strategy for operative repair is associated with better outcomes from these prospective studies (or large retrospective studies), most major centers do allow for a period of preoperative stabilization, with delayed repair of the diaphragmatic defect.[22,23] Criteria for stabilization vary, and some centers undertake early repair with use of ECMO in infants who receive respiratory support in the first hours of life. From a pulmonary function standpoint, there is evidence for delaying surgery; Sakai and colleagues[17] reported worsening respiratory system compliance (Crs) following surgery in 7/9 infants who underwent repair at less than 96 hours of age (median 20 hours), whereas Nakayama and associates[11] subsequently demonstrated improved Crs over a preoperative stabilization period. My colleagues and I[24] reported no substantial perioperative changes in Crs in a group of severely affected infants (fetal diagnosis with liver herniated into the chest), although after preoperative stabilization, Crs had decreased slightly from day 1, and it then improved 24 hours after surgery.

For babies with a prenatal diagnosis of CDH, most practitioners immediately intubate the trachea after delivery and rapidly place a decompressing orogastric tube to suction drainage. However, ongoing decompression of an infant with the stomach herniated into the chest can be challenging, because the tube placed from above may not advance beyond the distal esophagus without resistance (Fig. 20-1). Intraluminal gas in the stomach or the intestines can compress the ipsilateral lung and, potentially, the contralateral lung because of worsening mediastinal shift, so lung function may be further compromised. Pharmacologic paralysis will, of course, prevent the infant from swallowing air, and it has been advocated for patients with CDH through the time of operative repair. However, some effects of paralysis might be adverse in this situation, including a decreased ability to mobilize extracellular fluid and an inability to help clear airway secretions. Vagolytic effects of

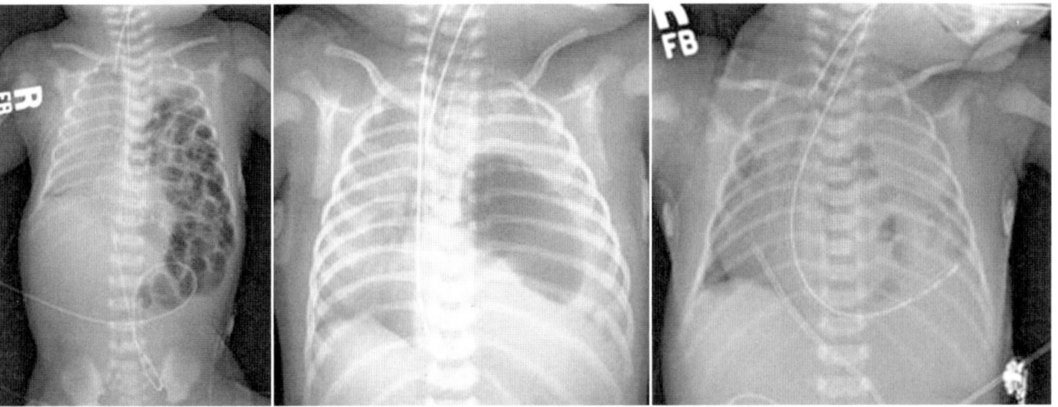

Figure 20-1 Chest radiographs of three infants with left-sided congenital diaphragmatic hernia prior to repair, with the stomach and liver herniated into the left hemithorax. **A,** Large amount of bowel gas in the chest and abdomen with mediastinum shifted severely to the right and a compressed right lung. Note the nasogastric tube in the distal esophagus, which was advanced until resistance was met. **B,** Persistent inflation of the intrathoracic stomach with severe mediastinal shift despite in situ nasogastric tube, which could not be advanced beyond the distal esophagus. **C,** Minimal intrathoracic bowel gas accumulated in an infant with the nasogastric tube advanced into the decompressed intrathoracic stomach.

pancuronium, which include tachycardia, are short-lived, in our experience. With respect to long-term outcomes, there is also some concern regarding the use of neuromuscular blockade in these patients, although later data do not support pancuronium as a causative agent in long-term morbidity (discussed later). Finally, allowing infants to breathe spontaneously enables them to contribute to their own ventilation, and offers an additional measure of clinical assessment, depending on the level of respiratory distress.

Another major evolution in the care of infants with CDH has been related to ventilation strategy. From the time of initial observations that hyperventilation could improve oxygenation in infants with persistent pulmonary hypertension of the newborn (PPHN), clinicians attempted to hyperventilate newborns with CDH. Hyperoxygenation, or high inspired oxygen concentrations (FIO_2), were also considered to be mainstays of treatment for pulmonary hypertension in infants with CDH. The result was poor survival to hospital discharge (31%-55%), with high rates of pneumothorax and early death.[22,23,25] Wung and colleagues[26] from Columbia University (New York, NY) reported an initial experience using a strategy of pressure limitation without hyperventilation or paralysis, with survival of 82% (52/63), at a single center. The goals of this approach were to protect the vulnerable hypoplastic lungs from ventilator-associated injury, allow for perinatal transition, and, ultimately, promote growth and recovery despite the physiologic limitations. At other centers, subsequent institution of permissive hypercapnia, with pressure limitation and permissive oxygenation, was associated with improvements in single-center survival rates to 69% to 93%.[23,25,27-29] Permissive oxygenation allows for persistence of a right-to-left shunt at the level of the ductus arteriosus (due to high pulmonary vascular resistance) while targeting preductal (usually right upper extremity) oxygen saturation (SpO_2) values as low as the 80s in severely affected newborns, accompanied by aggressive weaning from FIO_2 and peak inspiratory pressure (PIP).

Ventilator strategies and target oxygenation and ventilation described in studies from these centers are presented in Table 20-1. Generally, strategies from these centers with high survival rates have described limited ventilation pressures (maximum PIP 25-35 cm H_2O, usual PIP 20-25 cm H_2O) as part of the initial resuscitation and subsequent management of these infants. Infants are given a variable period to reach target preductal SpO_2 levels prior to escalation of therapy, as long as perfusion is adequate.[30] The use of high ventilator rates (60-100 breaths per

Table 20-1 MANAGEMENT STRATEGIES, STUDY PERIOD AND SURVIVAL RATES TO HOSPITAL DISCHARGE REPORTED FROM CENTERS DESCRIBING IMPROVED SURVIVAL WITH CHANGES IN TREATMENT OR MANAGEMENT STRATEGIES

Study(ies)*	Years	Survival (presenting < 6-12 hr), n	Selected Survival, n	Repair Timing	Ventilator and Ventilation Parameters	Oxygenation Parameters	ECMO Utilization, n	Weaning Support
Wung et al (1995)[26] / Boloker et al (2002)[30]	1983-95 1992-2000	52/63 = 83% 91/120 = 76%	91/114 = 80%[†]	"Minimal evidence" of pulmonary hypertension Ventilator support minimized	$Pa_{CO_2} \le 60$-65 "low rate": rate 40, Ti = 0.5, PIP 20, PEEP 5 "HFPPV": rate 100, Ti = 0.3, PIP 20, PEEP 0 Limit PIP to 25-30 HFOV if $Pa_{CO_2} > 65$ or decreased oxygenation	Pre-ductal Sp_{O_2} 90-95 or 80-89	14/63 = 22[‡] 16/120 = 13%[‡]	PIP for chest excursion FI_{O_2} weaning performed aggressively All extubated to nasal CPAP at 5
Frenckner et al (1997)[27]	1990-95	39/43 = 91%		24-96 hr "Adequate" blood gas values" No evidence of right-to-left shunt when $FI_{O_2} \le 0.40$	$Pa_{CO_2} < 60$-65 $PIP \le 35$	Post-ductal $Sp_{O_2} > 90$	7/43 = 16%	
Wilson et al (1997)[23]/ Downard et al (2003)[28]	1991-94 2000-02	51/74 = 69% 36/39 = 93%	36/43 = 84%[§]	Delayed repair	Permissive hypercapnia per Wung et al[26] $PIP \le 30$, PEEP 5, $P_{AW} \le 12$	Pre-ductal $Sp_{O_2} \ge 90$ Aggressive treatment of pulmonary hypertension with inhaled NO and other pulmonary vasodilators	43/74 = 53%	

Kays et al (1999)[25]	1992-98	47/67 = 70%	47/60 = 78%[‖]		PIP 20-24 PEEP 4-5 rate 40-80 Maximum PIP 25, occasional increase to 28 rate to 100, I:E 1:2 if rate > 30	Post-ductal SpO_2 > 97 Pre-ductal $SpO_2 \geq 85$	23/67 = 34%	FIO_2 weaning at 6 hr
Bohn (2002)[29]	1995-01	70/93 =75	70/83 = 84%[¶]	Low PIP and FIO_2 Minimal right-to-left shunting Transition to conventional ventilation if previously undergoing HFOV	$PaCO_2$ 45-55 pH > 7.3 PIP ≤ 25 HFOV if unable to be managed with limited PIP, $P_{AW} \leq 16$	Pre-ductal SpO_2 > 85 Trial of inhaled NO if elevated RV pressure	5/93 = 5%	

CPAP, continuous positive airway pressure (cm H_2O); ECMO, extracorporeal membrane oxygenation; FIO_2, inspired oxygen concentration; HFOV, high-frequency oscillatory ventilation; HFPPV, high frequency positive pressure ventilation; I:E, inspiratory-to-expiratory ratio; NO, nitric oxide; $PaCO_2$, arterial carbon dioxide tension (mm Hg); P_{AW}, mean airway pressure (cm H_2O); PEEP, positive end-expiratory pressure (cm H_2O); PIP, peak inspiratory pressure (cm H_2O); RV, right ventricle; SpO_2, oxygen saturation by pulse oximetry (%); Ti, inspiratory time (seconds).
*Timing of repair, ventilator, and oxygenation strategies is described for later studies from the same center, if the descriptions in the two publications differ.
†Lethal anomalies excluded.
‡Centers that have exclusion criteria for ECMO specific to severity of lung hypoplasia in congenital diaphragmatic hernia (CDH).
§Isolated CDH.
‖Lethal conditions excluded.
¶Major anomalies excluded.

minute) is physiologically appropriate, because these infants have restrictive lung disease due to lung hypoplasia, which is associated with low tidal volumes and high respiratory rates at later follow-up in infancy.[18,31] Even a short period of high–tidal volume ventilation increases pulmonary and extrapulmonary inflammation in the vulnerable lung,[32] and the literature in adults with acute lung injury supports the use of low–tidal volume ventilation (with compensatory higher ventilator rates to provide adequate ventilation).[33] In this population, a low–tidal volume ventilation strategy decreases lung injury and inflammation, extrapulmonary organ failure, and mortality.[34]

Rationale for additional ventilator management includes the use of relatively short inspiratory times, which are usually sufficient because of the short time constants of the lung. Low positive end-expiratory pressure (PEEP) set on the ventilator compensates for the intrinsic PEEP associated with higher ventilator rates.[33] In fact, lower PEEP (1-3 cm H_2O) is associated with higher respiratory system compliance (compared with the standard PEEP of 4 cm H_2O) in newborns with CDH (R. Keller, unpublished data).[13] At the University of California San Francisco (UCSF), we routinely use a PEEP of 3 cm H_2O regardless of ventilator rate (rates are commonly 60-80 breaths per minute), and at Columbia University, zero PEEP is used at high ventilator rates (100 breaths per minute). The full current UCSF protocol is described in Table 20-2. In addition to increasing lung compliance and decreasing air trapping, these strategies may improve pulmonary blood flow through prevention of lung overdistention.

Consistent with these strategies, the lung recruitment approach to the use of high-frequency oscillatory ventilation (HFOV), wherein mean airway pressure is immediately or steadily increased from the settings on conventional ventilation, has not been successful at consistently improving oxygenation or enhancing survival in infants with CDH.[29,35] This strategy may also promote overdistention of the lung and impedance to pulmonary blood flow. HFOV has been used as a "rescue" technique for infants who are unable to meet oxygenation or ventilation criteria and in those who are exceeding PIP limits set for conventional ventilation.[29,30] However, it is difficult to radiographically assess appropriate mean airway pressure on HFOV in CDH, in which the shape of the lung is distorted. The best assessment of the appropriate lung volume may be the conformation of the hemidiaphragm contralateral to the hernia. A "domed" diaphragm indicates more appropriate mean airway pressure, whereas a flattened one indicates the mean airway pressure is excessive. A trial based in the Netherlands has been designed to test whether or not primary support with HFOV (versus conventional ventilation) improves survival and respiratory outcomes at 28 and 56 days of age, although the trial is not actively recruiting as of yet.[35a] Centers that adhere to pressure limitation guidelines will offer ECMO support for infants who cannot demonstrate adequate oxygen delivery on their maximal settings, if exclusion criteria are not met.

Consistency of clinical care and decision-making within an institution may be the most critical factor in centers reporting high survival rates. Logan and colleagues summarized 13 reports from 11 institutions. Although most centers described permissive strategies for ventilation and oxygenation with pressure limitation, the target parameters were variable. These investigators subsequently reported the experience at their own center, following initiation of a protocol employing a standardized approach to ventilation management for CDH.[36] There was no description of the ventilator parameters from the pre-protocol period, but survival improved from 55% in the pre-protocol period to 85% in the protocol period. It may be that the most important factor in care of these infants is the interaction between the respiratory management and other aspects of care. A protocol that emphasizes active management of ventilator weaning allows for hemodynamic stability, weaning of sedation, and progression toward establishing enteral feeds (optimizing nonpharmacologic comfort measures)—all practices that limit the risk of late-onset nosocomial sepsis. In comparison, a nonprotocolized respiratory management approach might result in a situation in which infants are not actively weaned, requiring reactive responses to clinical decompensations and

Table 20-2 THE CURRENT (2011) PROTOCOL FOR RESPIRATORY MANAGEMENT OF INFANTS WITH CDH FROM THE UNIVERSITY OF CALIFORNIA SAN FRANCISCO (UCSF) BENIOFF CHILDREN'S HOSPITAL INTENSIVE CARE NURSERY, AS IMPLEMENTED FROM 2000 TO 2010

Survival, n	Repair Timing	Ventilator and Ventilation Parameters	Oxygenation Parameters	ECMO Utilization, n	Weaning Support
Overall: 125/188 = 66% Excluding limited care: 125/171 = 73%	Delayed repair, after weaning of FIO_2 until infants do not appear to be making substantial progress (usually FIO_2 0.30-0.60)	$PacO_2$ 45-65 pH > 7.20 PIP ≤ 25-26 PEEP 3, rate usually 60-80, as high as 100, rarely < 40 Short Ti 0.2-0.4, as appropriate for ventilator rate to limit air trapping HFOV if unable to ventilate adequately, P_{AW} ≤ 15 (usual P_{AW} 12-13)	"Weaning" infant: pre-ductal SpO_2 > 95 "Nonweaning" infant: pre-ductal SpO_2 ≥ 87 SpO_2 in mid-80s tolerated if lactic acidosis not increasing Ductal shunt tolerated and post-ductal SpO_2 and PaO_2 largely ignored except as indicators of mixed venous saturations Inhaled NO (20 ppm) initiated for hemodynamic compromise, persistent large pre- to post-ductal SpO_2 difference (> 5) or inability to achieve pre-ductal SpO_2 > 92	Overall: 22/188 = 12% Excluding limited care: 22/171 = 13%	FIO_2, PIP, and P_{AW} weaning performed initially. Rate weaned preoperatively following steady PIP weaning or attainment of minimum PIP (16-20). Pressure-support mode utilized postoperatively once infants have recovered enough to consistently trigger ventilator. Demand flow allows infant to determine own rate, Ti, and tidal volume. Pressure support is weaned and work of breathing assessed to determine tolerance of weaning.

ECMO, extracorporeal membrane oxygenation; FIO_2, inspired oxygen concentration; HFOV, high-frequency oscillatory ventilation; NO, nitric oxide; $PacO_2$, arterial carbon dioxide tension (mm Hg); P_{AW}, mean airway pressure (cm H_2O); PaO_2, arterial oxygen tension (mm Hg); PEEP, positive end-expiratory pressure (cm H_2O); PIP, peak inspiratory pressure (cm H_2O); ppm, parts per million; SpO_2, oxygen saturation by pulse oximetry(%); Ti, inspiratory time.

resulting in persistent respiratory support needs, hemodynamic compromise, additional sedation, and delayed establishment of enteral feeds—practices that increase the risk of nosocomial infection. There is some data from both animal studies and adults with acute lung injury that may be relevant to newborns with CDH. Even a brief period of high–tidal volume ventilation establishes pulmonary and systemic inflammation in premature lambs,[32] and markers of decreased inflammation are associated with lower–tidal volume ventilation, decreased extrapulmonary organ system dysfunction, and mortality in acute lung injury.[34] Standardized protocols can address the avoidance of these scenarios when assisted ventilation is applied.

Although these single-center studies and experimental data present a persuasive argument in favor of lung protection strategies, it remains difficult to interpret data from retrospective single-center studies. In contrast to the early reports of high single-center survival, contemporaneous (1991-2001) population-based studies present survival rates of approximately 55% in the United Kingdom and Australia.[37,38] A similar study from a population-based registry in California (1989-1997) demonstrated an overall survival of 61% with a diagnosis of CDH, with an improvement in survival over the study period by approximately 8% per year, from 53% to 72%.[39] However, a later US hospital-based study (1997-2004) of infants admitted at less than 8 days of age described a survival of only 67%.[40] A French population-based study (1986-2003) demonstrated improved survival rates over their study period, but only for cases of isolated CDH with no associated anomalies, and survival varied substantially from year to year.[41] Interestingly, population-based survival in Ontario, Canada, was 42% (96/229) in data from 1992-1999, whereas institution-based survival from the regional pediatric surgery centers over the same period was 68%, indicating that center-specific data are subject to a "hidden mortality" originally described by Harrison and colleagues.[42,43] Harrison and associates[41] reported data from Norway (1969-1975), and surprisingly, institution-based survival was 70% (23/33), whereas population-based survival was 34% (24/70). No differences in hidden mortality or overall survival were found in the Canadian study over time, but in single-center studies, there may be variable differences in rates of prenatal diagnosis[41] and changes in referral patterns in the prenatal and postnatal periods, making comparisons between periods and centers challenging.[44] To this point, although some of the described improvements in survival from single-center studies are substantial, they have occurred in the setting of increased institutional referrals.[23,25] Other researchers have reported higher survival rates in infants transferred after birth (outborn infants), indicating that some of the more severely affected infants might not survive to present at these institutions or that fetuses with additional anomalies (more frequently diagnosed with fetal CDH and higher mortality rates) might not be referred for delivery at a referral center owing to their poor prognosis.[30,41]

A direct piece of physiologic data that does lend credence to the lung protection approach is from the experience of Kays and associates.[25] These investigators reported increasing average PIP over the first 5 days of life during the era when there was no attention to pressure limitation during the attempt to achieve hyperventilation and hyperoxygenation. During the subsequent era of hyperventilation, with lower targets for oxygenation and some pressure limitation, mean PIP was lower but remained essentially unchanged over 5 days. Finally, in the era of permissive hypercapnia, with pressure limitation and permissive oxygenation, mean PIP was even lower and steadily declined over 5 days. Thus, more permissive targets with pressure limitation allow for additional weaning, indicating improving, rather than deteriorating, lung function. Further lending credence to the latter approach is growing support from experimental models that demonstrate lung injury and inflammation, alveolar simplification, impaired microvascular development, and pulmonary hypertensive changes in animals with vulnerable lungs exposed to chronic ventilation and hyperoxia.[45-47]

Additional evidence of the adverse effects of aggressive ventilation strategies is shown by the occurrence of pneumothorax related to active air leak. Pneumothorax is an acute marker of ventilator-associated lung injury. Its occurrence is associated with increased need for ECMO support and mortality.[22,38,40,48] The incidences of pneumothorax in two multicenter hospital-based reports were 20% and 38%.[38,40] Kays and associates[25] reported a decreasing incidence of pneumothorax, from 83% to 2%, as ventilator pressures were reduced with lowered ventilation and oxygenation targets. In contrast, the Columbia University group reported a preoperative pneumothorax rate of 18% despite the use of permissive strategies and pressure limitation.[30] However, they explicitly describe the use of nonsynchronized ventilation without paralysis, which may contribute to this acute risk in an infant with substantial respiratory distress.

Finally, the management of ventilation practices after diaphragmatic repair is less widely described in the literature. However, the approach to separation from mechanical support is important to consider, because infants with CDH have lung hypoplasia, some degree of lung injury, and abnormal diaphragmatic function, regardless of whether or not a primary repair has been accomplished. Following repair of the diaphragmatic defect, stimulated and spontaneous transdiaphragmatic pressures have been lower bilaterally in infants with CDH studied in the newborn period than in normal control infants, although the difference in spontaneous measurements did not reach statistical significance.[19] A follow-up study from the same investigators showed increased phrenic nerve latency and decreased stimulated pressure generation ipsilateral to the hernia when compared with contralateral measures, indicating that both nerve and muscle dysfunction are present.[49] Later studies of diaphragmatic function in survivors with left CDH have demonstrated decreased ipsilateral diaphragm excursion at 5 to 26 years of age with primary repair of the diaphragm,[20] and smaller contribution of the left lung to total tidal volume than in healthy controls at 6- to 18 years.[50] In consideration of these findings, it is useful to expect that infants with CDH must be able to tolerate lower ventilator settings than children without CDH prior to elective extubation of the trachea and successful separation from mechanical ventilation. Alternatively, routine extubation to higher levels of support might be indicated, such as the aggressive extubation to nasal CPAP described by the Columbia University group.[30] At UCSF, we transition to pressure-support ventilation as soon as the infant is able to maintain consistent respiratory effort and ventilate adequately. This practice allows the patient to control her or his own ventilation and inspiratory time, leading to greater comfort and potentially less need for sedatives. The infant is also able to assist the ventilator, a critically important feature because this assistance requires the use of accessory thoracic muscles, which are important for respiratory system function in the setting of abnormal diaphragmatic function.

Pulmonary Toilet

Mucous plugging can cause significant problems during mechanical ventilation, because major airway branches are reduced in caliber in infants with CDH, particularly ipsilateral to the hernia.[51] Thus, pulmonary toilet is very important, particularly in infants receiving ECMO support (see later discussion of this treatment). Assistance in clearing airway secretions may be one of the most important benefits of maintaining nonparalysis in an infant with CDH in the preoperative period. In addition, inhaled β-agonists may increase mucociliary clearance,[52] an effect that could be beneficial in infants with CDH. Airway obstruction has been demonstrated in CDH in infants younger than 6 months,[18] with bronchodilator responsiveness documented in ventilated infants at younger than 1 month.[53] Airway smooth muscle thickness has been shown to be increased only in infants receiving high levels of support (PIP = 25 mm Hg and $FIO_2 = 0.90$) for at least 24 hours.[54] Thus, there is a rationale for use of inhaled β-agonists in this patient population, particularly if the drug can be administered without removing the infant from mechanical support, and even early in the clinical course for infants exhibiting significant lability in ventilation and oxygenation.

Surfactant

Because of abnormalities in surfactant production in the ovine model of CDH, there has long been concern about surfactant deficiency in infants with CDH, regardless of gestational age at birth.[55] Fetal studies have shown that ontogeny of surfactant production and the quantity of its components (normalized to lung size) in infants with CDH are similar to those in controls.[55] Clinical studies in human infants with CDH have variably shown abnormalities of surfactant content, synthesis, and metabolism.[56-59] However, retrospective multicenter studies of selective administration of surfactant to both preterm and term newborns have shown no benefit of surfactant administration on any clinical outcome, including duration of mechanical ventilation, duration of ECMO support, and survival.[60-62] Prospective studies have not been reported. At UCSF, for infants of 34 weeks or less gestational age, we routinely administer prophylactic surfactant at birth in the delivery room, because of concern about potential exacerbation of lung injury if even mild surfactant deficiency (due to prematurity) is present. Further doses of surfactant are administered only if there is radiographic evidence of hyaline membrane disease.

Extracorporeal Membrane Oxygenation Support

C

CDH is currently the most common indication for ECMO support for neonatal respiratory failure.[63] Data from the Extracorporeal Life Support Organization (ELSO) registry demonstrate that survival to discharge for infants with CDH receiving ECMO support decreased from 60% in 1990 to 40% in 2003, likely indicating that generally, infants with more severe lung hypoplasia are being started on ECMO support. The Cochrane review of ECMO therapy for newborns with CDH and respiratory failure demonstrated a benefit to survival for ECMO over conventional treatment.[64] However, there are some limitations to these findings overall numbers were low (total n = 35); data were from the United Kingdom ECMO trial, in which infants receiving conventional therapy were managed at outlying hospitals whereas those with ECMO were managed at a single institution; and traditional criteria for ECMO initiation were used, including oxygenation index >40, a value that is less useful when pressure limitation is used. In North America, some centers that target gentle ventilation report very low utilization of ECMO in the CDH population (6%-19%, with the rate in outborn infants somewhat higher), and survival figures of 3/6 and 7/10 in inborn and outborn infants, respectively.[29,30] These reports also describe specific selection criteria for which the institutions do not offer ECMO, namely the inability to achieve a preductal Spo_2 above 85% or 90%. Other centers report higher ECMO utilization rates (43%) in association with survival rates that are generally higher than average (83%).[25] This variability in utilization and survival indicates that selection criteria likely differ between centers, with some centers using ECMO as a "last resort" rescue therapy and others using it earlier in the clinical course, explicitly for lung protection. Factors other than lung hypoplasia may contribute to a poor response to initial therapy. In data from one institution that serves only an outborn population, pneumothorax was the single independent predictor of the need for ECMO, and survival to discharge or transfer was 53% (8/15) following ECMO.[48] In this scenario, ECMO may be rescuing infants with an acute deterioration in status. Other potential reasons for decrements in lung function below the physiologic potential include retained fetal lung fluid, particularly in the setting of a cesarean section delivery without labor. Folkesson and colleagues[65] described two infants with CDH who demonstrated very low lung liquid absorption rates, 5% or less (normal rate is 11%-55%), during an attempt at liquid distention of the lung during ECMO support.[65] In translational studies in the rodent CDH lung, the investigators demonstrated a failure of perinatal transition from the fetal secretory state to the neonatal absorptive state owing to a deficiency in pulmonary epithelial sodium channel (ENaC) production.

It is unclear what degree of lung hypoplasia is lethal in the modern era. Although significant lung hypoplasia at autopsy (lung weight <5th percentile) has been described in infants who are not offered ECMO owing to an inability to transiently achieve acceptable oxygenation,[26] the ability to rescue infants who cannot achieve these criteria has not been described. Antunes and coworkers[12] measured functional residual capacity (FRC) preoperatively and post-operatively in infants with CDH. FRC was lower in nonsurvivors despite ECMO support than in survivors with and without ECMO; a preoperative FRC of 9 mL/kg (approximately 1/3 normal lung volume) was a good discriminator between survivors and nonsurvivors among infants who received ECMO support. Although all nonsurvivors (10/10) had FRC values less than 9 mL/kg (mean 4.5 ± 1 mL/kg), 13% (2/15) of survivors also had FRC values less than 9 mL/kg (mean 12.3 ± 5.4 mL/kg). Several other studies have examined the clinical predictors of mortality despite ECMO support in infants with CDH. Hoffman and colleagues[66] at Children's National Medical Center in Washington, DC, reported an overall survival of 50% among 62 infants requiring ECMO

(1993-2007). Nonsurvivors had higher pre-ECMO minimum $PaCO_2$ values, consistent with more severe lung hypoplasia; 27% survived with a minimum pre-ECMO $PaCO_2$ of 60 mm Hg or higher, and 0/5 survived with minimum $PaCO_2$ values of 70 mm Hg or higher. It is important to note that these outcomes were not from infants specifically managed with permissive hypercapnia, although the escalation of ventilator support beyond appropriate limits to transiently achieve values below these cutoffs is unlikely to improve outcomes (as Kays and colleagues[25] previously demonstrated). In the cohort described by Hoffman and colleagues,[66] nonsurvivors were also more likely to have a right-sided CDH, to be started on ECMO support earlier, and to remain on ECMO support longer. Tiruvoipati and associates[67] described their experience with ECMO for CDH in the United Kingdom (Glenfield Hospital, Leicester) from 1991 to 2004.[67] Survival among the 52 infants in this study was 58%. Infants were less likely to survive if they underwent prolonged ECMO or had renal insufficiency requiring hemofiltration; only 28% (2/11) of patients receiving ECMO duration for 14 days or more and only 22% (4/18) of patients with renal insufficiency survived. No pre-ECMO parameters differed between survivors and nonsurvivors in this cohort.

20

In our center, we offer ECMO for infants unable to achieve even transient acceptable oxygenation and ventilation with reasonable ventilator settings, unless a syndrome with poor prognosis or other life-threatening anomalies are present. We do not routinely proceed to emergency ECMO support in infants who cannot be resuscitated in the delivery room, however, and we do not recommend ECMO to families of infants in whom acceptable oxygenation has never been achieved. However, there are circumstances in which we cannot distinguish those babies with lethal lung hypoplasia from others with a reversible problem compounding respiratory insufficiency, as outlined previously, or in whom the less hypoplastic contralateral lung cannot be fully recruited. These babies may benefit from the temporary support that ECMO can provide.

Some centers have tried to identify fetuses with markers of severe CDH and high likelihood of requiring ECMO support, offering a trial of ventilation during an EXIT (ex utero intrapartum) procedure. This protocol entails a ventilation trial while the fetus remains on placental support, followed by cesarean section delivery with or without direct cannulation for ECMO support. The results of the use of this strategy at Boston Children's Hospital have been reported.[68] Fetuses with liver herniated into the thorax and a low lung-to-head ratio (LHR; area of contralateral lung divided by biparietal head circumference) on ultrasound,[69,70] a low percentage of predicted lung volume (PPLV) on magnetic resonance imaging (MRI),[71] or the presence of significant structural heart disease were eligible for delivery by EXIT procedure. Eleven of 14 fetuses were started directly on ECMO support, usually after a failed trial of ventilation (unable to achieve preductal $SpO_2 > 90\%$), and 7 survived (64%). This strategy has not been widely adopted, however.

Strategies for management of the infant with CDH undergoing ECMO support are not widely published, but they seem quite variable, on the basis of informal discourse over email list servers and at ECMO-focused conferences. Some centers keep babies on HFOV during ECMO, hoping to achieve greater lung protection. Other centers use identical resting settings (e.g., 15/5) for all babies regardless of whether or not the patients are supported with venoarterial or venovenous ECMO, and others use somewhat higher settings to attempt to maintain some lung inflation, particularly in the setting of venovenous ECMO, in which the right ventricle is pumping against a high pulmonary vascular resistance (PVR), which is further elevated in the setting of total lung collapse.[63] As with all patient populations receiving ECMO, a failure to reinflate the lung during weaning from ECMO support is a sign of poor lung compliance. However, in our experience, the small caliber of the airways in infants with CDH can increase the challenge of inflating the lungs, owing to inspissated mucous and airway debris. We use predominantly venovenous ECMO and attempt to maintain even minimal lung inflation with the conventional ventilator with the following settings: PEEP 5 cm H_2O, PIP 25-28 cm H_2O, rate 12 breaths/min, and a prolonged inspiratory time of 1 second. Much attention is paid to pulmonary toilet, with endotracheal suctioning and hand ventilation every 4 hours, often preceded by bronchodilator treatments and occasionally accompanied by DNase (Pulmozyme) treatments, both therapies administered to help clear secretions. Infants are also not paralyzed during ECMO support unless absolutely necessary for patient care.

C

Infants who are supported with ECMO prior to CDH repair either need to be weaned from ECMO support prior to surgical repair or must undergo repair while on ECMO, with an accompanying increase in the risk of hemorrhagic complications.[72] Clotting is also exacerbated by the interventions taken to limit bleeding, particularly in circuits that have been in use for some time. Many surgeons routinely load such a patient with aminocaproic acid just prior to the repair and initiate an aminocaproic acid infusion over 24 to 48 hours following surgery, until evidence of bleeding has resolved (loading dose 100 mg/kg followed by a 20-30 mg/kg/hr infusion). Because of concerns about bleeding and clotting, if repair is to be undertaken with use of ECMO support, it is important to have a circuit with minimal evidence of consumption and clot. At times, a change of circuit and recovery from this procedure may be required before the repair is undertaken. Thus, performing a surgical repair with the infant still on ECMO support may prolong the duration of ECMO and increase the incidence of complications. An analysis of data from the Congenital Diaphragmatic Hernia Study Group[73] demonstrated an increased mortality hazard of 1.4 for infants repaired while on ECMO support, despite the exclusion of infants who were unable to ultimately be weaned from ECMO support. This was a large study involving 636 infants managed in multiple centers from 1995 to 2005, allowing for adjustment for potential confounding factors, so, although it cannot account for all differences among centers, the data do suggest that outcomes are more favorable if CDH repair is undertaken after decannulation and normalization of coagulation status. For the infant undergoing surgical repair while on ECMO support, it is very important to consider placement of a thoracostomy tube, because hemothorax ipsilateral to the more hypoplastic lung may be difficult to detect postoperatively until it is severe.

Cardiopulmonary Interactions in Infants with CDH

Little data have been reported on cardiopulmonary interactions in infants with CDH. However, acute systemic-to-suprasystemic pulmonary hypertension, or PPHN, was prevalent in clinical series from the 1980s (46% and 79% despite exposure to FIO_2 1.0).[74,75] We reported a later cohort (2002-2005) of 39 infants managed with permissive hypercapnia and aggressive weaning from FIO_2.[76] The prevalence of PPHN based on echocardiograms obtained in the first 48 hours of life was 56% (22/39). This unchanged prevalence of PPHN despite less aggressive therapy for PPHN suggests that the less aggressive strategy is not harmful to the pathophysiology of PPHN. In fact, data from experimental models has demonstrated that exposure to FIO_2 1.0 for as little as 30 minutes in normal pulmonary vessels results in an augmented response to vasoconstrictive stimuli and increased expression and activity of phosphodiesterase-5 (PDE-5, the enzyme that hydrolyzes cyclic guanosine monophosphate, the second messenger for nitric oxide) in smooth muscle cells.[77,78] Similarly, smooth muscle cells from lambs with PPHN exhibited oxidant stress, increased PDE-5 activity, and decreased response to nitric oxide (NO).[79]

The association of renal insufficiency and greater mortality despite ECMO support is consistent with the importance of cardiopulmonary interactions in CDH.[67] Careful management of the ventilator to optimize systemic venous return and prevent tamponade of pulmonary blood flow, aggressive weaning of FIO_2 to attenuate abnormal vasoreactivity, and the avoidance of excessive tidal volumes to limit the systemic inflammatory response[34] may improve oxygenation and oxygen delivery in infants with CDH, allowing for further weaning. However, maintaining more generous SpO_2 values (>95%) at safer levels of FIO_2 (approximately <0.50 delivered or effective FIO_2) can enhance pulmonary vasodilation and consequently lower resting pulmonary vascular tone.[80-83]

Assessment and Management of Pulmonary Hypertension

Assessment of Pulmonary Hypertension

The clinical assessment of systemic-to-suprasystemic pulmonary hypertension is fairly straightforward if the ductus arteriosus is open, because continuous preductal and postductal SpO_2 monitoring will be diagnostic. However, even modest changes in the shunt may result in resolution of the preductal and postductal saturation differential and may represent only minor decreases in PVR. In addition, if the ductus arteriosus closes, the SpO_2 differential is no longer present. Therefore, reliance on the clinical assessment of a ductal level right-to-left shunt as the primary assessment of pulmonary hypertension in these infants is problematic. As such, routine monitoring of the infants with echocardiography can be very useful. We recommend an initial echocardiogram in the first 48 hours, followed by weekly studies, which can then be interpreted in the context of the infant's overall course with respect to level of cardiopulmonary support (mechanical ventilation, FIO_2, inotropic agents, and vasodilator therapy). We continue to monitor infants echocardiographically until findings are normal with all support withdrawn, although after 4 weeks of age, studies may be obtained less frequently, depending on a patient's overall status and how rapidly the findings have been changing. Additional studies may be obtained for significant decompensations or for specific therapeutic decisions, but the weekly studies give the best sense of the trajectory of the infant's course. This information is particularly important in the assessment of prolonged, near-systemic pulmonary hypertension, which may be difficult to detect until right heart failure develops. In this scenario, the physiologic change from PVR that is just subsystemic to PVR that is just suprasystemic is not large, although the clinical difference in the patient's oxygenation may be substantial.

The interpretation of echocardiographic studies requires multiple findings from the examination. Mourani and colleagues[84] described the sensitivity and specificity of echocardiogram for the diagnosis of pulmonary hypertension documented by cardiac catheterization in infants and young children with lung disease. Tricuspid regurgitant (TR) jet velocity (v) can estimate right ventricular systolic pressure (RVsp) with the Bernoulli equation, when there is also an estimate of right atrial pressure (RAp), as follows:

$$RVsp = 4 \times v^2 + RAp$$

Relative RV and left ventricle (LV) pressure can be assessed by the position of the interventricular septum (IVS). In the normal relationship, RV pressure is less than 50% of LV pressure. If the septum is flattened, the RV pressure is at least 50% of systemic pressure, and if it is significantly flattened, RV pressure is at least ⅔ systemic pressure. A D-shaped LV is present when RV pressure is suprasystemic.[85] Mourani and colleagues assessed echocardiographic measurements using an estimated cutoff RVsp of 40 mm Hg (TR velocity $\geq$ 3.2 m/s, assuming RAp = 0 mm Hg), a flattened LV septum, and other findings such as RA and RV dilation and RV hypertrophy. Use of the TR jet velocity alone had only an 88% sensitivity and a 33% specificity for the diagnosis of pulmonary hypertension. When combined with IVS flattening, sensitivity increased to 100%, but specificity remained low. This finding is concerning, because it could result in the unnecessary treatment of many children. The best specificity (100%) was the combination of a significant TR jet velocity and RV hypertrophy, with absence of these findings indicative of the failure to meet criteria for pulmonary hypertension at cardiac catheterization, although the confidence interval for this estimate was wide (44%-100%). The findings in these analyses were insensitive to varying RAp estimates.

We have used a hierarchy of findings to interpret echocardiograms in newborns with CDH, allowing us to classify pulmonary pressure estimates with respect to systemic pressure.[76] The ductal shunt is the best comparison of systemic and pulmonary vascular resistances. Thus the direction and velocity of the shunt, if present, has the highest priority for estimate of pulmonary hypertension. The next level of consideration is the IVS position, followed by the TR jet velocity. We were able to prospectively classify 140 of 144 echocardiograms using this system, but we found that studies were less likely to have a measureable TR jet with lower estimates of pulmonary pressure. Of course, the consideration of any additional findings in the interpretation of an echocardiogram is also important, including biventricular function, atrial or ventricular level shunts, any contribution of valvar or peripheral pulmonary artery stenosis, and pulmonary vein abnormalities.

Although pulmonary hypertension has been traditionally defined by pressure estimates, the assessment of PVR is the critical component in infants with CDH. Infants with significant pulmonary vascular disease likely have pulmonary hypertension (elevated pressure), but the converse is not necessarily true. We proceed to cardiac catheterization to improve our assessment of pulmonary vascular disease in the setting of persistent elevations in pulmonary artery pressure estimates at 1½ to 2 months of age. We believe that any additional contributors to our echocardiographic assessment of pulmonary hypertension at this age need to be more thoroughly assessed (shunt or obstruction), and long-term therapy for pulmonary vascular disease would be indicated in an infant who still has significant disease. The procedure thus allows us to consider the management of concomitant structural heart disease (suspected or unsuspected), and PVR can be estimated at baseline conditions and in response to a pulmonary vasodilator challenge (most commonly increased FIO_2 and/or inhaled nitric oxide). This evaluation allows for assessment of the components of elevated pulmonary arterial pressure in these patients—restriction (due the small pulmonary vascular bed) and constriction (due to elevated pulmonary vascular tone)—as well as the influence of any shunt or other obstruction (e.g., pulmonary artery or vein stenosis) that may be present. The information gained, therefore, allows us to most appropriately recommend long-term therapy, if indicated. Although it has commonly been stated that there is not a significant reactive component to pulmonary hypertension in infants with CDH, we have previously demonstrated vascular reactivity with exposure to vasodilator challenge in infants and children during cardiac catheterization.[82]

Elevated pulmonary vascular tone in infants with CDH may be present for multiple reasons. In a prospective study, we found that 1/12 (8%) infants who were discharged breathing room air and 14/19 (74%) infants who were discharged on oxygen support or died had an elevated estimated pulmonary-to-systemic pressure ratio that was at least ⅔ systemic pressure by echocardiogram.[76] Plasma endothelin-1 (a potent vasoconstrictor) levels at this time point were directly related to the extent of elevation in pulmonary pressure. These data suggest that biochemical abnormalities in the pulmonary vasculature contribute to persistent elevations in pulmonary vascular tone in infants with CDH. Other factors, including low pH due to poorly compensated respiratory acidosis or non-ideal lung volume (areas of collapse or hyperinflation), may contribute to elevated PVR in this patient population and may or may not be reversible with vasodilator challenge.

Management of Pulmonary Hypertension

Although infants with CDH can present with PPHN during the acute period, the greater concern in these children is their chronic elevations in PVR, which cause right heart strain, high shear stress in the pulmonary vascular bed, and ongoing vascular injury. Owing to a lack of improvement in oxygenation documented in randomized clinical trials of inhaled nitric oxide (iNO, described later), who should be treated for pulmonary hypertension and how they should be treated are not completely straightforward. In general, at UCSF, we have had both early (acute) criteria, and later (chronic) criteria, with generally different goals for treatment. In the acute stage, when stabilization and weaning of the patient is the primary goal of treatment, we use iNO if any of the following conditions exist: persistently low preductal SpO_2, large ductal level right-to-left shunt with an inability to significantly wean from FIO_2 or diminished ventricular function with evidence of elevated pulmonary pressure. Two studies did demonstrate decreased RV function in infants with CDH, measured by Tei index and tissue Doppler imaging.[86,87] Impaired LV output, if present, is likely due to decreased pulmonary venous return and/or interventricular dependence with abnormal RV conformation affecting LV function.[86] In this phase of management, clinically significant pulmonary hypertension resolves in the majority of infants by 2 to 4 weeks of age with an aggressive ventilator weaning protocol.[76] In fact, at 2 weeks of age, 15/16 infants (94%; 95% confidence interval 70% to 100%) with a low estimated pulmonary-to-systemic pressure ratio at 2 weeks went on to survive, and 11/16 infants (69%; 95% confidence interval 41% to 89%) were discharged breathing room air. These infants, from our institution, were treated with either supportive therapy only or inhaled NO up to the time of that assessment.

We consider evaluation by cardiac catheterization in anticipation of the transition to or addition of long-term therapy in infants in whom pulmonary hypertension has not resolved by 1½ to 2 months of age, because data suggest that these infants are unlikely to normalize their pressure on their own. Dillon and colleagues[88] described a retrospective cohort of infants with CDH cared for in the 1990s, with all echocardiographic pressure estimates based on TR jet velocity. Eight infants had estimates of persistent elevated systemic-to-suprasystemic pressure at 6 weeks of age, and all expired. In addition, all seven infants with elevated pulmonary pressure estimates of at least 50% systemic at 2 months of age still had elevated pressure estimates at discharge (as did ⅔ of infants requiring mechanical ventilation or supplemental oxygen at that time). In unpublished data from our prospective UCSF cohort, nine infants had at least 50% systemic pressure estimates at more than 1 month of age.[76] Four infants expired prior to discharge, all with estimated pulmonary artery pressures at least ⅔ systemic pressure. Five infants survived to discharge, all were discharged on supplemental oxygen, one still had persistent systemic-to-suprasystemic pressure (by echocardiogram and cardiac catheterization), and four had echocardiographic evidence of resolution of elevated pulmonary artery pressure, although in two of these infants, discharge followed prolonged hospitalization with long-term antihypertensive therapy.

In the acute setting, iNO is the best initial therapy for pulmonary hypertension in CDH because it can enhance ventilation-perfusion matching. Two randomized studies assessing the oxygenation response to inhaled NO have been conducted.[35,89] Although these studies demonstrated low rates of improvement in oxygenation, they were in the setting of either attempted alkalosis or without permissive hypercapnia and with prolonged exposure to FIO_2 1.0. Thus, the pulmonary vessels exposed to iNO in these studies may have been maximally dilated, whereas in the current era of permissive hypercapnia with more acid pH, vascular tone may be relatively higher, allowing iNO to provide some vasorelaxation. Further, autopsy data demonstrate decreased endothelial nitric oxide synthase (eNOS) expression in the lungs of fetuses with CDH throughout gestation, so endogenous NO production may be relatively deficient in these infants, with exogenous iNO replacing this deficiency.[90] Finally, as previously noted, prolonged high FIO_2 exposure may impair vasoreactivity; in the lamb with PPHN exposed to FIO_2 1.0 for 24 hours, PDE-5 expression and activity are restored after treatment with superoxide dismutase or iNO.[91] So although iNO may not have immediate or pronounced effects on oxygenation in infants with CDH, it may be beneficial to the pulmonary vasculature. Kinsella and associates[92] also described the longer-term noninvasive administration of iNO via nasal cannula in infants with CDH who were successfully extubated but still had echocardiographic evidence of elevated pulmonary artery pressure after discontinuation of the drug. Infants were treated from 5 to 60 days (until resolution of pulmonary hypertension following withdrawal of iNO), and 9/10 survived to 1 year of age. Nasopharyngeal measurements demonstrated NO concentrations at approximately 50% of the delivered dose, with nasal cannula flow at 1 L/min. On the basis of this report, when we initiate longer-term iNO therapy with nasal cannula support at UCSF, we maintain a nasal cannula flow of no less than 2 L/min and double our intended iNO dose from the delivery system. When using nasal CPAP, we continue the same dose as we administer from the ventilator.

Permissive oxygenation in CDH, allowing for a ductal level right-to-left shunt in the setting of suprasystemic PVR, may be a cardioprotective strategy, because it allows the right heart to pump against systemic rather than pulmonary vascular resistance. Often, with modest improvements in respiratory status, there is an increase in left-to-right shunting that may then lead to ductal constriction. Initiating a prostaglandin E_1 (PGE_1) infusion to relax the ductus arteriosus may be beneficial to the infant's hemodynamics,[29,93,94] although an increase in right-to-left shunt with greater ductal diameter may result in a reduced postductal SpO_2. Clinical signs of worsening cardiopulmonary status with ductal constriction in the setting of persistently elevated PVR include (1) increased lability in oxygenation without changes in ventilation or lung volume on chest radiograph, (2) difficulty achieving diuresis, persistent edema, or uremia out of proportion to diuretic therapy, and (3) new-onset or worsening peripheral systemic vasoconstriction with a pulmonary hypertensive crisis. Other problems, particularly infection, must be considered and treated, if present, so it is critical to confirm the clinical suspicion with an echocardiogram demonstrating new ductal constriction or closure as well as to maintain a high index of suspicion for infectious complications. Routine weekly echocardiograms also may detect this problem before it becomes clinically evident: Diminished right heart function in the setting of a decreased ductus arteriosus caliber with right-to-left or bidirectional flow should prompt consideration of a PGE_1 infusion, particularly in a severely affected infant who is likely to have chronic elevations in PVR. In our experience, a dose of 0.0125-0.05 mcg/kg/min is adequate to relax the ductus, depending on its level of constriction prior to drug initiation. One retrospective series from Japan demonstrated no difference in survival in infants with CDH between the use of PGE_1 and iNO and the use of iNO alone.[95] However, there was no requirement for clinical decompensation prior to initiation of PGE_1 infusion in this study, only a diagnosis of pulmonary hypertension, so infants who may have improved and recovered on their own were also treated. At UCSF, we have used PGE_1 in a more prophylactic manner only for infants undergoing venovenous ECMO support, because they often have very high PVR with atelectatic lungs, and more highly oxygenated blood pumped from the RV is diverted across the patent ductus arteriosus resulting in ductal constriction.

There are various published case reports of transient improvements in oxygenation and/or hemodynamic parameters in infants with CDH after systemic administration of vasodilator therapy. The latest reports have described the effects of intravenous prostacyclin and oral sildenafil.[94,96-98] In one series, there were increases in right ventricular output, along with nonsignificant decreases in systemic blood pressure and pulmonary vascular resistance estimates, following a single dose of sildenafil (1-2 mg/kg).[97] In general, systemic pulmonary vasodilator therapy in the setting of lung disease may improve oxygenation as a result of pulmonary vasodilation and increased output or, conversely, may worsen oxygenation by exacerbating the intrapulmonary shunt and ventilation-perfusion mismatch. Studies assessing intrapulmonary shunt and oxygenation in adults with lung disease have shown conflicting results for sildenafil.[99,100] However, PDE inhibitors may potentiate the effects of concurrent iNO, resulting in a more selective effect of the systemic drugs.[101,102] Further, a variety of drugs can result in more selective pulmonary vasodilation and may improve ventilation-perfusion matching if given via the inhaled route (iloprost and other prostacyclin analogs, and milrinone).[103,104]

Regardless, systemic pulmonary vasodilators should be given only with caution in the acute phase of critical illness in infants with CDH, and their effects must be monitored carefully. With short-acting intravenous therapy, such as epoprostenol ($t_{1/2}$ = 6 minutes), dose can be titrated to effect, and effects can be reversed rapidly. However, with longer-acting agents (e.g., sildenafil and milrinone, with $t_{1/2}$ = 3-4 hours), adverse effects are more difficult to reverse. As a continuous infusion, milrinone can also be titrated to effect, although the target dose is not clear. The target dose after cardiac surgery in children is 0.75 μg/kg/min, because that dose has been shown to decrease the incidence of low cardiac output syndrome in that patient population.[105] In infants with CDH receiving iNO who have persistent evidence of right heart failure, we initiate therapy with a continuous infusion of 0.25 μg/kg/min, and raise the dose to 0.5 μg/kg/min after several hours if systemic blood pressure and oxygenation are not further impaired. After several more hours, milrinone is again raised to our target dose of 0.75 μg/kg/min, unless a substantial improvement in the infant's condition has been seen.

There is similarly no direct data in support of a target dose for sildenafil. Raja and colleagues[102] studied 10 children with pulmonary hypertension following cardiac surgery who were receiving iNO. A drop in pulmonary artery pressure after initiation of sildenafil at a dose of 0.5 mg/kg was noted, and the pressure was not further decreased despite an increase of the dose to 2 mg/kg. In an infant with CDH, we described a reduction in the severity of pulmonary hypertension on echocardiogram with a dose of 0.3 mg/kg.[106] However, there is not broader data supporting a specific sildenafil dose in CDH, and Noori and associates[97] could not document a consistent response to a sildenafil dose of 1 to 2 mg/kg in infants with CDH receiving iNO. Even more uncertain is the dose of sildenafil for long-term treatment of pulmonary hypertension. Case series have reported dosing of 0.6 to 9 mg/kg/day in these infants.[82,97,98,106-108] However, such series still report significant mortality, and it is unclear what dose of sildenafil, if any, might improve outcome in infants with CDH. In fact, the most appropriate dose of sildenafil in adults with pulmonary hypertension is somewhat controversial. Although the oral dose approved by both US and European regulatory agencies is 20 mg three times daily, clinicians do raise the dose for patients with more severe disease.[109] Ahsman and coworkers[107] studied the pharmacokinetics of oral sildenafil in 11 infants from 2 to 121 days of age; there was great variability in plasma levels of sildenafil and its active metabolite. The investigators concluded that a dose of 4.2 mg/kg/day in infants would result in 24-hour levels comparable to the adult dose of 20 mg three times per day. However given the large variability in plasma levels, 24-hour levels of sildenafil and its metabolite at this dose could be as high as threefold or as low as one third of the comparable adult dose. An industry-sponsored (Pfizer Inc., New York, NY) sildenafil pediatric dose study (subjects 1-17 years of age) has been completed, although the results are not yet published (NCT00159913). Together, these studies might inform the appropriate chronic dose in infants with CDH.

Potential side effects of sildenafil are concerning in infants with CDH. There are dose-related symptoms of gastroesophageal reflux (GER) in adults, with mechanistic studies suggesting that both delayed gastric emptying and increased relaxation of the gastroesophageal junction influence these symptoms.[109-111] Although GER has not been widely reported as an adverse event in case series of children treated with sildenafil for pulmonary hypertension, it is an important comorbidity in infants and children with CDH that may contribute to pulmonary morbidity in this patient population.[112] There are also two serious idiosyncratic side effects reported in adults, acute vision and hearing losses.[113,114] It is not clear whether infants are at risk for these complications; a series of 22 term and near-term infants undergoing ophthalmologic examination following sildenafil treatment had no findings attributable to sildenafil exposure.[115] However, given that these are severe complications that may not be detected initially and may or may not be reversible, the risk-to-benefit ratio of treatment should be carefully considered. Finally, there are several reports of excessive bleeding and spontaneous intracranial hemorrhage in children and adults taking sildenafil without other known risk factors; sildenafil is a known inhibitor of platelet function.[116-119]

We have designed a study to evaluate the effects of early sildenafil in infants with CDH who are receiving mechanical ventilation with FIO_2 0.40 or higher or pulmonary arterial pressure (P_{PA}) estimated at least ⅔ systemic pressure, at 10 to 14 days of age (NCT00133679). Our preliminary data have suggested that these infants are at high risk for adverse outcome (death or discharge on supplemental oxygen)[76] (R. Keller, unpublished data). However, recruitment is challenging because the potential study population of patients is essentially bimodal: Many children have recovered by this time, and a good proportion of those who remain ill are so sick that their chances of survival are low.

There is good rationale for the use of endothelin-1 (ET-1) receptor antagonists in infants with CDH: Circulating levels of ET-1 are high in infants who ultimately

20

die or are discharged with oxygen support, and the expression of lung ET receptors is increased.[76,120] ET receptor antagonists have not been reported to have substantial vasodilating effects on the pulmonary vasculature, however, this therapy may be of benefit in infants with congenital heart disease and an obligate shunt (see later section on the approach to patients with congenital heart disease). An ET receptor antagonist may also be of use as an additional drug targeting a unique pathway in infants with more severe elevations in PVR or with failure of adequate response to single-drug therapy, or in infants with no substantial reactivity, because of the differences in the side effect profile from other treatment options. The largest pediatric experience in this class of drugs is with bosentan, a nonspecific ET receptor antagonist that binds both ET-A and ET-B receptors. Dose-for-weight ranges in older children that approximate 2 mg/kg per dose two times daily result in relatively low exposure to drug levels in comparison with standard adult dosing. However, a subsequent pharmacokinetic study demonstrated no difference in drug levels with a doubling of the dose, so the lower dose is recommended.[121,122] All ET receptor antagonists, including bosentan, undergo hepatic metabolism and carry a risk of a reversible increase in transaminases. Monthly monitoring of transaminases after drug administration is recommended, with the interval prolonged after 6 months if no adverse effects are seen. However, a report from a large European pediatric registry (subjects ages 2-11 years) suggests that increase in transaminases may be less common in children (approximately 3% incidence) than it is in adults; this difference may be related to the lower drug levels attained.[123] Owing to the limited experience with these drugs in infancy, we monitor transaminase levels weekly for the first month for inpatients. After the first month, or for outpatients, we monitor transaminases monthly for the first 6 months of therapy, and then less frequently if there have been no increases from pretreatment levels.

Inhaled iloprost may provide acute vasodilation and improve ventilation-perfusion matching.[103,124] Serum $t_{1/2}$ is less than 10 minutes, and drug levels peak within 5 minutes of completion of a 10-minute treatment.[103] Despite the limited vasodilation predicted by the pharmacokinetics, pharmacodynamic studies demonstrate that the half-life for vasodilatory effects is 25 minutes. However, of concern in infants with CDH is the increase in airflow obstruction and respiratory symptoms in some patients, despite the vasodilatory effects of the drug. Reichenberger and colleagues[125] found that four of eight adult patients with primary respiratory diagnoses discontinued the drug prematurely because of side effects. In another study, Ivy and associates[124] evaluated 13 pediatric patients without primary lung disease with spirometry before and after iloprost inhalation.[124] Five patients had substantial increases in expiratory obstruction following drug administration (decrease in FEF_{25-75} by at least 15%); two children were unable to start long-term therapy owing to acute respiratory symptoms, and two other children experienced symptomatic respiratory disease after several months of therapy, which was controlled with bronchodilators and inhaled steroids. The drug is dosed every 2 to 3 hours while the patient is awake, with 6 to 9 doses per day. For inpatients, we dose every 3 hours (8 doses per day), and for patients at home, we have families dose every 2 hours during awake periods (usually 6-7 doses per day). The target dose per treatment is the same as in adults, 5 μg; however, the delivery system approved for use with iloprost is an actuated, inhalation-only device (Adaptive Aerosol Delivery [AAD]). Conventional nebulizer devices are continuous-flow systems, and thus drug nebulized during exhalation is wasted (typically 60%), lowering the dose that is effectively delivered; the total dose may be increased to account for this loss.[103,126] Pneumatic nebulizers also have a relatively large dead volume (1-3 mL), which is problematic for low-volume medication delivery (≤0.5 mL for iloprost), although the use of an ultrasonic nebulizer with low dead volume addresses this problem to some extent. Modifications to AAD systems have been made to allow for drug delivery to young children, but they are not available in the United States.[127]

Generally, decisions about therapy in infants and young children with CDH need to be made carefully. The risk of long-term therapies in this young patient population is not known, and some children may respond to good supportive therapy and limited oxygen supplementation. Long-term morbidity is prevalent in these patients, with effects on neurologic development, hearing, growth and feeding, and pulmonary function. With the lack of randomized controlled trials and a thorough assessment of outcomes and adverse medication effects in these patients, the information gained from cardiac catheterization can only help in making optimal treatment decisions.

Approach to Patients with Congenital Heart Disease

Two retrospective studies have evaluated outcomes in children with CDH complicated by congenital heart disease (excluding patient ductus arteriosus and atrial septal defect/patent foramen ovale). Cohen and colleagues[128] reported single-center data from 24 liveborn infants with CDH and heart disease compared with 119 infants without heart disease. Ventricular septal defect (VSD) was the single most common lesion among liveborn infants (7/24, 29%), followed by aortic arch obstruction with or without VSD (5/24, 21%). Survival was significantly lower in infants with CDH and heart disease than it was in infants with CDH not complicated by heart disease (58% vs. 21%); 3/5 surviving infants had an isolated VSD. These data are in agreement with population-based studies that have consistently shown that postnatal survival is lower in infants with CDH and associated anomalies than in infants with isolated CDH.[39,41] A large series from the Congenital Diaphragmatic Hernia Study Group[129] had findings similar to those reported by Cohen and colleagues,[128] although with overall somewhat higher survival rates. The most common cardiac lesion was VSD (42%, 118/280), followed by aortic arch obstruction (15%, 42/280), and then hypoplastic left heart syndrome (14%, 38/280).[129] Survival was significantly higher in infants without heart disease than in those with heart disease (67% vs. 41%). Infants with VSD had the highest survival rates, at approximately 60%, and infants with single-ventricle physiology had the lowest survival rates, at approximately 5%.

Infants with congenital heart disease and CDH can pose difficult physiologic problems. Intracardiac communications with right-to-left shunting can result in hypoxemia in the setting of high PVR and diastolic dysfunction, common findings in infants with CDH and pulmonary hypertension.[86,87] Noori and associates[97] described the effects of sildenafil administration, as detected by echocardiography, on cardiac output measurements in four infants with CDH, one of whom had an atrial septal defect (ASD). This infant had no change in left ventricular output, with a 53% increase in RV output, owing to development of a left-to-right shunt following sildenafil administration. In the longer term, elevations in pulmonary-to-systemic blood flow will not be well-tolerated in an infant with lung hypoplasia. This becomes even more problematic in infants who require a PGE_1 infusion because of ductus-dependent systemic blood flow. If surgery is undertaken when PVR remains elevated, the effects of cardiopulmonary bypass on the vascular bed and the lung, combined with closure of the ductus arteriosus at the time of surgery, can result in severe pulmonary hypertension and ventricular dysfunction, which are associated with substantial perioperative morbidity and mortality.[130,131] Thus, the decision-making regarding the timing of surgery is complex.

Generally, repair of the diaphragmatic defect, with some period of recovery before heart surgery is undertaken, is the most rational initial approach, because reducing the hernia contents and closing the diaphragm will allow for further assessment of the infant's lung function, the degree of lung hypoplasia, and the ability to survive from a pulmonary perspective. Infants who can be weaned to low ventilator settings or from all mechanical support after CDH repair have the best opportunity to recover following cardiac surgery. In the absence of CDH, postoperative pulmonary hypertension is associated with prolonged hospitalization following surgery for congenital heart disease.[130] For infants who still have evidence of high PVR, one option is to proceed to cardiac surgery, provide extracorporeal support postoperatively as needed, and await recovery. Alternatively, one can provide support as needed while continuing the PGE_1 infusion, and await evidence of a decrease in PVR. Given the need to maintain ductal patency, and the left-sided obstruction, accurate assessment of PVR by echocardiogram can be challenging. Solely left-to-right ductal flow is reassuring, and when bidirectional flow is present, retrograde diastolic flow in the descending aorta is an encouraging sign of decreasing PVR. Cardiac catheterization again can be very helpful in these cases, to measure PVR and assess severity of pulmonary hypertension and vascular reactivity. For infants evaluated at more than 1 month of age who are not clearly candidates for cardiac surgery (on the basis of institutional thresholds for PVR elevation), initiation of bosentan therapy may help with the vascular remodeling process during the await for further evidence of appropriate surgical candidacy. Pulmonary vasodilation with bosentan is unlikely to be significant, yet there may be benefits to the vascular structure and reactivity over time. In contrast, the use of drugs that cause pulmonary vasodilation may increase pulmonary blood flow. Similarly, the pathophysiology in cases of arch obstruction with a VSD may be more complicated, because a prolonged waiting time for surgery may result in further deleterious pulmonary vascular remodeling if there is a left-to-right intracardiac shunt.

C

Longer-Term Issues in Survivors of CDH

Finally, there are multiple long-term morbidities in infants surviving with CDH. We have described that perinatal markers of anatomic and physiologic severity (liver herniation into the chest, need for nonprimary diaphragm repair, prolonged mechanical ventilation, and hospital discharge on supplemental oxygen) are associated with neurodevelopmental impairment, hearing loss, and gastrointestinal and pulmonary complications.[31,132] Hearing loss is of particular interest in relation to neonatal management. One study of children surviving with CDH from a single center in Canada found an association between sensorineural hearing loss and the use of pharmacologic paralysis with pancuronium.[133] However, because there is not a known mechanism for ototoxic effects of pancuronium, it is likely not a causative agent for hearing loss, but rather a concerning association related to the severity of the CDH.[134] Overall prevalence of hearing loss in this study was high (62%, 23 of 37 children), compared with 29% (26/90) found at 7 years of age in children with neonatal respiratory failure from diverse etiologies (with > 90% receiving paralytics).[135] An evaluation of children who were supported with ECMO in the neonatal period at Boston Children's Hospital described three independent factors for hearing loss (progressive in 21 of 29 cases): prolonged ECMO support (>160 hours, 14 days or more of exposure to aminoglycoside antibiotics, and a diagnosis of CDH.[136] Finally, in a later follow-up study from the Canadian group, prolonged exposure to loop diuretics (exceeding 14 days, the average length of treatment) was the strongest independent association with sensorineural hearing loss in 4-year-old survivors of neonatal respiratory failure, both with and without CDH, with no additional predictive value associated with pharmacologic paralysis.[137] Thus, the selection of potentially ototoxic medications during management of the critically ill or recovering newborn or infant with CDH, in combination with acute and chronic respiratory insufficiency, may contribute to longer-term morbidity. However, the broad patterns of hearing loss noted in children surviving with CDH[136] suggest that ototoxic medications are not the sole etiology of this morbidity. Specific modifiable neonatal factors influencing later neurodevelopmental impairment in survivors of CDH are also unknown, although commonalities are likely in the extremely preterm population, wherein illness complicated by an inflammatory state (such as infection and bronchopulmonary dysplasia) is associated with increased risk of impairment.[138,139]

Antenatal Therapies

Evidence from randomized trials of management strategies designed to improve survival in CDH is limited. In addition to the trials assessing timing of CDH repair, two randomized fetal trials have been undertaken: Our group performed a single-center study of tracheal occlusion to enhance fetal lung growth in fetuses with severe CDH, and the Congenital Diaphragmatic Hernia Study Group undertook a multicenter study of antenatal glucocorticoid administration in unselected fetuses with CDH and no associated anomalies.[140-143] Both of these studies failed to show a benefit. In the UCSF study, survival was higher than anticipated in the control group, who were all cared for at our institution.[140] In the antenatal glucocorticoid study, enrollment was low, and survival similar to that in the registry as a whole.[141] Selection of patients for intervention is important when survival and later morbidity are the outcomes of interest. Thus, there are clearly significant challenges in undertaking these studies, and for the most part, we are still left with making management decisions on the basis of overall physiology and the broad experience that is reported, albeit retrospectively.

References

1. Kitagawa M, Hislop A, Boyden EA, Reid L. Lung hypoplasia in congenital diaphragmatic hernia. *Br J Surg*. 1971;58:342-346.
2. Hislop A, Reid L. Persistent hypoplasia of the lung after repair of congenital diaphragmatic hernia. *Thorax*. 1976;31:450-455.
3. Geggel RL, Murphy JD, Langleban D, et al. Congenital diaphragmatic hernia: arterial structural changes and persistent pulmonary hypertension after surgical repair. *J Pediatr*. 1985;107:457-464.
4. Hislop AA. Airway and blood vessel interaction during lung development. *J Anat*. 2002;201:325-334.
5. Scarpelli EM. The lung, tracheal fluid, and lipid metabolism of the fetus. *Pediatrics*. 1967;40:951-961.
6. Alcorn D, Adamson TM, Lambert TF, et al. Morphological effects of chronic tracheal ligation and drainage in the fetal lamb lung. *J Anat*. 1977;123:649-660.
7. DiFiore JW, Fauza DO, Slavin R, et al. Experimental fetal tracheal ligation reverses the structural and physiological effects of pulmonary hypoplasia in congenital diaphragmatic hernia. *J Pediatr Surg*. 1994;29:248-257.
8. Sista AK, Filly RA. Paradoxical movements of abdominal contents indicating a congenital diaphragmatic hernia. *J Ultrasound Med*. 2007;27:497.
9. Comstock C, Bronsteen RA, Whitten A, Lee W. Paradoxical motion: a useful tool in the prenatal diagnosis of congenital diaphragmatic hernias and eventrations. *J Ultrasound Med*. 2009;28:1365-1367.
10. Langston C, Kida K, Reed M, Thurlbeck WM. Human lung growth in late gestation and in the neonate. *Am Rev Respir Dis*. 1984;129:607-613.
11. Nakayama DK, Motoyama EK, Tagge EM. Effect of preoperative stabilization on respiratory system compliance and outcome in newborn infants with congenital diaphragmatic hernia. *J Pediatr*. 1991;118:793-799.
12. Antunes MJ, Greenspan JS, Cullen JA, et al. Prognosis with preoperative pulmonary function and lung volume assessment in infants with congenital diaphragmatic hernia. *Pediatrics*. 1995;96:1117-1122.
13. Dinger J, Peter-Kern M, Goebel P, et al. Effect of PEEP and suction via chest drain on functional residual capacity and lung compliance after surgical repair of congenital diaphragmatic hernia: preliminary observations in 5 patients. *J Pediatr Surg*. 2000;35:1482-1488.
14. Barghorn A, Koslowski M, Kromminga R, et al. alpha-smooth muscle actin distribution in the pulmonary vasculature comparing hypoplastic and normal fetal lungs. *Pediatr Pathol Lab Med*. 1998;18:15-22.
15. Levin DL. Morphologic analysis of the pulmonary vascular bed in congenital left-sided diaphragmatic hernia. *J Pediatr*. 1978;92:805-809.
16. Naeye RL, Shochat SJ, Whitman V, Maisels MJ. Unsuspected pulmonary vascular abnormalities associated with diaphragmatic hernia. *Pediatrics*. 1976;58:902-906.
17. Sakai H, Tamura M, Hosokawa Y, et al. Effects of surgical repair on respiratory mechanics in congenital diaphragmatic hernia. *J Pediatr*. 1987;111:432-438.
18. Koumbourlis AC, Wung JT, Stolar CJ. Lung function in infants after repair of congenital diaphragmatic hernia. *J Pediatr Surg*. 2006;41:1716-1721.
19. Dimitriou G, Greenough A, Kavvadia V, et al. Diaphragmatic function in infants with surgically corrected anomalies. *Pediatr Res*. 2003;54:502-508.
20. Arena F, Romeo C, Calabro MP, et al. Long-term functional evaluation of diaphragmatic motility after repair of congenital diaphragmatic hernia. *J Pediatr Surg*. 2005;40:1078-1081.
21. Moyer V, Moya F, Tibboel R, et al. Late versus early surgical correction for congenital diaphragmatic hernia in newborn infants. *Cochrane Database Syst Rev*. 2002;(3):CD001695.
22. Azarow K, Messineo A, Pearl R, et al. Congenital diaphragmatic hernia—a tale of two cities: the Toronto experience. *J Pediatr Surg*. 1997;32:395-400.
23. Wilson JM, Lund DP, Lillehei CW, Vacanti JP. Congenital diaphragmatic hernia—a tale of two cities: the Boston experience. *J Pediatr Surg*. 1997;32:401-405.
24. Keller RL, Hawgood S, Neuhaus JM, et al. Infant pulmonary function in a randomized trial of fetal tracheal occlusion for severe congenital diaphragmatic hernia. *Pediatr Res*. 2004;56:818-825.

25. Kays DW, Langham MR, Ledbetter DJ, Talbert JL. Detrimental effects of standard medical therapy in congenital diaphragmatic hernia. *Ann Surg*. 1999;230:340-351.
26. Wung JT, Sahni R, Moffitt ST, et al. Congenital diaphragmatic hernia: survival treated with very delayed surgery, spontaneous respiration, and no chest tube. *J Pediatr Surg*. 1995;30:406-409.
27. Frenckner B, Ehrén H, Granholm T, et al. Improved results in patients who have congenital diaphragmatic hernia using preoperative stabilization, extracorporeal membrane oxygenation, and delayed surgery. *J Pediatr Surg*. 1997;32:1185-1189.
28. Downard CD, Jaksic T, Garza JJ, et al. Analysis of an improved survival rate for congenital diaphragmatic hernia. *J Pediatr Surg*. 2003;38:729-732.
29. Bohn D. Congenital diaphragmatic hernia. *Am J Respir Crit Care Med*. 2002;166:911-915.
30. Boloker J, Bateman DA, Wung JT, Stolar CJ. Congenital diaphragmatic hernia in 120 infants treated consecutively with permissive hypercapnia/spontaneous respiration/ elective repair. *J Pediatr Surg*. 2002;37:357-366.
31. Cortes RA, Keller RL, Townsend T, et al. Survival of severe congenital diaphragmatic hernia has morbid consequences. *J Pediatr Surg*. 2005;140:36-46.
32. Hillman NH, Moss TJ, Kallapur SG, et al. Brief, large tidal volume ventilation initiates lung injury and a systemic response in fetal sheep. *Am J Respir Crit Care Med*. 2007;176:575-581.
33. de Durante G, del Turco M, Rustichini L, et al. ARDSNet lower tidal volume ventilatory strategy may generate intrinsic positive end-expiratory pressure in patients with acute respiratory distress syndrome. *Am J Respir Crit Care Med*. 2002;165:1271-1274.
34. Frank JA, Parsons PE, Matthay MA. Pathogenetic significance of biological markers of ventilator-associated lung injury in experimental and clinical studies. *Chest*. 2006;130:1906-1914.
35. Kinsella JP, Truog WE, Walsh WF, et al. Randomized, multicenter trial of inhaled nitric oxide and high-frequency oscillatory ventilation in severe, persistent pulmonary hypertension of the newborn. *J Pediatr*. 1997;131:55-62.
35a. NTR1310. WHO International Clinical Trials Registry Platform. *http://apps.who.int/trialsearch/Trial.aspx*, accessed December 31, 2010.
35b. Logan JW, Rice HE, Goldberg RN, Cotten CM. Congenital diaphragmatic hernia: a systematic review and summary of best-evidence practice strategies. *J Perinatol*. 2007;27:535-549.
36. Tracy ET, Mears SE, Smith PB, et al. Protocolized approach to the management of congenital diaphragmatic hernia: benefits of reducing variability in care. *J Pediatr Surg*. 2010;45:1343-1348.
37. Stege G, Fenton A, Jaffray B. Nihilism in the 1990s: the true mortality of congenital diaphragmatic hernia. *Pediatrics*. 2003;112:532-535.
38. Levison J, Halliday R, Holland AJ, et al. Neonatal Intensive Care Units Study of the NSW Pregnancy and Newborn Services Network. A population-based study of congenital diaphragmatic hernia outcome in New South Wales and the Australian Capital Territory, Australia, 1992-2001. *J Pediatr Surg*. 2006;41:1049-1053.
39. Yang W, Carmichael SL, Harris JA, Shaw GM. Epidemiologic characteristics of congenital diaphragmatic hernia among 2.5 million California births, 1989-1997. *Birth Defects Res A Clin Mol Teratol*. 2006;76:170-174.
40. Aly H, Bianco-Batlles D, Mohamed MA, Hammad TA. Mortality in infants with congenital diaphragmatic hernia: a study of the United States National Database. *J Perinatol*. 2010;30:553-557.
41. Gallot D, Boda C, Ughetto S, et al. Prenatal detection and outcome of congenital diaphragmatic hernia: a French registry-based study. *Ultrasound Obstet Gynecol*. 2007;29:276-283.
42. Harrison MR, Bjordal RI, Langmark F, Knutrud O. Congenital diaphragmatic hernia: the hidden mortality. *J Pediatr Surg*. 1978;13:227-230.
43. Mah VK, Zamakhshary M, Mah DY, et al. Absolute vs relative improvements in congenital diaphragmatic hernia survival: what happened to "hidden mortality. *J Pediatr Surg*. 2009;44:877-882.
44. Ontario Congenital Anomalies Study Group. Apparent truth about congenital diaphragmatic hernia: a population-based database is needed to establish benchmarking for clinical outcomes for CDH. *J Pediatr Surg*. 2004;39:661-665.
45. Coalson JJ, Winter V, deLemos RA. Decreased alveolarization in baboon survivors with bronchopulmonary dysplasia. *Am J Respir Crit Care Med*. Aug 1995;152:640-646.
46. Coalson JJ, Winter VT, Siler-Khodr T, Yoder BA. Neonatal chronic lung disease in extremely immature baboons. *Am J Respir Crit Care Med*. 1999;160:1333-1346.
47. Bland RD, Albertine KH, Carlton DP, et al. Chronic lung injury in preterm lambs: abnormalities of the pulmonary circulation and lung fluid balance. *Pediatr Res*. Jul 2000;48:64-74.
48. Sebald M, Friedlich P, Burns C, et al. Risk of need for extracorporeal membrane oxygenation support in neonates with congenital diaphragmatic hernia treated with inhaled nitric oxide. *J Perinatol*. 2004;24:143-146.
49. Kassim Z, Jolley C, Moxham J, et al. Diaphragm electromyogram in infants with abdominal wall defects and congenital diaphragmatic hernia. *Eur Respir J*. 2011;37:143-149.
50. Abolmaali N, Koch A, Götzelt K, et al. Lung volumes, ventricular function and pulmonary arterial flow in children operated on for left-sided congenital diaphragmatic hernia: long-term results. *Eur Radiol*. 2010;20:1580-1589.
51. Areechon W, Reid L. Hypoplasia of lung with congenital diaphragmatic hernia. *Br Med J*. 1963;5325:230-233.
52. Sabater JR, Lee TA, Abraham WM. Comparative effects of salmeterol, albuterol, and ipratropium on normal and impaired mucociliary function in sheep. *Chest*. 2005;128:3743-3749.
53. Nakayama DK, Motoyama EK, Mutich RL, Koumbourlis AC. Pulmonary function in newborns after repair of congenital diaphragmatic hernia. *Pediatr Pulmonol*. 1991;11:49-55.

54. Broughton AR, Thibeault DW, Mabry SM, Truog WE. Airway muscle in infants with congenital diaphragmatic hernia: response to treatment. *J Pediatr Surg*. 1998;33:1471-1475.
55. Boucherat O, Benachi A, Chailley-Heu B, et al. Surfactant maturation is not delayed in human fetuses with diaphragmatic hernia. *PLoS Med*. 2007;4:e237.
56. Cogo PE, Zimmermann LJ, Rosso F, et al. Surfactant synthesis and kinetics in infants with congenital diaphragmatic hernia. *Am J Respir Crit Care Med*. 2002;166:154-158.
57. Cogo PE, Zimmermann LJ, Meneghini L, et al. Pulmonary surfactant disaturated-phosphatidylcholine (DSPC) turnover and pool size in newborn infants with congenital diaphragmatic hernia (CDH). *Pediatr Res*. 2003;54:653-658.
58. Janssen DJ, Tibboel D, Carnielli VP, et al. Surfactant phosphatidylcholine pool size in human neonates with congenital diaphragmatic hernia requiring ECMO. *J Pediatr*. 2003;142:247-252.
59. Janssen DJ, Zimmermann LJ, Cogo P, et al. Decreased surfactant phosphatidylcholine synthesis in neonates with congenital diaphragmatic hernia during extracorporeal membrane oxygenation. *Intensive Care Med*. 2009;35:1754-1760.
60. Colby CE, Lally KP, Hintz SR, et al, Congenital Diaphragmatic Hernia Study Group. Surfactant replacement therapy on ECMO does not improve outcome in neonates with congenital diaphragmatic hernia. *J Pediatr Surg*. 2004;39:1632-1637.
61. Lally KP, Lally PA, Langham MR, et al, Congenital Diaphragmatic Hernia Study Group. Surfactant does not improve survival rate in preterm infants with congenital diaphragmatic hernia. *J Pediatr Surg*. 2004;39:829-833.
62. Van Meurs K, Congenital Diaphragmatic Hernia Study Group. Is surfactant therapy beneficial in the treatment of the term newborn infant with congenital diaphragmatic hernia? *J Pediatr*. 2004;145:312-316.
63. Bahrami KR, Van Meurs KP. ECMO for neonatal respiratory failure. *Semin Perinatol*. 2005;29: 15-23.
64. Mugford M, Elbourne D, Field D. Extracorporeal membrane oxygenation for severe respiratory failure in newborn infants. *Cochrane Database Syst Rev*. 2008;(3):CD001340,.
65. Folkesson HG, Chapin CJ, Beard LL, et al. Congenital diaphragmatic hernia prevents absorption of distal air space fluid in late-gestation rat fetuses. *Am J Physiol Lung Cell Mol Physiol*. 2006;290:L478-L484.
66. Hoffman SB, Massaro AN, Gingalewski C, Short BL. Predictors of survival in congenital diaphragmatic hernia patients requiring extracorporeal membrane oxygenation: CNMC 15-year experience. *J Perinatol*. 2010;30:546-552.
67. Tiruvoipati R, Vinogradova Y, Faulkner G, et al. Predictors of outcome in patients with congenital diaphragmatic hernia requiring extracorporeal membrane oxygenation. *J Pediatr Surg*. 2007;42: 1345-1350.
68. Kunisaki SM, Barnewolt CE, Estroff JA, et al. Ex utero intrapartum treatment with extracorporeal membrane oxygenation for severe congenital diaphragmatic hernia. *J Pediatr Surg*. 2007;42: 98-104.
69. Metkus AP, Filly RA, Stringer MD, et al. Sonographic predictors of survival in fetal diaphragmatic hernia. *J Pediatr Surg*. 1996;31:148-152.
70. Lipshutz GS, Albanese CT, Feldstein VA, et al. Prospective analysis of lung-to-head ratio predicts survival for patients with prenatally diagnosed congenital diaphragmatic hernia. *J Pediatr Surg*. 1997;32:1634-1636.
71. Barnewolt CE, Kunisaki SM, Fauza DO, et al. Percent predicted lung volumes as measured on fetal magnetic resonance imaging: a useful biometric parameter for risk stratification in congenital diaphragmatic hernia. *J Pediatr Surg*. 2007;42:193-197.
72. Vazquez WD, Cheu HW. Hemorrhagic complications and repair of congenital diaphragmatic hernias: does timing of the repair make a difference? Data from the Extracorporeal Life Support Organization. *J Pediatr Surg*. 1994;29:1002-1005.
73. Congenital Diaphragmatic Hernia Study Group, Bryner BS, West BT, Hirschl RB, et al. Congenital diaphragmatic hernia requiring extracorporeal membrane oxygenation: does timing of repair matter? *J Pediatr Surg*. 2009;44:1165-1171.
74. Vacanti JP, Crone RK, Murphy JD, et al. The pulmonary hemodynamic response to perioperative anesthesia in the treatment of high-risk infants with congenital diaphragmatic hernia. *J Pediatr Surg*. 1984;19:672-678.
75. Bos AP, Tibboel D, Koot VCM, et al. Persistent pulmonary hypertension in high-risk congenital diaphragmatic hernia patients: incidence and vasodilator therapy. *J Pediatr Surg*. 1993;28: 1463-1465.
76. Keller RL, Tacy TA, Hendricks-Munoz K, et al. Congenital diaphragmatic hernia: Endothelin-1, pulmonary hypertension and disease severity. *Am J Respir Crit Care Med*. 2010;182:555-561.
77. Lakshminrusimha S, Russell JA, Steinhorn RH, et al. Pulmonary arterial contractility in neonatal lambs increases with 100% oxygen resuscitation. *Pediatr Res*. 2006;59:137-141.
78. Farrow KN, Lakshminrusimha S, Reda WJ, et al. Superoxide dismutase restores eNOS expression and function in resistance pulmonary arteries from neonatal lambs with persistent pulmonary hypertension. *Am J Physiol Lung Cell Mol Physiol*. 2008;295:L979-L987.
79. Farrow KN, Wedgwood S, Lee KJ, et al. Mitochondrial oxidant stress increases PDE5 activity in persistent pulmonary hypertension of the newborn. *Respir Physiol Neurobiol*. 2010;174: 272-281.
80. Abman S, Wolfe R, Accurso F, et al. Pulmonary vascular response to oxygen in infants with severe bronchopulmonary dysplasia. *Pediatrics*. 1985;75:80-84.

81. Kinsella JP, Ivy DD, Abman SH. Pulmonary vasodilator therapy in congenital diaphragmatic hernia: acute, late, and chronic pulmonary hypertension. *Semin Perinatol.* 2005;29:123-128.
82. Keller RL, Moore P, Teitel D, et al. Abnormal vascular tone in infants and children with lung hypoplasia: findings from cardiac catheterization and the response to therapy. *Ped Crit Care Med.* 2006;7:589-594.
83. Farrow KN, Groh BS, Schumacker PT, et al. Hyperoxia increases phosphodiesterase 5 expression and activity in ovine fetal pulmonary artery smooth muscle cells. *Circ Res.* 2008;102:226-233.
84. Mourani PM, Sontag MK, Younoszai A, et al. Clinical utility of echocardiography for the diagnosis and management of pulmonary vascular disease in young children with chronic lung disease. *Pediatrics.* 2008;121:317-325.
85. Reisner SA, Azzam Z, Halmann M, et al. Septal/free wall curvature ratio: a noninvasive index of pulmonary arterial pressure. *J Am Soc Echocardiogr.* 1994;7:27-35.
86. Baptista MJ, Rocha G, Clemente F, et al. *N*-terminal-pro-B type natriuretic peptide as a useful tool to evaluate pulmonary hypertension and cardiac function in CDH infants. *Neonatology.* 2008;94:22-30.
87. Patel N, Mills JF, Cheung MM. Assessment of right ventricular function using tissue Doppler imaging in infants with pulmonary hypertension. *Neonatology.* 2009;96:193-199.
88. Dillon PW, Cilley RE, Mauger D, et al. The relationship of pulmonary artery pressure and survival in congenital diaphragmatic hernia. *J Pediatr Surg.* 2004;39:307-312.
89. The Neonatal Inhaled Nitric Oxide Study Group. Inhaled nitric oxide and hypoxic respiratory failure in infants with congenital diaphragmatic hernia. *Pediatrics.* 1997;99:838-845.
90. Boucherat O, Franco-Montoya ML, Delacourt C, et al. Defective angiogenesis in hypoplastic human fetal lungs correlates with nitric oxide synthase deficiency that occurs despite enhanced angiopoietin-2 and VEGF. *Am J Physiol Lung Cell Mol Physiol.* 2010;298:L849-L856.
91. Farrow KN, Lakshminrusimha S, Czech L, et al. SOD and inhaled nitric oxide normalize phosphodiesterase 5 expression and activity in neonatal lambs with persistent pulmonary hypertension. *Am J Physiol Lung Cell Mol Physiol.* 2010;299:L109-L116.
92. Kinsella JP, Parker TA, Ivy DD, Abman SH. Noninvasive delivery of inhaled nitric oxide therapy for late pulmonary hypertension in newborn infants with congenital diaphragmatic hernia. *J Pediatr.* 2003;142:397-401.
93. Buss M, Williams G, Dilley A, Jones O. Prevention of heart failure in the management of congenital diaphragmatic hernia by maintaining ductal patency. A case report. *J Pediatr Surg.* 2006;41:e9-e11.
94. Filan PM, McDougall PN, Shekerdemian LS. Combination pharmacotherapy for severe neonatal pulmonary hypertension. *J Paediatr Child Health.* 2006;42:219-220.
95. Shiyanagi S, Okazaki T, Shoji H, et al. Management of pulmonary hypertension in congenital diaphragmatic hernia: nitric oxide with prostaglandin-E1 versus nitric oxide alone. *Pediatr Surg Int.* 2008;24:1101-1104.
96. De Luca D, Zecca E, Vento G, et al. Transient effect of epoprostenol and sildenafil combined with iNO for pulmonary hypertension in congenital diaphragmatic hernia. *Paediatr Anaesth.* 2006;16:597-598.
97. Noori S, Friedlich P, Wong P, et al. Cardiovascular effects of sildenafil in neonates and infants with congenital diaphragmatic hernia and pulmonary hypertension. *Neonatology.* 2007;91:92-100.
98. Hunter L, Richens T, Davis C, et al. Sildenafil use in congenital diaphragmatic hernia. *Arch Dis Child Fetal Neonatal Ed.* 2009;94:F467.
99. Ghofrani H, Wiedemann R, Rose F, et al. Sildenafil for treatment of lung fibrosis and pulmonary hypertension: a randomised controlled trial. *Lancet.* 2002;360:895-900.
100. Blanco I, Gimeno E, Munoz PA, et al. Hemodynamic and gas exchange effects of sildenafil in patients with chronic obstructive pulmonary disease and pulmonary hypertension. *Am J Respir Crit Care Med.* 2010;181:270-278.
101. McNamara PJ, Laique F, Muang-In S, Whyte HE. Milrinone improves oxygenation in neonates with severe persistent pulmonary hypertension of the newborn. *J Crit Care.* 2006;21:217-222.
102. Raja SG, Danton MD, MacArthur KJ, Pollock JC. Effects of escalating doses of sildenafil on hemodynamics and gas exchange in children with pulmonary hypertension and congenital cardiac defects. *J Cardiothorac Vasc Anesth.* 2007;21:203-207.
103. Olschewski H, Rohde B, Behr J, et al. Pharmacodynamics and pharmacokinetics of inhaled iloprost, aerosolized by three different devices, in severe pulmonary hypertension. *Chest.* 2003;124:1294-1304.
104. Haraldsson A, Kieler-Jensen N, Ricksten SE. The additive pulmonary vasodilatory effects of inhaled prostacyclin and inhaled milrinone in postcardiac surgical patients with pulmonary hypertension. *Anesth Analg.* 2001;93:1439-1445.
105. Hoffman TM, Wernovsky G, Atz AM, et al. Efficacy and safety of milrinone in preventing low cardiac output syndrome in infants and children after corrective surgery for congenital heart disease. *Circulation.* 2003;107:996-1002.
106. Keller RL, Hamrick SE, Kitterman JA, et al. Treatment of rebound and chronic pulmonary hypertension with oral sildenafil in an infant with congenital diaphragmatic hernia. *Pediatr Crit Care Med.* 2004;5:184-187.
107. Ahsman MJ, Witjes BC, Wildschut ED, et al. Sildenafil exposure in neonates with pulmonary hypertension after administration via a nasogastric tube. *Arch Dis Child Fetal Neonatal Ed.* 2010;95:F109-F114.

108. Humpl T, Reyes JT, Erickson S, et al. Sildenafil therapy for neonatal and childhood pulmonary hypertensive vascular disease. *Cardiol Young*. 2010;8:1-7.
109. Archer SL, Michelakis ED. Phosphodiesterase type 5 inhibitors for pulmonary arterial hypertension. *N Engl J Med*. 2009;361:1864-1871.
110. Sarnelli G, Sifrim D, Janssens J, Tack J. Influence of sildenafil on gastric sensorimotor function in humans. *Am J Physiol Gastrointest Liver Physiol*. 2004;287:G988-G992.
111. Kim HS, Conklin JL, Park H. The effect of sildenafil on segmental oesophageal motility and gastro-oesophageal reflux. *Aliment Pharmacol Ther*. 2006;24:1029-1036.
112. Huddleston AJ, Knoderer CA, Morris JL, Ebenroth ES. Sildenafil for the treatment of pulmonary hypertension in pediatric patients. *Pediatr Cardiol*. 2009;30:871-882.
113. Laties AM. Vision disorders and phosphodiesterase type 5 inhibitors: A review of the evidence to date. *Drug Safety*. 2009;32:1-18.
114. McGwin G. Phosphodiesterase type 5 inhibitor use and hearing impairment. *Arch Otolaryngol Head Neck Surg*. 2010;136:488-492.
115. Kehat R, Bonsall DJ, North R, Connors B. Ocular findings of oral sildenafil use in term and near-term neonates. *J AAPOS*. 2010;14:159-162.
116. Berkels R, Klotz T, Sticht G, et al. Modulation of human platelet aggregation by the phosphodiesterase type 5 inhibitor sildenafil. *J Cardiovasc Pharmacol*. 2001;37:413-421.
117. Gamboa D, Robbins D, Saba Z. Bleeding after circumcision in a newborn receiving sildenafil. *Clin Pediatr*. 2007;46:842-843.
118. Samada K, Shiraishi H, Aoyagi J, Momoi MY. Cerebral hemorrhage associated with sildenafil (Revatio) in an infant. *Pediatr Cardiol*. 2009;30:998-999.
119. Byoun HS, Lee YJ, Yi HJ. Subarachnoid hemorrhage and intracerebral hematoma due to sildenafil ingestion in a young adult. *J Korean Neurosurg Soc*. 2010;47:210-212.
120. de Lagausie P, de Buys-Roessingh A, Ferdadji L, et al. Endothelin receptor expression in human lungs of newborns with congenital diaphragmatic hernia. *J Pathol*. 2005;205:112-118.
121. Barst RJ, Ivy D, Dingemanse J, et al. Pharmacokinetics, safety, and efficacy of bosentan in pediatric patients with pulmonary arterial hypertension. *Clin Pharmacol Ther*. 2003;73:372-382.
122. Beghetti M, Haworth SG, Bonnet D, et al. Pharmacokinetic and clinical profile of a novel formulation of bosentan in children with pulmonary arterial hypertension: the FUTURE-1 study. *Br J Clin Pharmacol*. 2009;68:948-955.
123. Beghetti M, Hoeper MM, Kiely DG, et al. Safety experience with bosentan in 146 children 2-11 years old with pulmonary arterial hypertension: results from the European Postmarketing Surveillance program. *Pediatr Res*. 2008;64:200-204.
124. Ivy DD, Doran AK, Smith KJ, et al. Short- and long-term effects of inhaled iloprost therapy in children with pulmonary arterial hypertension. *J Am Coll Cardiol*. 2008;51:161-169.
125. Reichenberger F, Mainwood A, Doughty N, et al. Effects of nebulised iloprost on pulmonary function and gas exchange in severe pulmonary hypertension. *Respir Med*. 2007;101:217-222.
126. Denyer J, Nikander K, Smith NJ. Adaptive Aerosol Delivery (AAD) technology. *Expert Opin Drug Deliv*. 2004;1:165-176.
127. Nikander K, Arheden L, Denyer J, Cobos N. Parents' adherence with nebulizer treatment of their children when using an adaptive aerosol delivery (AAD) system. *J Aerosol Med*. 2003;16:273-281.
128. Cohen MS, Rychik J, Bush DM, et al. Influence of congenital heart disease on survival in children with congenital diaphragmatic hernia. *J Pediatr*. 2002;141:25-30.
129. Graziano JN, for the Congenital Diaphragmatic Hernia Study Group. Cardiac anomalies in patients with congenital diaphragmatic hernia and their prognosis: a report from the Congenital Diaphragmatic Hernia Study Group. *J Pediatr Surg*. 2005;40.
130. Brown KL, Ridout DA, Goldman AP, et al. Risk factors for long intensive care unit stay after cardiopulmonary bypass in children. *Crit Care Med*. 2003;31:28-33.
131. Ma M, Gauvreau K, Allan CK, et al. Causes of death after congenital heart surgery. *Ann Thorac Surg*. 2007;83:1438-1445.
132. Keller RL, Jancelewicz T, Vu L, et al. Perinatal anatomic and physiologic factors predict neurodevelopmental (ND) disability in congenital diaphragmatic hernia (CDH). *E-PAS*. 2008;635848:12.
133. Cheung PY, Tyebkhan JM, Peliowski A, et al. Prolonged use of pancuronium bromide and sensorineural hearing loss in childhood survivors of congenital diaphragmatic hernia. *J Pediatr*. 1999;135:233-239.
134. American Academy of Pediatrics Section on Surgery, American Academy of Pediatrics Committee on Fetus and Newborn, Lally KP, Engle W. Postdischarge follow-up of infants with congenital diaphragmatic hernia. *Pediatrics*. 2008;121:627-632.
135. McNally H, Bennett CC, Elbourne D, Field DJ, UK Collaborative ECMO Trial Group. United Kingdom collaborative randomized trial of neonatal extracorporeal membrane oxygenation: follow-up to age 7 years. *Pediatrics*. 2006;117:e845-e854.
136. Fligor BJ, Neault MW, Mullen CH, et al. Factors associated with sensorineural hearing loss among survivors of extracorporeal membrane oxygenation therapy. *Pediatrics*. 2005;115:1519-1528.
137. Robertson CM, Tyebkhan JM, Peliowski A, et al. Ototoxic drugs and sensorineural hearing loss following severe neonatal respiratory failure. *Acta Paediatr*. 2006;95:214-223.
138. Ehrenkranz RA, Walsh MC, Vohr BR, et al, National Institutes of Child Health and Human Development Neonatal Research Network. Validation of the National Institutes of Health consensus definition of bronchopulmonary dysplasia. *Pediatrics*. 2005;116:1353-1360.

139. Bassler D, Stoll BJ, Schmidt B, et al, Trial of Indomethacin Prophylaxis in Preterms Investigators. Using a count of neonatal morbidities to predict poor outcome in extremely low birth weight infants: added role of neonatal infection. *Pediatrics*. 2009;123:313-318.
140. Harrison MR, Keller RL, Hawgood SB, et al. A randomized trial of fetal endoscopic tracheal occlusion for severe fetal congenital diaphragmatic hernia. *N Engl J Med*. 2003;349:1916-1924.
141. Lally KP, Bagolan P, Hosie S, et al, Congenital Diaphragmatic Hernia Study Group. Corticosteroids for fetuses with congenital diaphragmatic hernia: can we show benefit? *J Pediatr Surg*. 2006;41:668-674.
142. Jani J, Keller RL, Benachi A, et al, on behalf of the Antenatal-CDH-Registry Group. Prenatal prediction of survival in isolated left-sided diaphragmatic hernia. *Ultrasound Obstet Gynecol*. 2006;27:18-22.
143. Jani J, Nicolaides KH, Keller RL, et al, Antenatal-CDH-Registry Group. Observed to expected lung area to head circumference ratio in the prediction of survival in fetuses with isolated diaphragmatic hernia. *Ultrasound Obstet Gynecol*. 2007;30:67-71.

CHAPTER 21

Management of the Infant with Severe Bronchopulmonary Dysplasia

Steven H. Abman, MD, and Leif D. Nelin, MD

21

- **Pathophysiology of Severe BPD**
- **Evaluation and Treatment of Severe BPD**
- **Long-Term Outcomes**

As first characterized by Northway and colleagues[1] nearly 45 years ago, bronchopulmonary dysplasia (BPD) is the chronic lung disease of infancy that follows preterm birth. This original report described severe respiratory morbidity and high mortality in relatively late-gestation preterm infants, which were largely due to the lack of surfactant therapy and insufficient neonatal ventilator care in that era. Improved obstetrical and neonatal care over time has improved survival of even the smallest of immature newborns, but BPD persists as a major problem, occurring in an estimated 10,000 to 15,000 infants per year in the United States alone. This disease has important health care implications, because infants with BPD require prolonged neonatal intensive care unit (NICU) courses; experience frequent readmissions during the first 2 years after discharge for respiratory infections, asthma, and related problems; and have persistent lung function abnormalities and exercise intolerance as adolescents and young adults.[2-8]

The overall incidence of BPD has not declined over the past decade,[8] but the respiratory course and number of infants with severe BPD have clearly changed with current clinical practice. Infants with chronic lung disease after premature birth have a different clinical course and pathology from those traditionally observed in infants dying with BPD during the pre-surfactant era.[6-12] The classic progressive stages of disease, including prominent fibroproliferative changes, that first characterized BPD are often absent now, and the disease has changed to being predominantly defined as a disruption of distal lung growth, referred to as "the new BPD."[5] In contrast with the past, the "new BPD" often develops in preterm newborns who may have required minimal or even no ventilator support and relatively low inspired oxygen concentrations during the early postnatal days.[6,7] At autopsy, the lung histology of infants who die with "the new BPD" displays more uniform and milder injury, but impairment of alveolar and vascular growth remains prominent. The "new BPD" is likely the result of disrupted antenatal and postnatal lung growth, leading to persistent abnormalities of lung architecture and function. The implications of how these changes in BPD alter long-term pulmonary outcomes remain uncertain.

Although marked improvements in care have led to milder respiratory courses for most preterm infants, infants with BPD can still experience severe chronic respiratory failure with marked cardiopulmonary impairment (Fig. 21-1). The current National Institutes of Health (NIH) classification system defines "*severe*" BPD as the need for supplemental oxygen greater than an FIO_2 (fraction of inspired oxygen) value of 0.30 with or without positive-pressure ventilation and continuous positive airway pressure (CPAP) at 36 weeks corrected post menstrual age (PMA).[13-19] Ehrenkranz and colleagues,[20] utilizing Eunice Kennedy Shriver National Institute of Child Health & Human Development (NICHD) Neonatal Research Network data found

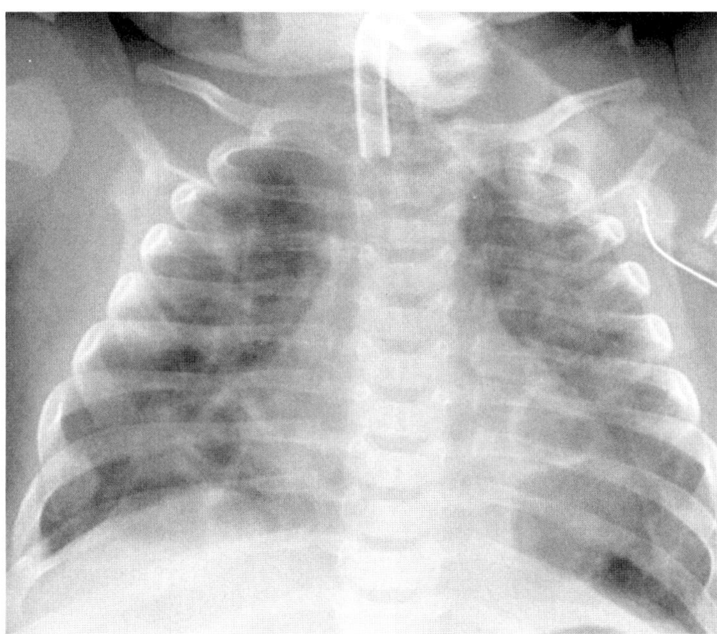

Figure 21-1 Chest radiograph showing features of severe, ventilator-dependent bronchopulmonary dysplasia.

that of 4866 infants born before 32 weeks of gestation (with a birth weight of 1000 g or less) who survived to 36 weeks or transfer, 16% demonstrated severe BPD.[20] A later study also using NICHD Neonatal Research Network data reported that the severity of BPD was inversely associated with gestational age and birth weight and that the incidence of severe BPD was greater in male infants and strongly related to need for mechanical ventilation, patent ductus arteriosus (PDA), sepsis and surgical necrotizing enterocolitis (NEC).[21] As Northway and colleagues[1] first observed, BPD has diverse, multifactorial etiologies, including hyperoxia, ventilator-induced lung injury, inflammation, and infection.[22,23] Animal and human studies suggest that lung injury due to each of these adverse stimuli is at least partly mediated through increased oxidative stress, which further augments inflammation, promotes lung injury, and impairs growth factor–signaling pathways.[24,25] Antenatal factors, such as chorioamnionitis, preeclampsia, and intrauterine growth restriction (IUGR), also contribute to the risk for severe BPD.[26-30] Another study suggests dose-related effects of antenatal endotoxin as a model for experimental chorioamnionitis on BPD severity and reports that moderate oxygen treatment actually improved lung structure rather than worsened outcomes.[31] Further studies are needed to determine how different etiologic mechanisms contribute to the development of severe BPD. Although severe BPD is less common than in the past, the subgroup of infants with the disease present persistent challenges, raising many questions about optimal strategies for enhancing outcomes, and at times, significant clinical and ethical dilemmas. This chapter discusses the pulmonary and cardiovascular pathophysiology of infants with severe BPD and current approaches to their management.

Pathophysiology of Severe BPD

Respiratory Function

Multiple abnormalities of lung structure and function contribute to late respiratory disease in BPD. Chronic respiratory signs in children with moderate and severe BPD include tachypnea with shallow breathing, retractions, and paradoxical breathing pattern; coarse rhonchi, rales, and wheezes are typically heard on auscultation. The increased respiratory rate and shallow breathing increase dead space ventilation. Non-uniform damage to the airways and distal lungs results in variable time constants for different areas of the lungs; inspired gas may be distributed to relatively poorly perfused lung, thereby worsening ventilation-perfusion matching. Decreased lung compliance appears to correlate strongly with morphologic and radiographic changes in the lung. Dynamic lung compliance is markedly reduced in infants with established BPD, even in those who no longer require oxygen therapy.[32] The reduction in dynamic compliance is due to small airway narrowing, interstitial fibrosis, edema, and atelectasis. Increased airway resistance can be demonstrated even during the first week after birth in preterm neonates at risk for BPD.[33] Infants with BPD at 28 days of age have an increased total respiratory and expiratory resistance with severe flow limitation, especially at low lung volumes.[34] The presence of tracheomalacia may also result in airflow limitation, which is worsened by bronchodilator therapy.[35] In the early stages, the functional lung volume is often reduced because of atelectasis, but during the later stages of BPD, there is gas trapping with hyperinflation. The use of pulmonary function testing to follow the progression of BPD and the response to therapeutic interventions has increased but is still not commonly applied in the clinical setting.[36-38]

Although the new BPD has been characterized as an arrest of lung and vascular growth, most of the observations were based on lung histology but evidence that provided direct physiologic data to support this finding was lacking. Tepper and colleagues, utilizing novel methods of assessing diffusion capacity, have demonstrated the important finding of reduced lung surface area in infants with BPD. Thus, established BPD is characterized primarily by reduced surface area and heterogeneous lung units, in which regional variations in airway resistance and tissue compliance lead to highly variable time constants throughout the lung. As a result, mechanical ventilation of infants with severe BPD requires strikingly different ventilator strategies from those commonly used early in infants with RDS to prevent BPD. Strategies for severe BPD generally favor longer inspiratory times, larger tidal volumes, higher positive end-expiratory pressure (PEEP), and lower rates to allow more effective gas exchange and respiratory function.[36]

Lung Mechanics

Diverse methods have been used to assess lung mechanics in infants with established BPD during tidal breathing. These include measurements of dynamic resistance and compliance of the lung with the use of esophageal pressure catheters; single-breath occlusion for measuring respiratory system resistance and compliance; plethysmography measurement of airway resistance; interrupter and forced oscillation methods for measuring respiratory system resistance; and multiple-occlusion and weighted methods of spirometry. Airway obstruction has also been determined from respiratory inductive plethysmography measurements of phase angle differences in chest wall and abdominal dimensions. These approaches have been reviewed in detail.[37,38] Normalized measures of lung compliance are reduced and lung elastic recoil is increased in severe BPD.[39-41] Resistance has consistently been shown to be high in infants with severe BPD.[40-43] Specific compliance and conductance generally improve in infants with severe BPD over the first 2 to 3 years of life.[40-43] However, concerns persist regarding limitations of infant pulmonary function testing. Measures of compliance and resistance can be variable because these values are generally determined over a limited tidal volume range and depend on the lung volume at which these measurements are made. For example, in patients with BPD and airway obstruction, measurements of compliance made during tidal breathing are markedly affected by respiratory rate (e.g., "frequency dependence"). Additional problems for assessing resistance and compliance as measured by the single-breath method include the substantial curvilinearity of the passive expiratory flow-volume relationship in infants with BPD. Jarriel and associates[44] have pointed out that respiratory system mechanics in these patients are much better characterized by a "two-compartment" rather than a linear "one-compartment" model (see later).

C

Lung Volumes

Functional residual capacity (FRC) has been measured in infants with BPD by body plethysmography and with nitrogen washout and gas dilution methods.[38] In contrast with plethysmography, washout and gas dilution methods measure only the gas that communicates with the conducting airways during tidal breathing. These measurements may underestimate the actual lung volume at FRC because they do not measure volumes of gas behind closed airways and can underestimate volumes in severely obstructed poorly ventilated areas.[45-48] Measurements made in patients younger than 1 year using gas dilution and washout methods have consistently reported reduced FRC in infants with both "old" and new BPD.[40,41,46,47] In contrast, plethysmography studies have demonstrated normal or elevated FRC values.[49,50] Reductions in gas dilution and nitrogen washout measurements of FRC probably reflect the amount of noncommunicating trapped gas not measured in infants with obstructive disease, rather than being indicative of a true restrictive defect. Reduction in the difference between the two methods is probably indicative of improvements in airway function, less gas trapping, and better gas exchange. Thus, functional abnormalities in infants with severe BPD are primarily obstructive rather than restrictive, but precise measurements are especially complicated in severe disease owing to heterogeneity of the airway and lung parenchymal abnormalities.

The use of the raised volume rapid thoracic compression (RVRTC) method of performing spirometry in sedated infants has now provided an alternative approach to measure fractional lung volumes, including total lung capacity (TLC) and residual volume (RV).[51] Robin and coworkers[50] reported the results of fractional lung volume measurements in 28 patients with new BPD.[50] Mean RV and RV/TLC ratio were found to be significantly higher in infants with BPD than in normal control infants, whereas mean TLC was in the normal range. In contrast, FRC as measured by plethysmography was found to be only marginally higher than in the normal control infants. In addition, TLC continues to increase over the second year of life in infants with BPD, yet the severity of air trapping, as reflected by the RV/TLC ratio, remains unchanged.[52] Thus, infants with "new BPD" have obstructive airway disease with gas trapping that persists over time and is strikingly abnormal in severe BPD.

Forced Flows

Measurements of forced flows have been made in infants with BPD, using the rapid thoracic compression (RTC) method to produce partial flow-volume curves and the forced deflation and RVRTC techniques to produce forced expiratory flows over the full range of vital capacity. The use of these tests in infants with BPD has been reviewed, and guidelines for the two RTC methods have been published.[53-55] As initially described by Tepper and colleagues,[35] the RTC technique to produce partial expiratory flow volume curves was applied to infants with BPD, demonstrating that average maximal flows measured at FRC ($V'max_{FRC}$) were approximately 50% lower than in normal infants.[35] A reduction in $V'max_{FRC}$ in infants with BPD has been a consistent finding in subsequent studies, and longitudinal measurements over the first 2 years of life demonstrated very modest increases in absolute flows in individual infants with BPD. On average, the rate of increase in peak flow for infants with BPD was substantially below that measured in normal infants over the same interval. Thus at follow-up, measurements of $V'max_{FRC}$ in the infants with BPD had fallen even farther below those measured in normal infants.

Lung Imaging

The chest radiographic characteristics of infants with BPD have changed substantially since the original description by Northway and colleagues.[1] Although the chest radiograph in BPD as classically described is still seen in infants with severe disease, radiographic changes in smaller, less mature infants with new BPD are much more variable and are often characterized by irregularly distributed areas of fine infiltrates and mild hyperlucency. Chest radiographs often underestimate and correlate poorly

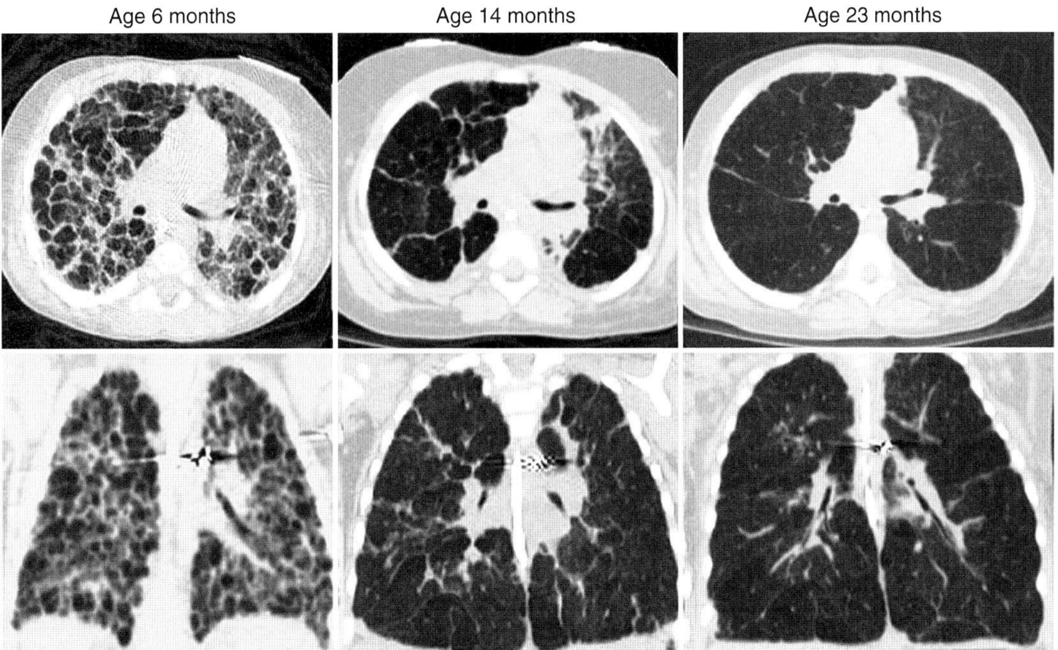

Figure 21-2 High-resolution computed tomography (HRCT) scans done at 25 cm H_2O during a breath-hold in the same patient with severe bronchopulmonary dysplasia (BPD) at three different ages. The *Top row*, transverse sections; *bottom row*, coronal sections taken from the same area. These scans demonstrate that despite ongoing mechanical ventilator support with lung growth and repair, the findings of HRCT improve over time, although the scan findings at 23 months of age remain abnormal.

21

with the extent of the pathologic changes in infants with established BPD.[56,57] High-resolution computed tomography (HRCT) is a more sensitive technique for detecting structural abnormalities in the lungs of patients with established BPD than plain chest radiography (Fig. 21-2).[58-63] Correlations between abnormalities seen on HRCT and measures of lung function and clinical severity suggest that HRCT may be useful in clinical management and as an outcome measure in this population.[36] CT is helpful for identifying unsuspected abnormalities in the lungs of individual patients with BPD, but its ultimate utility as a tool for clinical management and as an outcome measure for research investigations is not yet clear. Radiation exposure from CT is substantially greater than that with standard chest radiographs.[64] The development of novel scanning algorithms, however, has greatly reduced the radiation exposure from CT,[65-67] such that diagnostic HRCT in cystic fibrosis can be done at a radiation dose similar to that of a chest radiograph, and similar algorithm development is ongoing for patients with BPD.[67]

The Cardiovascular System

Acute lung injury also impairs growth, structure, and function of the developing pulmonary circulation after premature birth.[68,69] Endothelial cells are particularly susceptible to oxidant injury due to hyperoxia or inflammation. The media of small pulmonary arteries may also undergo striking changes, including smooth muscle cell proliferation, precocious maturation of immature pericytes into mature smooth muscle cells, and incorporation of fibroblasts into the vessel wall and surrounding adventitia.[70] Structural changes in the lung vasculature contribute to high pulmonary vascular resistance (PVR) owing to narrowing of the vessel diameter and decreased vascular compliance. Decreased angiogenesis may limit vascular surface area, causing further elevations of PVR, especially in response to high cardiac output with exercise or stress. The pulmonary circulation in patients with BPD is further characterized by abnormal vasoreactivity, which also increases PVR.[68,69] Abnormal pulmonary vasoreactivity is evidenced by a marked vasoconstrictor response to acute hypoxia.[69,70] Cardiac catheterization studies have shown that mild hypoxia causes marked elevations in pulmonary artery pressure, even in infants with modest basal levels of pulmonary hypertension (PH). Maintaining oxygen saturation levels above 92% to 94% effectively lowers the pulmonary artery pressure.[69] Strategies to lower pulmonary artery pressure or limit injury to the pulmonary vasculature may restrict the subsequent development of PH in BPD.

Early injury to the lung circulation leads to the rapid development of PH, which contributes significantly to the morbidity and mortality of severe BPD. Even in early reports of BPD, PH and cor pulmonale were recognized as being associated with high mortality.[71,72] Persistent echocardiographic evidence of PH beyond the first few months has been associated with up to 40% mortality in infants with BPD.[72] High mortality rates have also been reported in infants with BPD and severe PH, especially in those who require prolonged ventilator support.[73] In addition to the adverse effects of PH on the clinical course of infants with BPD, the lung circulation is further characterized by persistence of abnormal or "dysmorphic" growth of the pulmonary circulation, including a relative paucity of small pulmonary arteries with an altered pattern of distribution within the interstitium of the distal lung.[74-76] In infants with severe BPD, decreased vascular growth occurs in conjunction with marked reductions in alveoli, suggesting that the "new BPD" is characterized primarily by growth arrest of the developing lung. This reduction of alveolar-capillary surface area impairs gas exchange—thereby increasing the need for prolonged supplemental oxygen and ventilator therapy, causing marked hypoxemia with acute respiratory infections and late exercise intolerance—and further increases the risk for development of severe PH. Experimental studies have also shown that early injury to the developing lung can impair angiogenesis, which contributes to decreased alveolarization and simplification of distal lung air spaces (the "vascular hypothesis"[77-82]). Thus, not only are abnormalities of the lung circulation in BPD related to the presence or absence of PH, but more broadly, pulmonary vascular disease after premature birth as manifested by decreased vascular growth and structure also contributes to the pathogenesis and abnormal cardiopulmonary physiology of BPD.

In addition to pulmonary vascular disease and right ventricular hypertrophy, cardiovascular abnormalities associated with BPD include left ventricular hypertrophy (LVH), systemic hypertension, and the development of prominent systemic-to-pulmonary collateral vessels. Left ventricular hypertrophy can develop in infants with severe BPD without right ventricular hypertrophy. Systemic hypertension in BPD may be mild, transient, or striking and usually responds to medication.[83-85] The etiology remains obscure, but further evaluation of some affected infants reveals significant renal vascular or urinary tract disease. Interestingly, perinatal hyperoxia leads to late cardiovascular abnormalities in infant rats, suggesting that oxidative stress and related mechanisms cause chronic changes in the systemic circulation as well as the pulmonary vasculature.[86] Mourani and associates[87] showed that left ventricular diastolic dysfunction can contribute to lung edema, diuretic dependency, and PH in some infants with BPD. In addition, atrial septal defects commonly complicate the course of infants with BPD and make variable contributions to underlying disease severity. Prominent bronchial or other systemic-to-pulmonary collateral vessels were noted in early morphometric studies of infants with BPD and can be readily identified in many infants during cardiac catheterization. Although these collateral vessels are generally small, large collaterals may contribute to significant shunting of blood flow to the lung, resulting in edema and the need for higher levels of supplemental oxygen. Collateral vessels have been associated with high mortality in some patients with both severe BPD and PH. Some infants have improved after embolization of large collateral vessels, as reflected by a reduced need for supplemental oxygen, ventilator support, or diuretics. The contribution of collateral vessels to the pathophysiology of BPD, however, is poorly understood.

Box 21-1 GENERAL EVALUATION OF SEVERE BRONCHOPULMONARY DYSPLASIA

- Family needs and resources
- Neurodevelopment assessment
- Pulmonary status:
  - Chest radiograph for inflation, atelectasis, emphysematous changes, edema
  - Consider high-resolution CT for airway and parenchymal architecture
  - Pulmonary function testing, including testing for airway reactivity
- Respiratory needs:
  - Determination of supplemental oxygen needs
  - Frequency and character of hypoxemia episodes
  - Assessment of sleep
- Pulmonary hypertension:
  - Echocardiogram; repeat at reasonable intervals until pulmonary status improves
  - Consider cardiac catheterization if long-term therapy will be needed
- Nutritional status
- Gastroesophageal reflux (GER)

Evaluation and Treatment

A general evaluation (Box 21-1) and treatment plan (Box 21-2) for infants with significant BPD are described here. The initial clinical strategy for the management of severe BPD begins with assessing and treating the current state of the lung disease. A thorough evaluation of pulmonary status should be done starting with a chest radiograph to evaluate for dynamic hyperinflation, emphysematous changes, edema, and atelectasis. HRCT to evaluate airway and parenchymal architecture should be considered. Pulmonary function testing, including assessment of airway reactivity, should be performed. Furthermore, this thorough evaluation should assess for chronic gastroesophageal reflux (GER) and aspiration, structural airway abnormalities (such as tonsillar and adenoidal hypertrophy, vocal cord paralysis, subglottic

Box 21-2 GENERAL TREATMENT STRATEGIES FOR SEVERE BRONCHOPULMONARY DYSPLASIA (BPD)

- Family-centered chronic care model
- Focus on neurodevelopment:
  - Optimize pulmonary status/respiratory support
  - Long-term ventilator settings
  - Consider need for tracheostomy if long-term mechanical ventilation is necessary
  - Optimize oxygenation, targeting SpO_2 at 92%-95%
  - Use short courses of diuretics to treat episodes of pulmonary edema
  - Treat airway reactivity with inhaled bronchodilators and/or inhaled steroids
  - Reserve systemic steroids for acute deteriorations
- Pulmonary hypertension:
  - Avoid hypoxemia
  - Use inhaled nitric oxide (NO) for short-term therapy
  - Treatment will need to be long-term; sildenafil most studied
  - If response to sildenafil alone is poor, consider adding bosentan and/or prostacyclin
- Nutritional status:
  - Optimize nutrition: fluid restriction with high–caloric density feeds
- Gastroesophageal reflux (GER):
  - Medical management
  - Consider surgical management if severe or unresponsive to medical management

stenosis, tracheomalacia and other lesions), and any other potentially contributing factors. An assessment of the patient's respiratory needs and current therapies should also be undertaken. Periods of acute hypoxia, whether intermittent or prolonged, can often contribute to morbidities in BPD, including PH, agitation, and inability to partake in appropriate neurodevelopmental therapies. A sleep study may be necessary to look for noteworthy episodes of hypoxia and determine whether hypoxemia has predominantly obstructive, central, or mixed causes. Additional studies that may be required include flexible bronchoscopy for the diagnosis of anatomic and dynamic airway lesions (such as tracheomalacia) that may contribute to hypoxemia and poor clinical responses to oxygen therapy. For patients with severe BPD who cannot maintain ventilation or require high levels of FIO_2 despite conservative treatment, strong consideration should be given to tracheostomy and long-term mechanical ventilatory support.

An important consideration in the treatment of severe BPD is that recovery from this disease will be relatively slow, that is, will take months to years rather than days to weeks. Therefore, patience is required in the care of these complicated patients. In other words, management of infants with severe BPD requires a long-term care model, which is strikingly different in philosophy and treatment goals than the approach used in the acute care model that is generally followed in the NICU. This long-term model includes strategies for weaning from mechanical ventilation, assessing the need for long-term ventilator support, the role of tracheostomy, and related issues.

Supplemental oxygen remains a mainstay of therapy for infants with BPD, yet the most appropriate target for oxygen saturation levels remains controversial. Growing concerns regarding the adverse effects of even moderate levels of oxygen therapy have led many neonatologists to accept oxygen saturations below 85% to 90% early after birth of preterm newborns. However, it should also be kept in mind that patients with severe BPD are usually more than 36 weeks postmenstrual age past the time when retinopathy of prematurity is a major concern. Currently, most pulmonologists recommend maintaining infants with established BPD at oxygen saturations around 92%, with slightly higher levels for infants with BPD and growth failure, recurrent respiratory exacerbations, or PH. Prolonged monitoring of oxygenation while the infant is awake and asleep, and during feeds ensures the avoidance of hypoxia and is necessary while oxygen therapy is being adjusted. We recommend targeting higher levels of O_2 saturation (92%-95%) in infants with severe BPD to provide more consistent treatment of underlying PH, to minimize lability and cyanotic episodes, and to enhance growth.

In most NICUs, nasal CPAP (nCPAP) or high-flow nasal cannula therapy is used to maintain adequate oxygenation and ventilation while avoiding the need for prolonged ventilation or reintubation for ventilator support. Whereas several studies have examined the role of early nCPAP in lieu of endotracheal intubation during the first week after birth, there are no studies regarding benefits of the prolonged use of nCPAP in established BPD with chronic respiratory failure. In some infants with BPD, signs of severe respiratory distress persist despite nCPAP or high-flow nasal cannula therapy, including marked dyspnea, head bobbing, retractions, tachypnea, intermittent cyanosis, and CO_2 retention. These infants may benefit from reintubation and consideration of tracheostomy for long-term ventilator support if subsequent attempts at weaning are not successful. The timing and patient selection for tracheostomy and commitment to more prolonged ventilator support are highly variable among NICUs. Tracheostomy and long-term ventilator support may provide a stable airway to allow for more effective ventilation and less respiratory distress in order to enhance cardiopulmonary function, as reflected by lower oxygen requirements and less PH. Greater respiratory stability often improves tolerance of respiratory treatments, physical/occupational therapies, and handling by staff and family members, thereby improving maternal-infant interactions and neurodevelopmental outcomes. Successful management of children with long-term ventilator dependence requires well-organized, multidisciplinary teams to address the complexity of issues.

Table 21-1 VENTILATOR STRATEGIES IN BRONCHOPULMONARY DYSPLASIA

Early (prevention)	Strategies to prevent acute lung injury: 1. Low tidal volumes (5-8 mL/kg 2. Short inspiratory times 3. Increased PEEP as needed for lung recruitment without overdistention (as reflected by high peak airway pressures) 4. Achieve lower FIO_2 Goals for gas exchange: 1. Adjust FIO_2 to target lower O_2 saturations (88%-92%) 2. Permissive hypercapnia
Late (established BPD)	Strategies for effective gas exchange: 1. Marked regional heterogeneity: • Larger tidal volumes (10-12 mL/kg) • Longer inspiratory time (≥0.6 sec) 2. Airways obstruction: • Slower rates allow better emptying, especially with larger tidal volumes • Complex roles for PEEP with dynamic airway collapse 3. Interactive effects of vent strategies: • Changes in rate, tidal volume, inspiratory and expiratory times, pressure support are highly interdependent • Overdistention can increase agitation and paradoxically worsen ventilation 4. Permissive hypercapnia to facilitate weaning

PEEP, positive end-expiratory pressure.

21

Mechanical Ventilation

In contrast to an approach to acute RDS using a low tidal volume and high PEEP to minimize acute lung injury, most clinicians favor a strategy of larger tidal volumes delivered at slower rates with longer inspiratory and expiratory times in severe BPD (Table 21-1). This strategy is directly related to the striking differences in lung physiology that characterize newborns with acute respiratory failure from infants with severe BPD. Dramatic heterogeneity of lung disease, characterized by marked regional variability in time constants, provides the physiologic rationale for this strategy in severe BPD, to improve the distribution of ventilation, minimize physiologic dead space and gas trapping, and improve gas exchange. This represents a distinct change in strategy from the higher rates and lower tidal volumes commonly utilized early in the course of respiratory distress in the premature infant. It should be pointed out that no objective studies have been published to substantiate the newer strategy. Until such a time as other modes and/or modalities for ventilating patients with established BPD can be developed and studied, ventilation with a slow rate and long inspiratory time is the ventilation strategy that best provides for ventilation-perfusion matching and lung emptying. Furthermore, this ventilation strategy allows for interval lung growth, as demonstrated in the serial CT scans shown in Figure 21-2 from a patient with severe established BPD who was ventilated with a slow rate and long inspiratory time. The overall goal of this ventilator strategy is to provide support while preventing complications and optimizing lung growth and recovery for patients with the most severe form of BPD, that is, patients who continue to require intermittent positive pressure ventilation (IPPV) many weeks into their initial hospitalization.

Ventilation with larger tidal volumes and increased inspiratory times often improves the distribution of gas while minimizing dead space ventilation (Fig. 21-3). This strategy can reduce chronic retractions and respiratory distress and may decrease recurrent cyanotic spells in some patients. However, hyperinflation is typically present in severe, ventilator-dependent BPD. As a result, the patient is breathing on a relatively flat portion of the pressure-volume loop, such that generating large pressures results in only small changes in tidal volumes. Furthermore, lung hyperinflation will increase PVR because of compression of the alveolar vessels. Thus,

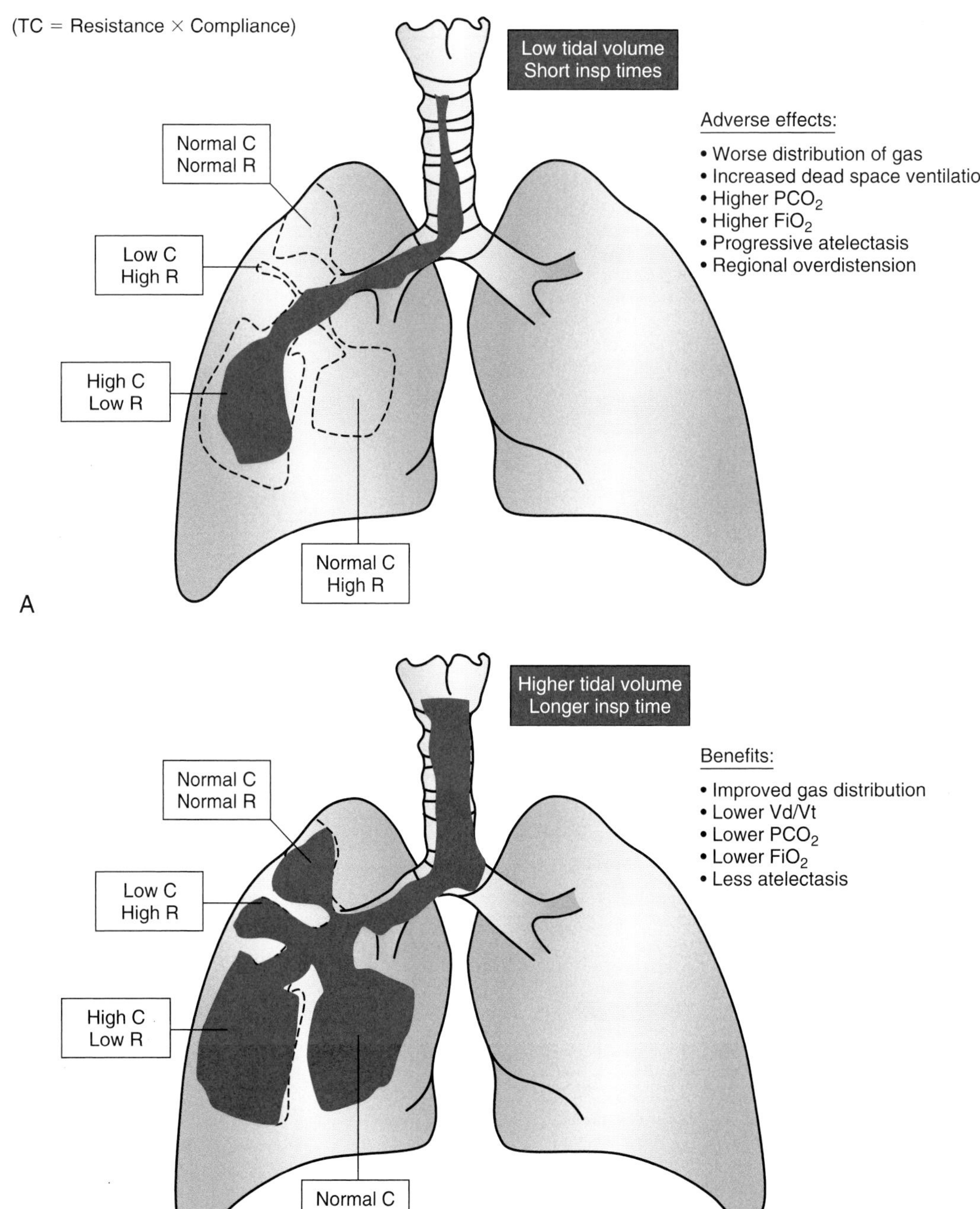

Figure 21-3 Theoretical effects of mechanical ventilator strategies for severe bronchopulmonary dysplasia (BPD). **A,** Small–tidal volume breaths often increase dead space ventilation, leading to atelectasis, hypercapnia, and high oxygen requirements in the setting of heterogenous lung disease in severe BPD. **B,** Increased tidal volumes and inspiratory (insp) times may enhance distribution of gas, leading to lower oxygen requirements, improved ventilation, and less atelectasis. C, compliance; R, resistance; TC, time constant.

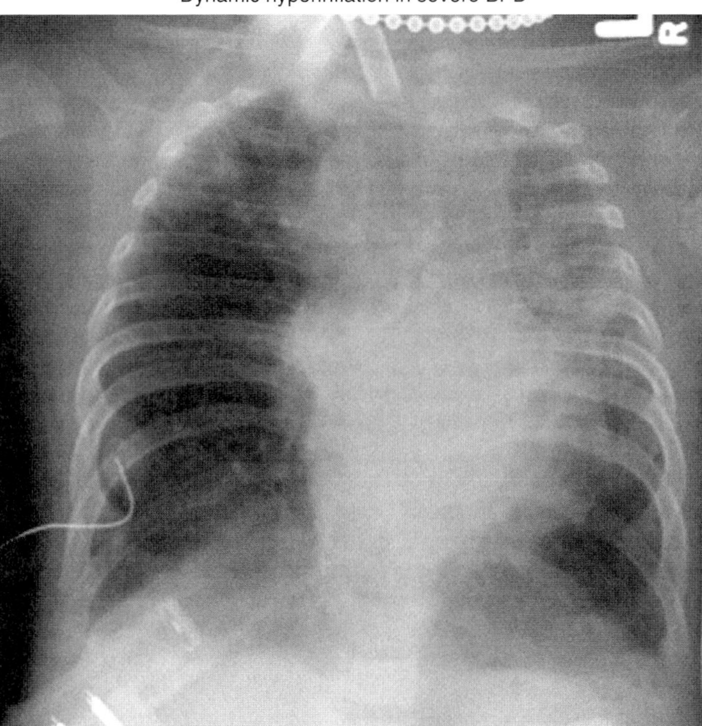

Figure 21-4 Chest radiograph demonstrating marked gas trapping and dynamic hyperinflation in severe bronchopulmonary dysplasia (BPD).

hyperinflation of the lung worsens ventilation-perfusion matching and pulmonary hemodynamics. To effectively reduce hyperinflation in severe BPD, strategies must also offer adequate time for exhalation in order to allow the lungs to empty with relatively lower ventilator rates and increased expiratory times. Thus, slower rates are needed to tolerate increases in tidal volume and inspiratory time, in order to avoid gas trapping, inadvertent PEEP, and dynamic hyperinflation (Fig. 21-4). Requirements for PEEP are highly variable among infants with ventilator-dependent BPD. Infants with severe BPD often have evidence of tracheomalacia or bronchomalacia, in which increased PEEP will decrease central airway closure. (Fig. 21-5) However, high PEEP can complicate gas trapping and may not be well tolerated without sufficient expiratory times and low ventilator rates.

Drug Therapies

Multiple pharmacologic therapies have been used in the management of BPD, including diuretics, bronchodilators, and steroids. In most cases, despite observations suggesting acute improvement with many of these interventions, data are limited regarding long-term safety and efficacy of many drugs used in infants with BPD.

Diuretics improve pulmonary compliance and airway resistance by reducing lung edema. Two Cochrane reviews assessed the effects of loop diuretics (furosemide) and diuretics acting on the distal renal tubule (thiazides and spironolactone) for preventing or treating BPD in preterm infants.[88,89] Long-term furosemide therapy can improve oxygenation and lung compliance in infants with BPD.[90] A small study suggested that furosemide (1 mg/kg 12 hourly intravenously or 2 mg/kg 12 hourly orally) can allow earlier weaning from the ventilator than placebo.[90] Aerosolized furosemide can acutely improve lung mechanics, but data are lacking regarding its long-term use.[91] Thiazides and spironolactone can improve lung function, but such improvement has not been a consistent finding.[92,93] The use of alternate-day

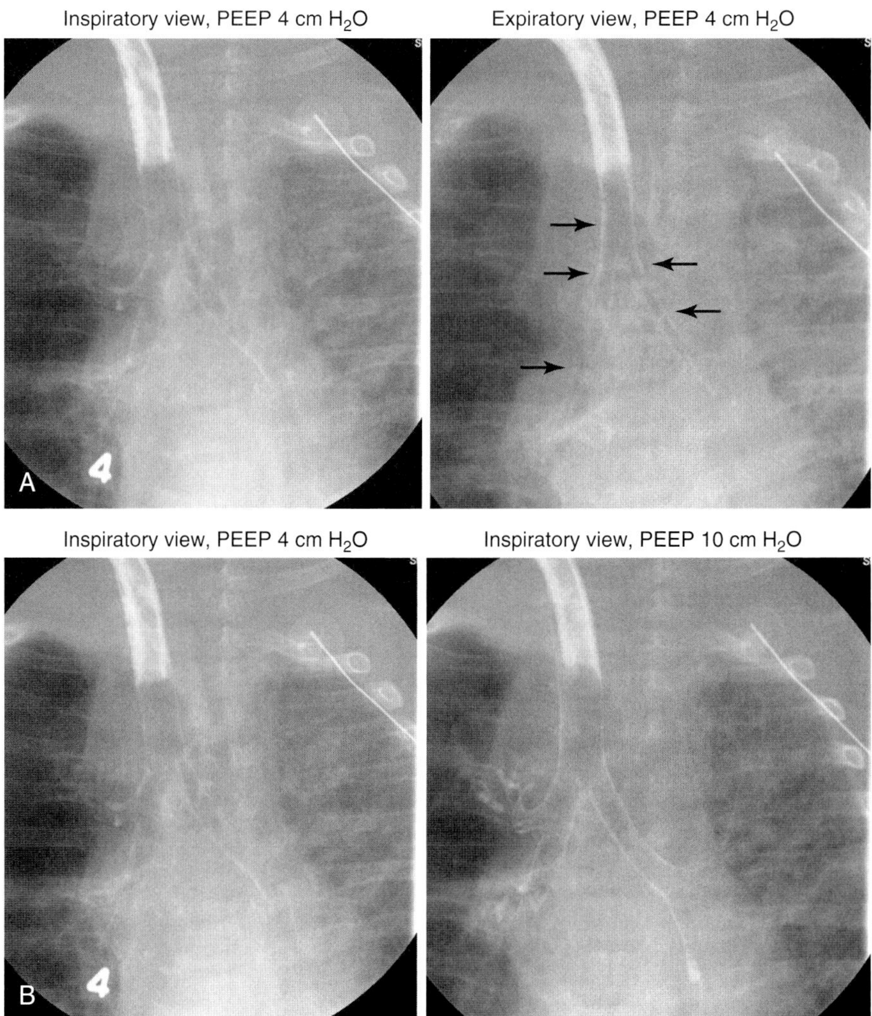

Figure 21-5 Bronchogram studies for assessing effects of positive end-expiratory pressure (PEEP) on central airway caliber. **A,** Low PEEP support is associated with small airway diameter on inspiration and expiratory airway closure (marked by *arrows*). **B,** Increased PEEP acutely enhances airway caliber on inspiration by preventing airway closure on expiration.

furosemide may sustain improvements in lung function while minimizing risks for electrolyte imbalance and nephrocalcinosis.[94] Although diuretics generally cause short-term improvements in lung compliance, there is little evidence of sustained reduction in ventilator support, length of hospital stay, and other long-term outcomes.

Infants with BPD have airway smooth muscle hypertrophy and often have signs of bronchial hyperreactivity that acutely improves with bronchodilator therapy, but response rates are variable.[95,96] Data showing a long-term benefit of bronchodilators, including β-agonists and anticholinergic agents, for the treatment of severe BPD are lacking.[97] In addition to their roles in apnea, aminophylline and caffeine can reduce airway resistance in infants with BPD and may have an additive effect with diuretics. Methylxanthines can improve weaning of infants from mechanical ventilation,[98] but jitteriness, seizures, and GER are known side effects.

Corticosteroid therapy, directed primarily at reducing lung inflammation, is one of the most controversial areas of BPD care.[99-101] The use of systemic corticosteroids to prevent BPD early in the course of care of preterm infants is currently discouraged by the American Academy of Pediatrics (AAP) because of their adverse effects on neurodevelopment. In established BPD, corticosteroids are generally used to reduce lung inflammation. The side effects, poor head growth and neurocognitive outcomes with early and prolonged high-dose strategies, are unacceptable risks for preterm infants at risk for BPD. However, steroid bursts (for example, methylprednisolone 1 mg/kg q6h for 2 days then 1 mg/kg q12h for 2 days then 1 mg/kg/day for 2 days[102]) may be helpful in the management of infants with severe BPD and acute deteriorations of lung function. Although commonly used in infants with asthma, inhaled steroids have not consistently showed improvement in lung function in BPD. However, one study demonstrated that inhaled steroids can improve the rate of successful extubation and reduce the need for systemic steroids.[103-105] The major effect of inhaled betamethasone in a multicenter randomized trial was to decrease the perceived need for the use of systemic steroids. Fluticasone propionate is a more potent steroid and when given by inhalation, was associated with a lower chest radiograph score but also led to a higher systolic blood pressure.

21

The contribution of GER to severe BPD remains controversial. Patients with severe BPD should be evaluated for GER with radiologic studies (barium swallow studies, upper gastrointestinal series), pH or impedance probes, and/or swallow studies. Because GER with chronic aspiration can contribute to ongoing lung injury, consideration should be given to gastrostomy with fundoplication in this fragile group of infants because of the high morbidity and mortality related to severe BPD. Many clinicians would also consider gastrostomy and fundoplication in the setting of severe BPD that is failing to improve if clinical suspicion remains high even though results of studies for GER are negative. Jadcherla and associates[106] reported that GER may cause symptoms in BPD even if the refluxate does not reach the pharynx and that the likelihood of symptoms was related to the clearance time of the acid refluxate.[106] These findings suggest that medical treatment of GER may improve symptoms in patients with BPD.

Treatment of Pulmonary Hypertension

Patients with severe BPD are at high risk for development of PH and cor pulmonale. Therefore, screening echocardiograms should be performed in patients with severe BPD. The weakness of screening echocardiography is that it depends on a tricuspid regurgitant jet to estimate right ventricular systolic pressure, and in cases without a clear and reproducible waveform, estimating pulmonary artery pressure (PAP) may be impossible. Some cases of PH might be missed with the use of echocardiography alone; nevertheless, it remains the best screening tool that we have to assess PH in severe BPD. This drawback, however, underscores the importance of cardiac catheterization to guide therapy, particularly in severe cases and in cases requiring long-term therapy. If the screening echocardiogram results are initially normal, screening echocardiograms should be performed at 1- to 2-month intervals until the respiratory status of the patient is significantly improved. If, on the other hand, the screening echocardiogram demonstrates PH, the initial clinical strategy for the management of PH in infants with BPD begins with optimizing the treatment of the underlying lung disease. Periods of acute hypoxemia whether intermittent or prolonged contribute to the pathogenesis of late PH in severe BPD and also exacerbate existing PH. Therefore, oxygen saturation limits may need to be changed to prevent periods of hypoxemia. Indeed, in patients with BPD and severe PH who are unable to maintain near-normal ventilation or require high levels of FIO_2 despite conservative treatment, strong consideration should be given to long-term mechanical ventilatory support and tracheostomy.

Despite the growing use of pulmonary vasodilator therapy for the treatment of PH in BPD, data demonstrating efficacy are extremely limited, and these agents should be used only after thorough diagnostic evaluations and aggressive management of the underlying lung disease. We strongly encourage cardiac catheterization prior to the initiation of long-term therapy. Current therapies used for PH therapy in infants with BPD generally include inhaled NO (iNO), sildenafil, endothelin receptor antagonists (ETRAs), and calcium channel blockers (CCBs). Mourani and colleagues,[107] in a study of 10 patients with severe BPD undergoing cardiac catheterization, found that iNO significantly decreased pulmonary artery pressure and the ratio of PVR to systemic vascular resistance. Calcium channel blockers (such as nifedipine) benefit some patients with PH, and short-term effects of these agents in infants with BPD have been reported.[108] In comparison with iNO reactivity in infants with BPD, the acute response to calcium channel blockers was poor and some infants demonstrated systemic hypotension.[107] In general, we use sildenafil or bosentan (an endothelin receptor antagonist) for long-term therapy of PH in infants with BPD. Sildenafil, a highly selective type 5 phosphodiesterase (PDE-5) inhibitor, augments cyclic guanosine monophosphate (GMP) content in vascular smooth muscle and has been shown to benefit adults with PH as monotherapy and in combination with standard treatment regimens.[109] In a study of 25 infants with chronic lung disease and PH (18 with BPD), prolonged sildenafil therapy as part of an aggressive program to treat PH was associated with improvement in PH on echocardiogram in most patients (88%) without significant rates of adverse events.[110] Although the time to improvement was variable, many patients were able to be weaned off mechanical ventilator support and other PH therapies, especially iNO, during the course of sildenafil treatment without worsening of PH. The recommended starting dose for sildenafil is 0.5 mg/kg/dose every 8 hours. If there is no evidence of systemic hypotension, this dose can be gradually increased over 2 weeks to achieve desired pulmonary hemodynamic effect or a maximum of 2 mg/kg/dose every 6 to 8 hours. Data on other agents, such as endothelin receptor antagonists and prostacyclin analogs, are largely lacking in infants with BPD that fails to respond to other approaches.

In summary, our approach to PH in severe BPD is to have a high index of suspicion and, when PH is found, to treat it aggressively (Box 21-3). Routine screening with echocardiography is important because the signs and symptoms of PH can mimic those of severe BPD until cor pulmonale has already developed. Once PH is diagnosed, respiratory support should be optimized and iNO at 20 ppm may be started. Sildenafil can then be added and optimized as previously described. At this point, attempts should be made to wean the patient from iNO therapy. Many patients with severe BPD and PH require sildenafil treatment until their respiratory status is substantially improved, often for 2 to 6 months. Some patients with PH associated with severe BPD cannot tolerate weaning from iNO even with maximum doses of sildenafil. In these patients we suggest either continuing both the iNO and sildenafil

Box 21-3 PULMONARY HYPERTENSION (PH) IN SEVERE BRONCHOPULMONARY DYSPLASIA

- Screening echocardiography:
  - Septal flattening, tricuspid regurgitant jet velocity, cor pulmonale
- If no PH, perform echocardiography every 1-2 months until significant improvement in respiratory status
- If PH/cor pulmonale present:
  - Optimize respiratory support, avoid hypoxemia
  - Start inhaled nitric oxide (iNO) at 20 ppm
- Switch to sildenafil:
  - Start at 0.5 mg/kg q8h and advance as needed to 2 mg/kg q6h if no systemic hypotension
  - Wean patient off iNO
- If unable to wean patient off iNO:
  - Continue iNO and sildenafil or consider endothelin receptor antagonist (ETRA) or prostacyclin analog
- Cardiac catheterization:
  - Evaluate pulmonary artery pressure and response to vasodilators to guide long-term therapy

or considering the addition of either an endothelin receptor antagonist or a prostacyclin analog. It is imperative to effectively treat the PH in severe BPD to avoid mortality and significant morbidities. In patients with severe BPD in whom PH develops, we recommend cardiac catheterization to guide therapy.

Interdisciplinary Care

Severe BPD is associated with poor nutrition and neurodevelopmental outcomes and with family stress. Therefore, optimal care of infants with severe BPD should be given by a multidisciplinary team, including representatives from neonatology, pulmonology, respiratory therapy, nutrition, occupational therapy, speech therapy, physical therapy, social work, pharmacy, discharge planning, and other services. It is imperative to involve the family in the interdisciplinary care of the patient with severe BPD early in the hospitalization in order to improve the family's comfort with the disease process. Such family-centered care hastens discharge home, decreases need for rehospitalization, and improves family dynamics.[111] Regular team meetings should occur throughout the course of the patient's NICU stay.

Nutritional care is critical not only to maintain growth for the patient but also to foster lung healing and repair. We recommend displaying a growth chart at the bedside of a patient hospitalized with severe BPD, to facilitate the daily assessment of nutritional needs. The goal should be 15 to 20 g/kg/day for infants younger than 37 weeks PMA and 20 to 30 g/day for infants 37 weeks PMA or older. These patients are often fluid restricted, but they usually require 120 to 150 kcal/kg/day to achieve adequate growth and lung repair, such that high caloric density is needed. Whenever possible, the mothers' own breast milk should be used in these patients, even if it needs to be heavily fortified.

In patients with severe BPD, neurodevelopmental assessments and care are of obvious benefit in optimizing long-term outcomes. Developmental consultation and application of behavioral interventions are often important factors in many aspects of the care plan, including the decision about the need for placement of a tracheostomy for long-term mechanical ventilation. Patients with severe BPD who are receiving long-term nasal CPAP or who have persistent distress and recurrent cyanotic episodes with less invasive respiratory support are not be able to interact well with the environment or to develop their motor skills, so their care should include developmental therapies three to five times a week while they are hospitalized. These developmental treatments should focus on creating an age-appropriate sensory and social environment. A formal neurodevelopmental assessment should be carried out at approximately 40 weeks PMA, and therapies should be directed at improving specific areas of developmental delay.[111] Behavioral aspects of nursing care and routine handling may reduce the frequency or severity of recurrent cyanotic episodes and irritability with agitation. Noxious stimuli (for example, arterial and heel sticks) should be minimized in these patients, and opioids and sedatives should be used with caution.

Discharge and Follow-Up

The patient with severe BPD often has a prolonged hospitalization and special needs at discharge, so discharge planning needs to be an ongoing process. Discharge planning has to consider the needs of the patient (i.e., supplemental oxygen, feeding pumps, monitors, medications) and the resources of the family as well as the community. For example, a family who lives in a large metropolitan area will have ready access to resources that a family living in a rural setting will not. In terms of medical readiness for discharge, factors include amount and stability of supplemental oxygen need and ability to feed.[111] There are no gestational age or weight criteria for these complicated patients. The ability of patients with severe BPD to remain at home without frequent readmissions requires detailed communication and coordination with the primary care physician in the community. We recommend that the primary care physician see the patient within a day or two after discharge; optimally, we would like the primary care physician to be involved in care prior to the patient's discharge, but this arrangement has proved very difficult owing to distances and scheduling. There must also be close coordination with the home care company to avoid problems with the equipment that might necessitate readmission. Finally, follow-up must be carefully orchestrated to answer primary pediatric needs, respiratory needs, nutritional needs, family needs, as well as provide ongoing neurodevelopmental assessments and therapies. We have developed a multidisciplinary BPD outpatient clinic that offers neonatology, pulmonology, nutrition, social work, occupational therapy, physical therapy, and speech therapy services. The patient is scheduled for the first visit in the BPD clinic 2 to 4 weeks after discharge, and further visits depend on the patient's needs and status. Formal developmental assessments are made at 18 and 24 months, including a Bayley Scales of Infant and Toddler Development, 3rd edition (Bayley III), examination.

Long-Term Outcomes

There is a paucity of studies examining the long-term respiratory outcomes of patients with severe BPD. A study of 86 survivors of extreme preterm birth (<1000 g or gestational age ≤28 weeks) at 10 or 18 years of age found significantly higher HRCT scores as well as more opacities and hypoattenuated areas in subjects with a history of moderate or severe BPD than in those with a history of no or mild BPD.[112] Similarly, Wong and colleagues[113] described abnormal HRCT findings with emphysematous changes in 19 subjects aged 17 to 33 years who had been born weighing less than 1500 g between 1980 and 1987 and who had received a diagnosis of moderate to severe BPD; these abnormal HRCT findings were correlated with abnormalities in pulmonary function.[113] Thus, there is evidence that severe BPD is associated with lifelong changes in pulmonary structure and function. However, more studies are needed to accurately determine the long-term course of premature neonates with severe BPD and their relative contribution to the growing adult population with chronic obstructive pulmonary disease.

References

1. Northway Jr WH, Rosan RC, Porter DY. Pulmonary disease following respiratory therapy of hyaline membrane disease. *N Engl J Med.* 1967;276:357-368.
2. Bland RD, Coalson JJ. *Chronic lung disease in early infancy.* New York: Marcel Dekker; 2000.
3. Jobe AH, Bancalari E. Bronchopulmonary dysplasia. *Am J Respir Crit Care Med.* 2001;163: 1723-1729.
4. Bancalari E, Abdenour GE, Feller R, Gannon J. Bronchopulmonary dysplasia: clinical presentation. *J Pediatr.* 1979;95:819-823.
5. Jobe AH. The new BPD: an arrest of lung development. *Pediatr Res.* 1999;46:641-643.
6. Charafeddine L, D'Angio CT, Phelps DL. Atypical chronic lung disease patterns in neonates. *Pediatrics.* 1999;103:759-760.
7. Rojas MA, Gonzalez A, Bancalari E, et al. Changing trends in the epidemiology and pathogenesis of chronic lung disease. *J Pediatr.* 1995;126:605-610.
8. Laughton M, Alfred EN, Bose C, et al. Patterns of respiratory distress during the first 2 postnatal weeks in extremely premature infants. *Pediatrics.* 2010;123:1124-1131.
9. Smith VC, Zupancic JA, McCormick MC, et al. Trends in severe bronchopulmonary dysplasia rates between 1994 and 2002. *J Pediatr.* 2005;146:469-473.
10. Hussain AN, Siddiqui NH, Stocker JT. Pathology of arrested acinar development in postsurfactant bronchopulmonary dysplasia. *Hum Pathol.* 1998;29:710-717.
11. Bancalari E, Gonzalez A. Clinical course and lung function abnormalities during development of chronic lung disease. In: Bland RD, Coalson JJ, eds. *Chronic lung disease in early infancy.* New York: Marcel Dekker; 2000.
12. Coalson JJ. Pathology of chronic lung disease of early infancy. In: Bland RD, Coalson JJ, eds. *Chronic lung disease of early infancy.* New York: Marcel Dekker; 2000:85-124.
13. Jobe AH, Bancalari E. Bronchopulmonary dysplasia. NICHD-NHLBI-ORD Workshop. *Am J Respir Crit Care Med.* 2001;163:1723-1729.
14. Mourani PM, Sontag MK, Kerby GS, et al. Persistent impairment of lung function during infancy correlates with the severity of bronchopulmonary dysplasia at diagnosis. Presented at the 2010 American Thoracic Society International Conference, New Orleans, May 14-19, 2010.
15. Greenough A, Kavvadia V, Johnson A, et al. A simple chest radiograph score to predict chronic lung disease in prematurely born infants. *Br J Radiol.* 1999;72:530-533.
16. Thomas MR, Greenough A, Johnson A, et al. Frequent wheeze at follow up of very preterm infants—which factors are predictive? *Arch Dis Child Fetal Neonatal Ed.* 2003;88:F329-F332.
17. Ellsbury DL, Acarregui MJ, McGuiness GA, Klein JM. Variability in the use of supplemental oxygen for bronchopulmonary dysplasia. *J Pediatr.* 2002;149:247-249.

18. Walsh MC, Wilson-Costello D, Zadell A, et al. Safety, reliability and validity of a physiologic definition of BPD. *J Perinatol*. 2003;23:451-456.
19. Walsh MC. Definitions of BPD and the use of benchmarking to compare outcomes. In: Abman SH, ed. *Bronchopulmonary Dysplasia*. New York: Informa Health; 2010:267-279.
20. Ehrenkranz RA, Walsh MC, Vohr BR et al. Validation of the NIH consensus definition of BPD. *Pediatrics*. 2005;116:1353-1360.
21. Laughon MM, Langer JC, Bose CL, et al. Prediction of bronchopulmonary dysplasia by postnatal age in extremely premature infants. *Am J Respir Crit Care Med*. 2011;183:1715-1722
22. Bonikos DS, Bensch KG, Northway WH Jr. Oxygen toxicity in the newborn. The effect of chronic continuous 100% oxygen exposure on the lung of newborn mice. *Am J Pathol*. 1976;85:623-650.
23. Crapo JD, Peters-Golden M, Marsh-Salin J, et al. Pathologic changes in the lungs of oxygen-adapted rats. A morphometric analysis. *Lab Invest*. 1978;39:640-653.
24. Davis JM, Rosenfeld WN, Sanders RJ, Gonenne A. Prophylactic effects of recombinant human superoxide dismutase in neonatal lung injury. *J Appl Physiol*. 1993;74:2234-2241.
25. Davis JM, Parad RB, Michele T, et al. Pulmonary outcome at one year corrected age in premature infants treated at birth with recombinant CuZn superoxide dismutase. *Pediatrics*. 2003;111: 469-476.
26. Van Marter LJ, Leviton A, Kuban KC, et al. Maternal glucocorticoid therapy and reduced risk of bronchopulmonary dysplasia. *Pediatrics*. 1990;86:331-336.
27. Zeitlin J, El Ayoubi M, Jarreau PH, et al. Impact of fetal growth restriction on mortality and morbidity in a very preterm birth cohort. *J Pediatr*. 2010;157:733-739.
28. Bose C, van Marter LJ, Laughon M, et al. Fetal growth restriction and chronic lung disease among infants born before the 28(th) week of gestation. *Pediatrics*. 2009;124:e450-e458.
29. Lee HJ, Kim EK, Kim HS, et al. Chorioamnionitis, respiratory distress syndrome and BPD in extremely low birth weight infants. *J Perinatol*. 2010;31(3):166-170.
30. Hansen AR, Barnes CM, Folkman J, McElrath TF. Maternal preeclampsia predicts the development of BPD. *J Pediatr*. 2010;156:532-536.
31. Tang JR, Seedorf G, Muehlethaler V, et al. Moderate hyperoxia accelerates lung growth and attenuates pulmonary hypertension in infant rats after exposure to intra-amniotic endotoxin. *Am J Physiol: Lung*. 2010;299:L735-L748.
32. Bryan MH, Hardie MJ, Reilly BJ, Swyer PR. Pulmonary function studies during the first year of life in infants recovering from respiratory distress syndrome. *Pediatrics*. 1973;52:169.
33. Goldman SL, Gerhardt T, Sonni R, et al. Early prediction of chronic lung disease by pulmonary function testing. *J Pediatr*. 1883;102:613-617.
34. Wolfson MR, Bhutani BK, Shaffer TH, Bowen Jr FW. Mechanics and energetics of breathing helium in infants with bronchopulmonary dysplasia. *J Pediatr*. 1984;104:752-757.
35. Tepper RS, Morgan WJ, Cota K, Taussig LM. Expiratory flow limitation in infants with bronchopulmonary dysplasia. *J Pediatr*. 1986;109:1040-1046.
36. Castile RG, Nelin LD. Lung function, structure and the physiologic basis for mechanical ventilation of infants with established BPD. In: Abman SH, ed. *Bronchopulmonary Dysplasia*. New York: Informa Health; 2010:328-346.
37. Balinotti JE, Chakr VC, Tiller C, et al. Growth of lung parenchyma in infants and toddlers with chronic lung disease of infancy. *Am J Respir Crit Care Med*. 2010;181:1093-1097.
38. Gappa M, Pillow J, Allen J, et al. Lung function tests in neonates and infants with chronic lung disease: lung and chest-wall mechanics. *Pediatr Pulmonol*. 2006;41:291-317.
39. Tepper RS, Pagtakhan RD, Taussig LM. Noninvasive determination of total respiratory system compliance in infants by the weighted-spirometer method. *Am Rev Respir Dis*. 1984;130: 461-466.
40. Gerhardt T, Hehre D, Feller R, et al. Serial determination of pulmonary function in infants with chronic lung disease. *J Pediatr*. 1987;110:448-456.
41. Baraldi E, Filippone M, Trevisanuto D, et al. Pulmonary function until two years of life in infants with bronchopulmonary dysplasia. *Am J Respir Crit Care Med*. 1997;155:149-155.
42. Moriette G, Gaudebout C, Clement A, et al. Pulmonary function at 1 year of age in survivors of neonatal respiratory distress: a multivariate analysis of factors associated with sequelae. *Pediatr Pulmonol*. 1987;3:242-250.
43. Farstad T, Brockmeier F, Bratlid D. Cardiopulmonary function in premature infants with bronchopulmonary dysplasia—a 2 year follow up. *Eur J Pediatr*. 1995;154:853-858.
44. Jarriel WS, Richardson P, Knapp RD, Hansen TN. A nonlinear regression analysis of nonlinear, passive-deflation flow-volume plots. *Pediatr Pulmonol*. 1993;15:175-182.
45. Mead J. Contribution of compliance of airways to frequency-dependent behavior of lungs. *J Appl Physiol*. 1969;26:670-673.
46. Hulskamp G, Pillow JJ, Dinger J, Stocks J. Lung function in infants and young children with chronic lung disease of infancy: functional residual capacity. *Pediatr Pulmonol*. 2006;41:1-22.
47. Stocks J, Godfrey S, Beardsmore C, et al. Standards for infant pulmonary function testing: Plethysmographic measurements of lung volume and airway resistance. *Eur Respir J*. 2001;17:302-312.
48. Morris MG, Gustafsson P, Tepper R, et al. ERS/ATS task force on standards for infant respiratory function testing. The bias flow nitrogen washout technique for measuring the functional residual capacity in infants. *Eur Respir J*. 2001;17:529-536.
49. Hofhuis W, Huysman MW, van der Wiel EC, et al. Worsening of V'_{maxFRC} in infants with chronic lung disease in the first year of life: a more favorable outcome after high-frequency oscillation ventilation. *Am J Respir Crit Care Med*. 2002;166:1539-1544.

21

50. Robin B, Kim YJ, Huth J, et al. Pulmonary function in bronchopulmonary dysplasia. *Pediatr Pulmonol.* 2004;37:236.
51. Castile R, Filbrun D, Flucke R, et al. Adult-type pulmonary function tests in infants without respiratory disease. *Pediatr Pulmonol.* 2000;30:215-227.
52. Filbrun AG, Linn MJ, McIntosh NA, Hershenson MB. Longitudinal measures of lung function in infants with bronchopulmonary dysplasia. *Am J Respir Crit Care Med.* 2007;175:A92.
53. Lum S, Hulskamp G, Merkus P, et al. Lung function tests in neonates and infants with chronic lung disease: forced expiratory maneuvers. *Pediatr Pulmonol.* 2006;41:199-214.
54. Sly PD, Tepper, R, Henschen, M, et al. Tidal forced expirations. ERS/ATS Task Force on Standards for Infant Respiratory Function Testing. European Respiratory Society/American Thoracic Society. *Eur Respir J.* 2000;16:741-748.
55. Lum S, Stocks J, Castile RG, et al. ATS/ERS Statement: Raised volume forced expirations in infants: guidelines for current practice. *Am J Respir Crit Care Med.* 2005;172:1463-1471.
56. Opperman HC, Wille L, Bleyl U, Obladen M. Bronchopulmonary dysplasia in premature infants. A radiological and pathological correlation. *Pediatr Radiol.* 1977;5:137-141.
57. Edwards DK, Colby TV, Northway WH. Radiographic-pathologic correlation in bronchopulmonary dysplasia. *J Pediatr.* 1979;95:834-836.
58. Mahut B, De Blic J, Emond S, et al. Chest computed tomography findings in bronchopulmonary dysplasia and correlation with lung function. *Arch Dis Child.* 2007;92:F459-F464.
59. Kubota J, Ohki Y, Inoue T, et al. Ultrafast CT scoring system for assessing bronchopulmonary dysplasia: reproducibility and clinical correlation. *Radiat Med.* 1998;16:167-174.
60. Oppenheim C, Mamou-Mani T, Sayegh N, et al. Bronchopulmonary dysplasia: value of CT in identifying pulmonary sequelae. *Am J Roentgenol.* 1994;163:169-172.
61. Aquino SL, Schechter MS, Chiles C, et al. High-resolution inspiratory and expiratory CT in older children and adult with bronchopulmonary dysplasia. *Am J Roentgenol.* 1999;173:963-967.
62. Howling SJ, Northway WJ, Hansel DM, et al. Pulmonary sequelae of bronchopulmonary dysplasia survivors: high-resolution CT findings. *Am J Roentgenol.* 2000;174:1323-1326.
63. Aukland SM, Halvorsen T, Fosse KR, et al. High-resolution CT of the chest in children and young adults who were born prematurely: findings in a population based study, *Am J Roentgenol.* 2006;187:1012-1018.
64. Raman P, Raman R, Newman B, et al. Development and validation of automated 2D-3D bronchial airway matching to track changes in regional bronchial morphology using serial low-dose chest CT scans in children with chronic lung disease. *J Digit Imaging.* 2010;23:744-754.
65. de Jong PA, Long FR, Nakano Y. Computed tomography dose and variability of airway dimension measurements: how low can we go? *Pediatr Radiol.* 2006 Oct;36:1043-1047.
66. Long FR. High-resolution computed tomography of the lung in children with cystic fibrosis: technical factors. *Proc Am Thorac Soc.* 2007;4:306-309.
67. de González AB, Kim KP, Samet JM. Radiation-induced cancer risk from annual computed tomography for patients with cystic fibrosis. *Am J Respir Crit Care Med.* 2007;176:970-973.
68. Abman SH. Pulmonary hypertension in chronic lung disease of infancy. Pathogenesis, pathophysiology and treatment. In: Bland RD, Coalson JJ, eds. *Chronic Lung Disease of Infancy.* New York: Marcel Dekker; 2000:619-668.
69. Parker TA, Abman SH. The pulmonary circulation in BPD. *Sem Neonatol.* 2003;8:51-62.
70. Tomashefski JF, Opperman HC, Vawter GF. Bronchopulmonary dysplasia, a morphometric study with emphasis on the pulmonary vasculature. *Pediatr Pathol.* 1984;2:469-487.
71. Halliday HL, Dumpit FM, Brady JP. Effects of inspired oxygen on echocardiographic assessment of pulmonary vascular resistance and myocardial contractility in bronchopulmonary dysplasia. *Pediatrics.* 1980;65:536-540.
72. Abman SH, Wolfe TT, Accurso FJ, et al. Pulmonary vascular response to oxygen in infants with severe bronchopulmonary dysplasia. *Pediatrics.* 1985;75:80-84.
73. Mourani PM, Ivy DD, Gao D, Abman SH. Pulmonary vascular effects of inhaled nitric oxide and oxygen tension in bronchopulmonary dysplasia. *Am J Respir Crit Care Med.* 2004;170:1006-1013.
74. Walther FJ, Bender FJ, Leighton JO. Persistent pulmonary hypertension in premature neonates with severe RDS. *Pediatrics.* 1992;90:899-904.
75. Fouron JC, LeGuennec JC, Villemont D, et al. Value of echocardiography in assessing outcome of BPD. *Pediatrics.* 1980;65:529-535.
76. Khemani E, McElhinney DB, Rhein L, et al. Pulmonary artery hypertension in formerly premature infants with bronchopulmonary dysplasia: clinical features and outcomes in the surfactant era. *Pediatrics.* 2007;120:1260-1269.
77. Coalson JJ. Pathology of chronic lung disease of early infancy. In: Bland RD, Coalson JJ, eds. *Chronic lung disease of early infancy.* New York: Marcel Dekker; 2000:85-124.
78. Jakkula M, Le Cras TD, Gebb S, et al. Inhibition of angiogenesis decreases alveolarization in the developing rat lung. *Am J Physiol Lung Cell Mol Physiol.* 2000;279:L600-L607.
79. Bhatt AJ, Pryhuber GS, Huyck H, et al. Disrupted pulmonary vasculature and decreased VEGF, flt-1 and Tie 2 in human infants dying with bronchopulmonary dysplasia. *Am J Respir Crit Care Med.* 2000;164:1971-1980.
80. Abman SH. BPD: a vascular hypothesis. *Am J Resp Crit Care Med.* 2001;164:1755-1756.
81. De Paepe ME, Mao Q, Powell J, et al. Growth of pulmonary microvasculature in ventilated preterm infants. *Am J Respir Crit Care Med.* 2006;173:204-211.
82. Hussain AN, Siddiqui NH, Stocker JT. Pathology of arrested acinar development in postsurfactant BPD. *Hum Pathol.* 1998;29:710-717.

83. Abman SH, Schaffer M, Wiggins J, et al. Pulmonary vascular extraction of circulating norepinephrine in infants with bronchopulmonary dysplasia. *Pediatr Pulmonology*. 1987;3:386-391.
84. Abman SH, Warady BA, Lum GM, Koops Bl. Systemic hypertension in infants with BPD. *J Pediatr*. 1984;104:928-931.
85. Anderson AH, Warady BA, Daily DK, et al. Systemic hypertension in infants with severe bronchopulmonary dysplasia: associated clinical factors. *Am J Perinatol*. 1993;10:190-193.
86. Yzdorczyk C, Comte B, Cambonie G, et al. Neonatal oxygen exposure in rats leads to cardiovascular and renal alterations in adulthood. *Hypertension*. 2008;52:889-895.
87. Mourani PM, Ivy DD, Rosenberg AA, et al. Left ventricular diastolic dysfunction in bronchopulmonary dysplasia. *J Pediatr*. 2008;152:291-293.
88. Brion LP, Primhak RA. Intravenous or enteral loop diuretics for preterm infants with (or developing) chronic lung disease. *Cochrane Database Syst Rev*. 2002;(1):CD001453.
89. Brion LP, Primhak RA, Ambrosio-Perez I. Diuretics acting on the distal renal tubule for preterm infants with (or developing) chronic lung disease. *Cochrane Database Syst Rev*. 2002;(1):CD001817.
90. McCann EM, Lewis K, Deming DD, et al. Controlled trial of furosemide therapy in infants with chronic lung disease. *J Pediatr*. 1985;106:957-962.
91. Brion LP, Primhak RA, Yong W. Aerosolized diuretics for preterm infants with (or developing) chronic lung disease. *Cochrane Database Syst Rev*. 2001;(2):CD001694.
92. Kao LC, Warburton D, Cheng MH, et al. Effect of oral diuretics on pulmonary mechanics in infants with chronic bronchopulmonary dysplasia: results of a double-blind crossover sequential trial. *Pediatrics*. 1984;74:37-44.
93. Kao LC, Durand DJ, McCrea RC, et al. Randomized trial of long-term diuretic therapy for infants with oxygen-dependent bronchopulmonary dysplasia. *J Pediatr*. 1994;124:772-781.
94. Rush MG, Engelhardt B, Parker RA, Hazinski TA. Double-blind, placebo-controlled trial of alternate-day furosemide in infants with chronic bronchopulmonary dysplasia. *J Pediatr*. 1990;117:112-118.
95. Sosulski R, Abbasi S, Bhutani VK, et al. Physiologic effects of terbutaline on pulmonary function of infants with bronchopulmonary dysplasia. *Pediatr Pulmonol*. 1986;2:269-273.
96. Wilkie RA, Bryan MH. Effect of bronchodilators on airway resistance in ventilator-dependent neonates with chronic lung disease. *J Pediatr*. 1987;111:278-282.
97. D'Angio CT, Maniscalco WM. Bronchopulmonary dysplasia in preterm infants: pathophysiology and management strategies. *Pediatr Drugs*. 2004;6:303-333.
98. Henderson-Smart DJ, Davis PG. Prophylactic methylxanthines for extubation in preterm infants. *Cochrane Database Syst Rev*. 2003;(1):CD000139.
99. Halliday HL, Ehrenkranz RA, Doyle LW. Early postnatal (<96 hours) corticosteroids for preventing chronic lung disease in preterm infants. *Cochrane Database Syst Rev*. 2003;(1):CD001146.
100. Halliday HL, Ehrenkranz RA, Doyle LW. Moderately early (7-14 days) postnatal corticosteroids for preventing chronic lung disease in preterm infants. *Cochrane Database Syst Rev*. 2003;(1):CD001144.
101. Halliday HL, Ehrenkranz RA, Doyle LW. Delayed (>3 weeks) postnatal corticosteroids for chronic lung disease in preterm infants. *Cochrane Database Syst Rev*. 2003;(1):CD001145.
102. Greir DG, Halliday HL. Management of bronchopulmonary dysplasia in infants: guidelines for corticosteroid use. *Drugs*. 2005;65:15-29.
103. Lister P, Iles R, Shaw B. Inhaled steroids for neonatal chronic lung disease. *Cochrane Database Syst Rev*. 2000;(3):CD002311.
104. Shah SS, Ohlsson A, Halliday H, et al. Inhaled versus systemic corticosteroids for the treatment of chronic lung disease in ventilated very low birth weight preterm infants. *Cochrane Database Syst Rev*. 2003;(2):CD002057.
105. Shah SS, Ohlsson A, Halliday H, et al. Inhaled versus systemic corticosteroids for preventing chronic lung disease in ventilated very low birth weight preterm neonates. *Cochrane Database Syst Rev*. 2003;(1):CD002058.
106. Jadcherla SR, Gupta A, Fernandez S, et al. Spatiotemporal characteristics of acid refluxate and relationship to symptoms in premature and term infants with chronic lung disease. *Am J Gastroenterol*. 2008;103:720-728.
107. Mourani PM, Ivy DD, Gao D, et al. Pulmonary vascular effects of inhaled NO and oxygen tension in BPD. *Am J Respir Crit Care Med*. 2004;170:1006-1013.
108. Johnson CE, Beekman RH, Kostychak DA, et al. Pharmacokinetics and pharmacodynamics of nifedipine in children with BPD and pulmonary hypertension. *Pediatr Res*. 1988;24:186-190.
109. Galie N, Ghofrani HA, Torbicki A, et al. Sildenafil citrate therapy for pulmonary arterial hypertension. *N Engl J Med*. 2005;353:2148-2157.
110. Mourani PM, Sontag MK, Lui G, et al. Effects of long-term sildenafil treatment for pulmonary hypertension in infants with chronic lung disease. *J Pediatr*. 2009;154:379-384.
111. Shepherd EG, Knupp AM, Welty SE, et al. An interdisciplinary bronchopulmonary dysplasia program is associated with improved neurodevelopmental outcomes and fewer rehospitalizations. *J Perinatol*. May, 2011, doi:10.1038/jp.2011.45.
112. Aukland SM, Rosendahl K, Owens CM, et al. Neonatal bronchopulmonary dysplasia predicts abnormal pulmonary HRCT scans in long-term survivors of extreme preterm birth. *Thorax*. 2009;64:405-410.
113. Wong PM, Lees AN, Louw J, et al. Emphysema in young adult survivors of moderate-to-severe bronchopulmonary dysplasia. *Eur Respir J*. 2008;32:321-328.

Index

Note: Page numbers followed by f, t, and b indicate figures, tables, and boxes, respectively.

A

ABCA3, in respiratory distress syndrome, 37
N-Acetylcysteine, for bronchopulmonary dysplasia, 223-224
Acidosis, bicarbonate for, 260
Acute hypoxic vasoconstriction, 96
Adaptive mechanical backup ventilation, 372
Adhesion molecules, in bronchopulmonary dysplasia, 43-44
Adolescents, respiratory function in, 238-240, 238t
Adrenal insufficiency
  bronchopulmonary dysplasia and, 184-185
  patent ductus arteriosus and, 184-185
Adult stem cells, 198-199. *See also* Stem cell(s).
Adulthood, early, respiratory function in, 238-240, 238t
Agonal gasping, 250
Air leaks
  infant-ventilator asynchrony and, 340-341
  pneumothorax and, in congenital diaphragmatic hernia, 388
Air-blood barrier, postnatal maintenance of, 121, 125
Airway clearance
  in congenital diaphragmatic hernia, 389
  in resuscitation, 250
Airway devices, 248
Airway, laryngeal mask, 254
Airway obstruction. *See also* Reactive airway disease.
  in congenital diaphragmatic hernia, 389
  after very preterm birth, 237, 237t
Airway resistance, in bronchopulmonary dysplasia, 408-409
  assessment of, 409
Albumin, 172
Alcohol use, maternal, lung development and, 84
Alk3, 30
Alladin NCPAP Infant Flow System, 274, 274f
Allopurinol, for bronchopulmonary dysplasia, 223-224
Alveolar epithelial cells
  endogenous, 206-208, 206f
  exogenous, 199-200
Alveolar fluid balance, undernutrition and, 167t, 170
Alveolar septation, 11-12, 12f
  timing of, 58-59
Alveolarization
  in bronchopulmonary dysplasia, 164, 220-221
  in congenital diaphragmatic hernia, 381
  in patent ductus arteriosus, 185-186
Alveolocapillary barrier, postnatal maturation of, 3
Alveologenesis, 5f, 6
  angiogenesis and, 12-13, 17f, 111-114, 113f, 113t
  elastin deposition in, 11-12, 12f
  epithelial-endothelial crosstalk in, 12-13, 17f, 111-114, 113f, 113t
  myofibroblast differentiation in, 11-12, 12f
  regulation of, 11-13, 12f, 17f
Amino acids, 172, 175
Aminocaproic acid, for congenital diaphragmatic hernia, 392
Aminophylline
  for bronchopulmonary dysplasia, 418-419
  for ventilator weaning, 357
Amniotic fluid culture, 65
Amniotic membranes
  culture of, 65
  rupture of
    chorioamnionitis and, 67-69. *See also* Chorioamnionitis.
    respiratory distress syndrome and, 67-69
    Ureaplasma infection and, 141-142, 143t
Angiogenesis, 13-16, 111-112. *See also* Vascular development.
  signaling in, 111-112, 113f, 113t, 114-115
Angiopoietins, 14-15, 113t, 114-115
  in lung injury, 39
Angiotensin 1, 113t, 114-115
Angiotensin 2, 113t, 114-115
  reactive oxygen species and, 92-93
Angiotensin-converting enzyme (ACE), in bronchopulmonary dysplasia, 46
Antenatal infections, 65-84, 135-151. *See also* Chorioamnionitis.
  in animal models, 69-72, 70f-71f
  bronchopulmonary dysplasia and, 135-151, 219-220. *See also* Bronchopulmonary dysplasia, chorioamnionitis and.
  causative organisms in, 65-66, 135-137
  clinical outcomes in, 67-69, 68t, 69f, 137-139
  immune response in, 72-73, 73t, 76-78, 77f
  overview of, 65
  types of, 65

Antenatal inflammation, 65-84. *See also* Inflammation.
 chronic, adaptation to, 75-76
 immune response in, 72-73, 73t, 76-78, 77f
 lung maturation and, 69-72
  animal models of, 69-72, 70f-71f
  in chronic chorioamnionitis, 75-76, 76f
  gestational age and, 73
  inflammatory mediators in, 72-73, 73t
  mechanisms of, 73-75, 74f
Antenatal stress, lung maturation and, 81
Antibiotics, for *Ureaplasma* infection, 150
Anti–CD18 antibody, in lung maturation, 74-75, 74f
Antigen, ureaplasmal Mb, 141
Antioxidants, 95
 endogenous, 310
  brain injury and, 310
  in bronchopulmonary dysplasia, 44
  expression of, 95
  hyperoxia and, 169
  impaired activity of, 95
  types of, 95
  undernutrition and, 169
 exogenous
  for bronchopulmonary dysplasia, 223-224
  for pulmonary hypertension, 103-105
Apnea backup ventilation, 372
Apnea of prematurity, 266
 nasal CPAP for, 266, 270
 nasal IPPV for, 270
Apnea, primary vs. secondary, 250, 250f
Arabella NCPAP Infant Flow System, 274, 274f
L-Arginine
 L-citrulline and, 103, 123
 nitric oxide synthase and, 123
Ascorbic acid, 165t, 174
Asphyxia, hypotension in, 258-260
Aspiration, meconium
 airway management in, 250
 surfactant for, 292-293
Aspiration pneumonia, ventilator-associated, 153-154
Assist-control ventilation, 344, 345f
Asthma
 bronchopulmonary dysplasia and, 154-155
 fibrocytes in, 208-209
 after late preterm birth, 236-237
 stem cell therapy for, 204-205
Asymmetric dimethyl arginine (ADMA), nitric oxide synthase and, 123
Atelectasis, in bronchopulmonary dysplasia, 408-409, 416f
ATP-binding cassette transporter A3
 in animal models, 29-30
 in bronchopulmonary dysplasia, 46
Atrial septal defects, in bronchopulmonary dysplasia, 412
Automatic mechanical ventilation, 367-380. *See also* Mechanical ventilation *and specific types.*
 weaning from, 362-363, 369-371
  supplemental oxygen and, 363
Azithromycin, for *Ureaplasma* infection, 150

B

Bags
 polyethylene, for warming, 249-250
 for positive-pressure ventilation, 248, 251
BAY 58-2667 (cinaciguat), for pulmonary hypertension, 103
Beractant, 285-286, 285t. *See also* Surfactant.
 budesonide with, 295
Beta-agonists, for congenital diaphragmatic hernia, 389
Betamethasone. *See also* Corticosteroids.
 antenatal, 61-64, 64t, 78-80
BH_4 (tetrahydrobiopterin), 102-103
 nitrous oxide synthase and, 123
Bicarbonate, in resuscitation, 260
Birth weight, ventilator-associated pneumonia and, 152-153
Bleomycin, pulmonary fibrosis due to, 203-204
Blindness. *See* Retinopathy of prematurity.
Bochdalek hernia. *See* Congenital diaphragmatic hernia.
Bone formation, undernutrition and, 168-169
Bone marrow–derived stem cells, 201-202. *See also* Stem cell(s).
Bone morphogenetic protein 4 (BMP4), 30, 32
Bone morphogenetic protein(s) (BMPs), in branching morphogenesis, 8-9, 9f, 30
Bone morphogenetic protein receptor type 1A (BMPR-1A), 30
BOOST Trials, 315-316, 320-321
Bosentan, for pulmonary hypertension, in congenital diaphragmatic hernia, 397-400
Bovactant, 285, 285t. *See also* Surfactant.
Bovine lipid extract surfactant, 285t. *See also* Surfactant.
Brain death, 260
Brain injury
 hypoxemic, 334-335
 oxygen toxicity and, 310-311
  clinical outcomes and, 316-317
 steroids and, 227, 358
Branching morphogenesis, 8-11, 9f
 bone morphogenetic proteins in, 8-9, 9f, 30
 epithelium-mesenchyme interactions in, 8-11
 fibroblast growth factor in, 8, 9f
 nitric oxide in, 117
 sonic hedgehog in, 8, 9f
 Sprouty in, 8, 9f
 transforming growth factor-ß in, 9-10
 Wnt in, 9-10
Breathing control, undernutrition and, 167t, 170
Bronchial vasculature, 13
Bronchoalveolar stem cells, 206-207, 206f
Bronchodilators, for bronchopulmonary dysplasia, 418
Bronchopulmonary dysplasia
 adrenal insufficiency and, 184-185
 asthma and, 154-155, 204-205
 chorioamnionitis and, 67-72, 68t, 69f, 135-162, 219-220. *See also* Chorioamnionitis.
  acute vs. subacute, 138-139
  duration of exposure in, 138-139
  fetal inflammatory response and, 139
  gestational age and, 136f
  maternal stage and, 138-139, 138f
  postnatal lung injury and, 139
  severity of, 68-69, 69f, 138-139, 138f
  steroid response and, 139
 clinical presentation of, 217-218
 etiology and pathogenesis of, 407-408
 fibrosis in. *See* Pulmonary fibrosis.
 fluid intake and, 165t, 170-171

Bronchopulmonary dysplasia *(Continued)*
genetic influences in, 42-50, 48t-49t, 222. *See also* Genetic influences, in bronchopulmonary dysplasia.
animal models of, 39-42
clinical context for, 42-50
gestational age and, 218f, 220
gram-negative organisms in, 150-151
in growth-restricted/small for gestational age infants, 81-83, 82f
immune response in, 148-149
incidence of, 163-164, 217, 218f, 407
long-term outcomes in, 236-240, 422. *See also* Long-term pulmonary outcomes.
lung repair in, nitric oxide in, 117-123, 120f
mechanical ventilation in, 415-417, 415t, 416f
long-term, 414
tracheostomy for, 413-414
mesenchymal stem cells in, 200-202
mild, 42
moderate, 42
neurodevelopment in, 421
"new", 217-218, 237-238, 407
patent ductus arteriosus and, 171, 186-187, 187f
pathogenesis of, 4, 16-20, 17f, 42, 43f, 217, 219f
altered signaling in, 16-19, 125-126, 139-140, 220-221
alveolarization in, 164, 220-221
antenatal infections in, 135-151, 219-220
central event in, 135
chronic hyperoxia in, 101-102
CTGF in, 17f, 18, 40
growth factors in, 220-221
hyperoxia in, 221, 311
hypoxia in, 221
inflammation in, 139-140, 144-148, 184-185, 219-220
matrix metalloproteins in, 19-20
postnatal infections in, 151-155, 220
TGF-ß in, 16-19, 17f
vascular hypothesis for, 220-221
VEGF in, 17f, 18-19, 47, 102, 125-126, 186, 220-221
pathophysiology of, 16, 408-412
PEEP for, 415-417, 418f
prevention of
antioxidants for, 223-224
mechanical ventilation and, 224-225
mesenchymal stem cells in, 228
nitric oxide in, 225
nutritional support in, 225-226
oxygen saturation levels and, 222-223
pentoxifylline in, 228
restrictive oxygen approach and, 313-314, 316
Ureaplasma eradication in, 150
pulmonary function tests in, 408-409
reactive airway disease and, 154-155, 204-205
retinol and, 173
severe, 42, 217-218, 407-425
cardiovascular system in, 411-412
course of, 414
definition of, 407-408
discharge and follow-up in, 421-422
drug therapy for, 417-419
etiology and pathogenesis of, 407-408
evaluation of, 413-414, 413b

Bronchopulmonary dysplasia *(Continued)*
forced flows in, 410
imaging studies in, 410-411, 411f
incidence of, 407
interdisciplinary care in, 421
long-term care model for, 414
lung mechanics in, 408-409
lung volumes in, 410
mechanical ventilation for, 414-417, 415t, 416f
nutritional support in, 421
oxygen therapy for, 414
pathophysiology of, 408-412
pulmonary hypertension in, 411-412, 419-421, 420b
radiographic appearance of, 407-408, 408f
respiratory function in, 408-409
stages of, 407
treatment of, 413-422, 413b
signaling in, 16-19, 125-126, 139-140
treatment of
antioxidants in, 223-224
caffeine in, 227-228, 418
CTGF antibody in, 18
developmental behavioral therapy in, 421
diuretics in, 417-418
interdisciplinary approach in, 421
methylxanthines in, 218-222, 228, 418
nasal CPAP in, 414
nitric oxide in, 117-123, 120f, 126-128, 127t, 128f, 225
nutritional support in, 225-226, 421
oxygen therapy in, 414
in severe disease, 413-422, 413b
stem cell therapy in. *See* Stem cell therapy.
steroids in, 61, 226-227, 418-419
TGF-ß antibody in, 17-18
tracheostomy in, 414
VEGF in, 18-19
twin studies of, 43
undernutrition and, 163-164, 167. *See also Under* nutrition.
Ureaplasma infection in, 143-148, 145f, 147f-148f. *See also Ureaplasma* infection.
viral infections and, 151
volume-targeted ventilation and, 370-371
Bubble CPAP, 275
Budesonide, with beractant, 295
Bulb suctioning. *See* Suctioning.

C

Caffeine
for bronchopulmonary dysplasia, 227-228, 418-419
for patent ductus arteriosus, 189
for ventilator weaning, 357
Calcium
in acute hypoxic vasoconstriction, 96
dietary, 165t, 174-175
Calcium channel blockers, for pulmonary hypertension, in bronchopulmonary dysplasia, 419-420
Calfactant, 285t, 286. *See also* Surfactant.
Caloric intake, 165t, 170
Canalicular stage, of lung development, 5-6, 5f
Capnography, during cardiac compressions, 258
Carbohydrates, 165t, 171
Carbon dioxide, retinopathy of prematurity and, 310

Cardiac catheterization
in congenital diaphragmatic hernia, 395, 399-400
for pulmonary hypertension, in bronchopulmonary dysplasia, 419-420, 420b
Cardiac compressions, 255-258
blood pressure during, 258-260, 259f
capnography during, 258
colorimetric $ETCO_2$ detectors during, 258
compression-to-ventilation ratio in, 257
compression-ventilation coordination in, 257-258
two-thumb technique for, 256, 257f
Cardiopulmonary resuscitation. *See* Resuscitation.
CARM 1, 30
Catalase, 95
for pulmonary hypertension, 103-104
ß-Catenin, in animal models, 30, 32
Catheter
esophageal, in neurally adjusted ventilatory assist, 375
intratracheal, surfactant administration via, 273-274, 292
Catheterization, cardiac, in congenital diaphragmatic hernia, 395, 399-400
CCAAT enhancer-binding protein α, 31
CD18, in lung maturation, 74-75, 74f
CD90, in lung injury, 41
Cebpa, 31
Cerebral ischemia, 260. *See also* Brain injury.
Cerebral palsy
oxygen therapy and, 317
steroids and, 227, 358
Cesarean section, antenatal steroids for, 64, 64t
cGMP. *See* Cyclic guanosine monophosphate (cGMP).
Children, respiratory function in, 236-240, 237t-238t
Chlamydial pneumonia, bronchopulmonary dysplasia and, 151
Chorioamnionitis, 65-84
acute vs. subacute, 138-139
in animal models, 69-72, 70f-71f
antenatal steroids for, 78-80, 78t, 79f-81f. *See also* Corticosteroids, antenatal.
asthma and, 154-155
bronchopulmonary dysplasia and, 135-151, 219-220. *See also* Bronchopulmonary dysplasia, chorioamnionitis and.
causative organisms in, 65-66, 135-137
clinical, 65, 66f
clinical outcomes in, 67-69, 68t, 137-139
in acute vs. subclinical infection, 68-69, 69f
cytokines in, 67-68
diagnosis of, 65-67, 66f
experimental chronic, 75-76, 76f
fetal inflammatory response in, 68t, 137, 139-140
funisitis and, 65, 67
grading of, 137
histologic, 65, 66f, 137
immune response in, 72-73, 73t, 76-78, 77f
inflammatory mediators in, 72-73, 73t
Mycoplasma hominis, 65-66
respiratory distress syndrome and, 67-69, 68t, 137-138
Chorioamnionitis *(Continued)*
severity of, 137-139
Toll-like receptors in, 72-73
Ureaplasma, 65-69, 72-73, 73t, 140-150. *See also Ureaplasma* infection.
Chronic lung disease. *See* Bronchopulmonary dysplasia.
Chronic obstructive pulmonary disease, stem cell therapy for, 205
Cigarette smoking, respiratory function and, 240
Cinaciguat (BAY 58-2667), for pulmonary hypertension, 103
Circulating stem cells, 207-209
L-Citrulline, 123
L-arginine and, 103, 123
for pulmonary hypertension, 103, 123
C-kit–positive cells, 207, 208f
Clara cells, 206-207, 206f
Coactivator-associated arginine methyltransferase 1 (CARM1), 30
Cognitive deficits
hypoxemia and, 334-335
oxygen therapy and, 317
Colfosceril palmitate, 285-286, 285t. *See also* Surfactant.
Collateral vessels, in bronchopulmonary dysplasia, 412
Color, in initial assessment, 248
Colorimetric $ETCO_2$ detectors, 258
Computed tomography, in bronchopulmonary dysplasia, 410-411, 411f
Computer-assisted weaning, 363
Congenital diaphragmatic hernia, 381-406
acute respiratory management of, 382-392
antenatal treatment of, 400-401
Bochdalek, 382
cardiopulmonary interactions in, 392
congenital heart disease and, 399-400
ductal shunts in, 387t, 395-396
ECMO for, 387t, 390-392, 415t
gastric decompression in, 382-383, 383f
hearing loss and, 400
inflammation in, 386-387
longer-term issues in, 400
lung hypoplasia in, 381-382, 390-391
lung protection strategies for, 386-388
lung recruitment approach for, 386
mechanical ventilation for, 382-389, 384t-385t, 387t
during EXIT procedure, 391
Morgagni, 382
neuromuscular blockade for, 382-383
obstetric delivery in, by EXIT procedure, 391
operative repair of
immediate vs. delayed, 382
preoperative stabilization for, 382
pathophysiology of, 381-382
presentation of, 382
pulmonary hypertension in, 393-399
assessment of, 393-394
cardiopulmonary interactions and, 392
management of, 394-399
pulmonary toilet in, 389
radiographic appearance of, 383f
radiography of, 383f
severity of, 400
surfactant for, 293-294, 389-390
survival rates for, 384t-385t, 386-388, 387t
Congenital heart disease
bronchopulmonary dysplasia and, 412
congenital diaphragmatic hernia and, 399-400

Congenital pneumonia, surfactant for, 293
Connective tissue growth factor (CTGF)
in bronchopulmonary dysplasia, 17f, 18, 40
in lung development, 18
in lung injury, 40
Continuous distending pressure, for respiratory distress syndrome, 271, 271f-272f
Continuous gas insufflation, 358
Continuous positive airway pressure (CPAP)
bubble, 275
historical perspective on, 266-267
for respiratory distress syndrome, criteria for, 60
in resuscitation, 252
surfactant and, 272, 288-289, 291-292
INSURE technique and, 290
with nasal CPAP, 272
vs. mechanical ventilation, 168
vs. oxygen therapy, for convalescent preterm infants, 318
weaning from, 277
Copper, dietary, 165t, 174
Copper/zinc superoxide dismutase, 95
for bronchopulmonary dysplasia, 223
Cor pulmonale, in pulmonary hypertension, in bronchopulmonary dysplasia, 419-421, 420b
Coronary perfusion pressure, in resuscitation, 258
Corticosteroids
antenatal, 60-64
adverse effects of, 64
for bronchopulmonary dysplasia, 61
for cesarean section, 64, 64t
for chorioamnionitis, 78-80, 78t, 79f-81f
for congenital diaphragmatic hernia, 400-401
for IUGR/SGA infants, 83
pneumothorax and, 61
pulmonary effects of, 60-61, 61t, 62f
regimens for, 61-64
for respiratory distress syndrome, 60-64
second courses of, 63-64
trials of, 63-64, 63t-64t
for bronchopulmonary dysplasia, 226-227, 418-419
antenatal administration of, 61
inhaled, 227
postnatal administration of, 226-227
cerebral palsy and, 227, 358
for patent ductus arteriosus, 182-183
for ventilator weaning, 357-358
Cortisol
in chorioamnionitis, 73, 73t
fetal stress and, 81
Cross-tolerance, 76-78
Cryotherapy, for retinopathy of prematurity, 316
Culture
amniotic fluid, 65
amniotic membrane, 65
Cu/Zn superoxide dismutase, 95
for bronchopulmonary dysplasia, 223
Cyclic guanosine monophosphate (cGMP)
in hyperoxia, 99-100
in lung development, 116-117, 116f
nitric oxide and, 124
Cyclic guanosine monophosphate modulators, for pulmonary hypertension, 103
Cysteine, supplemental, 175
Cytidylyltransferase-α, 31
Cytokines
in bronchopulmonary dysplasia, 144-148
in chorioamnionitis, 67-68
overexpression of, lung development and, 139-140
in respiratory distress syndrome, 39
in *Ureaplasma* infection, 144-148
Cytomegalovirus infection, bronchopulmonary dysplasia and, 151, 220

D

Dead space reduction, in ventilator weaning, 358
Deafness
and congenital diaphragmatic hernia, 400
pancuronium and, 400
sildenafil and, 397
Dexamethasone. *See also* Corticosteroids.
for bronchopulmonary dysplasia, 226-227
Diaphragm, undernutrition effects on, 167t, 168
Diaphragmatic hernia. *See* Congenital diaphragmatic hernia.
Diuretics, for bronchopulmonary dysplasia, 417-418
Drying and stimulation, in resuscitation, 250
Ductal shunts. *See* Shunts.
Dystroglycan, in bronchopulmonary dysplasia, 43-44

E

Echocardiography, of pulmonary hypertension
in bronchopulmonary dysplasia, 419, 420b
in congenital diaphragmatic hernia, 393-396
ECMO (extracorporeal membrane oxygen support), for congenital diaphragmatic hernia, 384t-385t, 387t, 390-392
Edema, pulmonary, patent ductus arteriosus and, 183-185
Elastic fiber density, *Ureaplasma* infection and, 144-145, 145f
Elastin, in alveologenesis, 11-12, 12f
Embryonic stage, of lung development, 4, 5f
Embryonic stem cells, 198-199
endogenous, 198-199
exogenous, 199-200
EME Infant Flow Nasal CPAP device, 274, 274f
Emphysema, nutritional, 167
Endoglin, 18-19
in bronchopulmonary dysplasia, 220-221
Endothelial colony-forming cells
in bronchopulmonary dysplasia, 220-221
therapeutic uses of, 200
Endothelial nitric oxide synthase, 31
in respiratory distress syndrome, 38
Endothelial progenitor cells, 202. *See also* Stem cell(s).
Endothelin receptor antagonists, for pulmonary hypertension, in bronchopulmonary dysplasia, 419-420
Endothelin-1, in patent ductus arteriosus, 185-186
Endothelin-1 receptor antagonists, for pulmonary hypertension, in congenital diaphragmatic hernia, 397-398
Endotoxin, antenatal, in bronchopulmonary dysplasia, 407-408
Endotoxin tolerance, 76-78

Endotracheal intubation, 252-254, 253f, 253t. *See also* Mechanical ventilation.
after failed nasal CPAP, 277
postextubation care and, nasal CPAP in, 267, 268f
with nasal IPPV, 268-270, 269f
routine, vs. nasal CPAP, 272-273
for surfactant administration, 290
vs. nasal CPAP, 273
vs. noninvasive respiratory support, 266
Energy intake, 165t, 170
Enteral nutrition, guidelines for, 165t. *See also* Nutritional support.
Enteroviral infection, bronchopulmonary dysplasia and, 151
Ephrins, in vascular development, 15
Epidermal growth factor receptor, 31
Epinephrine, in resuscitation, 258-259
Epithelial growth factor, in bronchopulmonary dysplasia, 221
Epithelial-endothelial interaction
in alveologenesis, 5f, 12-13, 17f, 111-114, 113f, 113t
in angiogenesis, 111-115, 113f, 113t
VEGF in, 114
Epithelial-vascular interactions, in lung development, 112-114
Epithelium-mesenchyme interactions, in branching morphogenesis, 8-11
Epoprostenol, for pulmonary hypertension, in congenital diaphragmatic hernia, 396-397
ErbB4, 32
Erythromycin, for *Ureaplasma* infection, 150
Erythropoietin, in bronchopulmonary dysplasia, 221
Escherichia coli, bronchopulmonary dysplasia and, 150-151
Esophageal catheter, in neurally adjusted ventilatory assist, 375
$ETCO_2$, during cardiac compressions, 258
Exercise tolerance, 240
EXIT procedure, for congenital diaphragmatic hernia, 391
Extracellular matrix, in lung development, 8-11
Extracorporeal membrane oxygen support (ECMO), for congenital diaphragmatic hernia, 384t-385t, 387t, 390-392
Extrauterine growth restriction/retardation, 163
bronchopulmonary dysplasia and, 167
definition of, 166
undernutrition and, 163, 166
Extubation, in ventilator weaning, 358. *See also* Mechanical ventilation, weaning from.
criteria for, 361-362, 362t
Eyes absent (Eya), 32

F

Face masks, 251
Factor VII, in bronchopulmonary dysplasia, 46
Factor XIII, in bronchopulmonary dysplasia, 46
Fas-ligand, in lung injury, 40
Fat emulsions, 165t, 171-172
for bronchopulmonary dysplasia, 225-226
Fatty acids, 165t, 171-172
Fetal hemoglobin, 304f-305f, 305-306
in fetal-to-neonatal transition, 307
Fetal inflammatory response, in chorioamnionitis, 68t, 137, 139-140
Fetal lung, in fetal-to-neonatal transition, 3. *See also* Transitional pulmonary vasculature.
Fetal membranes
culture of, 65
rupture of
chorioamnionitis and, 67-69. *See also* Chorioamnionitis.
respiratory distress syndrome and, 67-69
Ureaplasma infection and, 141-142, 143t
Fetal nutrient transfer, 164
Fetal oxygenation
critical threshold of, 306
during fetal-to-neonatal transition, 306-308
monitoring of, 306
Fetal P_{50}, 304f-305f, 305-306
Fetal partial pressure of oxygen (PO_2), 304f, 305-306
Fetal pulse oximetry, 306
Fetal pulse oxygen saturation ($FSpO_2$), 306
Fetal shunts. *See* Shunts.
Fetal-to-neonatal transition. *See also* Transitional pulmonary vasculature.
fetal hemoglobin in, 307
fetal lung in, 3
fetal oxygenation in, 306-308
hyperoxia in, 98-102
nitric oxide in, 125
oxygenation during, 306-308
transitional goal oxygen saturation in, 254, 254t
Fibroblast growth factor(s) (FGFs)
in bronchopulmonary dysplasia, 221
in lung development, 7, 32
in alveologenesis, 12, 12f
in branching morphogenesis, 8, 9f
in vascular development, 14, 113t, 114-115
in lung injury, 40
Fibroblast growth factor 3, in lung injury, 40
Fibroblast growth factor 4, in lung injury, 40
Fibroblast growth factor 8, 32
Fibroblast growth factor 18, 32
Fibroblast growth factor receptor 2, in lung injury, 40
Fibrocytes, 208-209
FIO_2, in oxygen therapy, 332-333, 333f
automatic adjustment of, 375-378, 377f-378f
Fish oil, 172
Fisher & Paykel Optiflow system, 277-278
Flk-1, 14
Flow-inflating bags, for positive-pressure ventilation, 248, 251
Flt-1, 14
Fluid intake, 165t, 170-171
Fluid resuscitation, 259-260. *See also* Resuscitation.
Fluticasone. *See also* Corticosteroids.
for bronchopulmonary dysplasia, 418-419
Forced flows, in bronchopulmonary dysplasia, 410
Forkhead box f1 (Foxf1), 32
Forkhead box m1 (Foxm1), 32
Fractures, rib, undernutrition and, 168-169
$FSpO_2$ (fetal pulse oxygen saturation), 306
Functional residual capacity, in bronchopulmonary dysplasia, 410
Funisitis, 65, 67
Furosemide, for bronchopulmonary dysplasia, 417-418

G

Gas exchange, nitric oxide in, 125
Gas leaks, in ventilator weaning, 358
Gasping, 250, 250f

Gastric aspirate analysis, for respiratory distress syndrome prediction, 294-295
Gastric aspiration, ventilator-associated pneumonia and, 153-154
Gastric decompression, in congenital diaphragmatic hernia, 382-383, 383f
Gastroesophageal reflux
  in bronchopulmonary dysplasia, 413-414, 419
  sildenafil and, 397
Gata6, 32-33
Genetic influences, 29-55
  animal models of, 29-37, 39-42
  in bronchopulmonary dysplasia, 42-50, 222
    adhesion molecules, 43-44
    angiotensin-converting enzyme, 46
    animal models of, 39-42
    antioxidants, 44
    ATP-binding cassette transporter A3, 46
    candidate genes, 43-47, 48t-49t
    clinical context for, 42-50
    dystroglycan, 43-44
    factor VII, 46
    factor XIII, 46
    glutathione-S-transferase, 44
    human leukocyte antigen A2, 46
    inflammatory mediators, 44-45
    insulin-like growth factor-1, 47
    interferon-γ, 44
    interleukin-4, 44
    interleukin-10, 44
    macrophage migration inhibitory factor, 45
    mannose-binding lectin 2, 44-45
    matrix metalloproteinase-16, 47
    5,10-methylenetetrahydrofolate reductase, 47
    microsomal epoxide hydrolases, 44
    monocyte chemoattractant protein-1, 45
    L-selectin, 44
    surfactant proteins, 45-46
    transforming growth factor-ß1, 45
    transporter associated with antigen processing, 47
    tumor necrosis factor, 45
    twin studies of, 43
    urokinase, 47
    VEGF, 47
  in lung development
    animal models of, 29-37
    ATP-binding cassette transporter A3, 29-37
    bone morphogenetic proteins, 30
    CARM1, 30
    ß-catenin, 30
    CCAAT enhancer-binding protein α, 31
    cytidylyltransferase-α, 31
    endothelial nitric oxide synthase, 31
    epidermal growth factor receptor, 31
    ErbB4, 32
    eyes absent, 32
    fibroblast growth factor 8, 32
    fibroblast growth factor 18, 32
    forkhead box f1, 32
    forkhead box m1, 32
    Gata6, 32-33
    GlcNac *N*-deacetylase/*N*-sulfotransferase-1, 34
    glucocorticoid receptor, 33
    G-protein–coupled receptor 4, 33
    hepatocyte nuclear factor-3ß, 33
    homeobox a-5, 33
    Kruppel-like factor, 33
Genetic influences *(Continued)*
    lysophosphatidylcholine acyltransferase 1, 34
    macrophage migration inhibitory factor, 34
    Nmyc, 34
    phenotype expression and, 36-37
    platelet-derived growth factor-A, 34
    platelet-derived growth factor-C, 34
    prophet of Pit 1, 34-35
    Pten, 35
    respiratory distress syndrome and, 37-39. *See also* Respiratory distress syndrome (RDS).
    retinoic acid receptor ß, 35
    sonic hedgehog, 35
    surfactant protein-B, 35
    thyroid transcription factor-1, 35
    transforming growth factor-ß receptor II, 36
    transforming growth factor-ß1, 35
    transforming growth factor-ß3, 36
    VEGF, 36
    wingless-Int7b, 36
  in lung injury, 39-42
    angiopoietin 1, 39
    animal models of, 39-42
    CTGF, 40
    Fas-ligand, 40
    fibroblast growth factor receptor 2, 40
    fibroblast growth factors 3 and 4, 40
    interferon-γ, 40
    interleukin-1ß, 40
    interleukin-6, 41
    interleukin-11, 41
    platelet-derived growth factor-A, 41
    stroma-derived factor 1, 41
    Thy-1 (CD90), 41
    thyroid transcription factor-1, 42
    tissue inhibitor of metalloproteinase 3, 41
    transforming growth factor-α, 41-42
    transforming growth factor-ß1, 42
    VEGF, 42
  in respiratory distress syndrome, 37-39
Genital mycoplasmas. *See also Ureaplasma* infection.
  lung injury and, 140-150
Gentle ventilation, 224-225
Gestational age
  bronchopulmonary dysplasia and, 218f, 220
  fetal lung development and, 58-59, 58f
    inflammation and, 73
  patent ductus arteriosus treatment and, 182, 182f
GlcNac *N*-deacetylase/*N*-sulfotransferase-1, 34
Gli genes, in lung development, 7
Glucocorticoid receptor, in lung development, 33
Glucose, recommended intake of, 165t, 171
Glutamine, supplemental, 175
Glutathione
  endogenous, as antioxidant, 310
  exogenous, for bronchopulmonary dysplasia, 223-224
Glutathione peroxidase, 95
Glutathione-S-transferase, in bronchopulmonary dysplasia, 44
N-G-monomethyl-L-arginine (L-NMMA), nitric oxide synthase and, 123
"Golden minute", 248
G-protein–coupled receptor A, in respiratory distress syndrome, 38

G-protein–coupled receptor 4, 33
Granulocyte macrophage colony-stimulating factor, in bronchopulmonary dysplasia, 221
Graseby pressure capsule, 343
Gremlin 1, 30
Group B streptococcal pneumonia, surfactant for, 293
Growth factors. *See also specific factors.*
  in bronchopulmonary dysplasia, 220-221
Growth restriction, extrauterine, 163
Growth retardation. *See* Intrauterine growth restriction (IUGR); Small for gestational age (SGA).
Guanosine monophosphate (GMP), in hyperoxia, 99-100
Guanosine monophosphate modulators, for pulmonary hypertension, 103
Guanosine triphosphate–cyclohydrolase (GTP-CH1), 102-103
Guanylate cyclase, soluble, in lung development, 116-117, 116f

H

Haemophilus influenzae infection, bronchopulmonary dysplasia and, 150-151
Hand hygiene, ventilator-associated pneumonia and, 154
Hearing loss
  and congenital diaphragmatic hernia, 400
  pancuronium and, 400
  sildenafil and, 397
Heart disease, congenital
  bronchopulmonary dysplasia and, 412
  congenital diaphragmatic hernia and, 399-400
Heart rate
  in initial assessment, 248
  in positive-pressure ventilation, 251-252
Heat loss prevention, 248-250
Hematopoietic stem cells, 197-198, 201-202. *See also* Stem cell(s).
Hemoglobin, fetal, 304f-305f, 305-306
  in fetal-to-neonatal transition, 307
Hemoglobin P_{50}, 304f-305f, 305-306
Hemorrhage, pulmonary
  patent ductus arteriosus and, 183-185
  surfactant for, 294
Hepatic nuclear factors, 124
Hepatocyte growth factor, in alveologenesis, 12-13
Hepatocyte nuclear factor-3ß, 33
Hering-Breuer reflex, infant-ventilator asynchrony and, 340-342, 340f
HIF-1α, nitric oxide synthase and, 124
High-flow nasal cannula (HFNC) ventilation, 277-278. *See also* Noninvasive respiratory support.
High-frequency ventilation, 224-225
  oscillatory, for congenital diaphragmatic hernia, 386, 391-392
    with ECMO, 391-392
  weaning from, 361
High-resolution computed tomography, in bronchopulmonary dysplasia, 410-411, 411f
Homeobox a-5, 33
Human amniotic fluid–derived surfactant, 285. *See also* Surfactant.
Human leukocyte antigen A2, in bronchopulmonary dysplasia, 46
Hydrocortisone. *See also* Corticosteroids.
  for bronchopulmonary dysplasia, 227
Hydrogen peroxide, 91-92, 95, 99-100
Hypercapnia, permissive, in ventilator weaning, 357
Hypercarbia, retinopathy of prematurity and, 310
Hyperoxia, 98-102, 254-255. *See also* Oxygen toxicity.
  brain injury and, 310-311, 316-317
  bronchopulmonary dysplasia and, 221, 311. *See also* Bronchopulmonary dysplasia.
  chronic, 101-102
  endothelial progenitor stem cells and, 202
  lung development and, 169
  mesenchymal stem cells and, 202-203, 203f
  monitoring for, 302f, 303
  prevention of, fatty acids for, 165t, 172
  reactive oxygen species and, 169
  retinopathy of prematurity and, 307f, 308-310. *See also* Retinopathy of prematurity.
  short-term effects of, 98-101, 99f
  sildenafil for, 103, 104f
  undernutrition and, 167t, 169
Hypertension
  pulmonary. *See* Pulmonary hypertension.
  systemic, in bronchopulmonary dysplasia, 412
Hyperthermia, 249-250
Hyperventilation, for congenital diaphragmatic hernia, 383
Hypotension, management of, 258-260
Hypothermia, prevention of, 248-250
Hypoventilation, in mechanical ventilation, 329-331, 330f
Hypovolemia, in resuscitation, 259-260
Hypoxemia. *See also* Hypoxia.
  in mechanical ventilation, 329-337
    behavioral disturbances and, 330-331, 333
    clinical outcomes and, 334-335
    FIO_2 and, 332-333, 333f
    lung development and, 335
    mechanisms of, 329-331, 330f
    postextubation, 333-334, 334f
    retinopathy of prematurity and, 335
    supplemental oxygen in, 332-333, 333f
    vascular development and, 335
    ventilatory strategies for, 331-332, 332f
Hypoxia, 96-98. *See also* Hypoxemia.
  acute vasoconstriction due to, 96
  in bronchopulmonary dysplasia, 221
  chronic, pulmonary hypertension and, 96-98
  resuscitation for, hyperoxia and, 98-101, 99f-100f
  retinopathy of prematurity and, 307f, 309-310
Hypoxia-inducible factors (HIFs), 36
  in bronchopulmonary dysplasia, 102
  in hyperoxia, 97
  nitric oxide and, 117, 124
  in pulmonary hypertension, 97
Hypoxic-ischemic encephalopathy, 260

I

Idiopathic pulmonary hypertension. *See* Pulmonary hypertension.
Iloprost, for pulmonary hypertension, in congenital diaphragmatic hernia, 398

Imaging studies
of bronchopulmonary dysplasia, 407-408, 408f, 410-411, 411f
of congenital diaphragmatic hernia, 383f
Immune response
in bronchopulmonary dysplasia, 148-149
in chorioamnionitis, 72-73, 73t, 76-78, 77f
undernutrition and, 169
in *Ureaplasma* infection, 148-149
Indomethacin, for patent ductus arteriosus, 184-185, 187-188
Induced pluripotent stem cells, 200
Infant Flow Driver, 274-275, 274f
Infant-ventilator asynchrony, 340-342, 340f-341f. *See also* Mechanical ventilation, infant-ventilator interaction in.
Infections
antenatal, 65-84, 135-151. *See also* Chorioamnionitis.
in animal models, 69-72, 70f-71f
bronchopulmonary dysplasia and, 135-151, 219-220. *See also* Bronchopulmonary dysplasia, chorioamnionitis and.
causative organisms in, 65-66, 135-137
clinical outcomes in, 67-69, 68t, 69f, 137-139
immune response in, 72-73, 73t, 76-78, 77f
overview of, 65
types of, 65
postnatal, bronchopulmonary dysplasia and, 151-155, 220
susceptibility to, undernutrition and, 167t, 169
Infertility, *Ureaplasma* infection and, 141-142, 143t
Inflammation
adrenal insufficiency and, 184-185
antenatal. *See* Antenatal inflammation.
in bronchopulmonary dysplasia, 139-140, 144-148, 184-185, 219-220
in chorioamnionitis, 68t, 137, 139-140
in congenital diaphragmatic hernia, 386-387
cytokines in. *See* Cytokines.
lung development and, 139-140
patent ductus arteriosus and, 184-185
Inositol
for bronchopulmonary dysplasia, 226
supplemental, 175
Insulin-like growth factor-1
in bronchopulmonary dysplasia, 47, 221
in respiratory muscle, undernutrition and, 168
in retinopathy of prematurity, 307f, 308-310
INSURE technique, 290
Intellectual deficits
hypoxemia and, 334-335
oxygen therapy and, 317
Interferon-γ
in bronchopulmonary dysplasia, 44
in lung injury, 40
Interleukin(s)
in bronchopulmonary dysplasia, 144-148, 145f
in lung development, 140
in lung injury, 41
in lung maturation, 74-75, 74f
in *Ureaplasma* infection, 144-148, 145f
Interleukin-1
in lung development, 140
in lung maturation, 74-75, 74f
Interleukin-1ß, in lung injury, 40
Interleukin-4, in bronchopulmonary dysplasia, 44
Interleukin-6
in lung development, 140
in lung injury, 41
in *Ureaplasma* infection, 146-148
Interleukin-10
in bronchopulmonary dysplasia, 44
in respiratory distress syndrome, 39
in *Ureaplasma* infection, 146-148
Interleukin-11
in lung development, 140
in lung injury, 41
Intermittent mandatory ventilation. *See also* Mechanical ventilation.
infant-ventilator asynchrony in, 340-342, 340f-341f
nasal, 349-351
synchronized, 344
Intermittent positive-pressure ventilation (IPPV)
with intubation. *See* Mechanical ventilation.
nasal. *See* Nasal intermittent positive-pressure ventilation (NIPPV).
Intra-amniotic surfactant, 291
Intratracheal catheter, surfactant administration via, 273-274, 292
Intrauterine growth restriction (IUGR)
antenatal steroids and, 83
bronchopulmonary dysplasia and, 81-83, 82f
lung development and, 83
respiratory distress syndrome and, 81, 82f
sudden infant death syndrome and, 170
Intrauterine infections. *See* Infections, antenatal.
Intravenous therapy, in resuscitation, 259-260
Intubation
endotracheal. *See* Endotracheal intubation.
nasogastric, in congenital diaphragmatic hernia, 382-383, 383f

K

Kruppel-like factor, 33

L

Labor, preterm-onset, *Ureaplasma* infection and, 141-142, 143t
Laryngeal mask airway, 254
Laryngoscopy, 252-254
Laser photocoagulation, for retinopathy of prematurity, 316
Left-to-right shunt. *See also* Shunts.
in patent ductus arteriosus, 183
Lipid emulsions, 165t, 171-172. *See also* Nutritional support.
in bronchopulmonary dysplasia, 225-226
Long-chain polyunsaturated fatty acids, 165t, 171-172
Long-term pulmonary outcomes, 235-243
controversies in, 235-236, 241
for late preterm infants, 236
for very preterm infants, 236-240
exercise tolerance, 240
exogenous surfactant and, 240
rehospitalization rates, 236-237

Long-term pulmonary outcomes *(Continued)*
respiratory problems
in adolescence and early adulthood, 238-240, 238t
in infancy and early childhood, 237
in later childhood, 237-238, 237t
smoking and, 240
Lucinactant, 285-286, 285t. *See also* Surfactant.
Lung
connective tissue scaffold of, 168
fetal, during fetal-to-neonatal transition, 3. *See also* Fetal-to-neonatal transition.
Lung bioengineering, 205-206
Lung bud initiation, 6-7
Lung compliance, in bronchopulmonary dysplasia, 408-409
assessment of, 409
Lung development, 3-27. *See also* Lung maturation.
alveolar septation in, 11-12, 12f
timing of, 58-59
branching morphogenesis in, 8-11, 9f, 111-112
in congenital diaphragmatic hernia, 381-382
connective tissue growth factor in, 18
cytokine overexpression and, 139-140
disruption of, 16-20
in bronchopulmonary dysplasia, 220-221
environmental factors in, 83-84
epithelial-endothelial crosstalk in, 12-13, 17f, 111-114, 113f, 113t
fetal, conceptual age and, 58-59, 58f
functional events in, 58-59
genetic influences in, 29-55. *See also* Genetic influences.
hyperoxia and, 101-102, 169
increased pulmonary blood flow and, 185-186
inflammation and, 139-140
in IUGR/SGA infants, 81-83
lung bud initiation in, 6-7
lung maturation and, 59-60
maternal alcohol use and, 84
maternal smoking and, 83-84
modulating factors in, 57, 58f
nitric oxide in, 111-114
branching morphogenesis and, 117
epithelial-endothelial crosstalk and, 111-116, 113f, 113t
oxygen tension and, 124
nitric oxide synthase in, oxygen tension and, 124
overview of, 3-4, 111-114
oxygen tension and, 124
perinatal events and, 57-90
gestational age and, 58-59, 58f
lung maturation and, 59-60
as substrate for adverse events, 58-59
postnatal, 3
hypoxemia and, 335
perinatal factors affecting, 57-90
pulmonary hypertension and, 185-186
signaling in, 6-7. *See also* Signaling.
bronchopulmonary dysplasia and, 125-126
stages of, 4-6, 5f, 29
alveolar, 6, 11-13, 12f, 17f, 29
canalicular, 5-6, 29
embryonic, 4, 29
pseudoglandular, 5, 29
saccular, 6, 29
structural events in, 58-59
Lung development *(Continued)*
tracheal-esophageal separation in, 6-7, 7f
undernutrition and, 166-167, 167t, 169
Ureaplasma infection and, 146, 147f
vascular. *See* Vascular development.
Lung function, undernutrition and, 168-169
Lung growth, compensatory, nitric oxide in, 117-121
Lung hypoplasia, in congenital diaphragmatic hernia, 381-382, 390-391
Lung imaging
in bronchopulmonary dysplasia, 407-408, 408f, 410-411, 411f
in congenital diaphragmatic hernia, 383f
Lung injury
genetic influences in, 39-42. *See also* Genetic influences, in lung injury.
neonatal. *See* Bronchopulmonary dysplasia.
stem cell therapy for, 202-203, 203f. *See also* Stem cell therapy.
Lung maturation, 59-60. *See also* Lung development.
antenatal inflammation and
animal models of, 69-72, 70f-71f
in chronic chorioamnionitis, 75-76, 76f
gestational age and, 73
immune response in, 72-73, 73t
antenatal steroids and, 60-64, 61t, 62f
evaluation of, 60
in growth restricted/small for gestational age infants, 81-83
inflammatory mediators in, 72-73, 73t
maternal smoking and, 83-84
Lung progenitor cells, 206-207, 206f, 208f
Lung repair, nitric oxide in, 117-123, 120f
Lung stem cells, 206-207, 206f, 208f
Lung surface area, in bronchopulmonary dysplasia, 409
Lung volume(s)
in bronchopulmonary dysplasia, 410
loss of, in mechanical ventilation, 329-331, 330f
Lysophosphatidylcholine acyltransferase 1, 34

M

Macrophage migration inhibitory factor, 34
in bronchopulmonary dysplasia, 45
Magnesium, for bronchopulmonary dysplasia, 223-224
Malnutrition. *See* Undernutrition.
Mandatory minute ventilation, 362-363, 372
weaning from, 362-363
Manganese, 165t, 174-175
dietary, 165t, 174-175
Mannose-binding lectin 2, in bronchopulmonary dysplasia, 44-45
Masks, face, 251
Matrix metalloproteins (MMPs), in bronchopulmonary dysplasia, 19-20, 47
Mb antigen, 141
Mechanical ventilation
adaptive mechanical backup, 372
adverse effects of, 266
air leaks in
infant-ventilator asynchrony and, 340-341
pneumothorax and, in congenital diaphragmatic hernia, 388
apnea backup, 372

Mechanical ventilation (*Continued*)
automatic, 367-380. *See also specific types.*
weaning from, 362-363, 369-371
supplemental oxygen and, 363
for bronchopulmonary dysplasia, 415-417, 415t, 416f
long-term, 414
tracheostomy for, 413-414
bronchopulmonary dysplasia due to, 217-218, 224-225. *See also* Bronchopulmonary dysplasia.
duration of
factors affecting, 368
pneumonia and, 152-153
forceful exhalations in, 329-331
gentle, 224-225
high-frequency, 224-225
oscillatory, for congenital diaphragmatic hernia, 386, 391-392
weaning from, 361
historical perspective on, 266-267
hypoventilation in, 329-331, 330f
hypoxemia in, 329-337. *See also* Hypoxemia.
infant-ventilator interaction in, 339-354, 340f-341f
asynchrony in, 340-342
in conventional mechanical ventilation, 339-342
in noninvasive ventilation, 349-351
in synchronized ventilation, 345-349
intermittent mandatory
infant-ventilator asynchrony in, 340-342, 340f-341f
nasal, 349-351
synchronized, 344
lung volume loss in, 329-331, 330f
mandatory minute, 362-363, 372
weaning from, 362-363
neurally adjusted ventilatory assist, 374-375
oxygen saturation in, 329-333, 330f
pneumonia and. *See* Ventilator-associated pneumonia.
postextubation care in, nasal CPAP in, 267, 268f
with nasal IPPV, 268-270, 269f
pressure-regulated–volume controlled, 369
pressure-support, 224-225, 344-345
in congenital diaphragmatic hernia, 389
proportional assist, 224-225, 373-374
respiratory distress syndrome and, 59-60
supplemental oxygen in. *See* Oxygen therapy.
supplemental vs. controlling, 342
surfactant administration during, 290
alternatives to, 291-292
synchronized, 342-349
advantages of, 342
airway pressure in, 343-344, 344f
assist/control, 344, 345f
autocycling in, 347-348
automatic termination in, 346-347, 347f
delayed triggering in, 347
end-inspiratory asynchrony in, 345-347
excessive PEEP in, 349
excessive/insufficient circuit flow in, 348
flow sensors for, 343, 343f
Graseby pressure capsule for, 343
intermittent mandatory, 344
limitations of, 345-349
long inspiration time in, 345-347, 346f
methods of, 342-344

Mechanical ventilation (*Continued*)
modalities of, 344-345
nasal, 349-351, 351f-352f
negative infant ventilator interaction in, 345-349
neurally adjusted ventilatory assist in, 374-375
peak inspiratory pressure, 348
pressure-support, 344-345
synchronized intermittent mandatory ventilation, 344
trigger failure in, 347
variable inspiration time in, 346-347, 347f
weaning from, 358-361, 359f-360f
targeted minute, 371-372, 372f-374f
weaning from, 362-363
Ureaplasma infection and, 144-148, 145f, 147f
volume guarantee, 368-369
volume-controlled, 224-225, 369
pressure-regulated, 369
volume-targeted, 224-225, 368-371, 369f-370f
hypoxemia and, 331-332
weaning from, 362, 369-370
vs. CPAP, 168
weaning from, 355-365, 368
automatic, 362-363, 369-371
supplemental oxygen and, 363
computer-assisted, 363
in congenital diaphragmatic hernia, 384t-385t, 386-387, 387t
continuous gas insufflation in, 358
continuous gas leaks in, 358
criteria for, 361-362, 362t
dead space reduction in, 358
FIO_2 in, 356
graduated steps in, 356
in high-frequency ventilation, 361
indications for, 361-362, 362t
mandatory minute ventilation in, 362-363
modes of ventilation and, 358-361
oxygen saturation in, 356
parameters for, 355-358
peak inspiratory pressure in, 356
PEEP in, 356
permissive hypercapnia in, 357
postextubation CPAP in
nasal, 267, 268f, 360
vs. intermittent ventilation, 358
postextubation nasal ventilation in, 360-361
pulse oximetry in, 356
respiratory center stimulants for, 357
spontaneous breathing test for, 361
steroids for, 357-358
strategies for, 361-362, 362t
from supplemental oxygen, 363
in synchronized ventilation, 358-361, 359f-360f
in targeted minute ventilation, 362-363
ventilator rate in, 356
from ventilator settings, 355-358
in volume-targeted ventilation, 362, 369-370
Meconium aspiration, surfactant for, 292-293
Meconium staining, airway management in, 250
Mesenchymal stem cells, 201-202. *See also* Stem cell(s).
therapeutic uses of, 200-205, 203f. *See also* Stem cell therapy.
for bronchopulmonary dysplasia, 228

Metabolic acidosis, bicarbonate for, 260
Metabolic bone disease, undernutrition and, 168-169
5,10-Methylenetetrahydrofolate reductase, in bronchopulmonary dysplasia, 47
Methylprednisolone. *See also* Corticosteroids.
  for bronchopulmonary dysplasia, 418-419
Methylxanthines
  for bronchopulmonary dysplasia, 218-222, 228, 418
  for patent ductus arteriosus, 189
Microsomal epoxide hydrolases, in bronchopulmonary dysplasia, 44
Milrinone, for pulmonary hypertension, in congenital diaphragmatic hernia, 396-397
Mitochondrial electron transport chain, 92-93
Mn superoxide dismutase, 95
Monocyte chemoattractant protein-1, 144-145
  in bronchopulmonary dysplasia, 45
Morgagni hernia, 382
MRSOPA mnemonic, 251-252
Mucous plugging, in congenital diaphragmatic hernia, 389
Multipotent stem cells, 197-198, 198f. *See also* Stem cell(s).
Muscles, respiratory, undernutrition and, 168
Mycoplasma genitalium, 140
Mycoplasma hominis chorioamnionitis, 65-66, 140
Mycoplasmas, genital. *See also Ureaplasma* infection.
  lung injury and, 140-150
Myofibroblasts, in alveologenesis, 11-12, 12f

N

NADPH oxidases. *See also under* Nox.
  reactive oxygen species and, 92-93
Nasal cannulas
  high-flow, 277-278
    for bronchopulmonary dysplasia, 414
  for nasal CPAP, 274-275, 274f-275f, 414
  skin trauma from, 276
Nasal continuous positive airway pressure (NCPAP). *See also* Noninvasive respiratory support.
  for apnea of prematurity, 266, 270
  for bronchopulmonary dysplasia, 414
  complications of, 276-277
  devices for, 274-275, 274f-275f
    trauma from, 276
  failure of, 277
  historical perspective on, 266-267
  infant-ventilator interaction in, 349-351
  postextubation, 267, 268f, 360
    with nasal IPPV, 268-270, 269f
  prophylactic surfactant and, 288-289
  for respiratory distress syndrome, 270-274
    continuous distending pressure and, 271, 271f-272f
    rationale for, 270-271
    surfactant administration and, 272-274
    in "surfactant era", 272
    vs. brief early intubation for surfactant, 273
  supporting pressure in, 275-276, 276f
  vs. high-flow nasal cannulas, 278
  vs. routine intubation, 272-273
  weaning from, 277
Nasal intermittent positive-pressure ventilation (NIPPV). *See also* Noninvasive respiratory support.
  in apnea of prematurity, 270
  infant-ventilator interaction in, 349-351
  with nasal CPAP, 268-270, 269f
  postextubation, 268-270, 269f
  in respiratory distress syndrome, 270
Nasal ventilation, postextubation, 360-361
Nasogastric decompression, in congenital diaphragmatic hernia, 382-383, 383f
Nasopharyngeal surfactant, 291
Near infra-red spectroscopy, in fetal oxygenation monitoring, 306
Nebulized surfactant, 291-292
Neonatal lung injury. *See* Bronchopulmonary dysplasia.
Neonatal resuscitation. *See* Resuscitation.
Neurally adjusted ventilatory assist, 374-375
Neurologic complications
  of hypoxemia, 334-335
  of oxygen therapy, 310-311
    clinical outcomes and, 316-317
  of steroids, 227, 358
Neuromuscular blockade, for congenital diaphragmatic hernia, 382-383
Niches, 198-199
Nitric oxide, 111-132. *See also* Reactive oxygen species (ROS).
  in air-blood interface maintenance, 121, 125
  in alveologenesis, 12-13, 111-114, 113f, 113t
  in angiogenesis, 12-13, 111-114
    angiogenic factors and receptors and, 113f, 113t, 114-115
  biologic availability of, 124
  in bronchopulmonary dysplasia, 117-121, 120f, 220-221
  cGMP and, 124
  expression of, 115-116
  in gas exchange, 125
  in hyperoxia
    acute, 98-101, 99f
    chronic, 94
  hypoxia-inducible factors and, 117, 124
  inhaled
    for bronchopulmonary dysplasia, 117-121, 120f, 126-128, 127t, 128f, 225, 419-420, 420b
    for pulmonary hypertension, 103, 419-420, 420b
      in bronchopulmonary dysplasia, 419-420, 420b
      in congenital diaphragmatic hernia, 387t, 394-396
  isoforms of, 115-116
  in lung development, 111-114
    branching morphogenesis and, 117
    epithelial-endothelial crosstalk and, 111-116, 113f, 113t
    oxygen tension and, 124
  in lung repair, 117-123, 120f
    in bronchopulmonary dysplasia, 117-123, 120f
    in nitric oxide synthase regulation, 121-123
  neurotoxicity of, 310
  in respiratory distress syndrome, 121
  superoxide dismutase and, 95, 124
  tetrahydrobiopterin and, 102-103
  transitional pulmonary vasculature and, 125
  in *Ureaplasma* infection, 146-148
  in VEGF-mediated angiogenesis, 12-13, 117

Nitric oxide synthase (NOS), 94, 97
L-arginine and, 103, 123
BH_4 and, 123
in bronchopulmonary dysplasia, 97, 220-221
catalytic function of, 121-123, 122f
HIF-1α and, 124
in lung development, 115-117, 116f, 118f, 121
in lung repair, 117-123, 122f
in nitric oxide synthesis, 115-116
oxygen tension and, 124
in pulmonary hypertension, 97, 102-103
TGF-ß and, 124
Nkx2.1, 6-7
Nmyc, 34
Noninvasive respiratory support, 265-282
for apnea of prematurity, 266, 270
benefits of, 266
high-flow nasal cannula ventilation in, 277-278
historical perspective on, 266-267
infant-ventilator interaction in, 349-351
nasal CPAP in. *See* Nasal continuous positive airway pressure (NCPAP).
nasal IPPV in. *See* Nasal intermittent positive-pressure ventilation (NIPPV).
vs. intubation, 266
Nox enzymes, 93-94
in bronchopulmonary dysplasia, 101
in chronic hyperoxia, 101
isoforms of, 93-94
in pulmonary hypertension, 96-97
Nox1, 93
Nox2, 93
Nox4, 93-94
Nuclear factor κB
hyperoxia and, 101
in *Ureaplasma* infection, 146-148
Nutrition, 163-180
bronchopulmonary dysplasia and, 163-164, 167
carbohydrates and, 165t, 171
energy intake and, 165t, 170
extrauterine growth restriction and, 163, 166
fats and, 165t, 171-172
fetal nutrient transfer and, 164
fluid intake and, 165t, 170-171
inadequate, 166-170. *See also* Undernutrition.
macronutrients and, 165t, 171-172
micronutrients and, 165t, 173-175
postnatal, recommendations for, 165t
prenatal, 164-166
fetal nutrient transfer and, 164
recommendations for, 164-166
proteins and, 165t, 172
trace elements and, 165t, 173
vitamins and, 165t, 173-174
Nutritional emphysema, 167
Nutritional support
in bronchopulmonary dysplasia, 225-226, 421
energy requirements for, 165t, 170
fluid intake in, 165t, 170-171
guidelines for, 165t
macronutrients in, 165t, 171-172
micronutrients in, 165t, 173-175

O

Obstetric complications, *Ureaplasma* infection and, 141-142, 143t
Obstetric delivery, by EXIT procedure, for congenital diaphragmatic hernia, 391
Oct-4–positive cells, 206-207
Oils
fish, 172
vegetable, 172
Ototoxicity
of pancuronium, 400
of sildenafil, 397
Oxidant signaling. *See also* Signaling.
acute hypoxic vasoconstriction and, 96
Oxidant stress. *See also* Reactive oxygen species (ROS).
in acute hyperoxia, 98-101
bronchopulmonary dysplasia and, 101-102
in chronic hyperoxia, 101-102
Oxygen
blended, 255
partial pressure of. *See* PO_2.
Oxygen hood, vs. nasal CPAP, in postextubation care, 267, 268f
Oxygen saturation (SpO_2)
fetal pulse, 306
in mechanical ventilation, 329-333, 330f
in weaning, 356
"normal" levels of, 311-312
in oxygen therapy, 96, 98-102, 99f-100f, 254-255, 254t, 316-317. *See also* Oxygen saturation.
automatic adjustment of, 375-378
bronchopulmonary dysplasia and, 222-223
optimal levels of
in neonatal period, 312-315, 312f, 313t
in post-neonatal period, 315-316
randomized trials for, 315-316, 319-323, 322t
shunt closure and, 307-308
vs. oxygen tension, in monitoring, 319-321
Oxygen tension, nitric oxide synthase and, 124
Oxygen therapy, 301-327
automatic adjustment of, 375-378
automatic weaning from, 363
benefits of, 312
blended oxygen in, 255
BOOST Trials for, 315-316, 320-321
for bronchopulmonary dysplasia, 414
complications of. *See* Oxygen toxicity.
controversies in, 317-319
optimal oxygen saturation and postnatal age, 319
oxygen saturation vs. oxygen tension in monitoring, 318-319
oxygen vs. CPAP for convalescent preterm infants, 318
fetal oxygenation and, 305-306, 305f
FIO_2 in, 332-333, 333f
automatic adjustment of, 375-378, 377f-378f
historical perspective on, 301-303
hyperoxia due to, 98-102. *See also* Hyperoxia.
"liberal approach" in, clinical outcomes and, 316-317
morbidity and, 316. *See also* Hypoxemia; Oxygen toxicity.
mortality and, 316
"normal" oxygenation levels in, 311-312
optimal oxygen levels in, 94-95, 312-317, 312f, 313t

Oxygen therapy *(Continued)*
oxygen saturation in. *See* Oxygen saturation (SpO_2), in oxygen therapy.
oxyhemoglobin dissociation curve, 303-305, 304f
P_{50} and, 304f-305f, 305-306
pulse oximetry in, 255, 302f, 303
restrictive oxygen approach in, 313-314, 313t, 314f
clinical outcomes and, 316-317
vs. liberal approach, 312-317, 312f, 313t, 314f
in resuscitation, 254-255
retinopathy of prematurity and. *See* Retinopathy of prematurity.
safe oxygen levels in, 302-303
SUPPORT Trial for, 320-323, 322t
$TcPO_2$ monitoring in, 303
undernutrition and, 169
Oxygen toxicity, 169, 254-255, 308-311. *See also* Hyperoxia.
cerebral, 310-311
ocular, 308-310. *See also* Retinopathy of prematurity.
pulmonary, 311. *See also* Bronchopulmonary dysplasia.
Oxygenation
fetal
critical threshold of, 306
monitoring of, 306
"normal" levels of, 304f, 311-312
during fetal-to-neonatal transition, 306-308
ductal closure and, 307-308
"normal" levels of
for fetuses, 304f, 311-312
for newborns, 311-312
for older infants, 311-312
permissive, in congenital diaphragmatic hernia, 383, 389-390
Oxyhemoglobin dissociation curve, 303-305, 304f

P

P_{50}, 304f-305f, 305-306
Pancuronium
for congenital diaphragmatic hernia, 382-383
ototoxicity of, 400
Pan-cytokeratin stem cells, 208f
Paracrine signaling, in stem cell therapy, 205
Parenteral nutrition. *See also* Nutritional support.
guidelines for, 165t
Partial pressure of oxygen. *See* PO_2.
Patent ductus arteriosus, 181-195
adrenal insufficiency and, 184-185
bronchopulmonary dysplasia and, 171, 186-187, 187f
etiology and pathogenesis of, 181
fluid intake and, 171
incidence of, 181
gestational age and, 182, 182f
infection and, 186-188
oxygen saturation and, 307-308
pulmonary consequences of, 183-186
acute, 183-185
alveolar development, 185-186
inflammation, 184-185
long-term, 185-186
vascular development, 185-186
Patent ductus arteriosus *(Continued)*
respiratory management of, 189-190
respiratory outcome in, 187-189
right-to-left shunt in
management of, 189-190
pulmonary effects of, 183-185
systemic effects of, 183
spontaneous closure in, 188
systemic consequences of, 183
treatment of, 182-183, 187-189
caffeine in, 189
corticosteroids in, 182-183
gestational age and, 182, 182f
indomethacin in, 184-185, 187-188
surfactant in, 183
surgical, 182, 182f, 188-189
Patient-triggered ventilation. *See* Mechanical ventilation, synchronized.
Patient-ventilator interaction. *See* Mechanical ventilation, infant-ventilator interaction in.
PECAM-1, in bronchopulmonary dysplasia, 220-221
Pentoxifylline, for bronchopulmonary dysplasia, 228
Perinatal events, lung development and, 57-90. *See also* Lung development, perinatal events and.
Periventricular leukomalacia, oxygen toxicity and, 310-311
Permissive hypercapnia
in congenital diaphragmatic hernia, 383
in ventilator weaning, 357
Permissive oxygenation, in congenital diaphragmatic hernia, 383, 395-396
Peroxiredoxin, 95
Peroxynitrite, 91-92, 94-95, 100-101, 103-104, 124
Phosphodiesterase, in hyperoxia, 99-101
Phosphodiesterase inhibitors, for pulmonary hypertension, 103
Phosphodiesterase-V, in lung development, 116-117, 116f
Phosphorus, dietary, 165t, 174-175
Photocoagulation, for retinopathy of prematurity, 316
Platelet-activating factor, in patent ductus arteriosus, 184
Platelet-derived growth factor (PDGF), in alveolar septation, 11-12, 12f
Platelet-derived growth factor-A, 34
in lung injury, 41
Platelet-derived growth factor-BB, in bronchopulmonary dysplasia, 221
Platelet-derived growth factor-C, 34
Platelet/endothelial cell adhesion molecule-1 (PECAM-1), in bronchopulmonary dysplasia, 220-221
Pluripotent stem cells, 197-198, 198f. *See also* Stem cell(s).
induced, 200
Pneumonia
chlamydial, bronchopulmonary dysplasia and, 151
congenital, surfactant for, 293
microbiology of, 151
Ureaplasma, 143, 144f, 145-146. *See also* *Ureaplasma* infection.
ventilator-associated. *See* Ventilator-associated pneumonia.
Pneumonitis, *Ureaplasma*, 143, 144f

Pneumothorax
antenatal steroids and, 61
in congenital diaphragmatic hernia, 388
from nasal CPAP, 276-277
PO_2 (partial pressure of oxygen)
fetal, 304f, 305-306
oxyhemoglobin dissociation curve and, 303-305, 304f
transcutaneous measurement of, 303
Polyethylene wrap, for warming, 249-250
Polymyxin B, with surfactant, for meconium aspiration, 292-293
Poractant alfa, 285-286, 285t. *See also* Surfactant.
doses for, 287
Positive end-expiratory pressure (PEEP)
in bronchopulmonary dysplasia, 415-417, 418f
for congenital diaphragmatic hernia, 386, 387t
excessive, 349
for patent ductus arteriosus, 189-190
in weaning, 356
Positive-pressure ventilation. *See* Resuscitation, positive-pressure ventilation in.
Postnatal growth retardation. *See* Extrauterine growth restriction/retardation.
Postnatal weight gain, recommended, 166-167
Premature rupture of membranes. *See* Amniotic membranes, rupture of.
Prenatal conditions. *See under* Antenatal.
Pressure-regulated–volume-controlled ventilation, 369
Pressure-support ventilation, 224-225, 344-345
in congenital diaphragmatic hernia, 389
Preterm birth, *Ureaplasma* infection and, 141-142, 143t
Preterm premature rupture of membranes. *See* Amniotic membranes, rupture of.
Preterm weight gain, recommended, 166-167
Preterm-onset labor, *Ureaplasma* infection and, 141-142, 143t
Proinflammatory cytokines. *See* Cytokines.
Prophet of Pit 1, 34-35
Proportional assist ventilation, 224-225, 373-374
Prostacyclin, for pulmonary hypertension, in congenital diaphragmatic hernia, 396
Prostaglandin E_1, for pulmonary hypertension, in congenital diaphragmatic hernia, 395-396
Protein, dietary, 165t, 172
Pseudoglandular stage, of lung development, 5, 5f
Pseudomonas aeruginosa infection, bronchopulmonary dysplasia and, 150-151
Pten, 35
Pulmonary artery
development of, 111-112. *See also* Vascular development.
in congenital diaphragmatic hernia, 381
remodeling of, in chronic hypoxia, 96-98
Pulmonary artery pressure, in bronchopulmonary dysplasia, 411-412
Pulmonary blood flow, increased, lung development and, 185-186
Pulmonary compliance, in bronchopulmonary dysplasia, 408-409
assessment of, 409
Pulmonary edema, patent ductus arteriosus and, 183-185
Pulmonary fibrosis
bleomycin-induced, 203-204
endothelial progenitor stem cells in, 202
fibrocytes in, 208-209
inflammation and, 139-140
stem cell therapy for, 203-204
Ureaplasma infection and, 144-145, 145f
Pulmonary function tests, in bronchopulmonary dysplasia, 408-409, 413-414
Pulmonary function, undernutrition and, 167t, 168-169
Pulmonary hemorrhage
patent ductus arteriosus and, 183-185
surfactant for, 294
Pulmonary hypertension
in bronchopulmonary dysplasia, 411-412
treatment of, 419-421, 420b
chronic hyperoxia and, 101-102
chronic hypoxia and, 96-98
in congenital diaphragmatic hernia, 392-399
assessment of, 393-394
management of, 394-399
echocardiography of
in bronchopulmonary dysplasia, 419, 420b
in congenital diaphragmatic hernia, 393-396
fibrocytes in, 208-209
impaired antioxidants and, 95
lung development and, 185-186
pathogenesis of, 95-98
prevention of, 102-105
resuscitation for, hyperoxia and, 98-101, 99f-100f
treatment of, 102-105
antioxidants in, 103-105
catalase in, 103-104
cGMP modulators in, 102-103
cinaciguat in, 103
L-citrulline in, 103
nitric oxide in, 103
phosphodiesterase inhibitors in, 103
sapropterin hydrochloride in, 102-103
sildenafil in, 103, 104f
stem cell therapy in, 204
superoxide dismutase in, 103-104
Pulmonary hypoplasia, surfactant for, 293-294
Pulmonary outcomes. *See* Long-term pulmonary outcomes.
Pulmonary vascular resistance
in bronchopulmonary dysplasia, 411-412
in congenital diaphragmatic hernia, 381
Pulmonary vasculature, 13-16
in bronchopulmonary dysplasia, 411-412
development of. *See* Vascular development.
transitional, 3
hyperoxic effects on, 98-103
Pulse oximetry, 255
fetal, 306
in oxygen therapy, 302f, 303
for automated FIO_2 control, 377-378
in resuscitation, 248
in ventilator weaning, 356
Pulse oxygen saturation, fetal, 306
Pumactant, 285t. *See also* Surfactant.

R

Radiant warmers, 249-250
Radiography
  of bronchopulmonary dysplasia, 407-408, 408f
  of congenital diaphragmatic hernia, 383f
Raised thoracic compression method, in bronchopulmonary dysplasia, 410
Raised volume rapid thoracic compression method, in bronchopulmonary dysplasia, 410
Reactive airway disease
  bronchopulmonary dysplasia and, 154-155
  fibrocytes in, 208-209
  after late preterm birth, 236-237
  stem cell therapy for, 204-205
Reactive oxygen species (ROS)
  acute hypoxic vasoconstriction and, 96
  cellular sources of, 91-95, 92f
    mitochondrial electron transport chain and, 92-93
    nitric oxide synthase, 94
    Nox enzymes, 93-94
    peroxynitrite, 94-95
    xanthine oxidase, 94
  functions of, 91
  in hyperoxia, 169
    acute, 98-101, 99f
    chronic, 101-102
  overview of, 91-95
  in pulmonary hypertension, 96-98
  undernutrition and, 169
Reactive oxygen species scavengers, 95
  vascular remodeling and, 96-98
Reflexes, respiratory, infant-ventilator asynchrony and, 340-342, 340f
Reflux
  in bronchopulmonary dysplasia, 413-414, 419
  sildenafil and, 397
Renal insufficiency, congenital diaphragmatic hernia and, 392
Residual volume, in bronchopulmonary dysplasia, 410
Respiratory assessment
  initial, 248, 251
  in positive-pressure ventilation, 251-252
Respiratory center stimulants, for ventilator weaning, 357
Respiratory colonization
  pulmonary outcomes and, 151-155
  with *Ureaplasma* spp., 143
    asthma and, 154-155
    bronchopulmonary dysplasia and, 143
    clinical manifestations of, 136f, 143
    pneumonia and, 143, 144f
Respiratory disorders
  after late preterm birth, 236, 238. *See also* Long-term pulmonary outcomes.
  after very preterm birth, 236-240. *See also* Long-term pulmonary outcomes.
Respiratory distress syndrome (RDS), 265-266
  chorioamnionitis and, 67-69, 68t, 137-138
  genetic influences in, 37-39
    candidate genes and, 37-39
    single-nucleotide polymorphisms/haplotypes and, 39
    twin studies of, 37
  in growth restricted/small for gestational age infants, 81, 82f
  lung maturation in, 59-60
Respiratory distress syndrome (RDS) *(Continued)*
  mechanical ventilation and, 59-60
  nasal IPPV for, 270
  nasal NCPAP for, 270-274. *See also* Nasal continuous positive airway pressure (NCPAP).
  patent ductus arteriosus and, 183
  pathogenesis of, 37
  predictors of, 294-295
  risk assessment for, 60
  treatment of
    antenatal steroids in, 60-64, 61t, 62f. *See also* Corticosteroids, antenatal.
    criteria for, 60, 60t
    inhaled nitric oxide in, 117-123, 120f, 126
    surfactant in, 60-61, 60t, 182-183, 182f, 272-274. *See also* Surfactant, exogenous.
  Ureaplasma infection and, 150-151
  VEGF in, 186
  volume-targeted ventilation for, 369-370
Respiratory effort, ventilatory support for, 342
Respiratory failure
  in congenital diaphragmatic hernia, ECMO for, 390-392
  hypoxemic, resuscitation for, 98-101, 99f-100f
  management of
    mechanical ventilation in. *See* Mechanical ventilation.
    resuscitation in. *See* Resuscitation.
  severe, surfactant for, 294
Respiratory muscles, undernutrition and, 167t, 168
Respiratory paralysis, pharmacologic, for congenital diaphragmatic hernia, 382-383
Respiratory reflexes, infant-ventilator asynchrony and, 340-342, 340f
Respiratory support. *See also* Mechanical ventilation.
  continuous distending pressure in, 271, 271f-272f
  noninvasive. *See* Noninvasive respiratory support.
  in resuscitation, 270-274
Respiratory syncytial virus infection
  bronchopulmonary dysplasia and, 220
  after late preterm birth, 236
Resuscitation, 247-263
  anticipating need for, 247-248
  cardiac compressions in, 255-258, 257f
  coronary perfusion pressure in, 258
  CPAP in, 252
  discontinuation of, 260
  epinephrine in, 258-259
  equipment for, 248
  fluid, 259-260
  "golden minute" in, 248
  hyperoxia and, 98-101, 99f-100f
  indications for, 260
  initial assessment in, 248
  intubation in, 252-254, 253f, 253t
  medications for, 258-260
  oxygen concentration/saturation in, 98-102
    bronchopulmonary dysplasia and, 222-223
    hyperoxia in, 98-102. *See also* Hyperoxia.
  positive-pressure ventilation in, 251-252
    assessment during, 251-252
    equipment for, 248, 251
    flow rate in, 252

Resuscitation *(Continued)*
inflation pressure in, 252
inflation time in, 252
ventilation rate in, 252
preparation for, 248
sodium bicarbonate in, 260
steps in, 249-251, 249f
clear airway, 250
dry and stimulate, 250
position, 250
provide warmth, 248-250
volume infusion in, 259-260
vs. routine care, 248
warming in, 249-251, 249f
Retinoic acid, in alveologenesis, 12
Retinoic acid receptor ß, 35
Retinol, 173
Retinopathy of prematurity, 308-310
clinical outcomes and, 316-317
long-term, 316-317
in neonatal period, 316
cryotherapy for, 316
historical perspective on, 302-303
hypoxemia and, 335
incidence of, 302, 302f
laser photocoagulation for, 316
neovascularization in, 309-310
pathogenesis of, 308-310, 309f
prevention of, restrictive oxygen approach and, 313-314, 316
pulse oximetry and, 302f, 303
$TcPO_2$ monitoring and, 303
threshold, treatment of, 316
Rib fractures, undernutrition and, 168-169
Right ventricular hypertrophy
in bronchopulmonary dysplasia, 412
in pulmonary hypertension, 96, 412
Right-to-left shunt, in patent ductus arteriosus. *See also* Shunts.
management of, 189-190
pulmonary effects of, 183-185
systemic effects of, 183
Rosiglitazone, for bronchopulmonary dysplasia, 17-18

S

Saccular stage, of lung development, 5f, 6
Sapropterin hydrochloride, for pulmonary hypertension, 102-103
L-Selectin, in bronchopulmonary dysplasia, 44
Selenium, 165t, 174
for bronchopulmonary dysplasia, 223-224
dietary, 165t, 174
Self-inflating bags, for positive-pressure ventilation, 248, 251
Septation, 11-12, 12f
timing of, 58-59
Shh. *See* Sonic hedgehog (Shh).
Shunts
closure of
failure of. *See* Patent ductus arteriosus.
oxygenation and, 307-308
in congenital diaphragmatic hernia, 387t, 395-396
left-to-right, in patent ductus arteriosus, 183
right-to-left, in patent ductus arteriosus
management of, 189-190
pulmonary effects of, 183-185
systemic effects of, 183
Signaling
in bronchopulmonary dysplasia, 16-19, 125-126, 139-140, 220-221
inflammation and, 139-140
in lung development, 6-7
in alveologenesis, 11-12, 12f
in branching morphogenesis, 8-11, 9f
in neonatal lung injury, 16-19
oxidant, acute hypoxic vasoconstriction and, 96
reactive oxygen species in, 91-95, 92f
in stem cell therapy, 205
in vascular development, 14-16, 111-115, 113f, 113t
Sildenafil, for pulmonary hypertension, 103, 104f
in bronchopulmonary dysplasia, 419-420, 420b
in congenital diaphragmatic hernia, 396-397, 399
Skin color, in initial assessment, 248
Small for gestational age (SGA) infants
antenatal steroids for, 83
bronchopulmonary dysplasia in, 81-83, 82f
lung development in, 83
respiratory distress syndrome in, 81, 82f
Smoking
maternal, lung development and, 83-84
respiratory function and, 240
Sodium bicarbonate, in resuscitation, 260
Soluble guanylate cyclase, in lung development, 116-117, 116f
Sonic hedgehog (Shh), 35
in lung development, 7
in branching morphogenesis, 8
Spirometry, raised volume rapid thoracic compression in, 410
Spironolactone, for bronchopulmonary dysplasia, 417-418
SpO_2. *See* Oxygen saturation (SpO_2).
Spontaneous breathing test, 361
Sprouty (Spry), in branching morphogenesis, 8, 9f
Stable microbubble test, 294-295
Stem cell(s), 197-216
adult, 198-199
bone marrow–derived, 201-202
bronchoalveolar, 206-207, 206f
division of, 197-198, 198f
embryonic, 198-199
endogenous
circulating, 207-209
lung, 206-207, 206f, 208f
endothelial progenitor, 202, 204
hematopoietic, 197-198, 201-202
in lung bioengineering, 205-206
mesenchymal, 201-202
therapeutic uses of, 200-205, 203f. *See also* Stem cell therapy.
for bronchopulmonary dysplasia, 228
multipotent, 197-198, 198f
niches for, 198-199
overview of, 197-199
pluripotent, 197-198, 198f
induced, 200
totipotent, 197-198, 198f
umbilical cord, 200-201

Stem cell therapy
  bone marrow–derived stem cells in, 201
    for COPD, 205
    endothelial progenitor, 202
    hematopoietic, 201-202
    for lung injury, 202-203, 203f
    mesenchymal, 201-205
    for pulmonary fibrosis, 203-204
    for pulmonary hypertension, 204
    for reactive airway disease, 204-205
    types of, 201-202
  cell types in, 201-202
  embryonic stem cells in, 199-200
  endothelial progenitor cells in, 202, 204
  engraftment in, 205
  induced pluripotent stem cells in, 200
  lung bioengineering and, 205-206
  paracrine signaling in, 205
  repair mechanisms in, 205
  umbilical cord stem cells in, 200-201
Stimulation, in resuscitation, 250
Stress, antenatal, lung maturation and, 81
Stroma-derived factor 1, in lung injury, 41
Suctioning, 250
  equipment for, 248
  in meconium staining, 250
  routine, 250
Sudden infant death syndrome
  intrauterine growth restriction and, 170
  undernutrition and, 167t, 170
Superoxide, 91-93. *See also* Reactive oxygen species.
  degradation to hydrogen peroxide, 95
  in pulmonary hypertension, 96-97
Superoxide dismutase (SOD), 91-92, 92f, 95
  actions of, 95
  Cu/Zn, 95
    for bronchopulmonary dysplasia, 223
  extracellular, 95
  in hyperoxia
    acute, 100-101
    chronic, 101
  isoforms of, 124
  Mn, 95
  nitric oxide and, 124
  for pulmonary hypertension, 103-104
  undernutrition and, 169
SUPPORT Trial, 320-323, 322t
Surfactant, 29, 283-299
  endogenous
    classes of, 168
    components of, 168
    deficiency of. *See* Respiratory distress syndrome (RSD).
    functions of, 168
    precursors of, 175
    undernutrition and, 168-169
  exogenous
    administration of, 273-274, 290
      by endotracheal tube, 290
      intra-amniotic, 291
      by intratracheal catheter, 273-274, 292
      nasopharyngeal, 291
      by nebulization, 291-292
      without intubation, 291-292
    antenatal steroids and, 61
    for congenital diaphragmatic hernia, 293-294, 389-390
    for congenital pneumonia, 293
Surfactant *(Continued)*
    CPAP and, 272, 288-289, 291-292
      INSURE technique and, 290
      nasal, 272
    doses for, 284t-285t, 286-287
      first, 284t, 287-289
      second/subsequent, 284t, 289-290
    future developments for, 294-295
    guidelines for use, 283-285, 284t
    INSURE technique for, 290
    long-term effects of, 240
    with mechanical ventilation vs. CPAP, 284t
    for meconium aspiration, 292-293
    natural, 284t-285t, 285-286
      vs. synthetic, 284t, 285-286, 295
    patent ductus arteriosus and, 183
    patient selection for, 60, 60t
    prophylactic, 284t
      CPAP and, 288-289, 291-292
      patient selection for, 287-289
      vs. rescue, 287-288
    for pulmonary hemorrhage, 294
    for pulmonary hypoplasia, 293-294
    rescue, vs. prophylactic, 287-288
    routine use of, 294
    for severe respiratory failure, 294
    synthetic, 285
      synthetic peptides in, 285-286
      vs. natural, 285-286, 285t, 295
    timing of
      for first dose, 284t, 287-289
      for second/subsequent dose, 284t, 289-290
    types of, 284-286, 284t-285t
Surfactant protein-A
  in bronchopulmonary dysplasia, 45-46
  in respiratory distress syndrome, 38, 38t
  in *Ureaplasma* infection, 148-149
Surfactant protein-B, 35
  in bronchopulmonary dysplasia, 45-46
  in respiratory distress syndrome, 38, 38t
Surfactant protein-C, in respiratory distress syndrome, 38
Surfactant protein-D
  in bronchopulmonary dysplasia, 45-46
  in respiratory distress syndrome, 38, 38t
Surfactant-TA, 285, 285t
Synchronized ventilation. *See* Mechanical ventilation, synchronized.

T

Targeted minute ventilation, 371-372, 372f-374f
  weaning from, 362-363
$TcPO_2$ monitoring, 303
Temperature maintenance, in resuscitation, 248
Tetrahydrobiopterin (BH_4), 102-103
  nitrous oxide synthase and, 123
Thiazide diuretics, for bronchopulmonary dysplasia, 417-418
Thoracic cage, undernutrition and, 168-169
Thy-1, in lung injury, 41
Thyroid transcription factor-1 (TTF-1), 6-7, 35
  in lung injury, 42
Tie1, 14-15, 114-115
Tie2, 14-15, 114-115
  in bronchopulmonary dysplasia, 220-221
Tissue engineering, 205-206
Tissue inhibitors of metalloproteinases (TIMPs)
  in bronchopulmonary dysplasia, 19-20
  in lung injury, 41

α-Tocopherol, 165t, 173-174
Toll-like receptors
in chorioamnionitis, 72-73, 76-78, 77f
in *Ureaplasma* infection, 149
Total lung capacity, in bronchopulmonary dysplasia, 410
Totipotent stem cells, 197-198, 198f. *See also* Stem cell(s).
Tracheal aspirates, in ventilator-associated pneumonia, 152
Tracheal occlusion, antenatal, for congenital diaphragmatic hernia, 400-401
Tracheal-esophageal separation, 6-7, 7f
Tracheostomy, for bronchopulmonary dysplasia, 413-414
Transcription factors. *See also* Signaling.
in lung development, 6-7
Transforming growth factor-α
in bronchopulmonary dysplasia, 221
in lung injury, 41-42
Transforming growth factor-ß
in alveolar development, 16-18
in branching morphogenesis, 9-10
in bronchopulmonary dysplasia, 16-18, 17f, 186, 221
in lung development, 186
in neonatal lung injury, 16-18
nitric oxide synthase and, 124
in patent ductus arteriosus, 186
Transforming growth factor-ß receptor II, 36
Transforming growth factor-ß1, 35
in bronchopulmonary dysplasia, 45, 144-148
in lung development, 139-140
in lung injury, 42
in *Ureaplasma* infection, 144-148
Transforming growth factor-ß3, 36
Transitional goal oxygen saturation, 254, 254t
Transitional pulmonary vasculature, 3
hyperoxic effects on, 98-102
nitric oxide and, 125
Transplantation, stem cell. *See* Stem cell therapy.
Transporter associated with antigen processing (TAP), in bronchopulmonary dysplasia, 47
Trans-scleral cryotherapy, for retinopathy of prematurity, 316
Tumor necrosis factor-α
in bronchopulmonary dysplasia, 144-148
in lung development, 140
in lung injury, 39
in patent ductus arteriosus, 184
in *Ureaplasma* infection, 144-148
Two-thumb technique, 256, 257f

U

Umbilical cord inflammation, 65
Umbilical cord stem cells, 200-201
Undernutrition, 166-170. *See also* Nutrition; Nutritional support.
alveolar fluid balance and, 167t, 170
bone formation and, 168-169
breathing control and, 167t, 170
bronchopulmonary dysplasia and, 163-164, 167
definition of, 166
extrauterine growth restriction and, 163, 166
hyperoxia and, 167t, 169
immune response and, 169
lung development and, 166-167, 167t
lung function and, 167t, 168-169
neurodevelopmental effects of, 166
Undernutrition *(Continued)*
nutritional emphysema and, 167
pulmonary effects of, 166-170, 167t
respiratory muscles and, 167t, 168
sudden infant death syndrome and, 167t, 170
susceptibility to infection and, 167t, 169
thoracic cage and, 168-169
Ureaplasma infection, 65-69. *See also* Chorioamnionitis.
animal models of, 142, 144-148
asthma and, 154-155
in bronchopulmonary dysplasia, 143-148, 145f, 147f-148f, 219-220
animal models of, 144-148
evidence for, 144-148
proposed model of, 148, 148f
diagnosis of, 149-150
immune response in, 72-73, 73t, 148-149
lung development and, 146, 147f
mechanical ventilation and, 144-148, 145f, 147f
obstetric complications and, 141-142, 143t
respiratory distress syndrome and, 150-151
subclinical, 142
surfactant protein-A in, 148-149
susceptibility to, 148-149
undernutrition and, 169
Toll-like receptors in, 149
treatment of, 150
virulence factors in, 141
Ureaplasma spp.
pathogenicity of, 141
respiratory colonization with, 143
bronchopulmonary dysplasia and, 143
clinical manifestations of, 136f, 143
pneumonia and, 143, 144f
postnatal, 151-155
Ureaplasmal Mb antigen, 141
Urokinase, in bronchopulmonary dysplasia, 47

V

Vapotherm system, 277-278
Variable-flow nasal CPAP device, 274, 274f
Variant Clara cells, 206-207, 206f
Vascular development, 13-16, 111-112. *See also* Lung development.
alveolarization and, 12-13, 17f, 111-114, 113f, 113t
angiogenesis in, 13-16, 111-115, 113f, 113t
angiopoietin in, 6-7
in bronchopulmonary dysplasia, 220-221
in congenital diaphragmatic hernia, 381
ephrins in, 7
epithelial-endothelial interaction in, 111-114, 113f
epithelial-mesenchymal interaction in, 111-112
fibroblast growth factors in, 14, 113t, 114-115
hypoxemia and, 335
morphogenesis in, 13-14
patent ductus arteriosus and, 185-186
postnatal, 111-112
of pulmonary artery, 111-112
in congenital diaphragmatic hernia, 381
signaling in, 14-16, 111-115, 113f, 113t
tie2 in, 6-7
vasculogenesis in, 13-16, 111-112, 114-115
VEGF in, 14, 112-114, 113f, 113t, 117, 186

Vascular endothelial growth factor (VEGF), 36
in air-blood interface maintenance, 121
in alveolarization, 12-13, 17f, 18-19, 112-115, 113f, 113t
angiopoietins and, 114-115
in bronchopulmonary dysplasia, 17f, 47, 102, 125-126, 186, 220-221
deficiency of, 36
deletion of, 114
hyperoxia and, 102
isoforms of, 114
in lung development, 36, 112-114, 113f, 113t
in lung injury, 42
in lung repair, 117-123
nitric oxide and, 114-115, 117
in patent ductus arteriosus, 186
prophylactic use of, 19
in respiratory distress syndrome, 186
in retinopathy of prematurity, 301-302, 309f
therapeutic use of, 19, 36
in *Ureaplasma* infection, 146-148
in vascular development, 14, 112-114, 113f, 113t, 117, 186
Vascular hypothesis, for bronchopulmonary dysplasia, 220-221
Vascular morphogenesis, 13-14, 111-112
Vasculature. *See also specific structures.*
bronchial, 13
pulmonary, 13-16
in bronchopulmonary dysplasia, 411-412
development of. *See* Vascular development.
transitional, 3
hyperoxic effects on, 98-103
Vasculogenesis, 13-16, 111-112. *See also* Vascular development.
VEGF in, 114-115
Vasoconstriction
acute hypoxic, 96
chronic hypoxic, pulmonary hypertension and, 96-98
hyperoxic
acute, 98-101, 99f-100f
chronic, 101-102
Vasodilators, for pulmonary hypertension
in bronchopulmonary dysplasia, 419-420
in congenital diaphragmatic hernia, 396-397, 399
Vegetable oils, 172
Ventilator-associated pneumonia, 151-155
aspiration, 153-154
birth weight and, 152-153
definition of, 151-152
diagnostic criteria for, 151-152
diagnostic procedures for, 152
microbiology of, 153
outcomes in, 154
Ventilator-associated pneumonia *(Continued)*
pathogenesis of, 153-154
prevention of, 154
risk factors for, 152-153
tracheal aspirates in, 152
ventilation duration and, 152-153
Ventricular septal defect, congenital diaphragmatic hernia and, 399-400
Viral infections, bronchopulmonary dysplasia and, 151, 219-220
Visual problems. *See also* Retinopathy of prematurity.
sildenafil and, 397
Vitamins, 165t, 173-174
vitamin A, 165t, 173
for bronchopulmonary dysplasia, 226
dietary, 165t
vitamin C, 165t, 174
vitamin D, 165t, 173
vitamin E, 165t, 173-174
Volume guarantee ventilation, 368-369
Volume infusion, in resuscitation, 259-260
Volume-controlled ventilation, 224-225, 369
pressure-regulated, 369
Volume-targeted ventilation, 224-225, 368-371, 369f-370f
hypoxemia and, 331-332
weaning from, 362, 369-370

W

Warming methods, 248-250
Water intake, 165t, 170-171
Weaning
from mechanical ventilation, 355-365. *See also* Mechanical ventilation, weaning from.
from nasal CPAP, 277
Weight, birth, ventilator-associated pneumonia and, 152-153
Weight gain
recommended postnatal, 166-167
recommended prenatal, 166-167
Wheezing. *See also* Reactive airway disease.
bronchopulmonary dysplasia and, 154-155
Wilson-Mikity syndrome, 75
Wingless-Int7b, 36
Wnt, in branching morphogenesis, 9-10

X

Xanthine oxidase, 94
in pulmonary hypertension, 97

Z

Zinc, dietary, 165t, 174